CLINICAL SIGNS RAPID REFERENCE

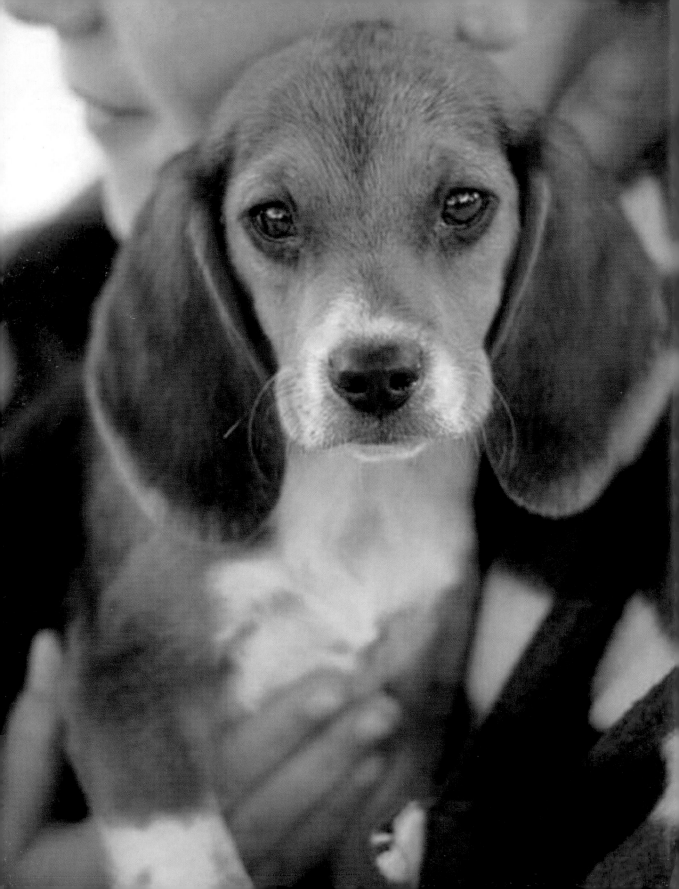

DR. BRUCE FOGLE

CARING

FOR YOUR

DOG

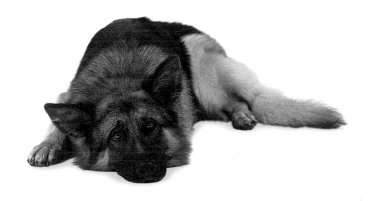

LONDON, NEW YORK, MUNICH,
MELBOURNE, DELHI

Managing Editor **Deirdre Headon**
Managing Art Editor **Lee Griffiths**
Senior Art Editor **Wendy Bartlet**
Art Editor **Jamie Hanson**
Design Assistant **Anna Plucinska**
Project Editors **Candida Frith-MacDonald,
Katie John, Heather Jones, Carla Masson**
Editors **Mary Davies, Robert Dinwiddie,
Alyson Lacewing, David Lloyd, Alison
Mackonochie, Pip Morgan, Amber Tokeley,
Gary Werner, Angela Wilkes**
Index **Hilary Bird**
DTP Designer **Louise Waller**
Production Manager **Lauren Britton**
Production Controller **Mandy Inness**
Picture Researcher **Sarah Duncan**
Picture Library **Hayley Smith**
Jacket Designer **Katy Wall**

Caring for your Dog provides general information
on a wide range of animal health and veterinary
topics. The book is not a substitute for advice from
a qualified veterinary practitioner. You are advised
always to consult your veterinary surgeon or other
appropriate expert if you have specific queries in
relation to your pet's health. Before administering
any medicine or any treatment to your pet, you
should ensure that you always read and follow the
instructions contained in the information leaflet. The
naming of any organization, product, or alternative
therapy in this book does not imply endorsement by
the publisher and the omission of any such names
does not indicate disapproval. The publisher regrets
it cannot accept any responsibility for acts or
omissions based on the information in this book.

2 4 6 8 10 9 7 5 3 1

First published in Great Britain in 2002
by Dorling Kindersley Limited,
80 Strand, London WC2R ORL
A Penguin Company

Copyright © 2002 Dorling Kindersley Limited,
London

A CIP catalogue record for this book is
available from the British Library.

ISBN 0-7513-3860-5

Colour reproduction by Colourscan, Singapore.
Printed and bound in Germany by Mohndruck

See our complete catalogue at
www.dk.com

CONTENTS

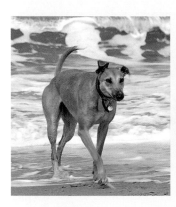
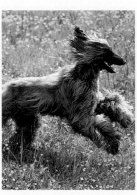
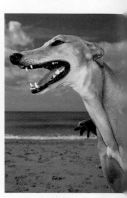

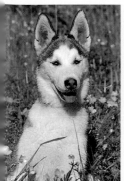
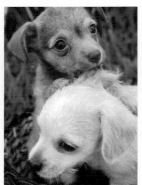
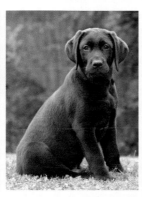
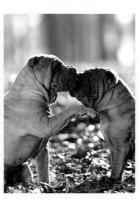
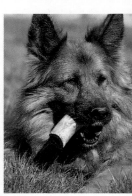

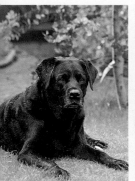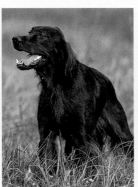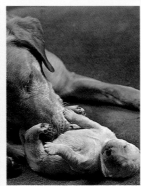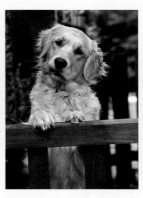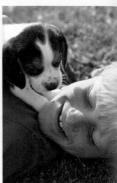

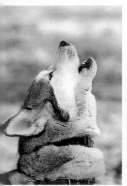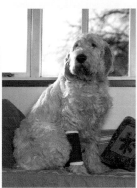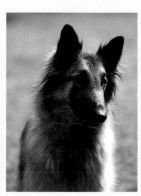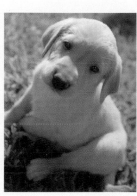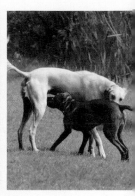

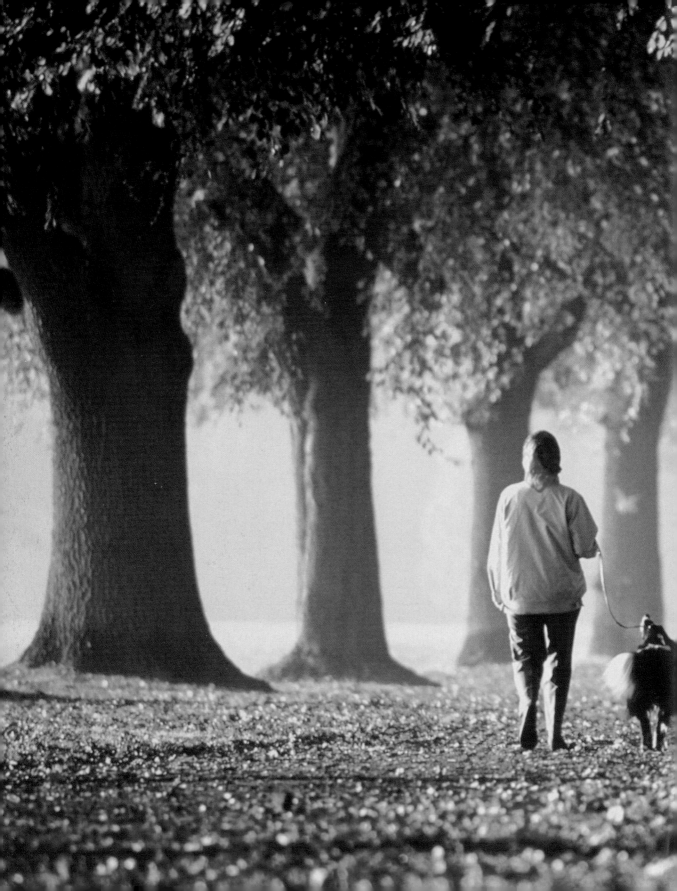

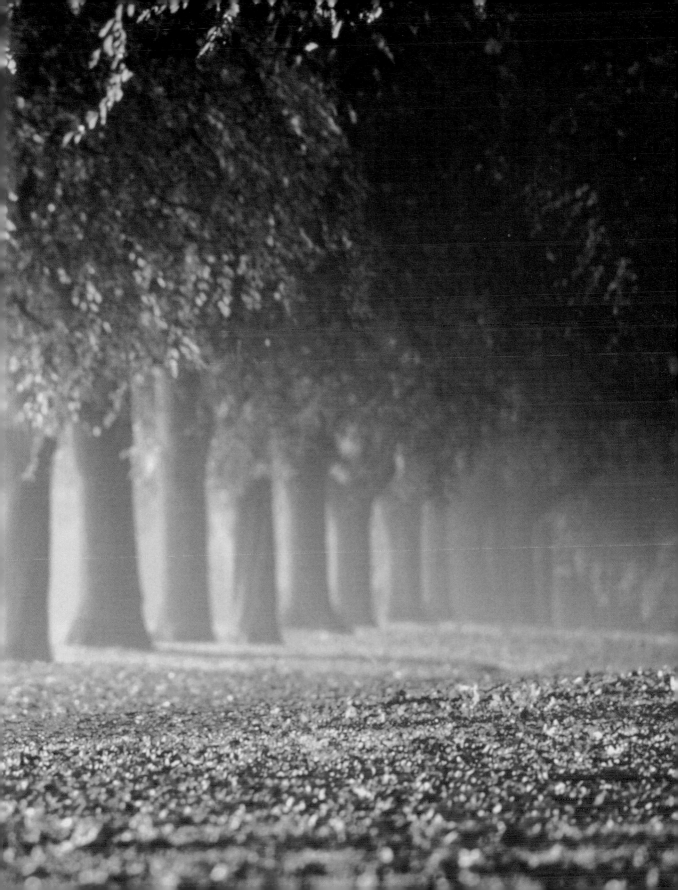

INTRODUCTION

If your dog is a typical family dog it relishes your presence, revels in activities with you, thrives on your touch, delights in hearing your voice, regrets your absence and probably warns you if it thinks there is imminent danger. Your dog treats you as a member of its very own family. Your dog cares for you – truly, deeply cares for you. I've lived with dogs since the day I was born, and as a practising vet I've attended to their medical welfare for over 30 years. Personally, I don't have any problems calling their behaviour "love".

Dogs develop a warm kinship with us and we do the same with them. We treat them as members of our family, not quite human but not as "animal" as all other animals. Over 20 years ago the American psychiatrist Aaron Katcher eloquently compared dogs to Peter Pan: forever caught between nature and culture, eternal children, wide-eyed, guileless, patently honest with their emotions.

In the relatively short time since I first picked up a stethoscope there has been a wonderfully positive trend in our attitude towards dogs, instigated by you, the dog owner. Your compassion, commitment and concern about your dog's physical and emotional welfare initiated the greatest ever advances in dog care and welfare. Veterinarians and pet-related health care businesses responded to your demands with effective vaccines, anti-parasitic drugs and nutritionally sound diets. These forms of preventative medicine are at the core of medically caring for your dog.

Today, virtually all diagnostics and treatments used in human medicine are available for dogs. For example, with new drugs, dogs with heart disease have longer and more comfortable lives. Advances in our understanding of kidney disease have led to foods being developed that prolong the working life of impaired kidneys. New surgical techniques have been perfected that can save damaged or diseased limbs that, previously, could only be treated by amputation.

While your veterinarian is important, the day-to-day health and happiness of your dog is in your hands. That's the reason for this book. It helps you to understand how dogs think, how to train and live with them, what they need to eat, and what medical problems they can get and how to prevent them. It shows you how to give first aid and how to make decisions about when to call in the vet. Principally, the book tells you how your vet will make a diagnosis and how your dog may be treated for its medical condition.

To ensure that what you read is as accurate as possible, internationally respected veterinary academics and teaching clinicians have reviewed and revised each chapter. The really good bits are due to them. The errors and omissions are all mine. As I write my young golden retriever, Macy, is asleep on my foot. I'm fortunate to have a healthy, happy human family but even so, Macy lying there, dreaming dumb dog dreams, brings a unique feeling of warmth and satisfaction to life. We're lucky that serendipity has given us such a bountiful relationship with such an honest, uncomplicated and kindred species.

DR BRUCE FOGLE
DVM, MRCVS

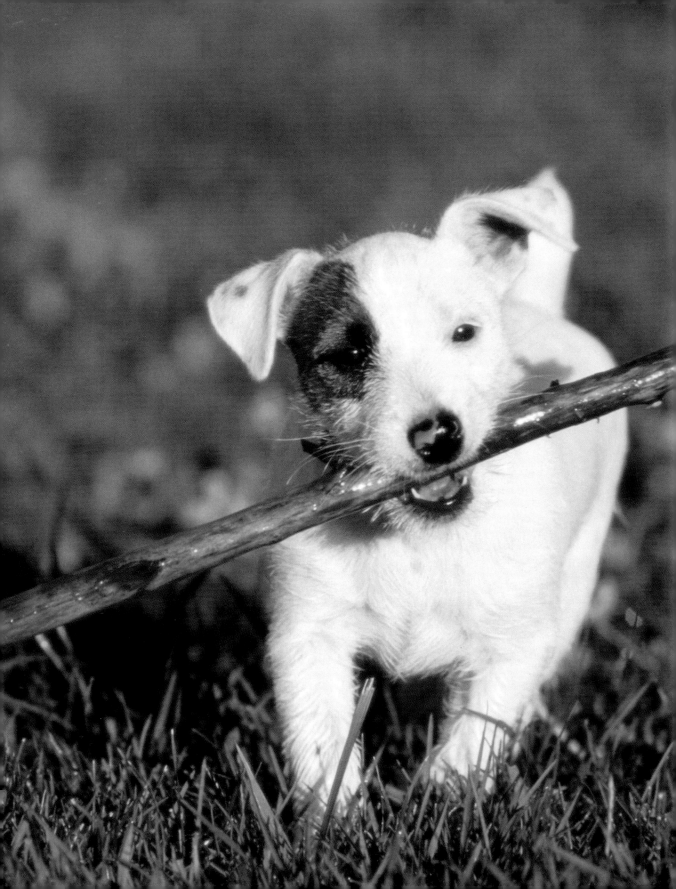

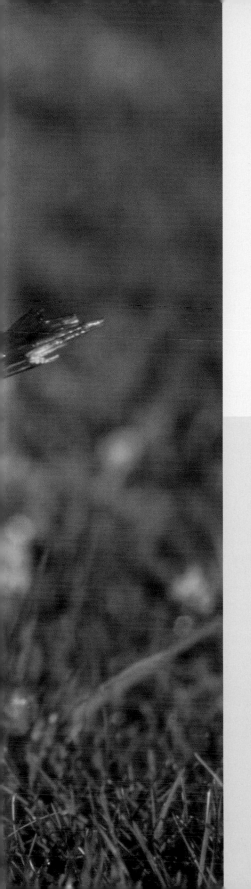

YOUR
FAMILY DOG

What is the most effective way to prolong your dog's life? Simply to acknowledge that your dog is not a person in cute disguise. By understanding how your dog thinks, like the pack canine it is, and by understanding its unique nutritional and training needs, you will begin to understand the responsibilities caring for your four-legged buddy. Choosing the right type of dog for your family's lifestyle is vital. Standard obedience training, including lead control, is probably the single most important factor in a dog's increased life expectancy. Dogs on leads seldom get into life-threatening situations. Simple obedience training is also at the heart of any remedial or advanced training or simply enjoying travel with your canine companion.

SELECTING A DOG
making the right choice

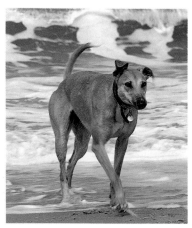

Your dog will need regular exercise

Owning a dog is a major decision, and a long-term commitment in both time and money. With the right decision, the rewards are enormous: activity, amusement, constancy, and fidelity, as well as protection. In curious ways the rewards of living with a family dog can be clearer and more achievable than living with other members of our own species. Choose carefully. Research what dog you want and understand why you want it. Be realistic. Your puppy will grow to become a good companion, but will always remain a dog – a wolf in disguise. When you have determined what type of dog is right for your family and where it will come from, make sure that your home and your family are well prepared for the new arrival.

NEW PUPS' NEEDS

A new puppy is time-consuming. It needs four meals a day and has to be taken to its toilet area each time it wakes, after each meal, and after each episode of activity and play. Until it is toilet trained there will be mess to clean up. Regardless of how careful you are, it will still find possessions to chew and destroy. It will need handling several times daily plus routine grooming. The more new and interesting experiences a pup has at an early age the less fearful it will be as an adult. Set aside time for your pup to meet children as well as adults, and other animals, such as cats and horses. Actively create situations for your pup to experience, from seeing an umbrella being opened or a bicycle going past to a short trip in the car. Your pup needs "time out", frequent, deep snoozes. This is when the growth hormone is most active, and pups need to grow quickly, especially compared to us.

ARE YOU RIGHT FOR A DOG?
If you have grown up with a dog and relish the joys of canine companionship, it is hard to live without one. It may be that through knowing families with dogs, you have seen the rewards they bring and want the same for your family.

Just wanting a family dog, however, is not enough. To put it bluntly: will a dog want to live with you? Bringing a dog into your home is a mutual venture. Before actually getting one, ask yourself these questions. Will I, both now and in the future, have the time to train, exercise, groom, and play with a dog? Will there be space in my home, and in the area where I live, to house and exercise a dog? Will I be able to afford the annual feeding and maintenance costs? Are there any family members who are intensely allergic or for other medical reasons should not live with a dog? Are there any local rules or regulations that prohibit me from keeping a dog or a specific breed of dog?

ARE YOU WILLING TO BE A RESPONSIBLE DOG OWNER?
Good intentions are not enough – you have to be honest with yourself and consider whether you are willing to be a responsible dog owner. Ask yourself the following questions:
• On streets and in parks, in your garden, and with your neighbours, will you keep your dog under control?
• Will you dog-proof your garden to prevent your dog from wandering?
• Are you willing to carry a "poop-scooper" with you and use it each time you take your dog out for play, training, or exercise?
• Will you control your dog's barking so as not to annoy your neighbours?

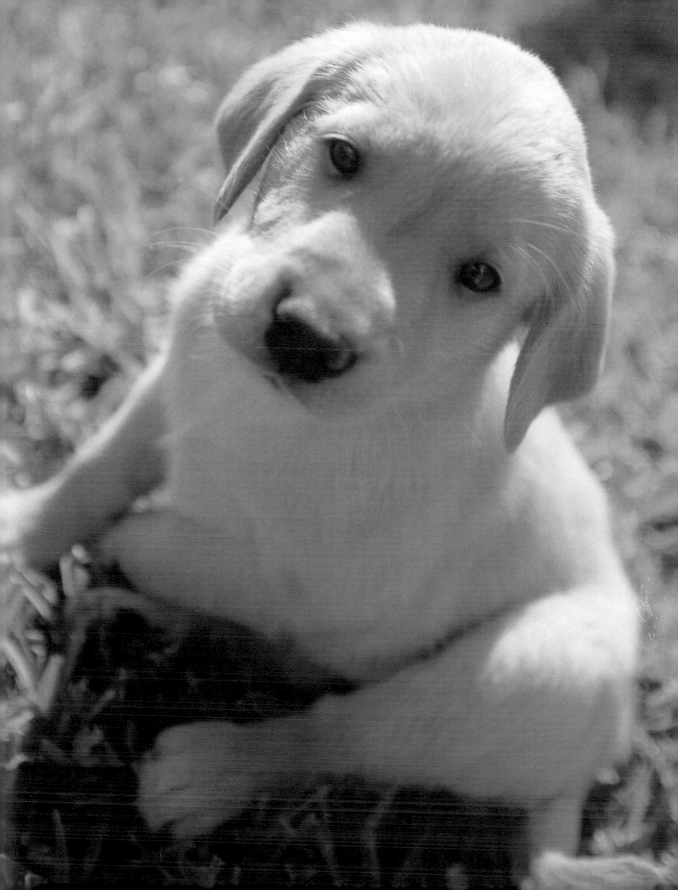

ESSENTIAL SUPPLIES

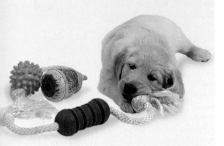

From food and bedding to toys, there are essential items your new dog will need.

- Puppy food
Continue feeding the food supplied by the breeder. Change gradually to your preferred food after your dog has settled into your home.

- Food bowl
Use non-slip ceramic or metal food and water bowls. Non-slip rubber bases are excellent. The best have sloped sides on the inside that are easy for a dog to lick clean.

- A place to sleep
Moulded plastic beds are relatively chew-proof and easy to clean. Use washable bedding with zip covers that can be removed for cleaning.

- Identification
Have an engraved ID tag ready, or a capsule ID container in which you write relevant details including your home and mobile telephone numbers.

- Collar
Lightweight and inexpensive braided nylon collars are ideal for puppies. Wait until your dog is physically mature before investing in an attractive design.

- Lead
Purchase a lightweight walking lead and also a long, lightweight houseline.

- Toys
Select three toys at most that your dog can use to chew on, squeak, or pull.

WHAT IS THE RIGHT DOG FOR YOU?

A good family dog is not just for you; it is a companion for both children and parents, a part of family life. Usually one family member takes charge of the daily responsibilities of feeding, training, and exercising a dog.

Large dogs and guarding breeds like the German Shepherd, Doberman Pinscher, and Rottweiler fit the stereotype image of "protectors", but before choosing a large breed think carefully about what you mean by "protection". Unless a dog is specifically trained for protection work, its true role is as a deterrent. In one survey, when police asked burglars about the greatest deterrent to breaking into a house, the most common answer was not a sophisticated burglar alarm system, but a barking dog – which means that in the opinion of at least one police force, an alert Yorkshire Terrier offers as much protection as a hulking Rottweiler.

All dogs (even breeds with a couch potato image) love activity, but some are better equipped for jogging with their owners than others. Choose a high-energy breed or individual only if you have the energy to meet its daily needs. If you are attracted to a specific breed, but want to be active with your dog, search out breeders who intentionally breed for activity (in the case of Dachshunds, for example, for longer "working" legs).

You may think that showing dogs is for the professionals, but it is strange what happens to us when we realize that our own dog is of "show quality". By the time a puppy is eight weeks old, breeders have a reasonable idea of its potential to become a show dog. Breed shows concentrate on dogs that are as close as possible to the breed standard of physical perfection; however, showing is not restricted to the beauty contest category. There are dog shows for everyone and every dog regardless of its background: shows for the best groomed dog, the waggiest tail, the happiest face, the most agile or obedient dog.

If you want a hunting companion, choose an individual that responds well to command training. All of the sporting breeds – the retrievers, setters, pointers, and spaniels – fit this category. Most, however, are bred as family companions, not for working. If you want a working dog, go to breeders who selectively breed for field trial work or hunting.

MALE OR FEMALE?

The two sexes differ in looks and temperament. As with most mammals, male dogs are bigger and more muscular than females. They are typically more active, demand more play time, and leave more urine scent marks where they walk than females. Males are naturally more aggressive with other dogs, likely to be more destructive, and have a greater inclination to wander. Untrained, they have a slightly greater risk of snapping at strangers.

Female dogs demand and give more affection and are more companionable than males. They are more willing to learn obedience (although no faster than males at learning) and are easier to house train.

These are typical sex characteristics, but it is very likely that your family dog, whether male or female, will be neutered. Neutering diminishes the sex differences (*see p.46*). Spaying a bitch eliminates the behaviour changes and social inconvenience of twice-yearly heat cycles. Medically speaking, spaying is life-enhancing. Spayed bitches live on average a year longer than unspayed ones. Castrating a male dog reduces urine marking, wandering, and aggression towards other male dogs, but does not prolong life-expectancy as in bitches.

MIXED, CROSS, OR PUREBRED?

Purebred dogs are usually intentionally produced to certain breed standards, such as shape, size, and temperament. This is the most important reason why choosing a specific breed is the most reliable way to find a dog with the temperament you want.

Crossbred dogs are mixes of two purebreds. For example, a Cocker Spaniel crossed with a Miniature Poodle is known as a "Cockerpoo". Most crossbreds are accidents, but usually glorious accidents. They also have reasonably predictable temperaments and needs derived from the known needs of their purebred parents.

Mongrels are mixed or random-bred dogs. Their ancestry is unknown, but that makes them no less valuable as family dogs. Mixed-breed dogs have a distinct advantage over purebreds. Most purebred dogs have developed from a small genetic base, which produces consistent size, shape, and personality, but also concentrates dangerous genes that increase medical risk. For example, Cavalier King Charles Spaniels are prone to heart disease, West Highland White Terriers to skin disorders, Golden Retrievers to hip and elbow conditions, German Shepherds to bowel complaints, and Bernese Mountain Dogs to cancer. Mongrels are just as prone to infection and injury as purebreds, but have a far lower risk of inherited diseases.

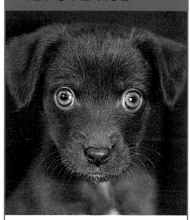

VET'S ADVICE

Before leaving the breeder's, remember the following:

• Obtain the puppy's pedigree and registration papers, its worming history (including the names of products used), and a vaccination certificate showing when its next inoculation is due.
• Pick up a diet sheet.
• Check over any guarantees before paying.
• Get a written statement that your purchase is based upon the puppy's good health and conformation and that this will be determined independently by your own vet, whom you should ask to examine the puppy within 36 hours.

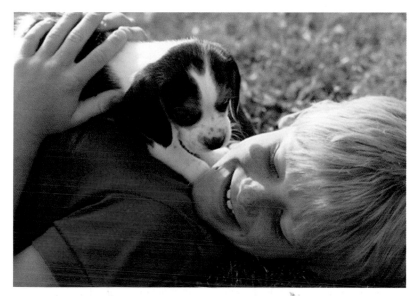

FAMILY COMPANION
In ideal circumstances a dog becomes a junior member of the family. In childhood a dog often becomes a best buddy, someone who understands when adults seem not to. If all goes well this puppy will be part of the family until its best friend leaves home.

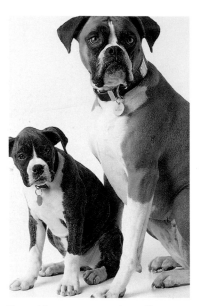

Expect to see your pup's mother

CHOOSING YOUR PUPPY

Choosing a puppy can be intensely emotional. You may instinctively be drawn to the underdog, the sad littermate that cowers and is trampled by its brothers and sisters. Or taken by the pup with the waggiest tail and biggest personality; the little tyke that barks at you when you try to examine it.

When making your final selection from the litter do so on the basis of the puppy's physical and apparent appearance. Investigate the breeder, the puppy's parents, and the puppy before making your choice. Breeders should willingly let you see the mother, but do not expect to see the father. Good breeders go outside their kennels for fathers. The puppies should also be housed in hygienic surroundings and have plenty of obvious contact with people.

OBSERVING BEHAVIOUR

If a puppy is struggling and biting, it may have a tendency towards dominance aggression. Shrinking, running away, or hiding are signs of extreme shyness and may develop into fearful behaviour – this puppy may not socialize well. If a puppy follows you with wagging tail held high, accepts petting, and struggles only temporarily when picked up, it has vitality and self-confidence. It will find the transition from the litter to your home easy.

WHAT TO LOOK FOR IN A PUPPY

Examine each puppy visually, looking for obvious signs of good health, such as bright eyes and easy movement with no obvious lameness. Compare one pup with another, looking at their heads, bodies, and limbs. All may appear the same at first but on careful inspection you will begin to notice the subtle differences within the litter.

Conscientious breeders will let you physically examine the litter. Each pup, even from the tiniest breed, should feel substantial. Inspect your puppy from head to toe even though your vet will examine it fully later. If you have not had a puppy previously, take a person experienced with dogs with you. Finally, ensure your purchase is contingent upon your vet's approval.

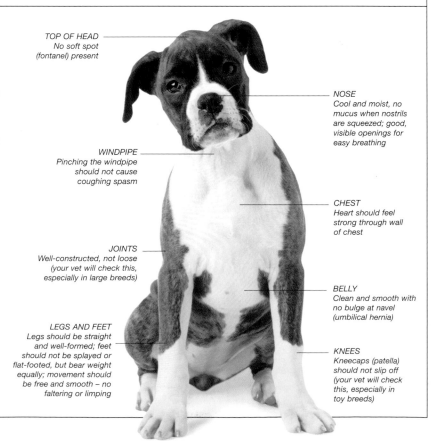

TOP OF HEAD
No soft spot (fontanel) present

NOSE
Cool and moist, no mucus when nostrils are squeezed; good, visible openings for easy breathing

WINDPIPE
Pinching the windpipe should not cause coughing spasm

CHEST
Heart should feel strong through wall of chest

JOINTS
Well-constructed, not loose (your vet will check this, especially in large breeds)

BELLY
Clean and smooth with no bulge at navel (umbilical hernia)

LEGS AND FEET
Legs should be straight and well-formed; feet should not be splayed or flat-footed, but bear weight equally; movement should be free and smooth – no faltering or limping

KNEES
Kneecaps (patella) should not slip off (your vet will check this, especially in toy breeds)

PHYSICAL EXAMINATION

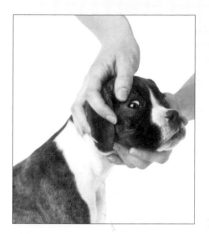

EYES
The eyes should be symmetrical and look straight ahead. There should be no tear staining below them, and the eyelids should neither roll in (entropion) nor hang loose (ectropion). There should be no extra eyelashes, inflammation, or discharge (conjunctivitis). The third eyelid may be visible but should not be inflamed or swollen.

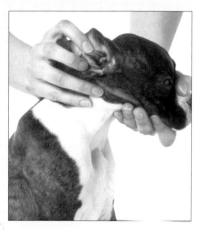

EARS
There should be no crust on the ear tips. Ears ought to have good hair cover. The ear canals should be clean and sweet-smelling, with no wax visible. The puppy should show no head-shaking or tenderness when you touch its ears. In breeds such as Dalmatians where deafness occurs, clap your hands and observe the speed of the dog's response.

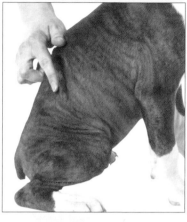

SKIN AND COAT
Hair texture, density and length should be appropriate for the breed with no thinning, balding or "moth-eaten" patches. There should be no scale, dandruff or flaking skin in the hair. On running your hands over the coat you should feel no unexpected bumps or crusty patches. There should be no skin damage nor signs of external parasites.

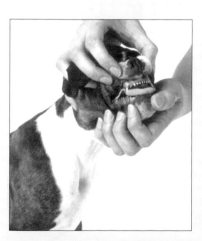

GUMS AND TEETH
The upper incisors must fit neatly over the lower incisors (scissors bite). If the upper incisors are too far forward it is overshot. In some short-nosed breeds like the Boxer, the lower incisors just overlap the upper incisors (undershot bite). Gums should be pink and healthy, and may have pigment spots.

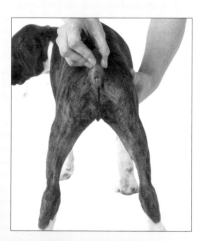

ANAL AND GENITAL AREA
The anal region should have no redness or hair loss. In a female, the vulva should have no inflammation, discharge, or "pasting" of hair (a sign of discharge and vaginitis). In a male, both testicles should be present in the scrotum, and the foreskin (prepuce) should slide back and forth easily with no sticking.

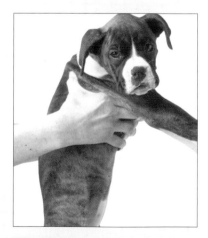

BEHAVIOUR
Temperament testing is not very accurate in young puppies. When picked up any puppy, regardless of breed or size, should feel "solid" with good muscle over the shoulders and no obviously extreme bony prominences. Excessive struggling or snappishness could indicate a dominant personality.

AGE IS IMPORTANT

The most impressionable period in a dog's life is its first 12 weeks. Weaning takes place at six weeks, but there is still much for the puppy to learn from its mother and littermates. Puppies should stay with their mothers until eight weeks old – a bit less for puppies from large litters and a bit more for puppies from small litters.

Around eight weeks is the ideal time for a puppy to move in with its new family. It certainly should do so before 11 or 12 weeks of age, to ensure that it is most receptive and relaxed in its new environment. Some breeders keep puppies on in their kennels, planning to show them; however, dogs raised in kennels do not always make good family dogs.

If you are getting an older puppy or adult dog, make sure it is house trained and used to living in a home with a family. A mature dog is more likely to suffer separation anxiety or have other behaviour problems.

WHERE TO GET A DOG

Breeders, neighbours, pet shops, dog shelters, and advertisements are all potential sources. The healthiest dogs come from neighbours, amateur breeders by accident or intent. Equally healthy puppies come from diligent, conscientious breeders who do what they do because they love their breed rather than because they want to make money from their endeavours.

Commercial breeding establishments seldom provide the enriched environment that puppies thrive on. Good breeders have the parents examined for health and possible hereditary problems before mating, and the puppies

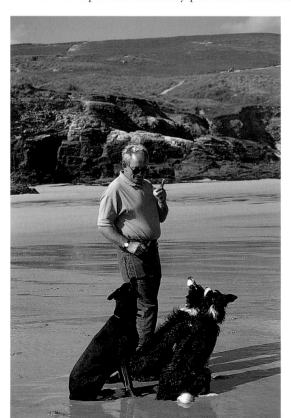

MULTIPLE-DOG FAMILIES
All dogs enjoy, or even thrive on, human companionship. We are excellent dog substitutes, but as good as we are, we are not as good as the real thing. The luckiest dogs have the opportunity to live with other dogs. If you enjoy canine companionship, consider getting a dog companion for your dog.

examined before sale. Honest and reliable breeders are also proud to show you the puppy's mother. If the mother is not there, be suspicious. Ask where the puppies live: those raised in a home develop better and faster than those raised in a kennels. Check the puppy's medical records and ask if the puppies have begun routine worming and inoculations.

Dog shelters and breed rescue associations always have dogs needing loving homes. When acquiring one of these dogs ask whether it was lost or handed in. Male strays often have a powerful "wanderlust". Ask about any known behaviour problems. Progressive rescue centres analyse and report on their residents' behaviour. The very best provide an "after-sales" service of continuing advice on behaviour problems.

As with pet shops and dog rescue centres, all locations where dogs from different sources are congregated are likely to have occasional infectious disease or parasite problems. The very best pet shops have specially designed ventilation and isolate puppies from different litters. While this reduces the risk of disease, it increases the sterility of life for puppies at one of the most important times in their lives. Avoid pet shops if you can.

Veterinary clinics are an excellent source of information on where to get a puppy, so feel free to enquire there. Clinic staff often know the best breeders or the best organized dog shelters.

PREPARING FOR THE NEW ARRIVAL

Puppies are extraordinarily inquisitive. Remove breakable and chewable items from your puppy's territory. Tape down electrical wires, or spray them with taste deterrents. Use baby-guards at the top or bottom of stairs to prevent access to areas not dog-proofed.

Keep outside doors closed and latched, and low windows closed, to prevent wandering. Keep toxic substances such as cleaning materials out of reach. Remove sentimental or valuable objects until your puppy is past its major chewing stage – usually by about 10 months.

MEETING OTHER HOUSEHOLD MEMBERS

Your puppy will be disorientated when it first arrives. Keep it in one room, but let it investigate to its heart's content. Keep human physical activity to a minimum. If you have children, explain to them the need to be quiet and calm. Avoid the temptation of playing "pass-the-parcel" with your new family member. Once it is more secure and confident – a matter of minutes for some but days for others – you can increase your activities with it.

An older dog may resent the arrival of a rambunctious newcomer. Let the resident make the first move; this is most successful when the new puppy is asleep. Open the door and allow your resident to enter and sniff the newcomer. Almost invariably, adult dogs recognize the smell of "youth" and when provoked by the newcomer will threaten rather than bite viciously.

Introduce the family cat in the same way. If your cat is dog-confident it will stand its ground and bat the face of an approaching puppy, the ideal way to establish ground rules. Make sure you move the cat's feeding bowl to a location inaccessible to your puppy.

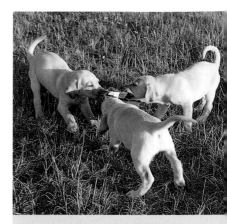

Q WHAT SHOULD I DO TO AVOID JEALOUSY BETWEEN MY OLDER DOG AND MY NEW PUP?

A Jealousy is as natural in dogs as it is in us and can sometimes lead to aggression. A new dog in your home will make your resident jealous. Make sure each dog has its own personal space. Ignore your resident dog when the new puppy is sleeping, but give lots of attention when the puppy is active; in this way your resident will learn to associate the puppy's presence with your increased attention. Make sure there is no eye contact between the dogs when they are fed. Do not let the new dog play with the resident's toys. Try to avoid giving bones. A bone for each will not work if they see each other – each will want both, and may fight to get them.

Q IS IT A GOOD IDEA TO GET TWO PUPPIES AT THE SAME TIME?

A This is a recipe for mayhem. House training two puppies at the same time is extremely difficult. If one dog listens while you train the other, you are unwittingly training the listener to pay no attention to you. If you want two puppies, it is best to get and train one before getting the next one.

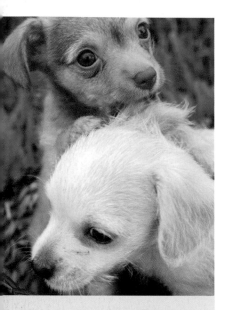

THE FIRST NIGHT

Where your puppy spends its first night is a personal decision. It does not need a special dog bed; a cardboard box makes an excellent first den. If you do buy a bed, make sure it is the right shape and measurements for the dog's eventual adult size and weight. Many puppies are kept in the kitchen.

Before leaving your puppy for the night, take it outside or to an area of floor protected by newspaper to relieve itself. Do not make a big fuss, but simply put it in its bed and leave quietly – no kissing good night. Ignore the protests – the stronger you are at ignoring them, the faster the puppy settles in to its new sleeping arrangements. If you have thin walls and light-sleeping neighbours, visit them with a box of chocolates, explaining what they might hear during the first few nights.

Consider using a dog crate. This can become your puppy's own personal space, a secure and comforting den. Have the crate ready when your puppy comes home, lined with newspaper and containing soft bedding and a toy. The toy, food, and water attract the puppy to walk in. During the day, keep the crate in a busy place such as the kitchen and leave the door open. Never use the crate to discipline a dog. In the evening after the final feed, play, and outdoor activity, introduce your puppy back to the crate and close the door. Set your alarm to get up during the night to let the puppy out of its crate to relieve itself.

I prefer to let new puppies sleep in their crate or cardboard bed in the bedroom with me. Having humans present overnight is less traumatic for a puppy that has just been taken from its mother. It is also easier to take it outside once during the night. There is a very important rule, though: never respond to soulful whimpering. It quickly teaches a puppy that this is a successful ploy for attention.

THE FIRST MEAL

Moving from where it has spent its entire life, with its mother and littermates, to its new home is the most stressful experience of a young puppy's life. The stress increases its risk of illness, especially gastrointestinal disorders. Regardless of what you plan to feed your puppy, always get a sample of what it has been fed. Avoid any new foods for the first few days, until your puppy is settled in and passing well-formed stools. At this time gradually, over a few days, switch to your preferred diet (*see Balanced Nutrition, pp.86–99*).

NAMING YOUR DOG

Your dog will respond best to a one- or two-syllable word that sounds different from words used in everyday conversation. If you choose a long name, make sure you have a short, sharp, familiar name to use when getting your dog's attention. Old-fashioned names like Rex are distinctive to a dog's ear. Always use your dog's name when getting its attention, but never call your dog for punishment – that only teaches it to worry when it hears its name. Ensure that all members of your family follow the same house rules with your dog – they should all use your dog's name first when they want its attention.

Q **IS OUTDOOR KENNELLING ALL RIGHT FOR MY DOG?**

A Outdoor kennelling is only appropriate for giant breed dogs that are too large to live permanently indoors. Be aware that it can interfere with proper socializing. If you have a giant breed puppy, plan for a combination of indoor-outdoor living, using the kitchen for routine activity. Treat the outdoor kennel as a large crate, including in it stimulating toys. Ensure your outdoors dog is played with by members of the family as often as if it were indoors and is never left alone for too long.

Q **CAN DOGS AND CATS LIVE TOGETHER?**

A Of course they can, but first lessons are vital. Do not put them nose to nose and expect them to be instant friends. Let your resident pet sniff your new puppy while it is in a deep sleep. This reduces your cat's natural fear. Allow your cat to hiss at your puppy. You want your dog to respect your cat and not to chase it. Do not leave them alone together until you are sure that your cat has the upper paw.

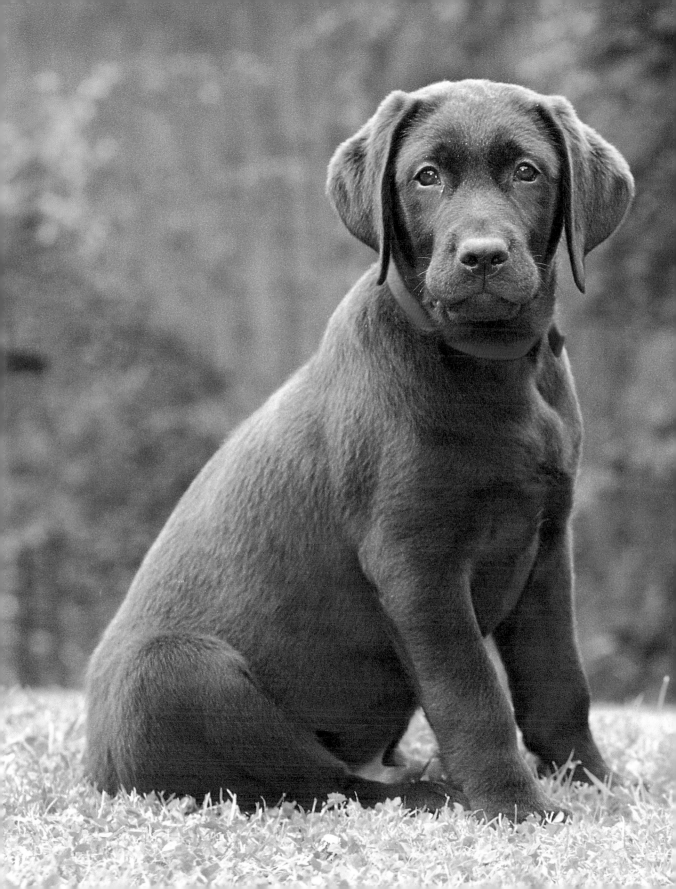

WHICH BREED?

Purebreds now account for the majority of dogs in North America, Europe, and Japan. The variety of sizes, shapes, and coats available appeals to virtually all conceivable tastes. While the appearance and mass of some dogs give us a feeling of security, the size and shape of others bring out our instinctive need to nurture. Most of us are drawn to particular breeds – because of our past experience with them or because their looks appeal to us.

A dog's looks should not be your only consideration. Just as important is its trainability, how noisy it can be, and how good it is with children. When you take these factors into consideration some breeds are excellent for any dog owner, while others are best in the homes of experienced dog people.

Remember that individual dogs are as different as individual people. The following charts, compiled from a worldwide survey of over 1,000 practising vets, show the average characteristics of the average dogs of each breed. On a scale of 1 to 5, 1 is the minimum level and 5 is the maximum for each feature.

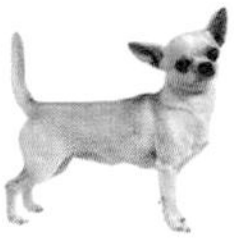

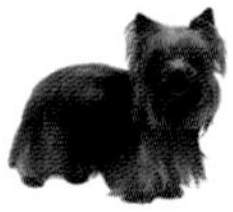

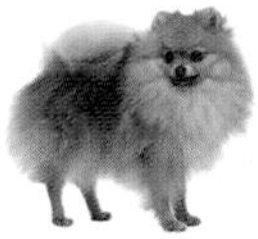

	CHIHUAHUA	YORKSHIRE TERRIER	POMERANIAN
GOOD FIRST DOG	NO	MAYBE	YES
SIZE	1	1	1
TRAINABILITY	2	1–2	3
NOISE	5	5	3
GOOD WITH CHILDREN	2	1	5

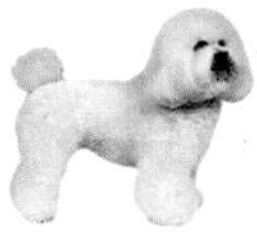

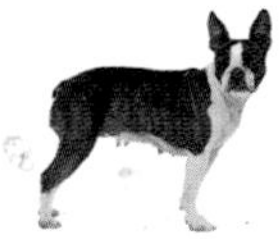

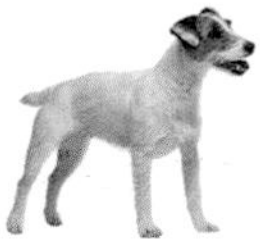

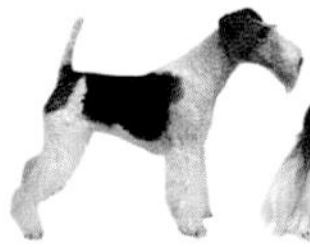

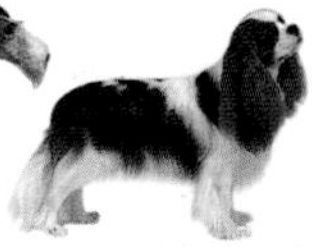

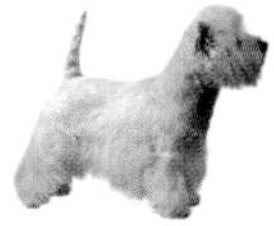

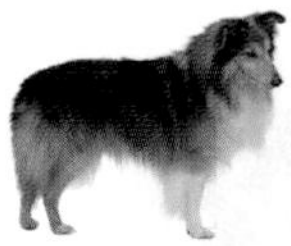

	BICHON FRISE	BOSTON TERRIER	JACK RUSSELL TERRIER	FOX TERRIER	CAVALIER KING CHARLES SPANIEL	WEST HIGHLAND WHITE TERRIER	SHETLAND SHEEPDOG
GOOD FIRST DOG	YES	YES	NO	NO	YES	MAYBE	YES
SIZE	2	2	2	2	2	2–3	2–3
TRAINABILITY	4	3	2	1	4	1–2	5
NOISE	5	4	5	5	3	5	4
GOOD WITH CHILDREN	5	4	1	1	5	1	4

MALTESE	PEKINGESE	SHIH TZU	DACHSHUND	POODLE (MINIATURE AND TOY)	CAIRN TERRIER	LHASA APSO	PUG
YES	MAYBE	YES	MAYBE	YES	YES	YES	YES
1	1	1–2	1–2	1–3	2	2	2
3	2	3	2	4–5	3	3	1
4	3	3	4	5	5	3	4
4	4	5	2	5	4	4	4

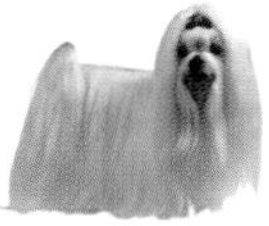

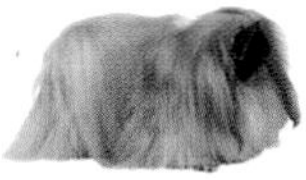

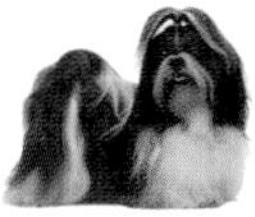

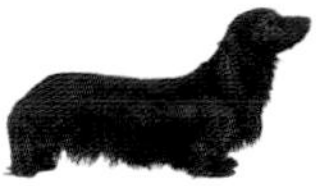

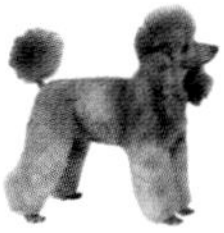

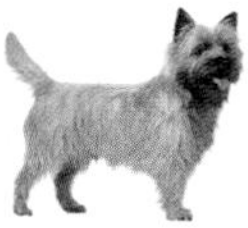

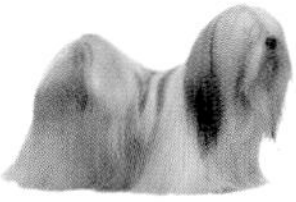

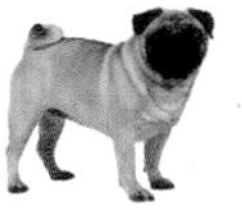

BEAGLE	COCKER SPANIEL (AMERICAN/ENGLISH)	ENGLISH SPRINGER SPANIEL	WELSH CORGI (CARDIGAN/PEMBROKE)	SCHNAUZER (MINIATURE)	SCOTTISH TERRIER	STAFFORDSHIRE BULL TERRIER	AIREDALE TERRIER
YES	YES	MAYBE	MAYBE	YES	MAYBE	MAYBE	NO
3	3	3	3	3	3	3	3–4
1	3–4	5	4	3–4	2	3	2
5	3	3	3	5	4	4	4
4	5	5	2	4	2	4	3

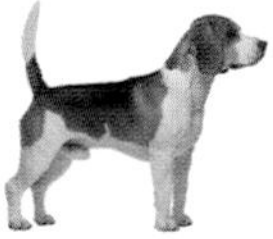

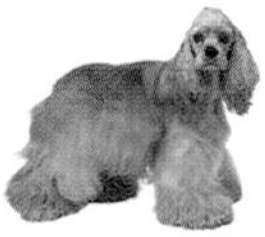

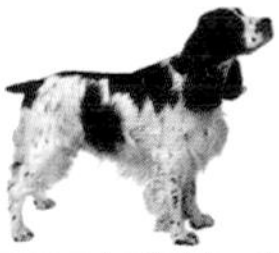

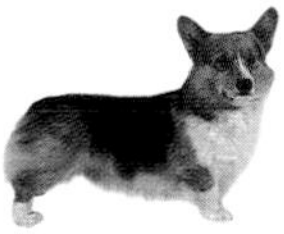

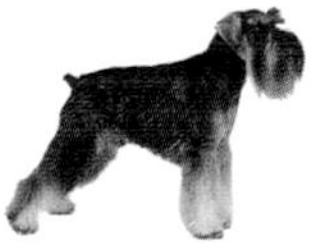

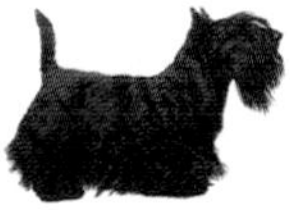

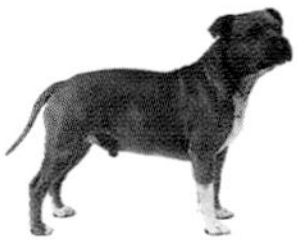

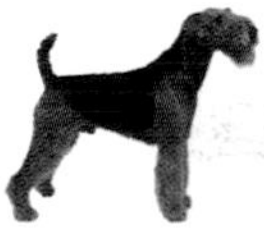

	BULLDOG	BORDER COLLIE	ALASKAN MALAMUTE	DOBERMAN PINSCHER	COLLIE (ROUGH)	DALMATIAN	CHOW CHOW
GOOD FIRST DOG	MAYBE	NO	MAYBE	MAYBE	YES	NO	NO
SIZE	3–4	3–4	3–4	4	4	4	4
TRAINABILITY	1	5	3	5	4	3	1
NOISE	2	3	1	2	2	3	1
GOOD WITH CHILDREN	4	2	3	3	5	2	1

	HUNGARIAN VIZSLA	SAMOYED	GERMAN SHORT-HAIRED POINTER	BASSET HOUND	BOXER	BLOODHOUND	AFGHAN HOUND
GOOD FIRST DOG	YES	MAYBE	YES	MAYBE	MAYBE	MAYBE	NO
SIZE	4	4	4	4	4	4	4
TRAINABILITY	4	2–3	3–4	1	3	2	1
NOISE	2	3	3	2	2	1	2
GOOD WITH CHILDREN	5	3	4	5	4	5	2

LABRADOR RETRIEVER	NORWEGIAN ELKHOUND	POODLE (STANDARD)	SIBERIAN HUSKY	WEIMARANER	GOLDEN RETRIEVER	SHAR PEI	SETTER (IRISH & ENGLISH)
YES	YES	YES	NO	MAYBE	YES	NO	YES
4	4	4	4	4	4	4	4
5	3–4	5	3	4	5	2	2
1	2	3	3	4	1	3	4
5	4	5	2	3	5	2	4

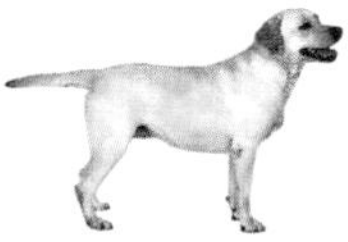

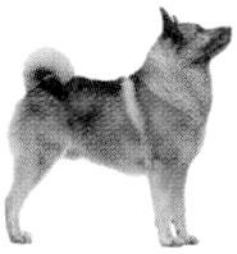

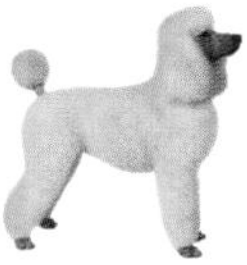

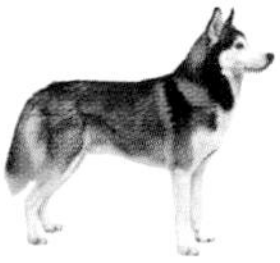

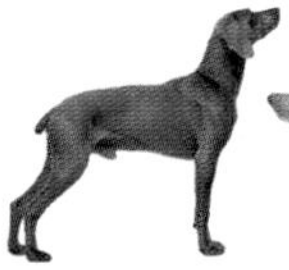

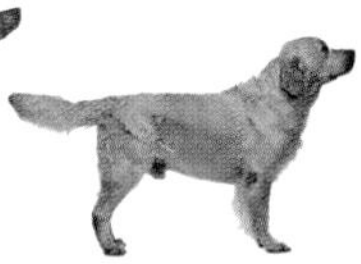

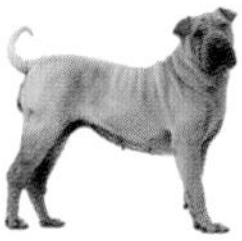

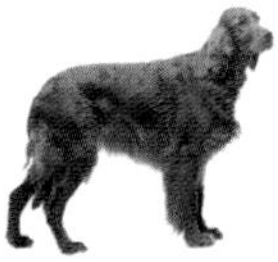

GERMAN SHEPHERD	CHESAPEAKE BAY RETRIEVER	ROTTWEILER	SAINT BERNARD	AKITA	NEWFOUNDLAND	OLD ENGLISH SHEEPDOG	GREAT DANE
NO	YES	NO	NO	NO	YES	NO	NO
4–5	4–5	4–5	5	5	5	5	5
5	5	3–4	2	3–4	3	2	3
3	1	1	1	1	1	1	1
3	5	2	4	2	5	3	4

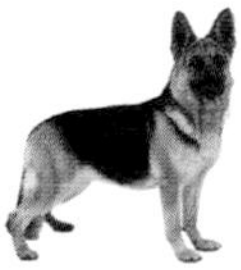

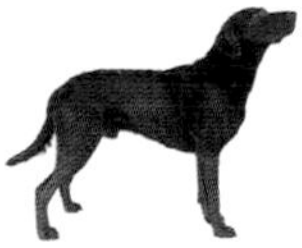

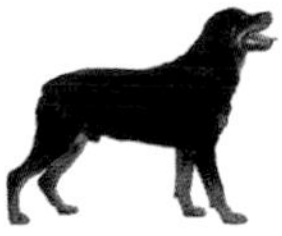

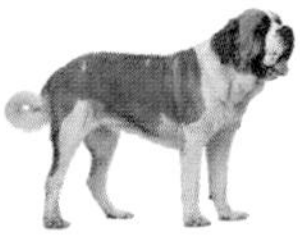

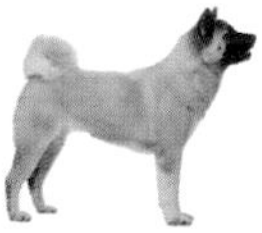

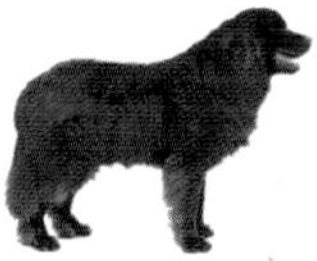

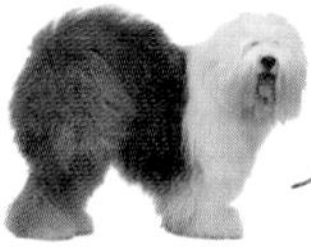

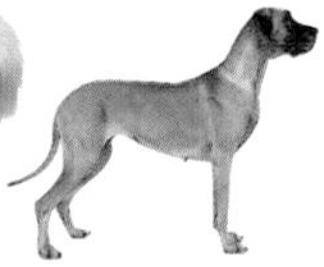

A SUCCESSFUL PARTNERSHIP
living with your dog

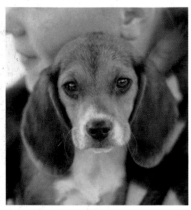

A beagle can be a popular companion

OBJECTIVES

Living with a dog offers a window into another world. Dog owners, by sharing their homes with another species, recognize that other species share with us a common range of needs and emotions, from security and constancy to jealousy and anger. The following are the simple objectives for integrating dogs into a productive and mutually satisfying partnership with us. Dogs should:

- socialize with humans, other dogs, and other animals;
- adapt to the human environment;
- enjoy human touch;
- accept restraint;
- learn to control their aggression;
- eliminate in designated areas;
- come when they are called;
- know how to walk on a lead;
- have good manners inside and outside the home;
- enjoy being home alone occasionally;
- trust people.

Caring for your dog is not just a matter of disease prevention or calling in the vet when problems develop. Good care means understanding your dog's psychological needs and at the same time integrating your canine companion into what is, from its evolutionary perspective, an alien environment. A dog has to learn to let strangers touch it, and to respond to the words used in training. You also have to take care of your dog's special needs, whether it travels with you or stays behind when you leave home. As your dog ages, you have to keep its best interests at heart – you are the one who will have to decide if and when to put your dog to sleep.

LIVING WITH US

It may sound attractive to let a dog do what it wants to do. After all, that gives it the ultimate freedom to act out its natural inclinations. This is, of course, as unrealistic for dogs as it is for us. We teach our children good manners, socially acceptable toilet habits, and how to control their natural aggression. We monitor their safety, channel their curiosity into constructive pursuits, and ask others who are more knowledgeable to help educate them. It should be the same with our canine family member.

A happy, contented dog has learned how to act responsibly with its own kind but also with other species, especially humans. It has learned to inhibit its inclination to bite, to respond positively to people, to enjoy being handled and accept restraint, and, for its own safety and security, to respond to our instructions. Simple obedience training is as important as any other factor in caring properly for our dogs.

THE ESSENCE OF TRAINING

Your dog is a pack animal, naturally inclined to respect and respond to the pack leader – that is, you. As a pack animal it enjoys contact with the rest of its pack, both their proximity and their touch. It thinks that food is the essence of life and loves to chew or just possess its own treasures. This gives you the basis for perfect rewards (food and toys) and natural discipline (isolation from you). A dog is acutely aware of body language and sounds, quickly learning to interpret your tone of voice and stance.

Be timely when using rewards and discipline. Have your reward at hand and let your dog know it is there. Give it, together with praise, the instant your dog responds. It will soon learn to respond to praise alone. Similarly, use discipline at the instant of disobedience. When using separation from you to discipline your dog, it should last less than a minute; it is purely symbolic.

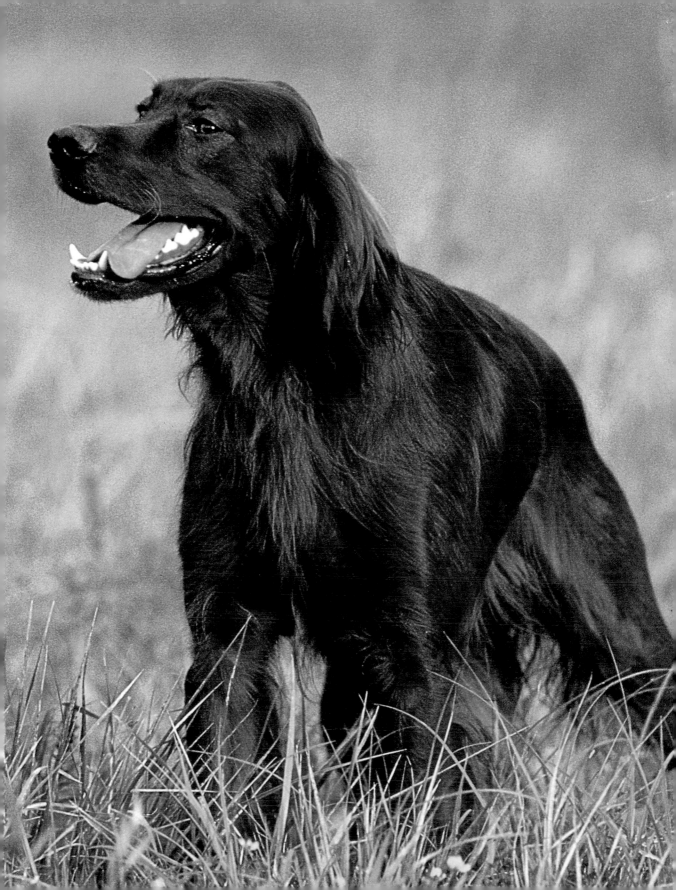

BASIC HOUSE TRAINING

1. Select a toileting area away from activity and distractions.

2. In the yard or a public place, choose an area that is easy to clean. Scooping is simpler from a hard surface than from grass.

3. Have scoops (such as a plastic bag) always available. Clean up immediately after your puppy relieves itself.

4. Take your puppy to relieve itself:
- after eating (within minutes);
- after play or exercise;
- after any excitement, such as a greeting;
- after waking up.

5. Watch your puppy's body language for these clues:
- sniffing the floor;
- circling;
- running with the nose to the floor;
- getting ready to squat.

When you see any of these activities, interrupt the puppy and take it outside. If you can, avoid picking it up; you want the puppy to learn it should walk to its toileting area when it wants to relieve itself.

6. Use word cues you will be happy to say in public. With time, your puppy will associate hearing these words with the need to go.

7. Accidents will happen. When you see your puppy relieving itself in the house, get its attention by shouting. You do this not to frighten or punish it, but rather to get its mind on you. As soon as you have the puppy's attention, call its name. You want to encourage it to follow you outside willingly where it will complete what it started earlier. When you return to the house, keep the puppy in another room while you clean up the mess.

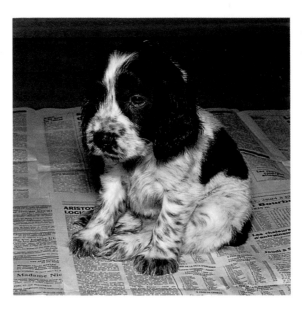

NEWSPAPER TRAINING
A puppy as young as this one urinates as soon as it feels a need to do so. Ensure that all areas the puppy has access to are covered with newspaper. The feel under foot is important. Within a few days a puppy will actively search out newspaper when it wants to empty its bladder.

HOUSE TRAINING
Dogs are instinctively clean animals, unwilling to soil their nest. Take advantage of this and teach your dog that your entire home is "the nest". The instinct not to soil the nest is already there in young puppies. Restrict a dog to its nest – a crate for example – and take it to the location that you want it to use for its toilet. Only then should the puppy, or adult dog, be given the reward of roaming elsewhere in your home. House training is simple, but it depends upon your vigilance.

TRAINING AN ADULT DOG
The basic principles of house training apply equally to older dogs. The important difference is that older dogs have to "unlearn" some toileting habits before learning new ones. To house train an older dog, tether it to you and do not allow it to roam the house freely until after it has relieved itself outdoors. If the dog starts to urinate or defecate, correct it with a sharp "No!", then immediately take it outside. Praise the dog with your most impressive "Good dog" when it performs where you want it to.

The key to success is to limit the chances of the dog's messing where you do not want it to mess. Accidents will happen, but keep your cool. If accidents happen frequently, it is an indication that you are not keeping a close enough eye on your dog. Any adult dog can learn the essence of house training within two weeks. If it is taking longer, contact your vet to ensure there are no medical problems, such as incontinence.

SUBMISSIVE URINATION
Dogs urinate when they are frightened, but more frequently they urinate as a sign of submission (females in particular). Do not mistake this for a lapse in house training. Urinating submissively is a natural way in which

a low-ranking dog appeases a higher-ranking one. This is why urinating when excited is more characteristic of a puppy than an adult problem.

If your puppy urinates when it sees you, do not reprimand it or show anger. On the other hand, do not stroke its head or reach down and touch it; these would be the actions of dominating high-rankers. Ignore the puppy and walk away, either to an area where there is newspaper on plastic sheeting, or out through the back door to where it can relieve itself.

Most puppies outgrow submissive urination as they mature and build confidence. Curiously, puppies with this habit are the easiest to obedience-train because they concentrate so intently on you, but it is absolutely imperative to avoid scolding or anger during training.

THE ESSENTIALS OF BASIC OBEDIENCE TRAINING

Training is easiest with puppies. Older dogs take longer to accept a new person as their leader, but if you show consistent behaviour a dog learns to respect you. Teaching good manners, or to come, sit, stay, or lie down, is surprisingly easy. Most dogs willingly carry out these activities because they want to please their leaders and because it is in their interest to do so.

Never punish your dog for something it has done earlier. Punishment when you return to a mess in the house is interpreted simply as inexplicable punishment. Your dog will not understand; all it will know is that you are angry with it. Your dog will respond by acting submissively to appease you. We make the mistake of thinking that its signs of appeasement are signs of guilt. They are not. Punishing after the fact is counterproductive.

Keep lessons short. A minute or two is perfect for a puppy. Five minutes is too long, but puppies are capable of concentrating on training several times during the day. Older dogs can concentrate for longer, but even dogs with the best mental stamina cannot concentrate on training for more than about 15 minutes at a time.

Keep lessons enjoyable. If your dog is not enjoying himself, forget about training. If it needs to release pent-up physical energy, let it. Once it has had some exercise your dog will concentrate more on what you are doing with it.

Train when your dog's mind is alert. An ideal time to train is before feeding time. With puppies that means you have three or four ready-prepared

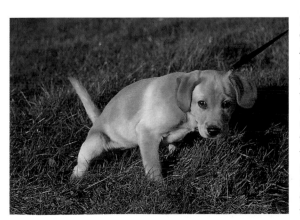

URINATING OUTDOORS

As soon as possible, introduce your puppy to the area outdoors where you want it to urinate. Most puppies naturally prefer the texture of grass, but at this age it is equally possible to train urban puppies with no gardens to urinate in the gutter.

Q MY DOG SEEMS TO HAVE FORGOTTEN ITS HOUSE TRAINING. WHY?

A Lapses in or loss of house training may occur in these circumstances:
- sex-related urine marking;
- sudden household activity, such as a party;
- changes in the primary "leader" of the dog's household;
- emotional turmoil in the family;
- the arrival of another pet;
- full training was never completed;
- submissive urination;
- fear, stress, or anxiety;
- high excitement;
- a medical problem.

Q SHOULD I USE A CHOKE CHAIN DURING TRAINING?

A Choke chains are used by disciplinarian trainers. As a dog pulls forward, the chain around its neck tightens until it hurts or the dog cannot breathe. If you put it on the wrong way, it does not loosen up when the dog stops pulling. A choke chain is unnecessary. Use a "half-check collar" instead. This collar is part fabric (usually braided nylon) and part choke; so nylon rather than metal links lie against the windpipe when a dog surges forward. It is impossible to put on backwards. For heel training use a head halter, body harness, or half check, not a choke collar.

Q WHAT FOOD TREATS ARE A GOOD IDEA DURING TRAINING?

A You have to "addict" your dog to the food treat you are using. Dried liver treats work very well because they are smelly. Yeast-based vitamin and mineral tablets are smelly and nutritious. If your dog is not interested in food, find a toy, usually a squeaky one, that triggers intense interest and use it as reward.

PUPPY CLASSES

Puppy classes are like preschool for children – an ideal environment for early learning and moulding behaviour. The best incorporate the following principles:

- There is a restricted puppy age group, preferably under 16 weeks old.

- The puppy's entire human family is encouraged to attend.

- Free play takes place amongst selected groups of puppies.

- Classes last about an hour, run for around six weeks, and cover a set curriculum.

- The class is recommended by your veterinary surgeon or the owner of a well-behaved dog.

When attending a puppy class, look for the following:

- Classes should be closely supervised, including free play.

- Children attending classes should also be closely supervised.

- Brash puppies should not be allowed to intimidate shy ones.

- Bold puppies should be selected for their own play group.

- All classes should end on a positive note for puppies and their owners.

- You should be sent home with homework to do before the next class.

training opportunities each day. As your puppy matures and the number of meals diminishes, train it shortly after it has awakened and after it has emptied its bladder and bowels.

At first always combine food rewards with praise. Eventually, only give the most powerful reward – food – intermittently. Giving rewards intermittently rather than constantly is the most effective way of reinforcing learning. Always finish formal training sessions on a high note. Do not save the most powerful reward for the end of the session; if you do, you are unwittingly training your dog to want the session to end so it can get hold of the potent reward.

Avoid distractions by beginning training inside your own home. This applies to simple obedience such as "Come", "Sit", "Stay", and "Down", but also to lead training or "walking-to-heel" training. A hallway is an excellent place to begin training. Once your dog reliably responds in that location, move on to a more distracting environment, such as the back garden. Only when your dog behaves well in this area should you advance to more complicated surroundings such as the street or a park.

Be consistent. Stand upright, use your dog's name to get its attention, and give verbal or hand signals only when you have eye-to-eye contact with it. Reward the dog as soon as it complies with your command, and do not issue a command unless you can enforce it. When disciplining your dog, use stern body language, lower your voice, and say "No" sharply. Teach the dog to respond to a combination of verbal and hand signals.

Do not get flustered. Avoid persistently repeating commands, because it will only confuse your dog. If training is not going well, stop. Think about what you are doing; the problem may be with you, not with your dog. Do not be bashful about asking for help – front-office staff at veterinary clinics are usually excellent people to ask for advice.

If more than one member of the family helps to do the training, make sure that everyone is using the same words and signals so as not to confuse the dog. Forget about trying to train several dogs at once – it is virtually impossible. If you have two dogs to train, take turns: keep one out of earshot while you train, reward, or discipline the other.

THE BASIC COMMANDS

The four basic commands are "Come", "Sit", "Stay", and "Lie down". Once your dog reliably understands basic obedience, it is ready for walking to heel. It must understand "Sit" because this is always the take-off point for walking to heel.

Traditionally, dogs are trained to walk by your left side. (The dog is always at the handler's heel, which, of course, is why training is called "heel" training.) It really does not matter whether you start heel training on or off the lead. It is not an issue of right or wrong, but rather what feels best for you and your dog. When a puppy follows you willingly off lead, it is easy to graduate to walking-to-heel training on a lead. Use a lead with a bolt-snap of appropriate weight for your dog. If you have not introduced the lead before, let your puppy look at it and smell it.

TEACHING YOUR DOG TO COME TO YOU

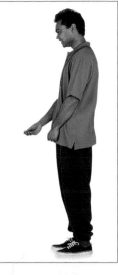

1 Stand a short distance away from the puppy, in a quiet room with no distractions. A hallway is an ideal location. With a food treat visible in your hand, speak the puppy's name and, as it begins to move forwards, give the command "Come".

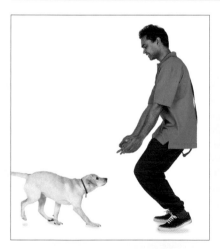

2 As the puppy moves towards you, praise it by saying the words "Good dog" using a bright and enthusiastic tone of voice. Encourage the puppy to come directly to you by bending your knees and opening your arms wide.

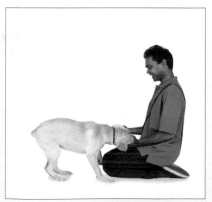

3 As the puppy approaches, kneel down to get closer to its level. Praise the puppy again with words, stroking as well as giving the food reward. In order to maintain the interest of the dog, vary the locations in which the training takes place.

TRAINING TIPS

Tips on teaching your dog to come to you:

• To ensure that your dog always complies with your instructions, use a thin houseline (or, when you are outdoors, the lead) to ensure you can always get your dog's attention. Do not use it like a fishing line, to reel in your dog. Instead, give a quick jerk on the lead to get its attention, then draw the dog to you with your reward, not with tension on the lead.

• Never say "Come" unless you are sure your dog will obey.

• Never use the "Come" command to call your dog from something exciting to something less interesting.

• Never use the word "Come" to call your dog to discipline.

• If your dog does not respond properly or does something wrong, avoid the word "No". Save that for more serious misdemeanours. Introduce a neutral word such as "Wrong" if it does not get the command right.

• If your dog loses concentration, you have probably chosen the wrong time or place for training. Try again when it is better prepared.

• Before training always let your dog play vigorously first to burn off excess energy.

TRAINING TIPS

Tips on teaching your dog to sit:

• Most dogs naturally assume a sitting position to keep an eye on something above them. If your dog does not, hold its collar in one hand and use your other hand to tuck its hindquarters into a sitting position. Give the command "Sit" as you do this and instantly reward the dog with a food treat and a verbal "Good dog". Eventually you will give the "Sit" command when you are walking with your dog and you stop, or when it is playing and you want its attention.

• Avoid overexcitement. If meals are so exciting that your dog cannot concentrate on your commands, do not use the meal as a reward. Train on a fuller stomach, using less stimulating but still interesting rewards.

• Never give a command without ensuring that your dog complies. If you do so, you are actively training your dog to disregard that command.

Tips on teaching your dog to stay:

• Train with your dog sitting at the base of a wall. That keeps it from sliding backwards.

• Avoid an abundance of praise after releasing your dog from "Stay". Too much praise on your part winds up your dog and teaches it to jump around and be exuberant at the end of a training session. Keep praise muted.

• Never try "Stay" training when circumstances make it hard for your dog to concentrate on what you are doing. If it is worried about the presence of other dogs or more interested in investigating other activities, its mind is elsewhere. During each short training session you want its full attention.

TEACHING YOUR DOG TO SIT

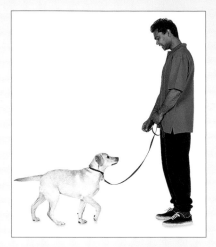

1 Facing the puppy, move away with the lead in your left hand and a food treat in your right. Keeping calm and trying not to excite the puppy, tell it to come to you as you show it the food.

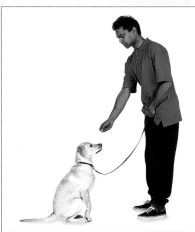

2 When the puppy reaches you, slowly move the treat up and over its head. The puppy will sit in order to keep its eyes on the food. Give the command "Sit" as it starts to bend its hind legs.

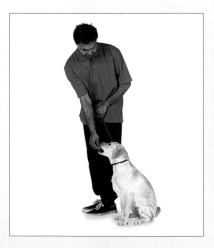

3 Reinforce the "Sit" command from the front and to the side of the puppy. Reward each response with verbal praise and food treats. Gradually reduce the food rewards until words alone are sufficient.

TEACHING YOUR DOG TO SIT AND STAY

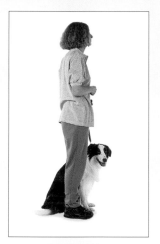

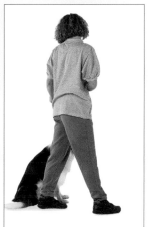

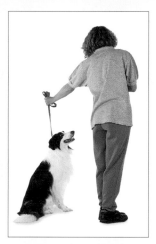

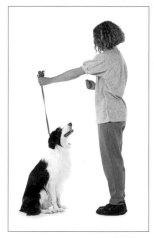

1 Hold the telescoped lead (folded so as to keep the tension) in your left hand and a treat in your right. As the dog sits, concentrating on the treat, command it to "Sit".

2 Maintaining tension on the lead, step forwards with your right foot. Give the "Stay" command as you begin to move forwards.

3 Move your left foot to join your right foot, remembering to maintain gentle eye contact with the dog at all times.

4 Exerting light pressure on the lead, held over the dog's head, turn to face the dog. Keep its attention by holding the food up high.

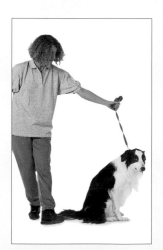

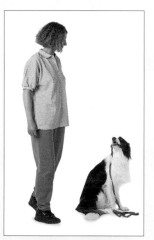

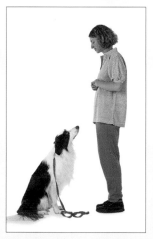

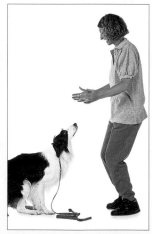

5 Reward the dog for staying. Now slowly walk around the dog, holding the lead above its head. Issue as few commands as possible, so that you do not confuse the dog.

6 After several sessions, the dog should sit and stay while on the lead. Now drop the lead and repeat each of the previous five steps, always praising the dog for good behaviour.

7 When the dog sits and stays with the lead dropped, give it the treat. Reward the dog while it is doing what it is told, not afterwards.

8 End the training by opening your arms and saying "OK". Always finish on a happy and positive note. Do not overexcite your dog with your own enthusiasm until the training period has ended.

TRAINING TIPS

Tips on teaching your dog to lie down:

• If your dog creeps forwards on its haunches rather than lying down, kneel beside it and, while it is sitting, put the palms of your hands under its forelegs, lift it gently into a begging position, then lower it into a lying position. Instantly reward it with praise and treats.

• If your dog refuses to stay down, use both hands to apply gentle pressure to its withers, the area above its shoulders. Reward it for lying down, then release it with the word "Finished".

Tips on teaching your dog to walk on a lead:

• If your boisterous dog tries to climb its lead, say "No!", move away, give the "Sit" command, and go back to the beginning of the exercise.

• If your dog chews the lead instead of walking along it, get an unpleasant-tasting but safe chew deterrent. Spray the parts of the lead likely to be chewed.

• If your dog is distracted, use your left hand on its collar to bring it back to the correct heel position, get its attention with the food treat, and continue. If a distraction is overwhelming, command it to do something you know it will do – a "Sit". Reward it with verbal praise and continue later when the distraction is no longer there.

TEACHING YOUR DOG TO LIE DOWN

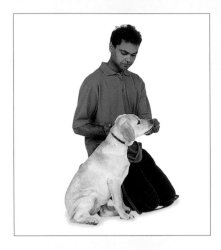

1 Once the puppy is sitting, kneel at its left side and hold its collar in your right hand. Holding a food treat in your left hand, place your hand on the puppy's nose before moving it downwards.

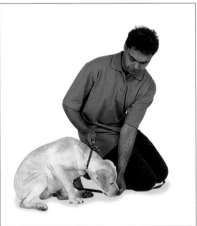

2 As the puppy's nose follows the treat, move it forwards to the front of its body. The moment the puppy starts to lie down, give the command "Down", but do not reward the puppy yet.

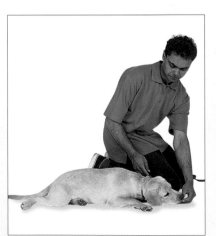

3 Move the food just far enough forwards to lure the puppy to lie down. Reward the puppy with praise and the food treat. Repeat the exercise frequently, until the puppy responds to words alone.

TEACHING YOUR DOG TO WALK ON A LEAD

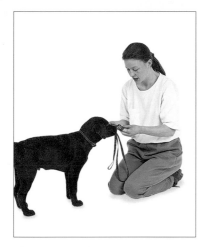

1 The training for this exercise should start indoors. The puppy should be wearing a comfortable, well-fitting collar. Let the puppy look at and smell the lead, then attach the lead to the collar.

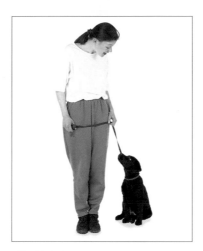

2 With the puppy on your left side, hold the lead and food reward in your right hand. Your left hand holds the slack, ready to slide down to the collar. Give the puppy the "Sit" command.

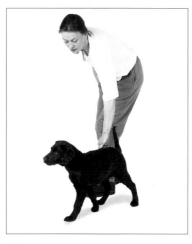

3 Begin to walk with your left foot first. As the puppy walks beside you, give the command "Heel". If the puppy surges forward, slide your left hand down the lead to its collar and gently pull backwards.

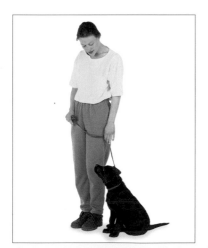

4 When the puppy is in the heel position, give the reward and verbal praise. Then give the command to sit. Slowly increase the distance you cover as the puppy obeys the sequence of commands.

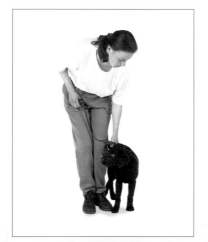

5 Once the puppy is able to walk to heel and sit obediently as you go in a straight line, you can train it to turn right. Guide it around to the right with your left hand, and give the command "Heel".

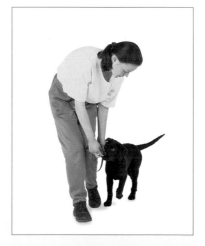

6 To make a left turn, increase your own speed and hold the food in front of the puppy's nose to slow it down. Keep the puppy close to your left leg and give the "Steady" command as it slows down.

HOME ALONE

The reality of modern living means that dogs can and should learn to be left alone occasionally for a few hours. This training is simple if you follow these guidelines to prevent boredom and separation anxiety.

• Crate-train your dog or dog-proof your home.

• Exercise your dog before leaving it home alone. Exhausted dogs are less likely to bark, dig, or destroy.

• Take your dog to relieve itself, then feed your dog before you leave. A dog naturally rests when its stomach is full.

• Provide your dog with its own "safe haven" at home, such as a comfortable basket or bed.

• Come and go without a fuss. That includes no petting or saying "Goodbye" to your dog when you depart and no exuberant greetings upon your return.

• Before you leave, rub a favourite toy in your hands to leave your scent, and give it to the dog.

• Hide other treats, such as dry food, in the house. This provides an opportunity for mental activity.

• Provide background noise such as that from the stereo, radio, or TV to filter out outdoor noises that your dog might find distracting.

• Drugs are available to help manage serious separation anxiety if it develops, but drugs do not cure the problem – training does.

• Never leave your dog at home alone all day. If you must leave it all day, get a friend to visit to take your dog for play and exercise. Alternatively, get a dog walker or take your pet to a dog day care centre (see p.49).

BEHAVIOUR PROBLEMS

Every dog will develop habits that you do not want it to have. Fortunately, most are minor and easy to live with, but some are sufficiently antisocial that they need to be changed. It helps to know what you are going to do when problems develop. First, minimize the chance that the problem will happen again and then try to understand the reason for the behaviour.

If your dog is chewing a shoe, train your family not to leave shoes about, but leave a chew toy instead. Take the initiative before your dog misbehaves by having it do something for you. If the dog jumps up to say hello, train it to sit when you come home and reward it for sitting rather than disciplining it for jumping. If it barks when it hears a noise, train it to fetch and carry. It is tough for a dog to bark effectively when its mouth is filled with a soft toy.

Unwanted behaviours fall into three categories: boredom problems, excitement problems, and aggression problems.

BOREDOM PROBLEMS

Boredom leads to anxiety, which leads to creativity on the dog's part, which produces mayhem. Separation anxiety is most common in rescued dogs or those that have become overly dependent on their owners. Signs of boredom are chewing, digging, howling, and barking, as well as fence-jumping or rhythmically pacing back and forth.

Dogs need to chew something. Apply taste deterrents to objects that you do not want chewed, and provide exciting chew toys.

If you have an instinctive digger, redirect its energy away from the flower beds or lawn to an acceptable area. Restrict the dog to a safe area of the garden, and give it a sand pit to dig in.

To turn off howling and barking, first train your dog to "Speak" on command. Attach your dog's lead to a fence, stand a few feet away, and tease it with a toy. When it barks from frustration, give it a food treat. Give the "Speak" command the moment it barks, then give the treat as a reward. When your dog consistently barks to the word "Speak" for the toy or food, switch to verbal rewards: "Good dog." Once it understands "Speak", give the command "Quiet" when it is barking and reward it with the toy or treat as soon as it stops. Be patient – this takes time.

Once it consistently stops barking when you say "Quiet", move a short distance away and repeat the exercise, returning to it initially with a food or toy reward. Eventually, switch to verbal rewards at a distance when it responds to your "Quiet" command. When the dog responds to verbal cues, set up mock departures, giving the "Quiet" command before you leave. Stand outside the door. If it barks, make a noise, for example by dropping an aluminium pan; you want to startle the dog into stopping barking. Return and praise it for being quiet.

For fence-jumpers, create obstacles. Tin cans strung on a rope about 30cm (1ft) from the fence and 90cm (3ft) off the ground make a nice, noisy, and natural deterrent. Chicken wire on the ground at take-off distance from the fence works well, but make sure the gauge of the wire is too small for one of your dog's feet to slip through. Chicken wire is also an excellent deterrent to digging.

EXCITEMENT PROBLEMS

Dogs show excitement in different ways. Some bark. Others pull on the lead. Many jump up, wanting to lick your face. Terriers often nip with excitement, while Bull Terriers in particular have a tendency to chase their tails. Activity and good basic obedience training are at the root of preventing over-excited behaviour. Plan ahead. If your dog jumps on visitors to greet them, for example, make sure it is on a lead or in another room when visitors come into your home.

Some dogs develop the common habit of pulling on the lead. If your dog has this problem, do not turn it into a tug of war – go back to basics until you are sure your dog follows basic obedience signals. Proceed to basic walking-to-heel retraining but now, with the dog on its lead at your left, slide your left hand down the lead to near its collar. If it pulls, pull back firmly and command it to "Sit". Start again, giving the "Heel" command. If the dog pulls, give another yank and command it to "Sit". Repeat this exercise until it walks quietly without pulling. Reward it with a food treat. Graduate to more distracting environments and circumstances.

Jumping up is also a common sign of excitement. It is better to use a positive command, such as "Sit", than a negative one such as "Off". Ignore flamboyant greetings. Avoid eye contact and go about your business. Do not raise your voice, wave your arms, or in any other way increase its excitement. When all four of the dog's feet are back on the

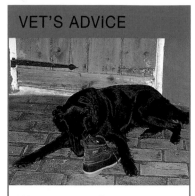

VET'S ADVICE

You can create circumstances where your dog learns automatically to stop doing something by itself, without your obvious involvement.

• Use a proprietary bitter spray, Tabasco sauce, or other safe but disagreeable tastes to prevent chewing where you do not want chewing.

• Use noise the same way. Inexpensive vibration-sensitive alarms for windows, available from most hardware stores, are ideal for putting on beds or sofas if you do not want your dog sleeping on these in your absence.

• Be creative and a little flamboyant with what dog trainers call "aversion therapy". It is a natural way for dogs to learn from a situation, rather than from your obvious intervention.

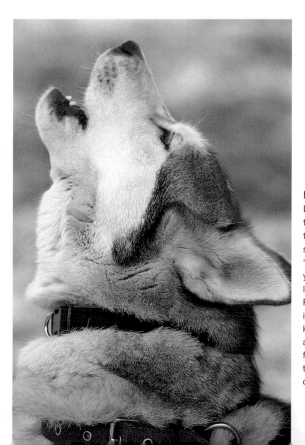

HOWLING
Dogs howl to "talk" to other members of the pack. Generally speaking a howl says "Where are you?" If your dog howls when left alone, it is bored. Rather than discipline it, review the way you keep your dog. Find alternatives – ranging from toys and activity to companionship – to overcome boredom.

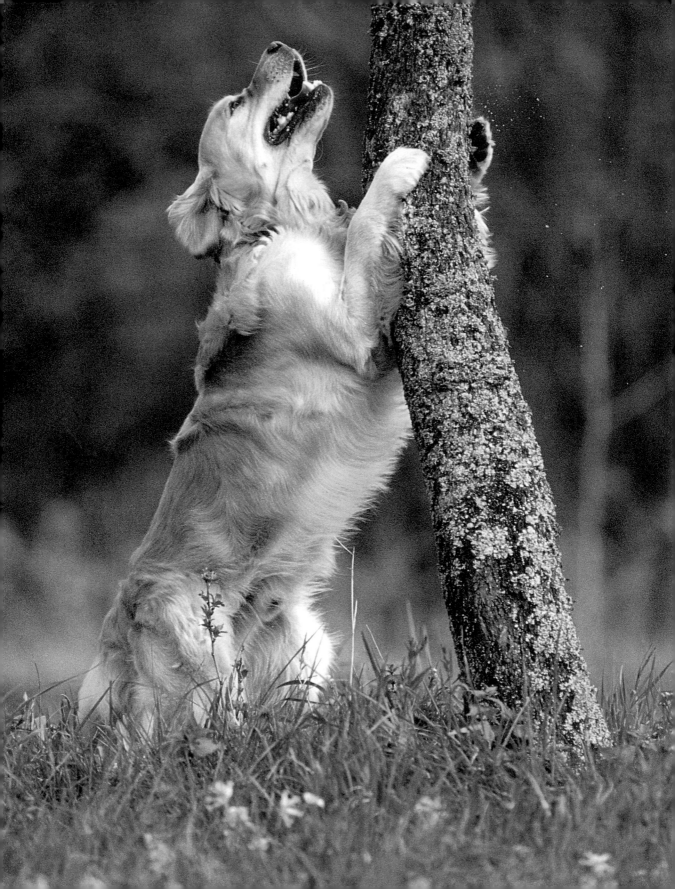

ground give the "Sit" command and reward your dog with a quiet "Hello". Praise all signs of calm obedience.

Terriers in particular tend to tug on clothes or nip when excited. Overcome this unpleasant habit by training your dog to carry a toy in its mouth. If it is preoccupied with one job, it is difficult to carry out another. Integrate toy-carrying with basic "Sit-Stay" obedience. Toy-carrying is also a wonderful way to muffle barking. To control barking itself, follow the procedure for controlling boredom barking (*see p.40*).

AGGRESSION PROBLEMS

Some dogs are born with a greater tendency to become aggressive, but problems only occur in homes that wittingly or unwittingly encourage the development of a dog's aggressive potential. Early socializing to the human family, to strangers, to other animals, and to a whole range of experiences reduces dramatically the likelihood that a dog will reach its "aggression potential".

There is always a reason for aggressive behaviour; a reason that is obvious to the dog, but not always obvious to us. It is important to understand exactly why your dog shows aggression. Once it develops, aggressive behaviour never disappears on its own: we have to contain it, reduce it, then eliminate it. Do not hesitate to get professional help.

Dominance aggression

This type of aggression is the most common reason why dogs growl at or bite their owners. Avoid physical punishment – it is provocative and may make matters worse. Use body posture, facial expression, and the tone of your voice to remind the dog that you are the leader of the pack. Reassert your authority over a pushy dog by attaching a lead to your dog's collar. Use this to move your dog to temporary (one-minute) isolation from the family. Do not hold a grudge, but review your relationship with your dog to determine why it thought it could challenge you. Remember, little things send big signals to your dog – you are the leader, so you eat first and you go through doorways first.

Dominance aggression between two dogs is more likely to occur when both are relatively equal – same sex, age, and size. Your instinct to comfort the underdog only increases the problem. Remember that the higher ranking dog eats first, is petted by you first, and goes out the door first. If aggression from the underdog is severe and this does not work, get your veterinary surgeon's help. Neutering a dog lowers its rank and this often cures the problem (*see p.46*). It may seem heartless to neuter the underdog, but this is usually enough to stop dominance fighting.

Sex-related aggression

Aggression related to sexual urges can occur in both sexes. It may occur only twice a year in females, when they are hormonally active. All females that have ovulated go through a two-month hormonal pregnancy (*see p.57*), and may become possessive over certain items such as shoes, soft toys, or socks. This is a form of maternal aggression.

RETRAINING RULES

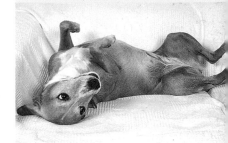

Although bad habits vary, almost all of them can be diminished or corrected following this basic programme.

● Go back to basic obedience. Make sure your dog understands all the basic commands.

● Ensure that your dog does something for you, such as sitting or lying down, before it receives any kind of reward, even a verbal "Hello".

● Avoid problems by making sure you can enforce obedience commands.

● Satisfy your dog's natural needs by creating acceptable outlets for natural behaviour.

● Eliminate the satisfaction that your dog gets from its unacceptable behaviour. Sometimes this will involve mild punishment.

● Persevere. Do not expect miracles overnight. Typically, it takes about three weeks to overcome most common behaviour problems.

● If you are unsure, or if aggression is involved, your veterinary clinic should be your first port of call if you have any questions about your dog's behaviour. They can recommend local dog trainers.

More common is male-to-male aggression, which may occur all year round. This is more likely to occur in dogs that as puppies were allowed to play rough games without correction. Do not let your puppy bite other dogs hard, put its paws on the other dog's back, or mount and thrust on any part of another dog. Tolerant, older family dogs often let a puppy get away with these activities, and it will try the same with unknown dogs.

Fearful aggression

Aggression due to fear is the most common reason why dogs bite strangers. Fear biting is most likely in dogs that as puppies did not have the opportunity to meet lots of people. Submissive wetters can turn into fear biters. Watch your dog for signs of fear such as body posture, growling, or teeth baring, and eliminate problems before they develop to fear biting.

Predatory aggression

This is a primitive and very basic form of aggression and is potentially there within all dogs. Dogs chase moving things. Certain breeds (such as terriers, herders, and sighthounds and scenthounds in particular) are genetically primed for chasing, pouncing, and biting after the pounce. Early socializing, and channelling a puppy's desire to chase toys, are the best forms of prevention.

Territorial aggression

Your dog is most self-confident on its own territory – in your home, garden, or car – and might show signs of territorial aggression if it thinks of strangers as possible threats. Prevent (or overcome) this problem by introducing your puppy to delivery people and others who visit.

There is nothing wrong with your dog alerting you when someone comes to your house, but it should not be compulsively protective of your shared territory. Use the same principle in your car. A car is a delightfully small territory, easy to protect.

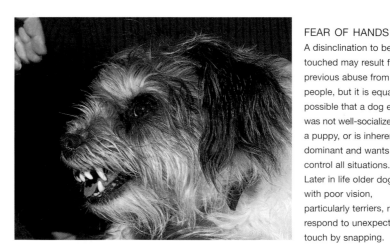

FEAR OF HANDS
A disinclination to be touched may result from previous abuse from people, but it is equally possible that a dog either was not well-socialized as a puppy, or is inherently dominant and wants to control all situations. Later in life older dogs with poor vision, particularly terriers, may respond to unexpected touch by snapping.

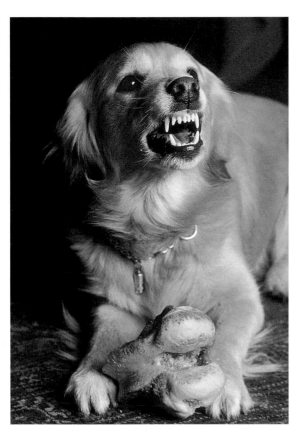

POSSESSIVE AGGRESSION
Some dogs growl and show their teeth as a theatrical threat to protect both toys and food. This is the most common form of aggression seen in Golden Retrievers. If theatrics are not enough, the dog fulfils the threat and bites. This form of aggression can be controlled within three weeks with proper professional help. Your vet can suggest a suitable dog trainer.

Food and toy aggression

Some dogs become possessive over food or toys. Teach your dog that being touched while eating is acceptable, non-threatening behaviour and that hands near the food bowl will not take food away. When you feed the dog, kneel down beside it while it is eating and offer it something even more tasty, such as a piece of meat or a liver treat. Once the dog is used to this, hide the treat in your hand, put your hand in its food bowl, and as the dog noses your hand, open it up and give the treat, then let the dog finish its meal. It will quickly learn to enjoy your presence rather than feel threatened.

Health-related aggression

If a dog is ill, it is natural for the animal to be grumpy or aggressive. If something hurts, the dog's natural response to pain is to bite. Be careful when touching or moving your sick or injured dog (*see pp.400–01*). Certain medical conditions, such as an underactive thyroid gland, are also known to be associated with aggression.

Learned aggression

Some people like to teach dogs to be aggressive. Learned aggression is hard to get rid of. If you want home protection, simply train your dog to bark fiercely and invest in an electronic burglar alarm.

Q HOW CAN I STOP MY DOG FROM CHASING JOGGERS AND CYCLISTS?

A Get friends, armed with water pistols, to help. When your dog chases, rather than rewarding the dog by running away, the jogger or cyclist stops and the dog gets an unexpected shot of water in its face.

Q MY DOG IS AGGRESSIVE TOWARDS DELIVERY PEOPLE. WHAT SHOULD I DO?

A Talk to your doorstep delivery people and leave food treats for them to leave with their deliveries. If your dog is in the garden when delivery people arrive, leave a favourite toy or food (in a weatherproof box) at your gate, with instructions for it to be given to your dog when the gate is opened.

Q I GOT MY DOG FOR SECURITY. HOW CAN I TRAIN IT TO PROTECT MY HOME?

A Train it to bark, not to bite. The proper security role of a dog is to deter threats – not to be used as a weapon. You are responsible for your dog's actions. If you knowingly train your dog to bite, and it does so, you are particularly culpable.

Q CAN I EVER TRUST MY DOG AGAIN IF IT HAS BITTEN A MEMBER OF MY FAMILY?

A It depends upon the cause of the bite, what form of aggression it was, and what you are doing to prevent it from happening again. Eliminate immediate risk by having your dog wear a muzzle. This gives you, your family, and your vet time to consider the situation and choose an effective course of action. In many instances, with prompt intervention, a dog can again become a reliable family member.

NEUTERING AND EFFECTS ON BEHAVIOUR

Neutering controls some forms of delinquency. This procedure involves removing the sex hormone-producing apparatus from the male or female. In males, the testicles are removed; in females, the ovaries and uterus. Neutering is still the procedure of choice for preventing unwanted puppies, but it also has effects on the behaviour of males and females.

Neutering eliminates (or to be more accurate, dramatically reduces) male hormones; it is likely to reduce a male dog's need to mark territory frequently with urine, to be aggressive towards other male dogs, and to wander over a large territory, preoccupied with sex scents left by other dogs. Female hormones affect a bitch's personality only during her heat cycles, but neutering eliminates the twice-yearly behaviour changes. In very rare circumstances, however, in naturally dominant females, the absence of the twice-yearly calming effect of progesterone can exaggerate her natural dominance.

Neutering has no effect, however, on house guarding, fear-biting, predatory aggression, or territorial aggression. It has no effect on other aspects of a dog's personality, except that dogs pay more attention to people because they are paying less attention to sex-related activity. If your male dog is aggressive towards other male dogs and you want to find out whether neutering will solve this problem, your vet can use hormones to "chemically castrate" your dog. This is a safe procedure when used in the short term, but the drugs may produce unwanted side effects if used over a prolonged period.

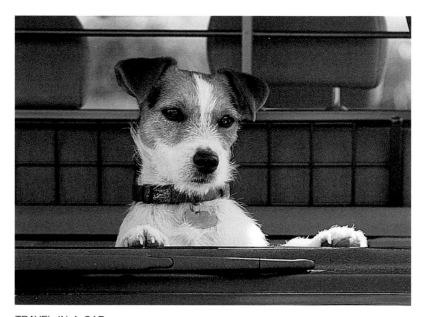

TRAVEL IN A CAR
Travel is an exciting event for most dogs. It relieves monotony and often ends in physical activity. Train your dog from an early age to settle down and be calm in the car, and not to become protectively territorial within it. Your vet can offer good advice on travel training.

TRAVEL WITH YOUR DOG

When travelling in a car, make sure your dog is safe and secure. Dogs should travel behind a dog barrier, ideally in a comfortable crate, or on the back seat equipped with a harness that attaches to the seat belt anchor and also allows it to lie down. During a journey, stop every two hours to let the dog exercise. Carry a bottle of water and water bowl. If travel sickness is a problem, discuss medication for motion sickness with your vet. If you travel frequently, most travel problems can be overcome within three weeks with proper, professionally approved training to break the habit.

Never ever leave your dog in your car in hot weather or direct sunshine. Heatstroke in hot cars is one of the most avoidable causes of death in dogs (*see pp.408-09*). Check whether local veterinary clinics provide day boarding facilities where dogs can be left on a short-term basis.

Do not let your dog hang its head out of the window, because eye injuries from dust and debris are common. Instead, open the window just enough to let the dog's nose inhale the excitement of speed.

TRAVELLING TO EUROPE WITH YOUR DOG

Many parts of Europe are downright dog friendly. Most forms of public transport accommodate dogs although there may be an additional fare to pay. In Belgium and France, your dog will be as welcome in many restaurants as you are, given its own food and water bowls under the table while you dine. Travelling with your dog to most countries in Europe is relatively simple. Each country has its own regulations but all stipulate that your dog is examined by a veterinarian and is healthy, free from infectious or contagious diseases and vaccinated against rabies, usually no less than 30 days or more than 365 days before your travel. The rabies-free regions of Europe – Norway, Sweden, Ireland, and the UK – impose restrictions on dogs entering their countries. These countries have Pet Travel Schemes permitting dogs from the rest of the Western Europe, and from rabies free regions of the world, such as Australia, New Zealand, Hawaii, and Japan, to visit. Dogs from elsewhere that reside in Western Europe for six months, can travel or live in Scandinavia or the British Isles by conforming to the needs of the individual country's Pet Travel Scheme. The UK's Scheme is being extended so that American and Canadian dogs will qualify to travel directly to the UK.

AIR, RAIL, AND SEA TRAVEL

Your home move or travel plans may include taking your dog on public transport. Ensure that your dog's travelling crate is secure, the right size for your dog, and meets the transport company's regulations. Your vet and the transport company will give you accurate guidelines.

Your dog should have two forms of ID: its tag and preferably a microchip as well. When flying, avoid hot sunny weather. It is rare, but each year there are fatal accidents when, because of runway delays, dogs suffer heatstroke in the holds of delayed aeroplanes. Whenever possible, book direct flights. Avoid tranquillizers – they may make you feel better, but they will increase your dog's risk of accidents. Some airlines allow toy-sized dogs to accompany you in the passenger cabin.

MISSING DOG

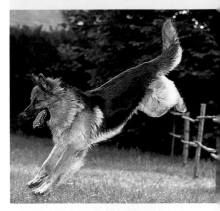

If you find that your dog has gone missing, remember the following.

• Do not panic. Think sensibly about what your dog may do if separated from you.

• Carry out an immediate search in your area, asking people if they have seen your dog.

• Contact the police, local dog shelter, your veterinary surgeon and other local vets. Give these people a description of your dog and at least two contact numbers for you – ideally your home phone and mobile number or e-mail address. Keep a phone number list of everyone you contact.

• Photocopy and post flyers where your dog went missing, with "LOST" and "REWARD" in large letters. A reward is an effective inducement. Include a picture of your dog on the flyers, for example the picture you keep in its emergency file.

• When the dog is safely returned, always contact the people on your phone list to give the good news and to thank them for their help.

Q WHAT DISEASES CAN A DOG PICK UP FROM KENNELS?

A The most likely contagious diseases are those transmitted in the air such as the canine or "kennel" cough viruses and bacteria. This is why all good kennels require up-to-date inoculation certificates. Internal parasites such as roundworms are a less likely hazard but external parasites, especially fleas, thrive where dogs congregate. If fleas are a problem in your area, treat your dog with an effective product (*see page 161*) before it is kennelled.

Q WON'T DOGS FIGHT IF THEY ALL EXERCISE TOGETHER?

A Good kennel staff or dog day care operators understand canine body language and effectively prevent most dog fights. And, fortunately, very few dogs feel the need to assert authority while in kennels or dog day care centres. Occasionally there will be disputes. Always ensure that whoever you leave your dog with has access to local veterinary care.

Q WHAT IF MY DOG IS ON MEDICATION AND NEEDS TO BE KENNELLED?

A As long as your dog's condition is stable, you explain what the condition is, and provide the kennel's vet with your vet's telephone number, there is usually no problem kennelling a dog on medication. Reliable kennel staff should have no difficulty giving medicines, although you cannot expect them to be as good as you at monitoring slight changes in your dog's condition.

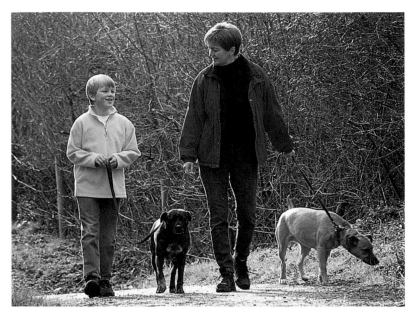

GOOD NEIGHBOURS
Friendships can develop between dog-owning neighbours who help each other when needs arise, but it remains a big responsibiliy to look after someone else's dog. A dog can be the glue to good neighbourly relations, but under the wrong circumstances it can also be the solvent.

BOARDING KENNELS

Good boarding kennels offer "home-away-from-home" facilities for your dog. Kennel facilities vary from basic to opulent. Some are veritable canine resorts offering individual sofas in each kennel, routine play activity, grooming, and even weight loss programmes. Generally speaking, the more you pay, the more personal attention your dog gets. Boarding kennel owners need a licence to operate a facility, but this licence does not necessarily ensure the facilities you want. When choosing boarding kennels, look for these signs of conscientious care:

- daily or weekly opportunities to inspect the facilities;
- requirements for up-to-date vaccination and worming;
- indoor/outdoor facilities offering each dog a choice of location;
- a raised platform in the kennel for a dog either to get on or under;
- comfortable, hygienic bedding;
- no unpleasant odour;
- routine twice-daily physical hands-on attention from the kennel staff;
- willingness to feed your dog what you want it to be fed;
- around-the-clock emergency veterinary care;
- two dogs housed together whenever practical.

If you plan to use boarding kennels for your dog, start using them as soon as your dog is properly toilet and obedience trained. Early learning that kennelling is part of life ensures that your dog will look forward to future visits. Remember to plan ahead. The best kennels are booked up months before busy seasons, especially at Christmas and New Year.

PET SITTERS AND WALKERS

If you plan to be away, no one is available at home to look after your dog, and you prefer not to use kennels, professional pet sitters are available. Use pet sitters from recognized organizations only, and ensure they are properly investigated and insured. Dog walkers are available to exercise your dog daily, but this is not sufficient when you are away. A dog should not be left alone even if a dog walker visits several times daily to exercise and feed it. Always ask for references from other dog owners before you use a dog walker.

DOG DAY CARE

Dog day care centres are available in urban locations. Look for the signs of proper canine care. The centre should have the right attitude towards dogs and training. It should be clean, safe, and secure. Dogs should be divided into groups not just by size, but by temperament and personality. When dogs are together, there should be constant supervision, and back-up arrangements should be in place in case you are unexpectedly detained.

MOVING HOME

If you have moved to a new home and you want your dog to use a specific area in the new garden as a toilet, bag a little earth from its previous toileting area and spread it in the new toileting area. Your dog may find it curious to come across its own scent, but this measure maximizes the likelihood that this is where the dog will pass waste. Before your dog is left alone in the garden, ensure that it is escape-proof. Rather than giving your dog the run of the entire new home, restrict it to a few rooms initially. This reduces the possibility that the dog will mark the territory with its urine.

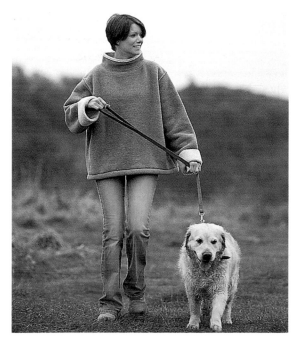

PET SITTERS
Someone living in your home while you are away is an expensive but excellent alternative to boarding your dog. A pet sitter is also a house sitter, someone to water your garden and, just as important, reduce the risk of burglary in your absence.

VET'S ADVICE

As our relationship with our pets intensifies, some people are increasingly reluctant to leave their dog because they feel the dog will not be able to cope with their absence. Not true! While some highly dependent dogs do experience temporary separation anxiety when their owners go on holiday, this is short-lived.

Dogs are a lot more fickle than some of us would like to think. When offered attention, contact comfort, security, tasty food, activity, and warmth virtually all dogs enjoy whoever they are with.

The one exception is the very elderly. Geriatric canines find it more difficult to accept temporary change. In your dog's twilight years it may be best to ensure it spends its time in your absence with someone it already knows. It may even be best to postpone a holiday – a slight inconvenience for you in return for years of devotion from your dog.

EUTHANASIA

When considering euthanasia, your choice is influenced by your culture. In the Judaeo-Christian tradition of Europe and North America, we have little difficulty taking on the responsibility for making such a decision on behalf of our dogs. In other cultures, for example the Buddhist-Shintoist tradition in Japan where all objects – animate like dogs and people, or inanimate like rocks – have souls, the decision to euthanize a dog is fraught with cultural conflict.

From the European/American tradition the following points are valid reasons for ending your dog's life:

- overwhelming physical injury;
- irreversible disease that has progressed to a point where distress or discomfort cannot be controlled;
- old age wear and tear that permanently affects your dog's "quality of life";
- physical injury, disease, or wear and tear resulting in permanent loss of control of body functions;
- incorrigible aggressiveness with risk to children, owners, or others;
- carrying untreatable disease dangerous to humans.

SAYING GOODBYE TO YOUR FRIEND

Whether death is unexpected or is the result of a decision that you and your vet take, the more caring the relationship you have had with your dog, the more difficult it will be to face. A feeling of loss is natural, as is the anger, denial, and pain of grieving. The stages of grieving, from denial to eventual acceptance and resolution, typically last for almost a year.

While passive euthanasia, that is not intervening to prevent death, is practiced in human medicine, in most parts of the world active euthanasia, the giving of a substance that causes death, is a uniquely veterinary consideration. Most dog owners feel that making this type of decision is the hardest aspect of owning a dog. Yet in North America and Europe active euthanasia is the most common cause of death in dogs over two years of age. Faced with the reality of making such a morally fraught decision, most dog owners, with a little advice from their vet, are capable of making sensible and sound decisions.

Any decision to euthanize your dog (*see pp.378-79*) should not be yours alone. Your dog is a member of your family and for this reason any decisions should be family decisions. Be honest and rational when thinking about what is best for your dog. Ask yourself these questions:

- Is the condition prolonged, recurring, or getting worse?
- Is the condition no longer responding to therapy?
- Is the dog in pain or otherwise suffering physically or mentally?
- Is it no longer possible to alleviate that pain or suffering?
- If your dog recovers, is it likely to be chronically ill, invalid, or unable to care for itself?
- If your dog recovers, will there be severe personality changes?
  If the answer to all these questions is "Yes", then euthanasia is the honest, simple, and humane option. If you answer "No" to several of these questions, then consider the following:
- Can you provide the necessary care?
- Will providing this care seriously interfere with or create serious problems for you and your family?
- Will the cost of treatment be unbearably expensive?

When there are other dogs in the family, the decision is especially problematic. The survivor does not know that its canine buddy has died. It only knows it is no longer there, and that routines have changed. For some dogs the absence is distressing, while for others it is exhilarating. If it is possible, there is certainly no harm in letting your other dog see and sniff the body of the dog that has just died.

Our grieving is perfectly natural although it is something that many find embarrassing. The emotional intensity of feelings of anger, denial, and pain may be directed at others or simply suppressed. As the bearers of bad news, most vets have experienced anger and grief directed at them. What more than compensates for these rare occasions is the gratitude that most dog owners feel for the care and consideration given to their dog, both in life and at the time of death. It is probably safe to say that vets get more letters of thanks for sympathetic euthanasia than for life-saving treatments.

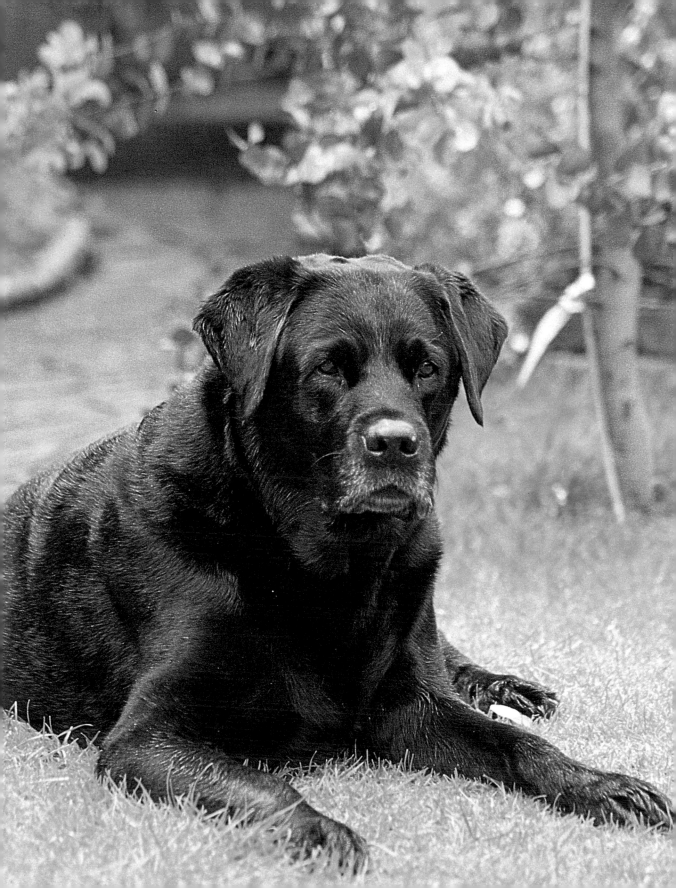

RESPONSIBLE BREEDING
breeding and puppy care

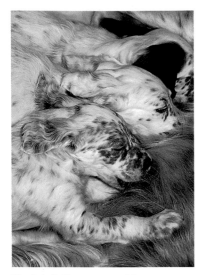

English Setter pups suckling

The arguments for breeding are self-evident. First, and most important to our hearts perhaps, we perpetuate our dogs. A dog's relatively short life span (typically just over 12 years) is the cause of the greatest sadness we have as dog owners. Breeding creates a continuity, almost an immortality. Second, again appealing to our hearts, breeding is "natural" – a dog should have the "right" to breed. We transpose our ethical values onto our dogs. Our attitude to breeding is influenced by our ethnic origins, religious values, or the country in which we live. Responsible dog breeding is a core concern within animal welfare and animal rights movements, with concerned individuals often taking diametrically opposing views. Letting a dog breed is the ideal. Yet deciding whether or not to let my dog have pups is a dilemma I go through each time a new dog joins my family.

ARTIFICIAL MATING

Purebred dogs are sometimes successfully bred by means of artificial insemination, or "AI". In this technique, vets collect semen (fluid containing sperm) from male dogs and then introduce the semen into a bitch's reproductive tract. Semen may be introduced into a bitch immediately; alternatively, it may be frozen and stored for transport or for use on a bitch at a later date.

The technique has, for example, permitted semen from proven, healthy stud dogs in one country to produce rapid improvements in the quality of stud dogs elsewhere. Kennel clubs have regulations concerning the registration of dogs produced by AI; if you wish to breed pups in this way, check out these regulations. Used properly, conception rates from AI are as good as from natural mating.

TO BREED OR NOT TO BREED

The arguments against breeding involve the mind rather than the heart. Be realistic. It might be "natural" to let our dogs breed, but is it "natural" that we keep them as companions at all? In a "natural" environment, would there ever be as great a congregation of unrelated dogs as there is in any city park in the morning? Is it "natural" to help runts survive, and thus to intervene in the survival of the fittest, which is what humans did when we created miniature or dwarfed breeds?

To my mind we cannot equate our dogs (or cats) with animals that fend for themselves. Dogs and humans have formed an integrated ecosystem, one that has been extraordinarily successful for dogs, when you see how they have spread throughout the world and increased in numbers beyond all other canids. This success has occurred in part because we make breeding decisions for them. Your decision whether or not to breed from your dog should be made on the basis of your dog's and its potential partner's inherited good health and temperament, and on your ability to ensure caring homes for the resulting litter.

NATURAL MATING BEHAVIOUR

The dog's natural ancestor, the wolf, comes into season only once each year, in the spring. Most domestic dog breeds, however, have at least two yearly seasons, when females are receptive to mating. Although the modern dog is well removed from its wolf origins, its mating rituals are similar to

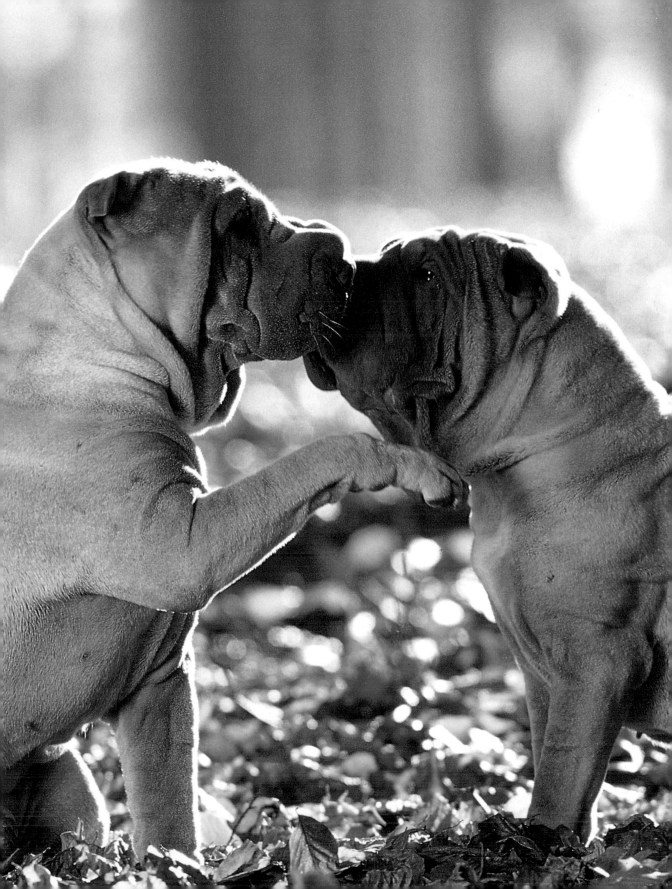

Q **HOW DO I KNOW IF MY BITCH IS READY FOR MOTHERHOOD?**

A Sexual maturity is reached long before emotional maturity. This latter state is obvious when a dog finally behaves as a serious adult, not as a young animal. Generally speaking, females will have reached adult emotional development by the second or third heat cycle. If your bitch is ready for breeding, your vet will examine her for good health and freedom from known inherited disorders.

Remember, do not breed from your dog simply "to satisfy nature". Pregnancy is riskier than not being pregnant. Helping to raise a young litter is a time-consuming and messy business. It may be more difficult than you think to find homes for the resulting pups.

Q **WHAT CAUSES INFERTILITY OR UNSUCCESSFUL MATING?**

A The usual cause of mating failure is poor timing on the handler's part rather than genuine infertility. In some cases, however, there may be physical conditions that prevent conception.

Infertility in male dogs can result from prostatic or testicular disease, an underactive thyroid, or even from a prolonged high fever. A male's fertility can be determined by sperm examination and count. Female infertility is more difficult to assess. Blood tests may be done during oestrus to measure levels of the sex hormones oestrogen, luteinizing hormone (LH), and progesterone. The ovaries can be examined by laparoscopy.

those of other social animals and are still rooted in the behaviour of a pack animal. Who mates with whom is dictated by the social structure of the pack. The dominant male rarely permits other males to mate with receptive females. Males willingly fight over females for the right to mate. Females do not necessarily choose the winner, however; they sometimes mate with a third party while the first two quarrel over rights.

Familiarity is also important; females rarely mate with unknown males. Given a ready supply of available and familiar males, females ovulate and then mate with their partners several times. The likelihood of pregnancy is very high. By contrast, in the rather unnatural circumstances of man-made mating rituals, the dog owner often takes a female to an unfamiliar male and expects her to mate willingly – something that many females are reluctant to do.

PREPARING TO BREED FROM YOUR DOG

If you do plan to breed from your dog or bitch, follow these guidelines. They will help ensure that your animal is both physically and mentally ready for reproduction, as well as being suitable for breeding.

• For a bitch, ensure that she is in good physical health, over 18 months old, and emotionally mature.

• If you have a male dog, check that he has both testicles descended in the scrotum. Recognize that if you use your dog for breeding he will be more interested in and successful at sex than he might otherwise have been.

• Train your dog so that it is well socialized to dogs as well as people (*see Puppy training, pp.31–39*). Intensely people-orientated dogs, denied an early opportunity to learn how to behave with other dogs, may be unwilling or unable to mate.

• Ensure that vaccinations and worming are up to date, especially for a female. Recent vaccination ensures that pups inherit good levels of maternal antibody protection against the common infectious diseases. Worm a female regularly before and during pregnancy – although some parasitologists say this does not make a difference to a pup's subsequent worm burden (*see Internal parasites, pp.166–75*).

• Choose your dog's partner by temperament and health, not simply by looks and bloodlines.

• If the dogs are purebreds, ensure that both partners are registered with a kennel club. Pups with documents are easier to home.

• If you are the owner of the female, always ensure that you have good homes for each pup in the litter.

• Check that you conform to local legal obligations concerning dog breeding.

• Have both dog and bitch examined by veterinary surgeons and certified healthy and free from known inherited diseases. In breeds that are known to suffer from inherited eye or joint diseases, have your breeding animals certified disease-free and registered with the appropriate organizations. To minimize the risk of diseases for which there are now genetic tests, such as progressive retinal atrophy in Irish Setters, have genetic screening tests carried out to ensure that the breeding dogs are not carriers.

• If brucellosis, a canine venereal disease, is a problem in your area, ensure that both the stud dog and the bitch have been checked and cleared. In addition, ask your vet about blood tests for herpes virus infection.
• During pro-oestrus and oestrus (*see p.315*), exercise your bitch only on her lead to eliminate any risk of mismating.
• Breeding is most successful when it occurs within two days of ovulation (when the female's ovary releases an egg). Ten days after the onset of oestrus, take your dog to your vet for vaginal cytology (examination of cells from the vagina) or measurement of blood progesterone. Cytology is simple and helps to show generally where she is in her oestrous cycle. Blood progesterone tests are more accurate, but these procedures are best done at referral laboratories.

VET'S ADVICE

• Do not even think of breeding from your dog unless you know you can find homes for the resulting litter.
• Do not expect the mother to carry out all the upbringing of her pups. It is your responsibility to ensure that pups are well socialized before they leave your home.
• Only breed from females that are emotionally as well as physically mature.
• Have your vet check both the male and female for the presence of any known inherited diseases.
• Do not breed from your dog, whether male or female, simply because it is "natural". It is actually unnatural to let your dog breed once, then expect it never to breed again.

THE BITCH'S REPRODUCTIVE CYCLE

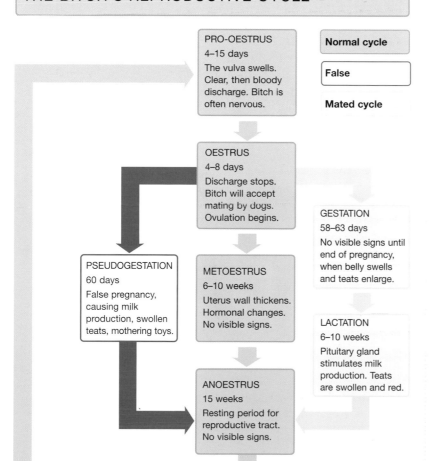

PRO-OESTRUS
4–15 days
The vulva swells. Clear, then bloody discharge. Bitch is often nervous.

Normal cycle

False

Mated cycle

OESTRUS
4–8 days
Discharge stops. Bitch will accept mating by dogs. Ovulation begins.

GESTATION
58–63 days
No visible signs until end of pregnancy, when belly swells and teats enlarge.

PSEUDOGESTATION
60 days
False pregnancy, causing milk production, swollen teats, mothering toys.

METOESTRUS
6–10 weeks
Uterus wall thickens. Hormonal changes. No visible signs.

LACTATION
6–10 weeks
Pituitary gland stimulates milk production. Teats are swollen and red.

ANOESTRUS
15 weeks
Resting period for reproductive tract. No visible signs.

Q WHY DO MATING DOGS GET "TIED" TOGETHER?

A The exact evolutionary reason for this curious phenomenon is not known; it is assumed that the male, by becoming "tied" to a receptive female, actively prevents other males from mating with her. (If this swelling occurs before sex, the penis will be unable to enter the vagina.) During a typical "tie", the male may lift his leg over the female so that they face away from each other. This may look uncomfortable, but it is probably an instinctive defensive position so that the partners can protect themselves while the tie lasts. Dogs do not appreciate jokes at this time.

Q WHAT SHOULD I DO IF MY DOG IS NOT IN THE MOOD FOR MATING?

A If the female shows signs of aggression and is unwilling to "stand" for the male, or if he shows no interest in her, it is likely that she is not ovulating and not ready to mate. Plan to repeat the procedure two days later. Do not persist! It is unfair on the dogs and will only lead to greater difficulties at the next try.

Q WILL MATINGS OVER SEVERAL DAYS RESULT IN PUPS OF DIFFERENT SIZES?

A Eggs are released and fertilized over a 1–3 day period. A litter may be fathered by several males if the female is mated to different dogs. The size of the developing pup (and its apparent maturity at birth) depends upon its genetic background, and on its overall health and position in the uterus, rather than on which day it was fertilized.

WHAT HAPPENS DURING MATING

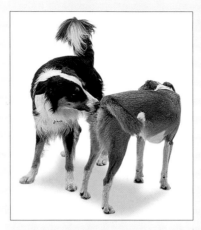

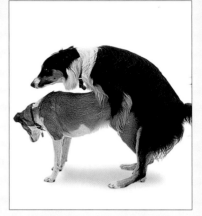

INITIAL CONTACT
Choose a suitable area; in hot weather, let the dogs meet and mate indoors. Minimize distractions. Keep people quiet and activity subdued. If the dogs show no signs of aggression towards each other, let them off their leads so that they can introduce themselves. A little romping, flirting, and mutual sniffing is a good predictor of successful mating.

MATING
If the bitch is ready to mate she obligingly holds her tail to the side and stands quietly. The dog then mounts her, clasping her hips with his paws to hold himself on, and inserts his penis into her vagina. Stand by to assist in case the dogs have any problems; inexperienced males may mount the wrong end of the female and could need guidance.

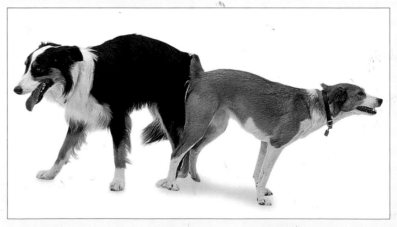

THE "TIE"
Ensure that a proper "tie" occurs. A "tie" occurs when the bulbourethral gland on the penis swells and the vulva contracts around it, preventing the dog from withdrawing his penis from the bitch's vagina. They are stuck, or "tied" together. The "tie" typically lasts for 20–40 minutes. A prolonged tie may be painful to the bitch; she may turn and snap at the male when it ends. A tie lasting a few minutes, however, seldom causes discomfort and is usually successful. After mating, both the male and female vigorously groom their genital regions by licking, an action that cleans away debris from the area and kills some harmful bacteria.

NORMAL MATING

For the best chance of success, arrange for two matings around the twelfth day of the female's oestrous cycle, one or two days apart. Bear in mind that each female has her own cycle; some ovulate as early as seven days into their cycle and others at up to 16 days after the onset of oestrus. The most common reason for unsuccessful mating is miscalculating ovulation times.

The bitch should be taken to the stud dog. Many dogs, however, have difficulty mating away from home; if your bitch is nervous or shy and the male is assertive, let him visit her territory. If you are the owner of the bitch, take her to your veterinary surgeon three weeks after the mating to confirm whether or not she is pregnant.

PREGNANCY AND FALSE PREGNANCY

Matings between dogs are repeated, and sperm can live for seven days in the female's genital tract. As a result, pregnancy almost always follows. After a bitch has been in oestrus, a unique sequence of events has evolved, which is different from all other domesticated species. Her hormonal system "assumes" that she will be pregnant each and every time she comes into season, regardless of mating. Even when not successfully mated, a female will still experience the full hormonal effects of pregnancy, with all the attendant physical and mental changes.

In pet dogs that have not been mated, the hormonal changes associated with oestrus create a "false" pregnancy. In this condition, the female goes through the hormonal and sometimes the physical changes of pregnancy. For some dogs, this even includes a degree of mild labour two months later. During her false pregnancy, a female can experience a dramatic variety of mood and sensory changes. These include rejecting her regular food, making a "den", and mothering objects such as toys. The most obvious consequence of a false pregnancy is milk production. Some behaviourists believe that this milk production evolved so that these female pack members could supplement the nutrition of pups born to higher-ranking females.

NOURISHING A PREGNANT MOTHER

Nutritionists discovered years ago that well-nourished mothers do not just produce puppies that are healthier than others. Their pups also crawl, walk, run, and play earlier, learn faster, and have fewer emotional problems than puppies from malnourished mothers. The effects of malnourishment can be perpetuated for generations; the young of poorly nourished mothers go on to become poor mothers themselves.

A dog's appetite increases only gradually in early pregnancy. During the first five weeks, she needs only a balanced diet with normal-sized meals (*see Nutrition, pp.86–99*). After the fifth week, increase her energy consumption (kilocalories) by 10 per cent per week until the birth.

Some animals, including those experiencing a false pregnancy, can suffer from morning sickness. Scientists think this is a natural way in which a mother minimizes her foetuses' exposure to toxins. Hormonal changes can also be the reason why some dogs develop food aversions in pregnancy. Be wary of all unnecessary drugs and chemicals during early pregnancy.

VET'S ADVICE

- Before the mating, ensure that both dogs are free from sexually transmitted diseases.
- Do not apply lubricants from an opened tube; they may be bacterially contaminated.
- Avoid actively trying to help a dog gain entry. Especially for a young, excited male, your helping hand is likely to lead to his ejaculating before entry.
- If a bitch has a very long coat, help by clipping hair from around the vulva beforehand, or by holding the hair to the side to enable the male to gain entry.
- Take care with large, possibly aggressive dogs. Use muzzles if you feel there is any risk to you or to the dogs themselves.
- Take your lead from the bitch's behaviour. If she totally lacks interest you probably have her ovulation date wrong. Try again a few days later.

ENERGY NEEDS

To meet a bitch's greater energy needs, increase her food intake from mid-way through her pregnancy. The chart below shows the maximum intake of energy (kilocalories) for pregnant bitches of different weights.

ADULT WEIGHT	AVERAGE DAILY NEEDS (KCAL)
2–5 kg	220–440
6–10 kg	505–740
11–20 kg	800–1250
21–30 kg	1295–1690
31–40 kg	1735–2100
41–50 kg	2140–2480

Q **IS A CALCIUM SUPPLEMENT FOR PREGNANT MOTHERS BENEFICIAL FOR THE PUPS' DEVELOPMENT?**

A No, it is not. Any good commercial dog foods, and well balanced home cooking, will already contain the right amounts of calcium and phosphorus, in the ideal ratio of 1.2 to 1.0. Excessive calcium in the diet will actually interfere with the absorption of zinc and manganese from food, and both of these minerals are essential for healthy puppy development in the womb. It may also predispose the mother to difficulties during labour (dystocia), and has been incriminated in predisposing the pups to developing bloat (gastric dilatation) after birth. Excessive calcium may even increase the risks of milk fever (eclampsia) – a serious, potentially fatal form of calcium deficiency in lactating mothers.

Q **ARE THERE ANY BENEFITS TO DOCKING PUPPIES' TAILS, REMOVING DEW CLAWS, OR CROPPING EARS?**

A In some parts of the world, it is customary to remove the dew claws and part or all of the tails from many breeds three days after birth. In some countries, the ears of breeds such as Boxers, Schnauzers, Dobermans, and Great Danes are also cropped. There is no reason to carry out these procedures on family pups. Contrary to what some breeders say, tail docking and ear cropping serve only human vanity. These procedures are unnecessary. Removing a pup's dewclaws may be beneficial for the dog later in life if it lives in a region with heavy snow in winter. The anatomy of the dewclaw makes it prone to injury from ice when a dog's feet penetrate through crusted snow.

HOW PUPS DEVELOP IN THE WOMB

After fertilization of eggs in the oviducts, embryos migrate over a period of 6–10 days to the womb (uterus). During the next 8–10 days they attach themselves to the uterine wall (endometrium). Natural chemicals called cytokines act to space the foetuses equally and symmetrically along each horn of the uterus to give roughly equal advantages to all of the foetuses. Position may, however, affect the health and size of the pups. The best positions are in the middle sections of each horn; these regions are the best sites for the placenta (which provides nourishment to the foetus) to develop. The larger and healthier the placental attachment, the better the nutrition of the developing puppy.

By day 35 after fertilization, all of the pup's body characteristics are apparent. By day 40, eyelids, claws, hair, and skin colour are visible. At 42–45 days, the pups' skeletons can be seen on X-rays. Most pregnancies last 62–65 days but there is considerable variation. Larger litters often have shorter gestations, with whelping as early as 57 days, while small litters may not be delivered until 67–68 days or even as late as 72 days after fertilization.

EMOTIONAL DEVELOPMENT IN THE WOMB

Through his research, Dr. T. Berry Brazelton at Harvard University has shown how human infants are influenced in the womb by their mother's lifestyle. The same applies to pups. What the mother eats and the emotions that she has will affect the emotional and physical development of the pups.

In dogs, there are additional influences on behaviour: where a pup finds itself positioned in the womb and who its neighbours are. Pups in the middle of each horn of the uterus are likely to receive the best nutrition (*see above*). More interesting is the influence of hormone produced by male pups while still in the womb. As a male pup's testes develop, they secrete bursts of the male sex hormone testosterone; the hormone travels to the developing brain, where it helps to forge connections that mould future male sexual characteristics such as dominance. Some researchers believe that female foetuses lying between two males are exposed to tiny amounts of male hormone, and as a result they are predisposed to develop a slightly masculinized brain and consequently a more dominant personality.

INFECTION RISKS FOR FOETUSES

Virtually all pups are born infected with roundworms. Heartworms and hookworms can also infect the foetuses in affected areas. Latent roundworm larvae in the mother become active around the 42nd day of pregnancy, when the bitch's natural immunity is suppressed by hormone changes related to this stage of her pregnancy. The larvae cross the placenta into the pups, settling in their livers. Some also migrate to the mother's mammary glands and pass to the pups in the first milk that they consume. Worming the mother with drugs such as fenbendazole on the 45th, 50th, 55th, and 60th days of pregnancy may reduce the worm load passed from mother to pups. Most heartworm preparations are safe to use during pregnancy and also prevent worm transmission to the pups. (*See also Internal parasites, pp.165–75.*)

DEVELOPMENT OF THE FOETUS

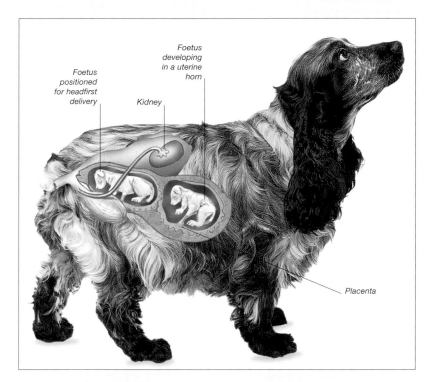

Foetus positioned for headfirst delivery

Foetus developing in a uterine horn

Kidney

Placenta

FROM EGG TO FOETUS

Fertilization takes place in the fallopian tubes (oviducts). During the following week the fertilized eggs (zygotes) migrate down the two tubes to the uterus. The dog's womb (uterus) consists of two pencil-thin tubes or "horns". Under the influence of minute amounts of body chemicals called cytokines, the zygotes become evenly spaced along each uterine horn. They implant into the wall of the uterus, then develop into two parts: embryos, which become foetuses, and placentas, which draw nutrients from the mother's bloodstream for the foetuses. The picture on the left shows the two horns of a pregnant female's uterus and the positioning of foetuses inside the uterine horns.

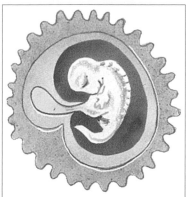

FIRST TWO WEEKS

During this time, embryo cells differentiate into all the cells needed for the body's development. Once an embryo has all of its main structures it is called a foetus. At two weeks, the foetus is minute but has a head, spine, limb buds, and tail. It is nourished by the yolk sac. This is the most critical stage of development; any drugs or diseases in the mother can severely damage foetuses.

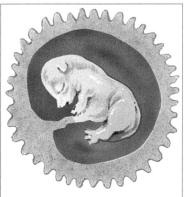

THREE WEEKS

By the end of three weeks, all of the tissues and organs necessary for life have developed. (This stage is roughly the equivalent of three months' development in a human foetus.) At three weeks, a vet can diagnose pregnancy in a lean-bodied female by feeling her abdomen and detecting individual developing foetuses through the abdominal wall.

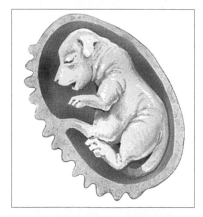

SIX WEEKS

By six weeks, the foetus has the form of a miniature dog. Skin colour, hair, claws, and eyelids are all distinct. The skeleton can be seen on X-ray, and skulls can be felt through the abdominal wall. From now until birth three weeks later, the foetus simply grows; however it still depends on nourishment via the placenta, and its lungs are not yet capable of taking in oxygen.

THE PROCESS OF WHELPING

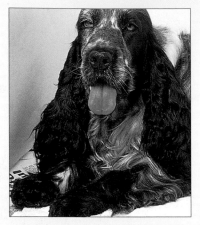

PREPARING FOR LABOUR
Like her wolf ancestors, the female finds a secluded den in which to deliver and raise her pups in maximum security. (Some females, especially terriers and other earth dogs, co-opt another animal's den.) Up to 36 hours before labour, she paces around, grows anxious, and builds a nest. She also stops eating, and may shiver or vomit.

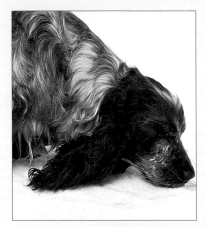

LABOUR AND DELIVERY
Signs of labour include contractions and straining. The dog may turn around in circles or may lie down for the delivery. A sac of fluid ("waters") containing a pup bulges through the vulva, then breaks; within two hours, the first pup is born. About 60 per cent of pups are born head first; the rest are born feet first.

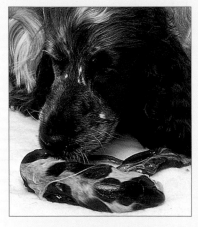

AFTER DELIVERING A PUP
The mother licks the membrane off the pup and severs the umbilical cord with her teeth. She also passes the afterbirth (placenta), together with a dark-green fluid. The mother instinctively eats the afterbirth from each pup to hide any evidence of her vulnerable newborns. Watch to ensure that she delivers one afterbirth for each pup.

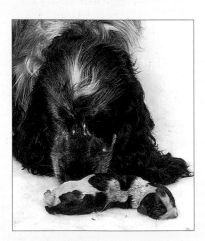

LICKING A PUP
The mother licks each newborn pup vigorously. This action dries and warms the pup, clears mucus away from its mouth and nose, and stimulates it to start breathing. In addition, licking produces chemical changes in the mother's brain, which help her to form an emotional bond with the pup.

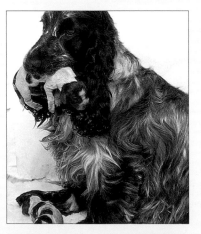

KEEPING THE LITTER TOGETHER
The first pup is born about an hour after labour starts; the rest are born at intervals of 10–80 minutes. Between births, the mother rests with her pups around her. If a pup moves too far away from her warmth, it may cry, prompting the mother to pick it up and bring it back. If a pup does not cry out, however, the mother may abandon it.

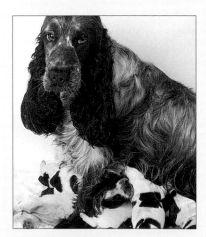

PUPS SUCKLING
Once all of the pups have been born, the mother will allow the litter to suckle for the first time. Once each pup has fed, the mother licks its anus and genitals, which stimulates it to pass urine and faeces. For the first few weeks she will consume all the pups' body waste; this instinctive act helps to hide them from danger.

GIVING BIRTH (WHELPING)

In a truly caring environment, owners and breeders can ensure healthy, natural births. We can do this most easily by feeding nourishing food, avoiding chemicals (including unknown herbs), and minimizing the risk of disease during pregnancy. Breeders can also help by selectively breeding not for the smallest-sized progeny or for the largest litters, but for ease of birth and litter sizes that mothers are able to feed and care for naturally.

A few weeks before the pups are due, make a whelping box, where the bitch can give birth and keep her pups for the first few weeks. Make the box 1.20–1.50 m (4–5 ft) square for a large dog and 60–90 cm (2–3 ft) square for a small dog. Make the front low so that the bitch can easily get in and out. Poles fitted 7.5–15 cm (3–6 in) from each side will enable pups to crawl underneath so that their mother does not lie on them. Position the box in a quiet, secluded place away from draughts. Line the base thickly with newspaper; cover this with a warm layer such as heavy towels or a mattress pad. Never use deep, loose bedding such as blankets – pups can smother in it. Two weeks before the birth, introduce the bitch to her box. Encourage her to sleep in it so that it becomes a familiar, secure place for her.

WHEN HELP MAY BE NEEDED

In dogs with "average" anatomy, birth is uncomplicated. Selective breeding, however, has led to physical and mental problems. If your bitch was mated with a larger male, she might have difficulty passing the pups through her birth canal. In breeds such as Bulldogs, the pups' heads are often too large to pass through the birth canal. In very small breeds, such as Yorkshire Terriers and Chihuahuas, pups must often be delivered by Caesarean section. In addition, some dogs become very distressed when in labour and virtually stop contracting, wanting to be on a lap rather than in the whelping pen. (Selective breeding has accelerated puberty in dogs; as a result, a female may be physically but not emotionally prepared to be a good mother.)

Before the delivery date, and especially if you anticipate any problems, assemble a kit for the birth, and keep it near the whelping box. Include disinfectant, towels, scissors (and matches for sterilizing them), and gauze. In addition, warn your vet beforehand so that help is available if needed.

LITTER SIZE

Generally, the larger the breed the bigger the litter. While Yorkshire Terriers usually have about three pups, Labrador Retrievers and German Shepherds typically have about eight. It is not unusual in some breeds, such as the Dalmatian, for a mother to have more pups than she has teats. In this situation, competition between pups for the most productive teats decides who is best nourished and grows fastest. Litter size also depends on the father's sperm count (see p.313); poor sperm counts result in smaller litters.

The pups should be about equal in size. The smallest in the litter (runt) may have invisible congenital defects or may have been poorly nourished in the womb. These are generally the pups at greatest risk after birth. While some breeders "leave it to nature" to decide whether runts survive, others intervene by hand-feeding (see p.64).

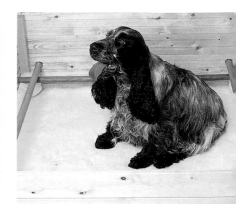

Q ARE ALL FEMALE DOGS GOOD MOTHERS?

A Not necessarily. There is no "maternal behaviour centre" in a female's brain, and such behaviour cannot be hormonally induced. A mother's behaviour does depend on hormones to some extent, but also depends on how well the dog was mothered by her own mother.

Q WILL A CAESARIAN SECTION INTERFERE WITH MY DOG'S MOTHERING BEHAVIOUR?

A Normally, the passage of a pup through the birth canal, and licking the pup just after birth, will trigger subtle chemical changes in the mother's brain that imprint the pup in her mind, which is necessary for good mothering. If neither event occurs, there is a greater risk that the mother will reject the pup.

Q WHY DO SOME MOTHERS EAT THEIR NEWBORN BABIES?

A Cannibalism of pups is rare in dogs. It occurs most often in Bull Terriers, especially in those that have had a Caesarian section. Some authorities claim that cannibalism of some pups, or the rejection of runts, is a realistic and sensible way for a mother to limit the number of mouths to feed and increase the chances of survival of the healthiest in her litter.

NEWBORNS

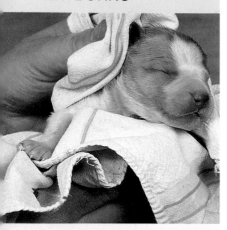

Experienced mothers instinctively lick off foetal membranes, chew off umbilical cords, and stimulate their pups, but immature or tired mothers may need your help.

• With a warm towel, wipe the birth membranes from the face, particularly the nose and mouth.

• Hold the pup securely upside-down in the towel, and gently but firmly swing it to drain birth fluids from its airway. Rub its chest with the towel. It should breathe spontaneously; if it does not, give artificial respiration (see p.385).

• Using gauze or thread, tie the umbilical cord 1 cm (½ in) from the pup's body. With sterilized, blunt-tipped scissors, sever it between the placenta and the tie.

• Place the pup in body contact with its mother. If this is not practical or if she rejects it, wrap it in a warm towel and temporarily keep it warm on a wrapped hot-water bottle containing water at body temperature.

• Once the pups are born, place each on one of its mother's teats. They should suckle successfully. If the mother cannot produce enough milk, the pups will need hand-feeding (see p.64).

DEALING WITH WHELPING PROBLEMS

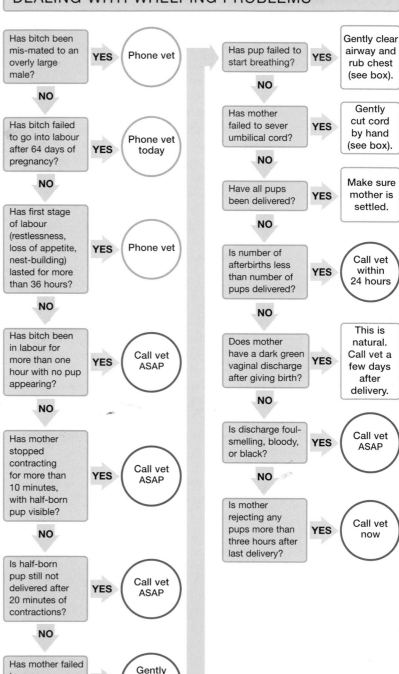

Has bitch been mis-mated to an overly large male? — **YES** → Phone vet

NO ↓

Has bitch failed to go into labour after 64 days of pregnancy? — **YES** → Phone vet today

NO ↓

Has first stage of labour (restlessness, loss of appetite, nest-building) lasted for more than 36 hours? — **YES** → Phone vet

NO ↓

Has bitch been in labour for more than one hour with no pup appearing? — **YES** → Call vet ASAP

NO ↓

Has mother stopped contracting for more than 10 minutes, with half-born pup visible? — **YES** → Call vet ASAP

NO ↓

Is half-born pup still not delivered after 20 minutes of contractions? — **YES** → Call vet ASAP

NO ↓

Has mother failed to remove membrane around pup? — **YES** → Gently remove it by hand

NO ↓

Has pup failed to start breathing? — **YES** → Gently clear airway and rub chest (see box).

NO ↓

Has mother failed to sever umbilical cord? — **YES** → Gently cut cord by hand (see box).

NO ↓

Have all pups been delivered? — **YES** → Make sure mother is settled.

NO ↓

Is number of afterbirths less than number of pups delivered? — **YES** → Call vet within 24 hours

NO ↓

Does mother have a dark green vaginal discharge after giving birth? — **YES** → This is natural. Call vet a few days after delivery.

NO ↓

Is discharge foul-smelling, bloody, or black? — **YES** → Call vet ASAP

NO ↓

Is mother rejecting any pups more than three hours after last delivery? — **YES** → Call vet now

THE FIRST FEW WEEKS OF LIFE

For domestic as well as wild canines, survival depends on the mother's ability to provide safety, security, and nourishment. Their mother has to feed them, clean them, and keep them warm. She also defends them from predators and, unwittingly, protects them from disease.

The first milk that the mother releases, called colostrum, is vitally important. It provides passive immunity (antibodies) against many of the diseases to which she has been exposed in her lifetime. This protection lasts for eight to twelve weeks, although protection against some diseases may persist for as long as 26 weeks. Vaccination during this time period provides continuing protection for developing pups (*see p.69*).

Newborn pups cannot generate or retain heat naturally by shivering or constricting their blood vessels. For the first week of life, therefore, contact with their mother is the only way to keep warm. A typical room temperature of 22°C (72°F) is not warm enough for newborn pups. If a mother leaves her pups for only half an hour in this environment, their body temperature drops from around 38°C (100°F) to a chilling 34.5–35°C (94–5°F).

A good mother stimulates her pups to feed by cleaning and licking. For the first few days she may prompt them to nurse, but soon they start feeding on their own. Later, the eruption of the pups' pin-sharp milk teeth (*see p.261*) will stimulate her to reduce her feeding periods. After 5–6 weeks, the mother weans the pups. Although they might like to suckle for as long as possible, suckling drains the mother's energy; good mothers always lose weight. Her objective is to wean her pups as soon as possible.

VACCINATION

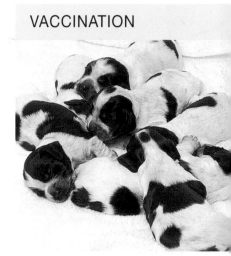

At birth, pups gain protection against diseases to which their mother has been exposed, because maternal antibodies against diseases are passed on to the pup in the first milk (colostrum). Never try to boost this natural protection, however, by vaccinating a dog while she is pregnant. Her immune system is already compromised because she is carrying "foreign protein" – her own pups – in her womb. In addition, never vaccinate any housemates of pregnant females, because vaccine virus can be shed by these dogs and passed on to the mother-to-be.

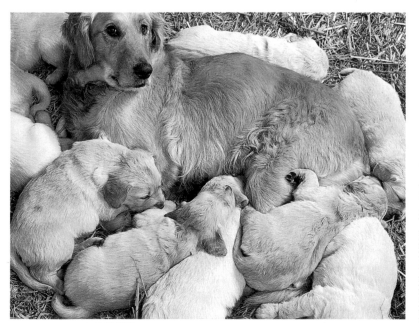

BENEFITS OF SUCKLING
Suckling is vital for bonding as well as feeding. Unlike cats and pigs, pups do not always use a specific nipple; however, dominant pups usually defend the most productive teats, of which there are several. Mothers find suckling relaxing and comforting.

MAKING UP FEEDS

If mother's milk is not available, you will have to feed pups using formula from your veterinary surgeon. When feeding a puppy by hand, take care not to over-feed it. Instead, allow the pup to decide how much food it wants to take.

Milk formula is available ready mixed or in powder form. To mix powder formula, boil some water, allow it to cool, then stir in the formula. Always feed formula at room temperature.

As a general rule, in each 24-hour period a pup needs about 15 ml (1 tablespoon) of formula for each 50 grams (2 ounces) of its body weight. A fuller guide is given below.

BODY WEIGHT	AMOUNT OF FORMULA PER DAY
115 g (4 oz)	2 tablespoons
225 g (8 oz)	4 tablespoons
340 g (12 oz)	6 tablespoons
450 g (16 oz)	8 tablespoons
570 g (20 oz)	10 tablespoons
680 g (24 oz)	12 tablespoons
795 g (28 oz)	14 tablespoons
910 g (32 oz)	16 tablespoons

In emergencies, use the following formula to feed newborn pups:

1 can condensed milk

an equal quantity of water

2 tablespoons yoghurt with active cultures (or 1 egg yolk)

2 tablespoons mayonnaise

2 tablespoons glucose powder or corn syrup

25 grams (1 ounce) gelatin powder.

Boil the water, whisk in gelatin until it has dissolved, then remove mixture from the heat. Add condensed milk, yoghurt (or egg yolk), mayonnaise, and glucose powder, whisking thoroughly. Allow to cool, then refrigerate it where the formula will thicken; bring back to liquid consistency by warming it in a microwave or using a double boiler.

REARING PUPPIES BY HAND

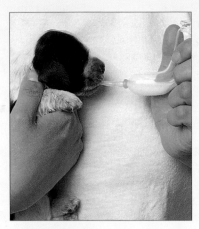

BOTTLE-FEEDING
Feed the pup every two hours. Ask your vet for a feeding bottle; in an emergency, you can use a clean eye dropper. Hold the puppy upright and insert the bottle teat into its mouth. Hold the bottle at a 45-degree angle to help prevent the pup from swallowing air, and keep a slight pull on it to encourage the pup to suck.

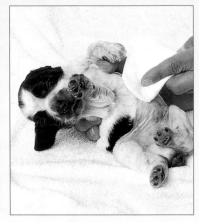

STIMULATING BODY FUNCTIONS
Feeds usually take about five minutes. After each feed, "burp" the puppy by gently rubbing or patting its back. Using clean, damp gauze, wipe away any spilt milk from its face and chest. In addition, clean around the genitals and anus, as the pup's mother would do, to stimulate it to pass urine or faeces.

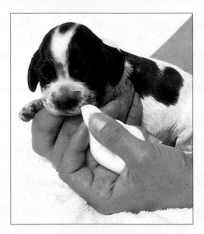

DAILY CARE
Handle the pups every day, but if they are still living with their mother take care not to upset her. Wash your hands before handling a very young puppy, to minimize the risk of passing on disease to it. If you are rearing the pup yourself, clean its eyes, ears, and mouth every day, using a piece of clean, damp gauze.

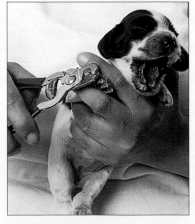

NAIL TRIMMING
Regularly check the puppy's claws. If it is still feeding from its mother, trim the claws if they are long or sharp. This is necessary because pups "knead" or "tread" the area around the teats with their paws as they suckle, as an instinctive way to aid milk flow. If they have sharp claws, they could hurt the mother's sensitive teats.

EARLY PHYSICAL DEVELOPMENT

Puppies are born with immature, still developing brains. A pup's best developed senses are heat and smell; it is also sensitive to touch, pain, and taste. Its hearing, sight, and temperature control, however, will not develop for another few weeks. A healthy pup spends 90 per cent of its time sleeping while the essential processes of growth take place. During these first weeks of life, the mother is the overwhelming influence on the pup's development; because its brain is still growing, it is not yet strongly influenced by the wider environment. Early development includes the following processes.

• During the first few days, the heart rate increases from around 160 beats per minute to just over 200 beats per minute. The breathing rate and body temperature also increase in the days just after birth.

• The eyes and ears, which are sealed at birth, start to open at ten to 16 days. At the same time, the body develops the ability to control its temperature. By 28 days, a pup's vision is as good as an adult's. Its hearing and ability to right itself also have reached adult abilities, although muscle coordination will take months to develop.

• At birth only a pup's head has highly developed touch reflexes, but by two weeks of age the front legs have touch reflexes and by three weeks so do the hind legs. This is why pups can sit up at two weeks and stand at three weeks. A few days more and they are walking and trotting.

• Pain sensation is present at birth but very slow. It may take a few seconds for the brain to register pain. By three weeks of age, the brain and nerves have both developed to register pain as quickly as those of an adult dog.

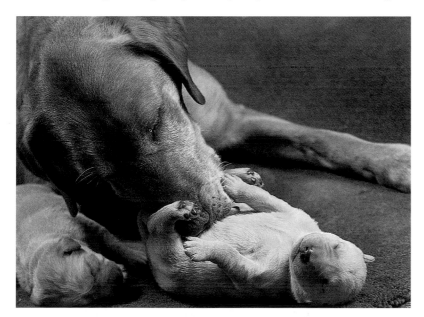

THE IMPORTANCE OF PHYSICAL CONTACT
Touch is as important to dogs as it is to us. A pup's earliest experiences are being licked by its mother, then lying in warm contact with its mother and littermates. Such comforting experiences may be the reason why our dogs enjoy being stroked and petted by us.

NURSING MOTHERS

Dogs' milk is naturally rich, with about 40 per cent more energy than cows' milk. To produce milk, a mother needs plenty of energy. Even when pups are weaned, her energy demands remain 50 per cent above what is needed to maintain her normal weight. This chart shows typical energy needs of lactating family dogs.

NORMAL WEIGHT	DAILY ENERGY NEEDS (KCAL)		
	wks 1–2	wks 3–4	wks 5–6
2–5 kg	370 – 735	555 – 1,105	370 – 735
6–10 kg	845 – 1,235	1255 – 1,855	845 – 1,235
11–20 kg	1,330 – 2,080	1,995 – 3,120	1,330 – 2,080
21–30 kg	2,160 – 2,820	3,235 – 4,230	2,160 – 2,820
31–40 kg	2,890 – 3,500	4,335 – 5,250	2,890 – 3,500
41–50 kg	3,565 – 4,135	5,345 – 6,205	3,565 – 4,135

VET'S ADVICE

Take the following steps to help the mother feed and care for her pups effectively.

• Do not be over-zealous about cleaning the mother's teats with soap and water, because this will make it more difficult for the pups to find the teats and feed.

• If a pup is not suckling, allow the mother to lick it. Encourage her to lick her teats (or apply some of her saliva to a teat) so that the area carries her smell, then put the pup on to a teat.

• If the mother has to leave the pups for meals, drinks, or toilet functions, use a hot-water bottle wrapped in a cloth or towel to keep the pups warm.

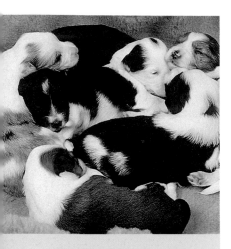

THE MOTHER–PUP RELATIONSHIP

The first days of life are crucial to a pup's mental and social development. The pup's first important relationship is with its mother. Its social life with its littermates, and with us, really begins only when its senses are mature and it can communicate by voice, posture, body language, and activities.

A pup needs its mother for survival, so its relationship with her is marked by dependency and care-seeking. At first, the newborn pup whines and roots around its mother, searching for food and warmth. As the senses develop, it learns to wag its tail, yelp, jump up and lick its mother's face, paw her, or simply follow her like a shadow.

These care-seeking actions provoke different responses from different mothers. Some mothers lick or nibble their pups to control them. Others threaten with their mouths, growl, or give inhibited bites to stop their pups pestering them. This is the pups' first experience with compromise. Benign mothers are more likely to "paw" their pups into compromise, grooming them afterwards as a reward for obedience. More aggressive mothers bite their pups with less inhibition, and may continue to discipline a pup even after it has withdrawn from her. These pups grow into dogs that are less socially gregarious with people than pups raised by benign mothers. In mental tests such as "fetch the tennis ball", these pups perform less well. The care-seeking behaviour of puppyhood eventually evolves into the subtleties of submissive behaviour.

THE START OF PACK BEHAVIOUR

From the security of the womb, where all needs were met, the pup must now find its food by searching for its mother's teats. Its littermates compete with it for this vital resource; this is its first active experience of living in a pack society. At the same time, however, the pups care for each other by huddling and sleeping together, providing warmth and contact comfort. In this way, pups start to learn about the importance of relationships and develop their particular position in the "pecking order".

The dog litter is a fascinating but temporary society. By playing with each other, the pups create their own social bonds and learn how to communicate with each other. In addition, each pup's social status first becomes apparent. Whether a pup develops a dominant, sub-dominant, or submissive personality depends, in part, on the relationships it develops with its littermates. For most family dogs, the seven to ten weeks it spends with its mother and littermates will be the only time in its life during which natural pack behaviour is allowed to develop and flourish. Later, when we intervene more actively in the pups' life, they will apply the knowledge they acquired in this pack environment to their relationships with their human family – their new "pack".

PRINCIPLES OF GOOD PUPPY CARE

Your dog's health and behaviour are deeply influenced by the way in which its breeder cared for it. Good breeders provide an enriched environment for their pups, ensuring that each animal begins its life in the best possible physical and mental health.

Q DOES LITTER SIZE AFFECT A DOG'S PERSONALITY?

A Yes, it does. Pups from very small litters may be less successful later in life in developing subtle social relationships with other dogs. Pups from large litters, who are able to interact with a wider range of personalities, gain more experience of relationships. Their environment makes it possible for them to learn the delicate nuances of body language faster.

Q DO MOTHERS EVER CAUSE HARM TO PUPS?

A Most mothers are devoted to their pups. A few, however, may put the pups' health at risk. A new mother may accidentally endanger her pups by abandoning or rejecting them due to fright or lack of experience. A mother may actively reject a pup if she senses there is something seriously wrong with it. Later in a pup's life, overly harsh discipline from the mother may adversely affect a pup's mental and social development.

A good breeder can compensate for these problems by hand-rearing the pup (see p.64) and later by careful training.

Breeders should ensure that pups do not suffer from internal or external parasites, and protect them against infectious diseases by maintaining a hygienic environment. In addition, breeders are responsible for weaning pups off their mother's milk and on to safe and nutritious solid food.

Breeders also stimulate mental development by gradually exposing pups to life in the real world, away from their mother. Pups are allowed to explore, play, and meet other dogs and other species – especially humans.

MENTAL STIMULATION AND LEARNING

How a dog grows and matures depends on its genetic inheritance and the behaviour of its mother, but also on the experiences that it acquires early in life. Numerous experiments show that an animal raised in an "enriched" environment, with plenty of chances for playing and socializing, has better mental development than an animal in a "deprived", bare environment. It grows a heavier brain with a thicker cerebral cortex (responsible for thinking), more connections between brain cells, and higher levels of brain chemical transmitter substances. The first three weeks are important but the next month of life, while the pup is still with the breeder, is also vital for the development of behaviour that makes an ideal family dog.

Playful behaviour is a lifelong activity. Dogs willingly play with other species such as cats, and especially with us, but always according to rules that they understand. When playing with a pup, the breeder must respond much as littermates do. In the litter, a pup learns to inhibit its bite during play when its littermate squeals and stops play or bites back. The equivalent is for the breeder to withdraw rewards or even play when a pup misbehaves. This means a theatrical "ouch" and an immediate end to play; however, the activity can resume a minute later when the pup has settled down (*see Time-out training, p.16*). Remember that excessively harsh discipline from the breeder or the mother inhibits a pup's social development.

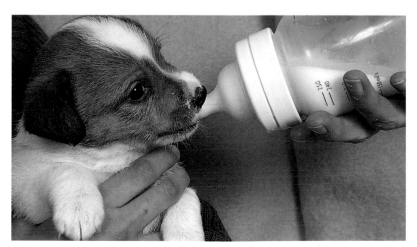

EMOTIONAL EFFECTS OF HAND-FEEDING
Routine hand-feeding accelerates and intensifies a pup's attachment to its human family. If a pup needs hand-feeding, it is important for its emotional development that it spends as much time as possible with its littermates and its mother.

Q HOW EFFECTIVE IS APTITUDE TESTING FOR DETERMINING A PUP'S LIKELY TEMPERAMENT ONCE IT IS MATURE?

A Various puppy aptitude tests are available, but so far the answer to this question is unclear. A puppy's personality and behaviour are affected by many factors, not simply inherited genes and what happens early in life. It is open to immense modification as the pup matures. The only consistently positive evidence from puppy aptitude tests concerns dominant aggression: pups that test positive for dominantly aggressive behaviour at eight weeks of age will probably mature into dominantly aggressive adults. General dominance is most readily predicted by size, sex, hormonal status, and breed.

Q CAN I DO ANYTHING TO GIVE PUPS A HEAD START IN LIFE?

A Of course, good health and nutrition are central to proper development, but at a more subtle level there are exercises you can undertake that may accelerate brain development. It was observed over 40 years ago that pups that are presented with gentle challenges early in life appear to be more adaptable as adults. Stimulants include being handled by a wide variety of people, gentle slopes to walk up and down, and simple obstacles such as broom handles on the floor to overcome. These exercises can begin as soon as a pup is brave enough to explore its surroundings, usually starting at around three weeks of age.

VET'S ADVICE

If you wish to wean your pups using alternatives to specially designed puppy foods, bear the following points in mind.

• Some breeders recommend alternatives such as prepared baby foods, mother's milk replacer, goat's milk, cooked egg yolk, cottage cheese, glucose powder, baby cereal, and breakfast cereal. All of these are good sources of nutrients but need careful balancing; consult your vet for detailed advice.

• Feeding dry foods can be difficult for pups whose milk teeth have not yet erupted; in some breeds, such as the Pekingese, Lhasa Apso, and Shih Tzu, eruption of milk teeth may be delayed until eight to ten weeks of age. Always soften dry food by mixing it with tepid water to make a "porridge", until the pup can efficiently chew and crush biscuits.

• There is no need to feed cows' milk to pups; other foods contain the nutrients available in milk. Very young pups produce an enzyme in their intestines to digest lactose (the sugar in milk); however, the quantity of this enzyme naturally diminishes as the pups mature, and in some dogs may be virtually gone by three months of age. Drinking milk will cause diarrhoea in dogs that lack the enzyme. If you like giving pups milk but it upsets their stomachs, feed them lactose-free milk, which is made for lactose-sensitive children and is available at supermarkets.

WEANING PUPPIES

Weaning is the process by which pups cease taking their mother's milk and start to eat solid food. It naturally happens at between three and six weeks of age. Even after weaning is completed, though, suckling for comfort may continue for a while. Some mothers may even allow pups to suckle until they leave their first home to join their new human families.

The pups need at least four meals a day as well as a constant supply of fresh water. For their first solid meals, mix equal parts of evaporated milk and baby cereal or good puppy food appropriate for the breed. If using dry food, mix it with warm water to make a sloppy porridge. Dip your finger in the mixture and let the pup suckle it. Once it learns to do so, lower your finger so that the pup has to reach down to it. Move on to giving meals in a saucer. When pups are willing to eat solid food, start to reduce the mother's food. At about six weeks the pups' milk teeth have erupted; this makes suckling uncomfortable for her. While pups want to keep suckling, she starts to shorten nursing periods; this change, with her reduced food intake, will reduce her milk supply and should encourage the pups to eat solid food.

AVOIDING OVERFEEDING

A plump, shiny-coated pup looks attractive, but there are health problems associated with plumpness. Nutritionists suspect that the number of fat cells a pup develops is directly related to the risk of obesity later in life. They say that a dog's metabolism "defends" this initial quantity of fat cells and, as a result, losing weight is much harder for dogs that were plump pups than for dogs that were lean. It is especially important not to overfeed large or giant breeds, because an excess energy intake during puppyhood (a time of rapid growth) contributes to bone and joint disorders such as hip dysplasia and osteochondrosis (*see pp.366–67*).

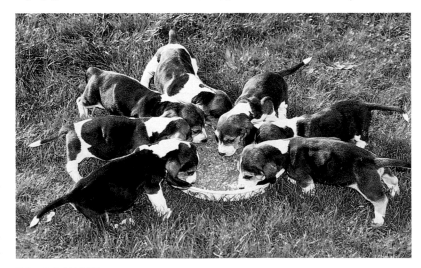

FEEDING HABITS
While there are great personality and even breed differences in dogs' desire to eat (Labrador Retrievers, like the French, live to eat while Yorkies, like the British, only eat to live), dogs evolved as competitive feeders.

PREVENTING INFECTION

Make sure that parasites such as ear mites, fleas, and intestinal worms do not have a chance to establish themselves. Examine pups' parents and canine visitors (the usual sources) for infestations. Breeding animals and family dogs should be routinely vaccinated against infectious diseases.

Pups inherit protection against infections that the mother has had or for which she has been vaccinated. The most common of these diseases are parvovirus, distemper, hepatitis, leptospirosis, adenovirus 2, and parainfluenza. Inherited protection wanes and disappears between six and 20 weeks of age, and usually before 12 weeks, leaving pups at risk of disease. Vaccinate against diseases that are prevalent where you live or where the pup will be moving. Unless disease risk is high, give the first inoculation at eight weeks.

Almost all pups inherit roundworms. To minimize their worm load and reduce the risk of reinfestation, give drugs such as fenbendazole at three, four, five, and eight weeks. Tell a pup's new family to repeat worming at 10 and 12 weeks, then every three months until the dog is mature.

WHEN TO CALL THE VET

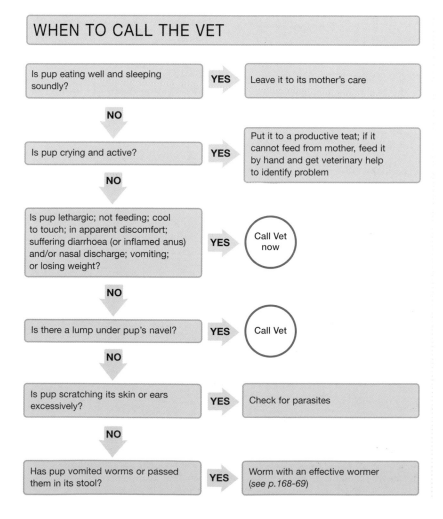

Is pup eating well and sleeping soundly?	**YES**	Leave it to its mother's care
↓ **NO**		
Is pup crying and active?	**YES**	Put it to a productive teat; if it cannot feed from mother, feed it by hand and get veterinary help to identify problem
↓ **NO**		
Is pup lethargic; not feeding; cool to touch; in apparent discomfort; suffering diarrhoea (or inflamed anus) and/or nasal discharge; vomiting; or losing weight?	**YES**	Call Vet now
↓ **NO**		
Is there a lump under pup's navel?	**YES**	Call Vet
↓ **NO**		
Is pup scratching its skin or ears excessively?	**YES**	Check for parasites
↓ **NO**		
Has pup vomited worms or passed them in its stool?	**YES**	Worm with an effective wormer (*see p.168-69*)

Q WHY DO MOTHERS EAT THEIR PUPPIES' BODY WASTE?

A During the first and most dangerous days of puppies' lives, the mother knows that their body waste provides a scent trail for predators and a breeding ground for germs. She reduces these risks by consuming her pups' urine and faeces. A newborn pup empties its bladder and bowels when its mother licks its anogenital area. As the pup discharges waste, the mother eats it. This natural waste disposal is not limited to mother dogs – many pups go through a normal stage of eating their own or other dogs' droppings.

Q WHY DO MOTHERS REGURGITATE FOOD FOR THEIR PUPS?

A Regurgitating food for pups is normal in wolves, but is less common in dogs (perhaps because early breeders found it unpleasant). A mother may start regurgitating food when her pups are about three weeks old. Pups beg for food by licking their mother's mouth; this is why our family dogs try to "kiss" us. (Pups can also trigger regurgitation from other adult dogs.) If the pups do not eat the food, the mother usually will. Later in life, it is natural for dogs to eat their own vomit.

Q WHY DO PUPPIES DIE AND HOW CAN I PREVENT IT?

A Regrettably, it is natural for some pups to die between birth and weaning. These individuals are born with visible defects, such as cleft palates, or serious internal conditions, such as heart defects. A normal pup just eats and sleeps for most of the time, and any crying will stop as soon as it suckles. If crying continues or if a pup is unusually restless, something is wrong.

MEDICAL DISORDERS IN PUPPIES

DISORDER	SIGNS AND CAUSES	PREVENTION AND TREATMENT
LOW BODY TEMPERATURE (hypothermia; *see also pp.410-11*)	The pup feels cool and is inactive and lethargic. This condition, a major cause of puppy death, is usually seen in pups rejected by their mother.	• Keep the room temperature above 24°C (76°F) for the first three weeks. Provide a covered hot-water bottle for the pups if the mother is away for more than 15 minutes. Prevent exposure to cold drafts or floors. • To treat a pup, gently warm it to "mother" temperature using your body heat or a hot-water bottle.
HERNIA (*see also p.70*)	The pup has a swelling at the navel (umbilicus) or at the groin (inguinal hernia). A reducible hernia can be pushed back in, but a strangulated hernia cannot. There is a strong genetic predisposition towards hernias in some families or in breeds such as the Lhasa Apso, Shih Tzu, and Yorkshire Terrier.	• Small hernias need no treatment. Larger hernias that you can poke your finger in need surgical correction. Your vet will recommend the best time to operate. • A hard, painful swelling at a typical hernia site is a serious emergency and needs immediate veterinary attention.
LOW BLOOD SUGAR (hypoglycaemia; *see also p.338*)	The blood sugar level drops, leading to weakness; possible tics and excessive salivating; convulsions; and finally death. Hypoglycaemia develops without warning, usually when a pup is stressed but also if it is ill or neglected. Some toy breeds, especially Yorkshire Terriers, inherit poor blood sugar control; affected dogs are between six and 14 weeks of age, and may be well muscled and well fed.	• Hand-feed poor feeders with a commercially produced milk replacer that contains adequate amounts of sugar. • Corn syrup, honey, or glucose powder can be given by mouth to a conscious pup. • Unconscious pups or those having convulsions need sugar (dextrose) intravenously as soon as possible.
DIARRHOEA	Pups dehydrate six times faster than adults. For them, even mild diarrhoea can lead to serious dehydration and possible death. The mother will clean away the diarrhoea, leaving no sign apart from a slightly inflamed anus. The most common cause is overfeeding, especially in hand-reared pups.	A dehydrated pup will need veterinary treatment with electrolyte solution and medications.
UNDERFEEDING	Competition can be fierce for the most productive teats. Underfed pups cry more and eventually become listless and cool to touch.	• Detect problems early by weighing all of the pups every day. • Weak pups need to be hand-fed.
RETAINED URINE AND FAECES	The mother normally prompts newborn pups to urinate and defecate by licking them. If she neglects to do so, urine and faeces are retained.	• Passing of body waste can be stimulated by gently massaging the genital area with cotton wool pads soaked in warm water. Do this after each feed and at least once between feeds.

DISORDER	SIGNS AND CAUSES	PREVENTION AND TREATMENT
BLEEDING (haemorrhagic syndrome)	This disorder is due to a lack of vitamin K, necessary for blood clotting. The vitamin is produced by intestinal bacteria. During the first few days of life a pup gets its vitamin K from its mother, until its intestines have been colonized by the bacteria. A malnourished mother can produce pups susceptible to bleeding from minor injuries.	• Affected pups need vitamin K by injection.
NAVEL INFECTIONS	The severed umbilical cord usually shrinks and falls off, leaving the navel. Sometimes the navel becomes infected and appears red and swollen. Pus may be present.	• Clean the area with warm water and a mild antiseptic. • Phone your vet for advice on whether to take in the affected pup.
BLOOD POISONING (septicaemia)	Bacteria may enter pups via the navel, or if the mother has an infected mammary gland (mastitis) that releases them into milk. Pups become restless and distressed, with diarrhoea, straining, or bloating. A red or blue tint to the skin shows lethal inflammation of the abdomen lining (peritonitis).	• Affected pups need urgent veterinary treatment. Thereafter, they need hand-feeding.
HERPES VIRUS	Herpes virus seldom causes clinical signs in the mother. If she passes it to her pups during birth, however, the pups will stop nursing, cry, develop diarrhoea, and be in considerable pain.	• Herpes virus survives best at around 36°C (98°F). Veterinary care, in which the pups are kept in an incubator heated to over 38.5°C (101°F) may help, but this infection is usually fatal. • Subsequent litters from a herpes-infected mother do not necessarily become ill with herpes virus.
FADING PUPPY SYNDROME	This is a general term for pups that are listless, do not feed well, become weak, do not gain weight, then fade away and die. There are many causes including birth defects; chilling; poor feeding; toxic milk from the mother; and herpes virus infection.	• Keep affected pups well-nourished and warm. • Mark a pup that you want to monitor by applying a spot of non-toxic ink to the coat or nail varnish to a few toes.
FLAT PUPPY SYNDROME (swimmers)	Affected pups have weak muscles. They appear flat-chested, looking much like swimming turtles. This occurs more frequently in giant breed pups, especially in overweight individuals.	• Encourage affected pups to sleep on their side by "hobbling" the forelegs together at the elbows while the pup sleeps. • Provide a gripping surface such as grass or carpet for walking exercise. • Most individuals recover to normal by mid-puppyhood.

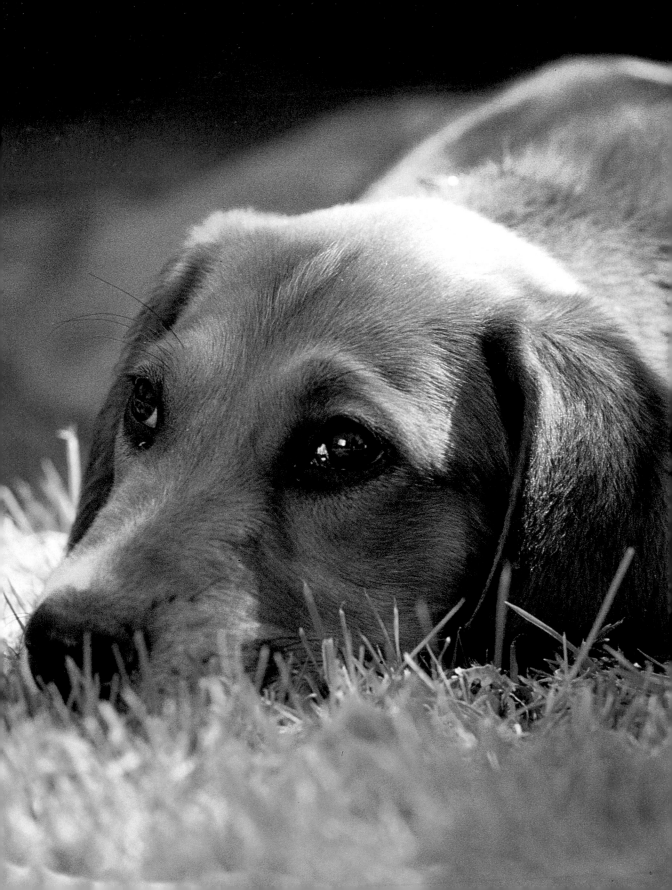

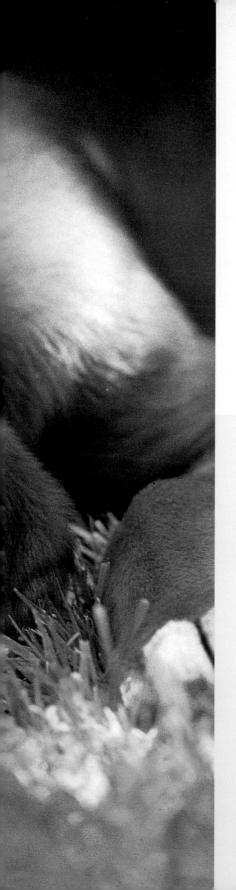

DISEASES
AND
DISORDERS

Your dog and your veterinarian both depend upon you for an accurate description of what you have seen, felt, heard, or smelled. What you tell your vet, and what he or she then ascertains from a physical examination and diagnostics is at the core of problem-oriented veterinary medicine. Although each chapter in this section of the book describes a specific part of the dog's body, common problems such as scratching, limping, coughing or vomiting, all of which may have their origins outside the part of the body obviously affected, are discussed from a problem-oriented viewpoint. In veterinary medicine observation is vital. We can only describe a dog's clinical signs, what we see. Technically, therefore, we can only guess at its symptoms, and how a dog feels.

THE HEALTHY DOG
how does your dog stay healthy?

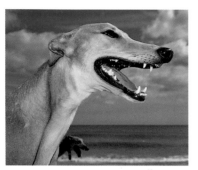

Good health means vitality

Most dogs remain in good health throughout their lives, and illness is extraordinarily rare. Many natural processes take place in your dog's body to help it to stay healthy and defend itself against disease and injury. During every second of every day of a dog's life, its body is identifying potential health problems, protecting itself, and repairing damage. To do this, the dog's body cells are constantly renewing and repairing themselves, instructed by several different chemicals and by the cells' genetic material.

Organs, cells, and even molecules are capable of self-diagnosis. Under normal circumstances, your dog's body will recognize damage at any of these levels and will then proceed to remove, repair, or replace the damaged area. It is extremely efficient at doing so, and constantly protects itself, diagnoses problems, and heals itself every day.

This constant self-regulation, maintaining the optimum conditions for life in a stable equilibrium or "homeostasis", is the basis of good health. Only when the body's self-diagnosis and homeostatic regulation fail does illness or disease follow.

Q   DO NUTRITIONAL SUPPLEMENTS HELP TO KEEP A DOG HEALTHY?

A   A dog's diet influences the levels of different fatty acids in its cell walls. Some nutritionists believe that cells with high levels of omega 3 fatty acids in their walls are less affected by inflammation than those with a majority of omega 6 fatty acids. Vitamins and minerals can also affect cell health (see pp.86–99).

Q   DOES A DOG'S STATE OF MIND HAVE AN EFFECT ON ITS HEALTH?

A   People who suffer the stress of bereavement have a dramatically higher incidence of infections, cancer, and heart disease in the years immediately following their loss. Our health can be powerfully influenced by our state of mind. It is very likely that the same is true for dogs.

HEALTH DEPENDS ON CELL REGENERATION
Your dog's body is constantly rebuilding itself. In areas such as the skin and the lining of the gut, cells are constantly being shed and replaced. For a wound to heal (see pp.392–97), new cells are required to grow over the damaged area.

The processes of cell repair and renewal are controlled by chemical regulators called cytokines: proteins so small and so scarce they are almost impossible to detect. Some cytokines stimulate cell growth, others inhibit it, and there is a natural, well-regulated balance between these opposing cytokines. Healing – a return to homeostasis – depends upon coordination of cytokine activity. If you consider that the entire lining of your dog's digestive system is renewed several times each week, this gives you an idea of the level of coordination required. The natural balance of cytokine activity is influenced by hormones produced by the pituitary, thyroid, and adrenal glands (see p.329). It is also affected by the nervous system (see pp.350–55) – by your dog's state of mind.

THE ROLE OF THE CELL WALL
The wall of a cell is to the cell what skin is to the body: its first and most important line of defence. The wall protects the contents of the cell and is the part of the cell most vulnerable to external attack and injury. It is not a permanent structure, but a membrane made up of proteins embedded in a fatty substance.

Cell walls are covered with special receptor sites that recognize certain nutrients, hormones, and other substances and bind them to the cell. When these chemicals bind to their receptor sites, they trigger signalling pathways within the cell, influencing the cell's activity. To ensure that the receptor sites are always working properly, parts of the cell wall are constantly being withdrawn into the cell, where they are examined, repaired if necessary, and then returned to the cell's surface. Inside the cell, scavengers called lysosomes recognize and eliminate defective sections of the cell wall.

GENETIC CONTROL OF CELL RENEWAL

The life span of most cells is short, and cells must be replaced when they become worn out. Dogs have trillions of cells in their bodies, and millions of these are replaced every single day.

Cells make new cells by passing on their DNA, the genetic information contained in their central nuclei, from one generation of cell to the next. DNA also copies information into another related molecule called RNA, which can travel out of the nucleus and into the cell fluid. There, RNA translates the information it acquired from DNA, directing cells to manufacture specific proteins that determine the form and function of all aspects of life. These are the most basic processes of life and are finely balanced or homeostatic.

VET'S ADVICE

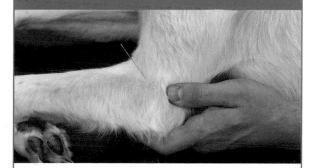

Given the right conditions, your dog will heal itself. Mind–body therapies may be beneficial for us, but these approaches have minimal value for dogs. However, certain complementary therapies, such as acupuncture (*above*), and chiropractic, are appropriate for use on dogs and may be helpful in treatment. Only use treatments that have been shown to be effective for dogs (*see pp.114–15*), and seek a vet who is qualified in this type of therapy.

OUR ROLE IN MAINTAINING HEALTH

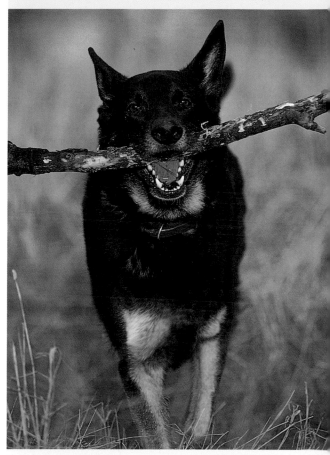

The roles of both owner and veterinary surgeon in caring for a dog are essentially to help it look after itself; to guard against and prevent injury or disease; and to aid recovery when illness occurs. Prevention is achieved through sensible training (*see pp.30–39*), good nutrition (*see pp.86–99*), and measures such as vaccination (*see p.106*). When good health falters and illness occurs, the job of the vet is to create the best conditions for your dog's body to repair itself. This may involve:
- recommending an appropriate diet;
- providing medicines to help the body overcome infection or organ failure (*see pp.104–113*);
- conducting surgical procedures that repair damaged tissue or remove things that are interfering with good health (*see pp.118–19*).

Owners can help by providing care and a good environment for healing, and by making sure that the dog gets both exercise and plenty of rest.

CHALLENGES TO GOOD HEALTH

Your dog's natural state is one of good health, a condition maintained by its physical, behavioural, and immunological defences. It is only when these defences fail, or accidents happen, that medical problems develop.

Many diseases in dogs are caused by the invasion of pathogens, such as viruses, bacteria, fungi, and animal parasites (*see pp.142–75*). Other problems, such as injuries and poisoning, are due to the environment in which a dog finds itself. For some medical conditions, such as certain forms of blindness, arthritis, and cancer, there is a genetic predisposition.

INFECTIOUS DISEASES

A common cause of disease in dogs is infection by microorganisms. Commonly known as pathogens, these organisms may enter the dog's body in a variety of ways. Some are breathed in or swallowed in food or water; others may gain entry through a break in the skin. Once disease-causing organisms have entered the body, they may spread through the bloodstream and affect many organs at once, or they may target and damage one particular organ, such as the liver or intestines. These organisms multiply within the body, disrupting the normal function of organs and tissues and causing the symptoms of illness.

Infections are more likely to develop if the number of infecting organisms is large or if the dog's immune resistance is reduced, which may be the case if the dog is elderly or already has a chronic disease. There are many types of disease-causing microorganisms; these can be grouped into viruses, bacteria, and fungi.

VIRUSES

Viruses are the smallest infectious organisms. They consist of a single or double strand of genetic material that is surrounded by a protein case, sometimes with a protective outer envelope. Viruses invade living cells and reproduce inside them by taking over the functions of the host cell.

Diseases such as rabies (*see p.144*) and distemper (*see p.147*) are caused by viruses. Since viral infections are difficult to treat with drugs, most vets recommend vaccination (*see p.106*) against the most common viral diseases.

BACTERIA

Bacteria are microscopic single-celled organisms. Some disease-causing bacteria invade body cells and reproduce inside them; others cause illness by secreting toxins that kill or disrupt cells.

Leptospirosis (*see p.151*), a serious condition of the liver and kidneys that can also affect humans, is caused by bacteria. Infections caused by bacteria are usually treated with antibiotics.

FUNGI

Fungi, particularly yeasts, can also cause disease in dogs. For example, in blastomycosis (*see p.157*), fungi are inhaled or enter the skin and spread throughout the body, producing coughs, skin lesions, and eye problems. Fungal infections are treated with antifungal drugs.

PARASITIC INFESTATION

Parasites vary in size from microscopic single-celled organisms through just-visible skin mites to intestinal tapeworms several metres long. Parasites have evolved to live on or in animals, deriving their nutrition from the animal's body and often reproducing inside it.

The dog's immune system has developed strategies to cope with parasites, and recent research suggests that exposure to parasites early in life may strengthen a dog's immune response to later infestation. Most

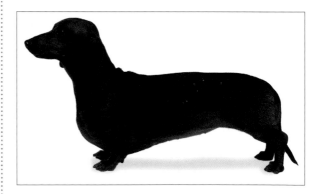

LONGER LIFE
Improvements in care and preventative medicine have extended the life span of domestic dogs. Size still plays a part, with larger breeds having a shorter life expectancy. Many smaller dogs, such as Dachshunds (above), now live on average for over 14 years.

parasitic infestations that affect dogs can be treated easily with the appropriate drugs.

ENVIRONMENTAL HAZARDS TO HEALTH

The dog evolved to live outdoors, within a pack, obtaining nourishment by hunting animals and grazing on vegetation. The nature of canine diseases changed when we moved dogs from their evolutionary environment into ours.

Mixing dogs from different packs increased the risk of transmissible diseases, and living in cities increased the risk of road traffic accidents, while in some places gunshot and arrow wounds are a common cause of traumatic injury. Simply living in our warm homes has created new challenges to canine health; in the temperate zone, fleas are a more important cause of disease in dogs than they have been in the past because fleas find our centrally heated homes an ideal habitat.

The dog's natural defences evolved over millennia to cope with the threats posed by its natural enemies. In the last 100 years, however, modern science has created unnatural enemies against which dogs have no defences. Nitrate food preservatives, heavy metals in water, dioxins produced by the manufacturing industry, the insecticide DDT – all of these substances are harmful because dogs do not have natural ways to

VET'S ADVICE

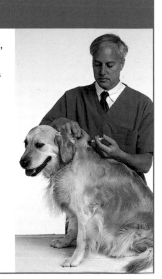

In addition to temperament, age, sex, breed, and environment, economics is a major factor in a dog's health and susceptibility to disease. Money often determines the level of preventative medicine, and also how early in a disease a dog receives treatment. A responsible owner must be prepared to face the expense involved in preventing and treating disease.

rid their bodies of these substances. Toxic chemicals, such as PCBs, are tasteless and odourless. Once ingested, they bind to fat, a body tissue only too abundant in many dogs, and accumulate, potentially disrupting hormonal balances. These toxic substances are never expelled from the body, because there are no natural enzymes to attack and destroy them.

GERIATRIC CONDITIONS

At one time, the average life expectancy of a domestic dog was the same as that of the wolf, typically about seven or eight years. Many individuals did live for longer, and the potential life expectancy was greater still, but the vagaries of life meant that few dogs got much past this average.

Disease control and balanced nutrition have enabled more dogs to reach their potential life expectancies. The median life expectancy for all dogs has increased to 12.8 years. Some breeds live two years longer.

With advancing years come inevitable changes in a dog's physical condition and its ability to combat disease. Geriatric medicine is a new field in veterinary science, ironically owing its existence at least in part to the successes of disease control, owner responsibility, and good nutrition. Older dogs are more likely to suffer from cancer, heart disease, hearing problems, and certain metabolic disorders than their younger counterparts, but advances in geriatric veterinary care mean that most dogs now remain healthy into old age.

GERIATRIC DOGS

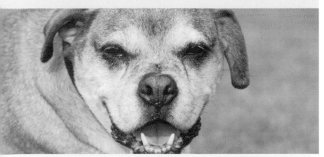

A wider range of age-related disorders is now being diagnosed in dogs than ever before: wear and tear, organ inefficiencies, metabolic disorders, and diseases that result from slow but steady accumulation of damage, such as cancer and heart disease. Even senile dementia, similar in many ways to Alzheimer's disease in people, occurs in dogs. Other typical conditions that affect elderly dogs include reduced hearing, muscle weakness, bowel sensitivity, and an inclination to bark absently, or "backwards", as it has been eloquently described.

CHANGING GENETIC PRESSURES

Mutations – spontaneous changes in the chemical make-up of genetic material – are constantly occurring in animals and in people. Mutations that occur in egg and sperm cells are passed on to the next generation, and some of these mutations produce changes in the physical appearance or condition of the offspring. In nature, "survival of the fittest" means that beneficial genetic mutations are retained, while harmful ones die out quickly. For example, in a cold climate, a dog with thick fur would survive to pass on its genes, but a mutation that produced fine fur would disappear from the genetic mix because individuals with this mutation would be more likely to die before reproductive age.

When we intervened in dog breeding, we influenced canine genetic pressures. Through beauty contests and breeding to circumscribed aesthetic standards, kennel clubs have unwittingly accelerated evolutionary genetic changes in dogs and in some cases created animals that would not have been selected for in nature. Many of our breeds today come from small genetic bases. Any genetic problem existing in that genetic base, such as

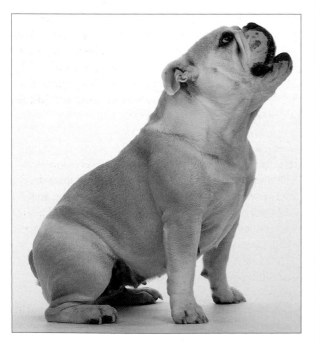

DANGEROUS CHANGES
Dogs naturally have long muzzles and wide-set eyes. Many breeds, such as this bulldog, have been selectively bred to have shortened or "brachycephalic" muzzles and frontal eyes: this gives a humanized face that appeals to owners, but carries health risks for the dog.

the West Highland White Terrier's predisposition to skin allergy, is magnified through the breed population. Other harmful genetic changes have occurred because of the success at dog shows of one individual in a particular breed; any unknown genetic defects in that dog will have been spread to a larger than normal population because of the dog's popularity for breeding.

SELECTIVE BREEDING

We increase the risk of disease for dogs through selective breeding. For example, the unnaturally flattened face of a Pekingese or a bulldog is associated with a greater risk of heart disease, eye injuries, choking, and facial skin infection in these breeds than were found in their ancestors. We also continue to perpetuate some medical problems, such as deafness in Dalmatians, which we would not do were they critical or life-threatening.

GENETIC DISEASES AND GENETIC TESTING

There is no question that hereditary or genetic diseases are a significant problem in pedigree dogs. Identifying which animals were carriers of genetic diseases, such as blindness-inducing progressive retinal atrophy or the bleeding disorder von Willebrand's disease, previously depended upon time-consuming test matings. Recent developments in genetics have enabled more precise detection and the treatment of many canine genetic diseases. The huge advance in human molecular genetics, fuelled by the Human Genome Project work to "map" the genetic blueprint of humans, has a smaller parallel in the Canine Genome Project. This is generating new information about canine genetics on an almost weekly basis.

Good breeders are increasingly aware of advances being made in genetic testing for inherited diseases, as are the breed associations. The best breeders and breed registry associations ensure that all practical tests are carried out on breeding stock and that results are available for potential puppy buyers. Anyone who intends to buy a purebred pup should read books and, if possible, visit websites devoted to the breed to learn as much as possible about the known genetic problems. In addition, talk to staff at the veterinary clinic; they are usually well informed about local breeders and genetic problems within particular breeds.

Genetic testing is simplest for diseases that have the same genetic cause in more than one species. For example, von Willebrand's disease affects both dogs and humans. The DNA sequence that causes the disease in people is already known, and with perseverance a similar mutation was eventually discovered in Scottish Terriers. Unfortunately for genetic research, most other canine genetic diseases that have been studied do not share a common genetic cause with their counterpart in humans. For genetic diseases for which the DNA sequence of the causative abnormal gene is not known, tests have been developed using genetic markers.

DNA TESTING FOR DISEASES

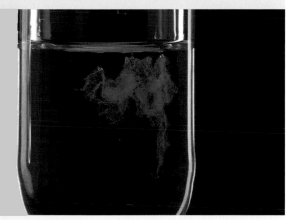

Canine genetic testing is a rapidly developing field. As well as identifying the risks of various diseases, it has produced a curious bonus for dog breeders: several breeds can be DNA tested for the coat colour genes they carry.

DISEASES THAT CAN BE TESTED FOR INCLUDE:

von Willebrand's Disease
Scottish Terrier
Shetland Sheepdog
Doberman (Toy)
Manchester Terrier
Pembroke Welsh Corgi
Poodle (all sizes)

Renal Dysplasia
Shih Tzu
Lhasa Apso
Soft-coated Wheaten Terrier

Progressive Retinal Atrophy
Irish Setter
Cardigan Welsh Corgi
Portuguese Water Dog
Chesapeake Bay Retriever
English Cocker Spaniel

Q DO GENETIC TESTS TELL US WHETHER A DOG WILL DEFINITELY GET A DISEASE?

A Looking for the genetic markers of a disease gives a probability, not a certainty. Geneticists suggest that most genetic tests are 95 per cent accurate.

Q HOW DOES GENE THERAPY WORK AND WHAT IS IT USED FOR?

A A gene carrying specific instructions, perhaps to destroy cancer cells, is "spliced" (integrated) into a benign (non-disease-causing) virus. The gene-containing virus is then inserted into the particular cells in the dog that are being targeted by the therapist, where they multiply. This technique is in the earliest stages of development.

A genetic marker is a short segment of identifiable DNA. Each of a dog's chromosomes consists of strings of sites called alleles, and a genetic marker must have at least two alleles. When the frequency of the most common component of an allele, within a specific population of dogs, is less than 95 per cent, that marker is described as "polymorphic". These markers almost always accompany a specific abnormal gene on the same chromosome. If the marker can be detected, it is likely that the abnormal gene is also present. Such tests indicate a probability, but not a certainty, of the presence or absence of a disease.

THE THREAT FROM WITHIN

The greatest "enemy within" is cancer. Every time a cell divides in two during the processes of growth and renewal, its DNA must be copied into the new cell. Overseeing DNA activity is an intricate selection of proteins called enzymes. Enzymes are the mechanics that carry out the DNA's instructions. They cut up DNA molecules, remove certain sections, add other sections, and put the molecules back together with amazing precision and speed. A great deal can go wrong, however. A DNA molecule might be damaged by radiation or by one of the hundreds of carcinogenic (cancer-causing) chemicals. When this happens, the DNA makes a mistake when it copies itself: the new cell is then "wrong". If this mistake is not detected, the "wrong"cell multiplies and the resulting abnormal cells become a cancer.

NATURAL DEFENCES
how the body fights off disease

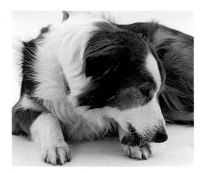

Dog grooming itself

Recruiting the body's own self-healing capacities, amplifying natural recuperative processes, and creating an environment conducive to wellbeing were once at the heart of medicine. With the development of modern drugs and technology, mainstream Western medicine temporarily lost sight of these principles of engendering good health, although they became (and in many cases still are) the defining aspect of complementary medicine. A shift in thinking is now restoring balance to veterinary care.

Healing takes place on many levels. Visible healing is obvious. If a dog suffers a skin tear, we can see the skin repairing itself over the next few weeks. All of us are familiar with the inflammation that occurs around a cut, the formation of a scab, and the growth of new skin under the scab to fill in the wound. At the same time, new cell formation begins at the margins of the wound. The new cells grow across the wound under the protection of the blood clot that has formed. At the same time, new blood vessels sprout from the closest intact vessels and grow with the new cells. The real repair work, however, is less visible.

NATURAL BARRIERS
Any part of the body connected to the outside world, and thus easily accessible to pathogens, has a natural ability to repair itself. Your dog's first line of defence is its skin: hair gives insulation and protection, while the skin forms a barrier to pathogens. The skin is also the primary organ in your dog's immune system – the network of organs, tissues, and cells that fights infection within the body *(see pp.120-29)*.

The lining of the gut, which is the second largest organ in the immune system, and the liver, which is linked to the gut, have also evolved sophisticated, highly effective powers of regeneration. Defensive actions take place throughout the gastrointestinal system: pathogens that have been ingested are killed by saliva in the mouth or by stomach acid, while toxic substances are denatured (chemically altered) in the stomach or intestines or detoxified by the liver.

Sometimes, foreign particles or pathogens can enter the body through the respiratory tract when a dog inhales. The airways of the respiratory system are lined with mucus, which traps invading particles and is then directed away from the lungs by tiny hairs called cilia.

MECHANICAL DEFENCE REACTIONS
Coughing, sneezing, vomiting, diarrhoea, frequent urination, and even scratching the skin are all natural defensive actions designed to rid the body of unwanted organisms or substances. Coughing, for example, is a

Q HOW DO YOU KNOW WHEN TO INTERVENE WITH A DOG'S NATURAL DEFENCES?

A In general, a gentle response from the body's natural defences is almost always beneficial to your dog, while an extreme response is not. For example, a mild fever of a degree or so above the usual temperature is normal during an infection, but seek your veterinary surgeon's advice if your dog develops a high fever, which may itself be damaging. Similarly, gentle coughing may be helpful, but not constant hacking. A brief bout of vomiting to rid the stomach of substances that should not be there can also be a good thing, but persistent vomiting upsets the acid-base balance (the natural balance between acidity and alkalinity in the body fluids and tissues). Your vet will advise you where to draw the line between useful and harmful natural responses.

complicated procedure involving a coordination of the diaphragm, chest muscles, and the voice box, which is designed to clear harmful material from the windpipe. When coughing is successful, the material can then be either spat out or swallowed and destroyed by stomach acids. Grooming, which includes simple scratching, rids the body of parasites. Many dog owners see these natural defences as the problem itself and want their dog's defences suppressed, but in fact eliminating the defence may create a greater problem.

UNDERSTANDING DEFENCE REACTIONS

When a pathogen tries to invade your dog's body, the body responds in specific ways that can sometimes be misinterpreted. The brain sets the body's thermostat at a higher level, resulting in fever. This is a natural defence, because the raised temperature creates a better internal environment for killing certain pathogens, but it has its costs. A moderate fever increases a dog's metabolic rate by about 20 per cent, and may even cause temporary male sterility, while a high fever can lead to seizures. Not eating is another natural defence. Bacteria need iron in order to survive and multiply, and temporary fasting reduces the amount of iron available to invading bacteria. During an infection, a chemical called leucocyte endogenous mediator (LEM) is released into the dog's bloodstream, and this further inhibits the absorption of iron from the gut.

VET'S ADVICE

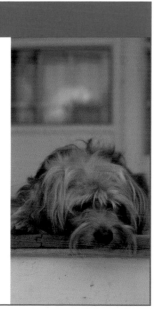

Dog owners commonly visit vets because their dog is not eating and is sleeping more than usual. These are not signs of specific illness but rather ways your dog conserves energy when it is feeling unwell. If you see that your dog is behaving in this way, it is a sensible idea to contact your vet for advice. Your vet can then find out what is causing your dog to behave as if unwell and offer treatment if needed.

DEFENCES CHECKLIST

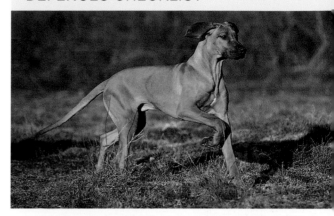

GOOD NATURAL DEFENCES AND HUMAN CARE

Cleanliness
Natural grooming and scratching help to remove parasites from the skin. Additional grooming, and maintaining a clean environment for your dog, reinforces this defence.

Maintaining healthy natural barriers
A healthy digestive tract repels attacking pathogens. In addition, a balanced, healthy diet will help to keep a dog's coat in good condition.

Avoiding of known pathogens
Train your dog to avoid close contact or fighting with unknown dogs and not to scavenge. In this way you will help to protect it from encountering pathogens.

HOW NATURAL DEFENCES FIGHT PATHOGENS

Attacking
Patrolling white blood cells will immediately converge on the invading pathogen to attack it (*see p.83*).

Poisoning
Certain white blood cells, called killer T-cells, secrete chemicals that kill pathogens (*see p.82*).

Starving
Fasting, and the release of chemicals in the body, deprive intestinal bacteria of the iron they need to grow and multiply.

Isolating
The connective tissue cells around the damaged area multiply to wall off the area from healthy tissue. This process results in the formation of pockets of infection, such as pustules and abscesses (*see pp.188, 194*).

THE IMMUNE RESPONSE

If a pathogen gets beyond the natural barriers of the skin, gut, or airways, and is not expelled mechanically, it is confronted by the dog's second line of defence: white blood cells.

The immune defence system is awe-inspiring. At all times, a variety of white blood cells circulate in the bloodstream, waiting for accidents and infections to happen. When an injury such as a skin puncture wound occurs, neutrophils (the body's most populous white blood cells) converge where the defensive barrier of the skin has been breached and attack and kill the invading germs. The action of the neutrophils creates debris, but other white blood cells arrive almost immediately to engulf and digest the debris; these cells are called macrophages (literally, "big eaters"). In addition, macrophages transport the pathogens to other white blood cells called B-lymphocytes. These cells, in turn, "paint" antibodies (chemical labels) on the pathogens, marking them out for attack by larger white blood cells called killer T-cells. These cells, as their name implies, secrete chemicals that destroy the pathogens.

To prevent the immune system from attacking the body's own cells, every cell in your dog's body carries its identity imprinted on its surface so that it is recognizable to white blood cells. This identification system is technically referred to as the major histocompatibility complex.

Only when the dog's sophisticated immune system fails or is overwhelmed do invaders get through. Even in these circumstances, back-up defence mechanisms are available. White blood cells called memory T-cells, which float in the dog's circulation, are capable of "remembering" past encounters with a particular pathogen. The memory T-cells activate a rapid response when they come across that pathogen a second time, stimulating B-cells to produce antibodies labelling the invader for immediate destruction. This process is the basis for effective biological vaccination against infectious diseases.

MOLECULAR MONITORS

Your dog's body has evolved to heal itself right down to the molecular level. Molecular mistakes in cells occur daily, and each one is a potential cancer. However, virtually all are caught in time. Molecular troops are present waiting for mistakes to happen. If DNA copying during cell replication goes wrong, or if a spontaneous genetic mutation occurs, special enzymes move in. They snip out the damaged section of DNA, fill the gap with a correct version, then paste the whole system back together.

CUNNING PATHOGENS

Unfortunately, pathogens have natural methods of defence and preservation, as well as cunning ways to propagate themselves. Some types of pathogen actively attack your dog's white blood cells. Others, such as intestinal worms, consume your dog's natural nutrients and thus weaken the dog. Certain pathogens use other agents, such as ticks, to gain access to your dog's body. Another group manipulates your dog's natural defences and uses immune responses such as sneezing or diarrhoea to spread themselves further. The adaptation of pathogens to overcome an organism's natural defences in this way is sometimes called the "co-evolutionary arms race".

INDIVIDUAL VARIATIONS IN RESPONSE

Most dogs are exposed to common causes of medical conditions in a uniform manner, but each individual responds in its own way. For example, every dog in a particular household may be exposed to fleas, but

Q **WHAT ARE THE MOST DANGEROUS EVERYDAY POLLUTANTS?**

A The greatest hazards are man-made chemicals against which dogs have no "evolutionary" defences, such as food preservatives, waste from manufacturing, and agricultural chemicals such as fertilizers and pesticides.

Q **CAN I DO ANYTHING TO HELP MY DOG'S IMMUNE SYSTEM FIGHT OFF ATTACK?**

A The best protection is to arm your dog's immune system. Your vet can give vaccinations to provide immune antibodies against serious infectious diseases. In addition, it is vital for you to give the dog a balanced diet with adequate antioxidants, vitamins, minerals, and fatty acids (see pp.86–99).

while one is not bothered by flea bites, another animal may be intensely irritated by a single flea having a single meal and develop hypersensitivity or an allergy (*see p.124*); that dog may also suffer a secondary bacterial infection or even a systemic disease (a disease that affects the whole body). The competence and reactivity of your dog's immune system ultimately determines what illnesses your dog gets and how its body copes with those illnesses.

GENETIC INFLUENCES ON DEFENCES

The efficiency of your dog's defences also varies according to its age, sex, and breed. Natural defences are most efficient when your dog is in its prime of life, but in time the immune defence system often begins to falter. This is why cancers and overwhelming infections increase in frequency with advancing years.

Some breeds inherit natural defences that are better or worse than average. For example, an infectious agent may challenge a number of dogs, but a Cocker Spaniel is more likely than other breeds to develop an autoimmune condition (a disorder in which the immune system attacks the body's own cells), such as the blood disorder autoimmune haemolytic anaemia, as a consequence of that challenge.

The natural defences may also be challenged by particular drugs, such as anaesthetics. As an example, all dogs can be safely anaesthetized with a fast-acting barbiturate drug but sighthounds such as Greyhounds take much longer to metabolize the barbiturate, and as a result take longer to recover from the anaesthetic.

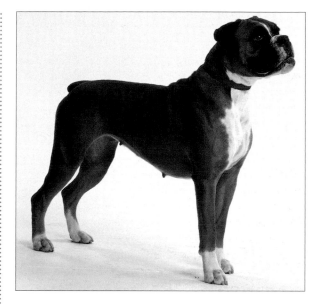

NATURAL VARIATION
Just as breeds vary in their susceptibility to different diseases, they also vary in their responses to drugs. Greater care must be taken, for example, when sedating Boxers than other breeds.

Similarly, acepromazine, a pre-anaesthetic sedative, is safe in all healthy dogs, but Boxers become more deeply sedated for longer periods than other dogs given the same amount on a body-weight basis.

It is important to find out whether your dog's breed makes it any more or less susceptible to infections or other medical conditions and whether it may require special care with particular kinds of treatment.

WHITE BLOOD CELL ATTACKING PATHOGEN

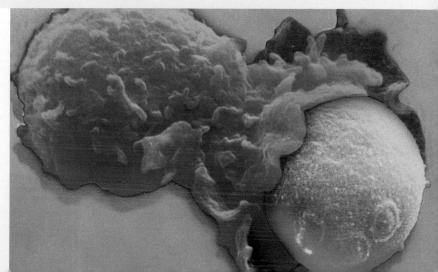

The defensive capabilities of white blood cells are still being unravelled. There are several types of white blood cell. The most numerous are neutrophils, seen here attacking an invading yeast cell. Macrophages are cells that wander the circulatory system searching for bacteria, debris, and even cancer cells to engulf. Killer T-cells release toxic proteins to destroy the infecting organisms. Helper T-cells aid the coordination of other cells involved in the immune response.

PAIN AS AN EARLY WARNING SYSTEM

Pain is not a disease or an illness but an early warning system. It has a vital protective function, because feeling pain causes a dog to avoid activities that could cause it harm. In addition, continued pain reduces the use of damaged tissues, allowing time and rest for repair, and inactivity as a result of pain may even encourage the immune response. Limping, for example, rests an injured leg and creates the best circumstances for natural repair.

Pain may have an obvious, visible source such as an injury, or may arise through damage to an internal organ. Nerve endings called receptors that are capable of receiving pain messages exist throughout the body – in muscles, joints, and especially concentrated in the skin. Nerve receptors are stimulated by temperature, pressure, or natural chemicals called prostaglandins, which are released by damaged cells. Messages are relayed from the receptors through the nerves to the brain, where they are interpreted as pain. The perception of pain differs from dog to dog, partly as a result of inheritance and partly of experience.

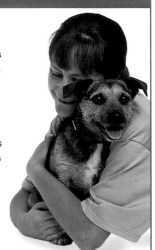

VET'S ADVICE

The touch of a familiar human may "damp down" or alleviate stress responses to pain in a dog. An owner's comforting presence and attention will help a dog to fight illness by promoting a relaxed state of mind, allowing its natural defences to work at their best. Unless your vet advises otherwise, physically comfort your dog with frequent stroking or petting.

ACUTE AND CHRONIC PAIN

Pain is the natural way in which a dog knows either that it should avoid something or that something has gone wrong. It can be either acute (short-term) or chronic (long-term). Acute pain may range from mild to so excruciating that it causes a dog to go into clinical shock (see p.388). Pain is considered chronic when it lasts longer than about six weeks and is continuous. Chronic pain is relentlessly uncomfortable, but most dogs affected will behave stoically. It may be that a dog's owner notices changes in behaviour, such as a reluctance to play as actively as before, difficulty climbing stairs, or irritability.

An episode of pain has two dimensions: intensity and unpleasantness. The sensation of pain is a constant, not affected by typical painkilling drugs, but the unpleasantness of pain can be reduced by drugs, by conditioning, or even by placebo. Acute pain can usually be relieved with appropriate painkillers (see p.108). Chronic pain does not respond as well to existing therapies and is often difficult to treat.

The amount of pain a dog feels is not related to the amount of damage that exists. Your dog's brain constantly monitors the influx of all information and sets a biological priority to a fraction of the data. If your dog suffers potentially painful penetrating

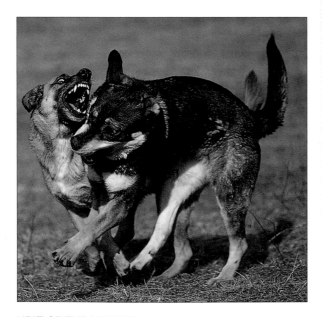

HEAT OF THE MOMENT
During the emotional intensity of a dog fight, there can be serious injuries, but dogs appear resistant to pain and keep fighting. On the other hand, the relatively mild discomfort of an injection may be overwhelmingly painful to a dog that anticipates that it may feel pain.

bite wounds from another dog, its immediate response may be to bite back, not to feel the pain. Conscious acute pain registers only after other priorities have been met. The dog with deep puncture wounds from a fight may appear pain-free until its brain registers different priorities and pain sensation develops.

According to the "gate control" theory, information from nerve receptors travelling to the brain has to pass through "gates", and a number of factors determine how wide these gates open. Emotion certainly affects the size of the opening – probably by altering the body's levels of natural painkillers, endorphins.

Narcotic painkillers like pethidine and morphine, used for severe pain associated with trauma, major surgery and some forms of cancer, mimic endorphins and act directly on the brain. Painkillers like aspirin and non-steroid anti-inflammatory drugs (NSAIDs), such as carprofen and meloxicam, work by inhibiting the production of inflammatory prostaglandins in body tissues. NSAIDS are commonly used for mild to moderate pain. Steroids are sometimes used when pain is associated with intense inflammation.

One thing that still surprises me is the way in which some people assume that if a dog walks away from even a severe accident (such as a road traffic accident) and does not complain, it is not in pain. Dogs are far more stoic than we are. They do not dwell on their pain; they just get on with life.

While acute pain may cause a dog to shriek or cry out, chronic or insidious pain seldom does. There may be a grunt when the dog moves, but otherwise its behaviour may seem almost normal even though it is in considerable discomfort. As a general rule, it is wise to assume that anything that causes us pain will do the same, and with the same intensity, to a dog.

IMPORTANCE OF TOUCH

Interacting with your dog may have a beneficial influence on its physical and psychological response to pain. Clues as to how this occurs come from research on dogs that was carried out in the 1960s by Dr James J. Lynch, author of *The Broken Heart: The Medical Consequences of Loneliness*. (While admiring Dr Lynch's contribution to our understanding of the importance of touch, one cannot help but feel deeply disturbed by the research methods that he and other Pavlovian researchers used in their work.) In a scientific paper entitled "The Effect of Petting on a Classically Conditioned Emotional Response", Lynch showed that when alone, a dog hearing a tone warning that it would soon receive an electric shock had an increase in heart rate and then a greater increase in heart rate when it received the shock. When the dog was petted, however, there was no increase in heart rate either at the tone or when the electric shock was administered. Physical contact with a person made an enormous difference to the dog's perception of pain.

"STATE OF MIND" AND DISEASE RESISTANCE

Certain brain chemicals, called neuropeptides, are released to relieve pain. These chemicals also have powerful effects on your dog's health, the level of the animal's energy, its general constitution, and natural resistance to disease. Neuropeptides act like an invisible chemical nervous system that forms a bridge between the dog's mind and its body.

In terms of resistance to disease, a dog's psychological defences can be as important as its physical state and its environment. Careful training to teach your dog how to cope with stress can enhance its natural defences and wellbeing.

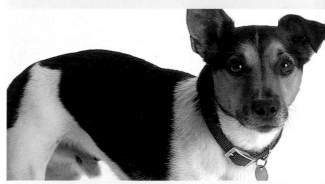

RELATIVE PAIN RESPONSE

The perception of pain varies enormously between individual dogs. As well as individual variations, there are breed differences, too. Most Bull Terriers, for example, appear to be less sensitive to pain than most small spaniels. Perhaps these differences can be traced back to the origin of the breeds: a high level of pain resistance would be prized in terriers bred for fighting, while a dependent, "soft" temperament would be desired in a pet. The Jack Russell (*above*) is renowned for its ability to withstand pain.

BALANCED NUTRITION
the vital role of a healthy diet

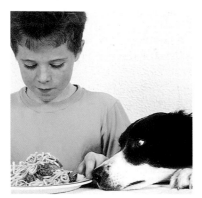
Ignore your dog if it begs for food

Feeding dogs is similar to feeding babies, in that neither has much say in what they eat; they depend on us to make the right decisions. A well-balanced diet is vital for good health. Specialized veterinary diets are available to help prevent or treat illness or to compensate for age-related needs. The easiest way to provide a balanced diet is to use a premium food, containing high-quality nutrients, from a reputable manufacturer. The alternative is to cook for your dog; if you decide to do this, make sure you understand the principles of good canine nutrition. Ensure that your dog's diet is appropriate for its age, size, and energy level.

WHY DOGS EAT LIKE DOGS

Hunger is a dog's natural state. Dogs are competitive feeders – they evolved to eat whatever is available and to eat it quickly. Watch puppies at a food bowl and you will see that the drive to eat is overwhelmingly potent. From birth, each pup is in competition with its siblings for its mother's milk and then for solid food: eat first, eat fast, eat most. This is an excellent gambit when food is scarce, but for dogs fed by us, this brain-driven need to eat whatever is available is at the root of the most common nutritional "disease" today – obesity due to over-nutrition.

DIET, DOGS, AND US

Good nutrition for dogs is not the same as for us. Dogs are scavenging carnivores, preferring meat; humans are omnivores, able to digest almost any food. If meat is not available dogs are moderately good omnivores, but this is not ideal for their digestion. You need to consider certain differences between human and canine nutrition.
• Insoluble fibre from whole grains may help prevent colon cancer in humans, but grains have never been a natural part of the dog's diet except in conditions of extreme starvation.
• Megadoses of vitamin C may be beneficial for humans under stress because we cannot make this vitamin ourselves. Dogs, however, can make their own vitamin C (*see box, p.89*).
• Chocolate may lift our spirits, but excessive amounts can poison dogs or even kill small ones (*see p.99*).

Energy comes from the protein, fat, and carbohydrate that your dog eats. Meat and fat are the basis of life for dogs and contain all the essential amino acids, essential fatty acids, vitamins, and minerals they need. Never feed your dog a meat-only diet, however; it might seem natural to you but plain meat lacks balance in its calcium:phosphorus ratio and can cause illness due to nutrient imbalance (*see Hormonal system, pp.328–39*). Vitamins and minerals are essential for energy conversion, enzyme activity, and bone growth. Fibre is needed to promote good digestion and solid stools. Finally, clean water is the very essence of life.

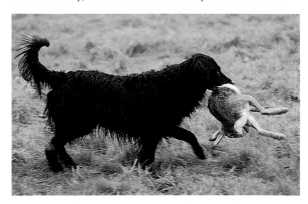

PROS AND CONS OF FRESHLY KILLED FOOD
A whole rabbit is probably the most natural food, providing protein, fat, vitamins, minerals, and fibre. However, rabbits carry germs, bones may damage the dog's intestines, and fur might cause a blockage.

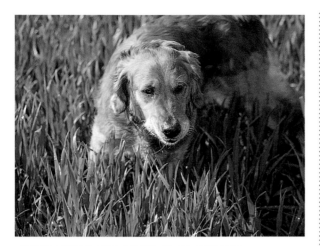

EATING GRASS AND OTHER PLANT MATTER
Some dogs like eating grass; however, grass, vegetables, roots, and berries are difficult for dogs to digest and eaten only in emergencies. Cooked vegetables provide more nutrients than raw plant matter.

Inside your dog's intestines is a dynamic ecosystem; a variety of "good" bacteria vie with each other and ultimately strike a balance amongst themselves. The first of these bacteria come from mother's milk. As the dog grows it continues to receive new bacteria from different foods. Most of these bacterial "guests" are transient and die within a few days, but some stay longer to create a stable environment for digesting nutrients from food. This balanced homeostatic environment is necessary for optimum digestion of nutrients. The components of food and the good gut bacteria also help to build an efficient immune system that protects your dog from illness and infection (*see Natural defences, pp.80–81*).

CHANGING NEEDS THROUGHOUT LIFE

Your dog's nutritional needs gradually change throughout its life, and switching from one source of nutrients to another should be carried out in an equally gradual way. Plan diet changes to occur over a 5- to 10-day period, because the digestive enzymes need time to adjust to new food and diarrhoea can occur if you abruptly change from one food to another. Begin by adding a little of the new food to your dog's existing diet, then gradually increase the proportion of new food over the following days. Any bowel problems, or signs that the dog is going on hunger-strike because of smell, taste, or texture, should become obvious before these potential problems become serious.

Q   **WHAT IS A NATURAL DIET AND HOW SHOULD IT BE FED?**

A   Our "natural diet" is raw meat, worms, roots, berries, and cockroaches. (We produce an enzyme in our intestines that digests chitin, the building component of cockroach shells.) Over time we found that cooked food is often tastier. It is the same with dogs. Their natural diet is meat and all other body parts, including fur, bones, and the contents of their prey's intestines. Raw meat is not really necessary for them. In fact, because of the risks of bacterial contamination and, in some regions, parasites, raw meat for your dog is generally more dangerous than cooked meat.

Q   **I AM A VEGETARIAN; CAN I SAFELY FEED MY DOG A VEGETARIAN DIET?**

A   A dog is able to survive on a well-balanced vegetarian diet but this is a path no dog willingly follows. Dogs are designed to eat best as carnivores. Vegetarianism is a human ethical decision. If you think it is important that your dog shares your ethical principles about meat-eating make sure you get excellent nutritional advice on how to create a balanced vegetarian diet for your dog. Alternatively, buy a balanced manufactured veggie diet. (Never try this with cats. A cat must eat meat to live. If it is fed only a vegetarian diet, it will eventually die from deficiencies in amino acids and other essential nutrients.)

Q   **ARE "LITE" AND "LOW-CALORIE" DOG FOODS GOOD FOR MY DOG?**

A   Manufacturers seldom state the calorie content of their dog food, even when it is promoted as "lite" or "lean". (In the EU it is not permitted to state the energy content on the majority of dog foods!) As a rule of thumb, assume that a "lite" food has 15–25 per cent fewer calories than the average from that manufacturer. If a label does not explain the metabolisable energy per kilogramme of product, reputable manufacturers will provide you with this important information.

INGREDIENTS OF A HEALTHY DIET

The essential components of a healthy canine diet are protein and fat. Proteins are complex molecules made up of a variety of amino acids. These chemicals are the building blocks of all body tissues and of the enzymes that support the body's chemical reactions. The most natural source of protein is meat, but like us, dogs can get all the essential amino acids they need for sustaining life from vegetable protein.

Dogs also need fat. This substance contains essential fatty acids, or EFAs (*see box, opposite*). It is the most energy-dense form of nutrient, with more than twice as many calories per gram as protein or carbohydrate. Fat also transports the fat-soluble vitamins A, D, E, and K around the body. In addition, it helps to make food more palatable.

Fibre is a perfectly natural part of a dog's diet, consumed when it eats the fur or intestine contents of other mammals. It stimulates the production of saliva and gastric juices. In addition, it is potentially beneficial for preventing or treating constipation, sugar diabetes, obesity, inflammatory bowel disease, and excess fat in the bloodstream. There are many types of fibre. They fall into two main groups: water-soluble and insoluble. Water-soluble fibre, found in foods such as cooked vegetables and rice, increases the stickiness of food. As a result, it keeps food in the stomach longer, and slows down digestion and absorption of nutrients in the small intestine. Insoluble fibre, such as bran and animal fur, retains water and makes the faeces more bulky, helping waste matter to pass through the intestines more quickly and easily. Some types of fibre ferment, creating substances in the intestines that may inhibit harmful bacteria. Beet pulp, chicory, rice bran, unprocessed bran, and breakfast cereals containing bran are common sources of fermentable and non-fermentable fibre. The amount of fibre that your dog needs varies with its age and lifestyle; older dogs sometimes benefit from an increase in both soluble and insoluble fibre in their diet, to aid bowel function.

Water is the largest component of most of the cells of the dog's body. It carries the water-soluble vitamins (the B group of vitamins, folic acid, and vitamin C) and is absorbed by fibre to add beneficial bulk to your dog's diet. Always provide fresh, clean, easily accessible water.

ESSENTIAL FATTY ACIDS

Nutritional studies show that fats do more than simply provide energy. During the 1990s, it was found that essential fatty acids (EFAs) have several vital roles. They are involved in controlling a range of problems, such as allergies, arthritis, dermatitis, inflammation, heart disease, flea bite hypersensitivity, auto-immune disease, kidney and nervous system problems, and even cancer.

There are two main groups of these fats: Omega 6 and Omega 3 EFAs. The larger group, Omega 6 EFAs, enable cell membranes to function properly; however, they are also associated with cell inflammation and may suppress the immune system. Omega 3 EFAs are associated with reduced cell inflammation. Generally speaking, these fatty acids do not suppress the immune system; in fact, working at the cellular level, they may enhance the efficiency of the immune system.

Dogs need a good supply of linoleic acid, an Omega 6 EFA. This substances aids growth, wound healing, liver function, and other essential activities. Dogs can convert linoleic acid to arachidonic acid, which is necessary for effective blood clotting, good coat condition, maintaining the health of the heart and eyes, and efficient reproduction. They also use omega 3 EFAs, such as docosahexaenoic acid (DHA) and eicosapentaenoic acid (EPA), to help maintain the structure of cell walls. Supplements containing omega 3

VET'S ADVICE

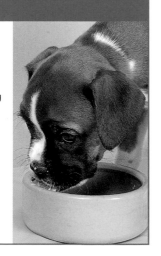

Excess vitamin C is dangerous. Although this vitamin is normally beneficial because it acts as an antioxidant, capturing damaging "free radicals", when given in excess it is excreted in the urine as a substance called oxalate. This material can form into bladder sand or stones. Too much vitamin C can also cause loose stools in puppies.

VITAMINS

FAT-SOLUBLE VITAMINS

VITAMIN A

Vitamin A has many roles, including helping to maintain healthy skin and eyesight. Dogs can manufacture it from substances called carotenoids, found in plant cells. They obtain most of their supplies, however, from eating the liver of another animal. Fish oils, milk, and egg yolk are also good sources of this vitamin. Some Cocker Spaniels may be unable to manufacture enough vitamin A, and as a result may develop oily skin conditions. Long-term supplementation may help these dogs; it is also reported to produce skin improvements in the Labrador Retriever and the Miniature Schnauzer.

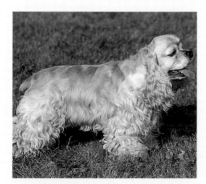

Cocker Spaniel

VITAMIN D

This vitamin helps the body to balance its calcium and phosphate levels, and aids the formation of healthy bones and teeth. Dogs synthesize it in their skin and obtain the essentials for this activity from the diet. Heavy coats can reduce a dog's ability to make the precursor of this essential vitamin. Deficiency, which causes rickets, is now rare because virtually all diets contain enough vitamin D. Excess vitamin D is more common; it leads to calcium deposits in soft tissue and to skeletal deformities.

VITAMIN E

This vitamin, together with the mineral selenium, acts as an antioxidant and thus neutralizes "free radicals" (atoms or molecules that destroy cell membranes). Supplementation seems to aid anti-inflammatory activity for some dogs with skin disorders, and in particular for Dachshunds with acanthosis nigricans (a condition causing hair loss and increased skin pigmentation). It may also be of benefit for vascular, heart, or neurological conditions. Dogs with the skin parasite *Demodex*, and stressed or hard-working dogs, may also benefit from vitamin E supplements.

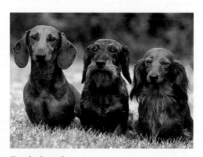

Dachshunds

VITAMIN K

This vitamin plays an essential part in the blood-clotting process. Some vitamin K is manufactured by bacteria in the dog's intestines. Dogs that have been on antibiotics for long periods may have reduced vitamin K levels if the drugs have destroyed some of these "good" bacteria. Deficiencies in vitamin K rarely occur; however, eating a rodent killed with the anti-blood-clotting rodenticide warfarin (or the even more lethal chemical coumarin) may create a sudden and unattainable demand for vitamin K in the body. As a result, the dog may suffer life-threatening internal bleeding and will need emergency veterinary help (*see "Poisons", pp.418–23*).

WATER-SOLUBLE VITAMINS

B COMPLEX VITAMINS

This group includes B1 (thiamine), B2 (riboflavin), niacin, pantothenic acid, B6 (pyridoxine), and vitamin H (biotin). They are important parts of the enzymes that regulate most cellular processes. Many of the B vitamins are synthesized by bacteria in the intestines. Antibiotics may interfere with these bacteria; if your dog needs prolonged antibiotic treatment it might benefit from a safe supplement such as yeast-based tablets.

VITAMIN B12

The roles of vitamin B12 include aiding the development of red blood cells in bone marrow and the utilization of folic acid (see below) and carbohydrates, and ensuring healthy nervous system function. It is absorbed from foods such as liver, kidneys, and other meat; eggs; and dairy products. Some Giant Schnauzers have an inherited condition that interferes with vitamin B12 absorption, and need injections of B12.

FOLIC ACID

This substance is also a B vitamin. In dogs, it is manufactured by bacteria in the intestines. Dogs that are fed on good commercial foods are unlikely to develop folic acid deficiency; however, a supplement may benefit those with cardiovascular or skin problems.

VITAMIN C

This vitamin is important for the function of various enzymes. Dogs manufacture their own supplies from glucose in their liver. It is thought that dogs under stress may be able to increase their production of vitamin C, so dogs should not need supplements. Excessive amounts in the diet may be harmful (*see box, opposite*).

MINERALS

CALCIUM AND PHOSPHORUS

These minerals are necessary for the growth and maintenance of the skeleton and for healthy cell membrane and neuromuscular function. Ideally, there should be marginally more calcium than phosphorus, in the ratio of 1.2–1.4 : 1. The availability of these minerals varies with different types of food. A meat-only diet (low in calcium), especially in young dogs, can cause over-stimulation of the parathyroid glands (see p.333) and eventually lead to swollen, painful joints and deformed, easily broken bones. In females with young puppies, normal lactation can result in low blood calcium, leading to convulsive seizures, or eclampsia (see p.314). Feeding females diets that are too high in calcium during pregnancy may actually increase the risk of eclampsia during lactation. Excess dietary calcium over a long period may induce zinc deficiency; in giant, fast-growing dog breeds, it can cause bony malformations.

MAGNESIUM

Magnesium helps to maintain a normal balance of calcium, phosphorus, and potassium levels. It also aids muscle contraction and nerve impulses. Giant-breed dogs, especially those on heart medication, may have heart arrhythmias due to low magnesium levels.

SELENIUM

This is an essential part of the enzyme systems that maintain healthy body tissue such as heart muscle. As a free-radical scavenger it may also play a role in the immune system, helping to neutralize environmental and dietary carcinogens. In addition, selenium may be involved in reproduction. The mineral interacts with other antioxidants such as vitamins A, C, and E, and with the trace minerals zinc, manganese, and copper. Selenium is a heavy metal and can be toxic at relatively low levels. Only trace levels are needed in the diet.

COPPER AND IRON

Copper is stored in the liver. Together with iron, it is involved in transporting oxygen around the body in red blood cells. Some Bedlington Terriers may have an inherited copper storage disease that leads to copper poisoning. Doberman Pinschers, West Highland White Terriers (below), and Cocker Spaniels may suffer from a copper build-up in the liver that is secondary to other liver disease (see p.296). This problem causes loss of appetite, lethargy, vomiting, and abdominal pain. It can be controlled by restricting the amount of copper in the diet.

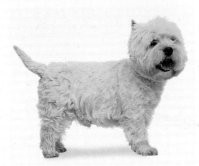

West Highland White Terrier

ZINC

Zinc is essential for healthy skin and taste buds and for an efficient immune system. It is also vital for the effective functioning of many enzymes, and is involved with detoxifying ammonia waste. Zinc deficiency in the diet can lead to a poor skin and coat. This deficiency has been called "generic dry dog food disease" because it used to be associated with poorly formulated dry dog foods with a low meat and high cereal content, which had low available zinc levels. Too much calcium in the diet can also compete with zinc, resulting in the same poor skin and coat conditions, especially in fast-growing large and giant breed puppies. Some Alaskan Malamutes (below) and Siberian Huskies have an inherited zinc metabolism disorder in which their bodies cannot absorb sufficient amounts of zinc. This disorder causes scaling, crusting skin and a dull, dry coat. It does, however, improve with zinc supplementation. In addition, all well-balanced commercial dog foods from reputable manufacturers should have adequate zinc levels for these breeds.

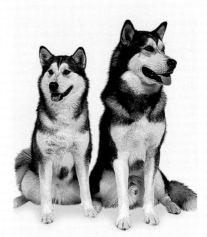

Alaskan Malamutes

IODINE

Iodine is necessary to enable the thyroid gland to produce sufficient hormones. Underactivity of the thyroid gland (see p.331) results in a lack of thyroid hormones. Although this condition is probably the most common hormonal imbalance that dogs suffer from, it is rarely associated with a natural deficiency of iodine in the diet.

EFAs can reduce skin itchiness in some dogs. Evening primrose, fish, and linseed oils all are naturally high in omega 3 EFAs; these substances can all be effective in the long-term control of allergic dermatitis.

VITAMINS AND MINERALS

Food is converted into energy though cascades of chemical reactions. These processes (metabolism) turn protein, fat, and carbohydrate, the "macronutrients" of food, into simple chemical compounds that the body can use or store. Such reactions (and various other vital body functions, such as blood clotting) rely on tiny quantities of vitamins and minerals, the "micronutrients". Extra micronutrients may be useful for a dog whose body is stressed as a result of illness, medication, or advancing years.

Vitamins are divided into fat-soluble and water-soluble groups (*see box, p.89*). The body obtains the fat-soluble vitamins (A, D, E, and K) from fat in food and stores them in the liver. If too much of these vitamins is stored they may have a toxic effect and the dog may become ill. The water-soluble vitamins (the B complex vitamins, vitamin B12, folic acid, and vitamin C) may be obtained from a variety of foods. Only limited amounts are stored in the body; any excess is excreted in urine. For this reason, there is virtually no risk of overdosing with these vitamins.

About four per cent of your dog consists of basic chemical elements called minerals (*see box, opposite*). The main minerals are calcium and phosphorus, which are found in bone and in the circulation. Like vitamins, minerals perform several vital functions in body cells.

COMMERCIAL DOG FOOD STANDARDS

The best dog food manufacturers use only nutrients fit for human consumption. Their premium products are made to fixed formulas. The ingredients are always the same. At the next price level down, foods are made from a varying supply of ingredients to set nutritional and quality standards. While the nutritional value of these foods remains constant, the ingredients vary. This is important to know if you have a dog with a tricky tummy or fixed taste preferences. In the late 1990s, veterinary nutritionists realized that by carefully balancing the type of fibre in dog food they could encourage healthy digestion. This balance is now a fixed feature of the best foods. The best diets, with carefully balanced fibre content, nourish beneficial gut

Q DOES MY DOG NEED CARBOHYDRATES IN ITS DIET?

A Carbohydrates are not a natural energy source for dogs, but dogs are able to convert them into glucose. This sugar is used to produce glycogen, which is stored in muscle for later energy use. (Greyhounds are particularly good at storing glycogen.) There is some evidence that carbohydrates are a good energy source for pregnant and lactating dogs. Starch is the most common source of carbohydrate for dogs, and cooked starch such as potato is easily digested.

Q WHAT ARE ANTIOXIDANTS, AND DOES MY DOG NEED THEM?

A An antioxidant is a substance that destroys free radicals – molecules and atoms that destroy cell membranes. Antioxidants include vitamins C and E, and substances called "carotenoids", such as lutein or beta-carotene. Dogs have their own natural free-radical scavenging systems; however, food containing antioxidants may boost these natural systems. Pet food manufacturers claim that their added antioxidants significantly improve the immune systems of mature dogs, restoring them to the efficiency levels of youth.

Q CAN I SUPPLEMENT MY DOG'S DIET WITH VITAMINS AND MINERALS?

A Take great care if you decide to give vitamin and mineral supplements. Higher levels of some nutrients reduce the absorption of others. It is potentially dangerous to give large amounts of any single mineral. When a higher dose of a nutrient is needed, use a broad-spectrum vitamin and mineral supplement formulated for dogs. This helps to maintain a proper balance by raising the nutritional levels of other nutrients as well.

Q WHAT ARE "NUTRACEUTICAL" SUBSTANCES, AND DOES MY DOG NEED THEM?

A The increasing acceptance that certain nutrients, such as fatty acids, can be therapeutic resulted in the development of the term "nutraceuticals" to describe food substances with proposed therapeutic activity. A North American Veterinary Nutraceutical Council has been formed to ensure that products contain the ingredients on the label, are safely manufactured to high standards, and do what the labels claim they do. Until standards are set, nutraceuticals can be marketed as "miracle cures". Be wary of all miracle supplements: miracles seldom happen.

UNDERSTANDING FOOD LABELS

Nutrient levels

Comparing protein, fat, or fibre levels in different foods just by reading labels is pointless because levels vary according to the food's water content. To compare foods accurately, you have to convert the data to a "dry-matter" basis – what remains if all moisture is removed. Pet food manufacturers will gladly provide this information; you can also find it yourself.

A typical canned food label might say: protein 6.5%; oil 3.5%; fibre 0.5%; moisture 81%. This food is 81 per cent moisture so it is 19 per cent dry matter. You can calculate the true levels of protein, fat, and fibre using this formula.

Dry matter nutrient content = The label's nutrient percentage x 100 ÷ Dry-matter content percentage. Therefore:

Protein = 6.5x100÷19 = 34.2%

Oil (fat) = 3.5x100÷19 = 18.4%

Fibre = 0.5x100÷19 = 2.6%

Extra information

Labelling laws often prevent dog food manufacturers from putting explicit information about ingredients on the label. The information that is there often needs interpretation or an explanation direct from the manufacturer. It may include:

- Typical or guaranteed analysis

This list usually shows the minimum amount of protein and fat and the maximum amount of fibre and moisture. It says little about the quality of a product.

- Ingredients

This gives more information on quality but usually fails to be specific. Items are listed in descending order of weight. "Meat" is muscle. "Meat by-products or derivatives" are viscera, bone, and marrow. "Meat meal" means dry products rendered from animal tissues. If a food "contains permitted colourant, flavours, and preservatives", the manufacturer's consumer services will tell you what these are if you ask.

- Feeding guidelines

These recommendations are only suggestions, based on the needs of an average dog in average weather and assuming ideal body composition. Your dog may need more or, often, less than what is recommended.

- Nutritional adequacy statement

This statement, on North American foods, specifies the canine life stages appropriate for the food. Look for the phrase "animal feeding tests". If the text says instead, "formulated to meet the nutritional profiles..." the manufacturer is relying on laboratory analysis, not real-life feeding trials, to determine the food's nutritional content.

bacteria and at the same time inhibit the development of harmful bacteria.

Most of the world's commercial dog foods are made to standards set in North America or Europe. In the United States, dog foods and their labels conform to regulations prepared by the Association of American Feed Control Officials (AAFCO). Label information is more extensive than in other parts of the world, in that the "Guaranteed Analysis" includes minimums for protein and fat and maximums for fibre and moisture, but labels do not state the amount in the package. In Canada there is a voluntary certification scheme monitored by the Canadian Veterinary Medical Association. Manufacturers who comply with these standards provide more information on food labels and must substantiate any claims they make. European foods are labelled according to EC directives, which state what preservatives have been added but do not require that any preservatives in "preprocessed" ingredients to be listed. All European dog foods include a "best before" date, which usually corresponds to the shelf life of the fat-soluble vitamins in the product.

If you plan to feed your dog a commercial food, it is wise to do some homework. If you have Internet access, visit the manufacturer's website, a good source of additional information. Prepare your list of questions. Reliable dog food producers will tell you everything you want to know; unreliable ones will not.

DRY AND MOIST DOG FOODS

The convenience of all-in-one dry food has made this form of canine nourishment the most popular type of dog food in North America. These foods are cooked under pressure and then dried. Fat is sprayed on the particles for palatability, but because fat can turn rancid, a preservative must be added. Antioxidants are excellent preservatives. Some food manufacturers have switched the type of preservative from "synthetics" to vitamins C and E. They made this change, however, because of public pressure – not because of scientific evidence that these vitamins are better as antioxidants. Curiously, natural antioxidants do not last as long as synthetic ones. If you choose a dry food that is "naturally" preserved, buy it from a retailer with a high inventory turnover and, once you have opened it, store it in a sealed container in a dry, cool location. Whenever possible, use dry food products within six months of their manufacture date.

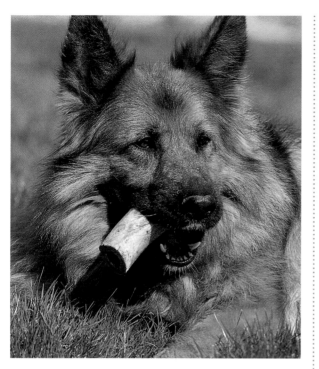

FEEDING BONES
Take care to give your dog hard bones, which will not splinter when bitten. Do not let your dog become possessive over them. Like toys, bones belong to you (*see p.45*).

Canned (moist) food, mixed with dry food, remains the most popular form of dog food in Britain and elsewhere in Europe. Heat sterilization and vacuum sealing prevent spoilage of canned or vacuum-packed foods, so no preservative is needed. These foods are highly palatable, and most are nutritionally complete; however, they provide no exercise for the teeth and gums and are prone to contamination if not eaten immediately. As a guideline, assume that a standard 400-gram (1-lb) can contains about 400 kilocalories.

Manufacturing processes make foods safer, but can involve certain risks. First, foods may be exposed to stresses such as heat pasteurization, which can destroy micronutrients. Good manufacturers compensate for this by adding vitamin and mineral supplements to their products. Second, mistakes can happen, such as a wrong substance being included. Dry food can spoil in the package after it leaves the factory. Lastly, the processes can change foods in unknown ways. These potential problems are inversely related to the degree of quality control that a manufacturer employs.

HOME COOKING

If you wish to cook for your dog, remember not to feed muscle meat alone, because this type of diet is low in vitamins A and D and in calcium. Dogs are not solely "meat eaters" – their natural diet includes both meat and items such as plant matter from prey animals' intestines. Mix meat with other foods, such as rice (see below).

Avoid tofu and other bean products as food sources, especially if you have a deep-chested breed such as a Great Dane or any type of setter. These foods stimulate gas production and may increase the risk of stomach bloat (*see p.277*), which can be life-threatening.

Take care with dairy products. Puppies produce an enzyme called lactose that digests milk, but by adulthood in some dogs little of that enzyme is still produced. If cow's milk causes diarrhoea in your dog but you still want to feed milk, give the dog lactose-free milk, which is available at your supermarket for lactose-sensitive people.

Take great care when feeding bones. Like every vet in the country, I have had to open up dogs' bellies to repair the damage that bones cause. They are also perhaps the most common cause of broken teeth, although gnawing on them does massage the gums and keep the teeth clean. If you plan to feed bones, introduce them as early as possible in the dog's life, so that it learns "responsible bone eating". Offer only the hardest bones (beef bones). As an excellent alternative give your dog highly compacted dog biscuits. These are intentionally manufactured to offer hours of chewing.

Here is a sample balanced home-made diet for an adult dog:

Chicken	70 g (2½ oz)
Liver	30 g (1 oz)
Uncooked rice	140 g (5 oz)
Sterilized bone meal	10 g (³/₈ oz)
Iodised salt	pinch
Sunflower or corn oil	2 g (½ tsp)

Cook the rice, bone meal, salt, and sunflower oil in twice the volume of water. Simmer for 20 minutes, then add the chicken and liver, simmering for another 10 minutes. Cool before feeding. This recipe produces about 800 kcal of energy, enough to feed an active 10-kg (22-lb) dog for a day.

Energy is in this form on a dry-matter basis.

Protein	17%
Fat	31%
Carbohydrate	53%

ENERGY NEEDS THROUGHOUT LIFE

Each dog has its own energy needs. These are based on its metabolic rate and its level of activity. They change with age and activity level, sexual activity, and even with the seasons of the year. As with us, who its parents are also predetermines a dog's metabolic rate. Some individuals, and some breeds, are born with a tendency to be lean or to get fat.

PUPPIES

During puppyhood, dogs need a lot of energy in order to grow and mature. A puppy's diet should contain around 22 per cent protein and 5 per cent fat on a dry-matter basis (*see box, p.92*). If puppies ingest too much energy-dense food they may be heading towards life-long obesity, because the excess energy creates a larger than normal number of fat cells in the adult. It is harder to reduce the number of fat cells than to reduce their size. Avoid allowing a pup grow too plump – it may look cute but it is not healthy in the long term.

From birth until a puppy reaches half its adult size, it needs about twice the amount of energy needed for adults, and during the rest of its growth it needs 50 per cent more than for adults. The growth phase of a dog's life varies according to breed: small dogs stop growing much earlier than giant breeds. For simplicity, assume that dogs up to 5.5 kg (12 lb) finish growing by six months of age. Those up to 9 kg (20 lb) finish by nine months, and those up to 20.5 kg (45 lb) at 15 months. Larger dogs take up to two years to finish growing.

Calculate the kilocalories needed according to the breed's weight and your pup's activity level. Double this standard allowance for the first half of a puppy's growing period, then feed only 50 per cent more than the standard until it is mature. At this stage, reduce its intake to the normal adult level. Reduce the number of meals for pups from four times down to twice daily.

ADULT DOGS

On a dry-matter basis, feed your adult dog a diet containing at least 18 per cent protein and 5 per cent fat. Many commercially produced foods contain far more than enough nutrients, and are very tasty. If these nutrient-rich diets are fed freely, obesity is the natural outcome. By some estimates, about one third of all pet dogs are obese; that is, they weigh 15 per cent or more above their ideal body weight (*see Obesity, p.96*).

HIGHLY ACTIVE DOGS

Working dogs that herd, guard, search, race, or are otherwise active need one-and-a-half to two-and-a-half times more food energy than pet dogs. If the weather is cold, energy demands can go up another 50 per cent. (Simply living in an unheated kennel in winter leads to a 25 per cent increase in food need.) Greyhounds and other dogs working in short sprints benefit from increased carbohydrates, while endurance dogs need to have increased fat in their diet to give them the stamina needed for hard work. In the most extreme circumstances of winter sled dog races, a sled dog may need 10,000 kilocalories per day.

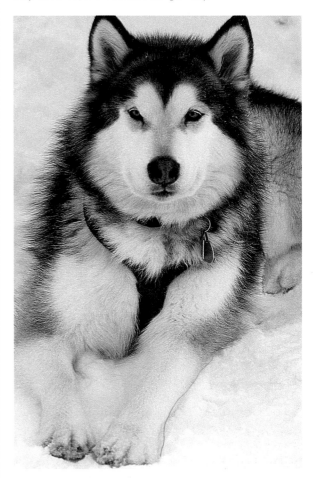

WORKING DOGS AND THEIR ENERGY NEEDS
Working sheepdogs, gundogs, and hounds often need 50 per cent more energy while active than they do at rest. Sled dogs, like the one shown above, may need double their resting energy needs.

If your dog is used for work, feed a high-fat, highly digestible, energy-dense diet. Give two or more meals daily, with a small meal about one hour before work and the largest meal an hour after hard work. Dogs involved in endurance activities, which demand a lot of energy and stamina, may also need small amounts of high-fat, high-protein food while they are working.

SEXUAL ACTIVITY AND BREEDING

All reproductive activities take up energy – not just the act of mating. While some dogs lose their appetite while looking for sex, others have increased energy demands. For male dogs in particular, just looking for sex is energy-consuming. It means more wandering, more leg-lifting, more creating and defending of territory, and more fighting. Male and female sex hormones also affect metabolism. When these hormones are reduced, through neutering or advancing years, about one third of dogs develop a tendency to get fat. To prevent any weight gain after neutering, find out your dog's weight beforehand and reduce food consumption by 20 per cent. Chances are your dog will retain its preoperative weight. If it is losing weight on the new diet, return to the former meal size.

Pregnant dogs require very little increase in food until late in pregnancy (see Reproduction, p.57). A female's energy needs, however, soar when she is producing milk for her pups. At the height of lactation she will need three times her normal food intake. Even after her pups reduce their milk consumption, she will continue to need 50 per cent more than normal just to return to her standard condition. A puppy or performance food is ideal for females at this time.

AGING DOGS

Generally speaking, dogs start to show signs of aging in the last third of their life span. Large breeds with shorter life spans age earlier than small breeds with longer life expectancies. In my veterinary practice, I recommend elective health check-ups as early as seven years old for some dogs but not until over ten years for others. In two per cent of the inspections, blood tests reveal that kidney or liver function or intestinal absorption has become inefficient.

Aging is not an illness, but loss of homeostasis can develop into clinical disease. The effects of aging, or age-related health problems, may demand subtle modifications to the existing diet. Some older dogs gain weight because the energy that we supply them is not being used up through exercise. In certain cases, however, this weight gain is caused by an underactive thyroid gland (see Hypothyroidism, p.331). If your elderly dog is gaining or losing weight, make sure that it has a clean bill of health before adjusting its diet.

Most older dogs thrive on their adult diet simply reduced slightly in quantity and augmented with extra vitamins and minerals. Some may benefit from special "senior" diets; such diets contain high-quality, easily digested nutrients and extra antioxidants to help the immune system, and extra nutrients for skin and gut health. Overweight elderlies should be slimmed down gradually, while underweight dogs or those recovering from illness benefit from increased-energy food.

If your aging dog is fussy with its food, it may have a health problem. Gum disease, deteriorating teeth, diminished taste or smell, or underlying disease are common causes of finicky eating. Seek veterinary help. At the same time, encourage your dog to eat by warming its food. Warmth enhances flavour and smell, which are the most powerful appetite stimulants.

DIFFERENCES IN ENERGY NEEDS

Here are average daily kilocalorie (kcal) requirements for different body weights, life styles, and ages. Dogs in colder climates need a slightly higher energy intake according to the amount of time they spend outside.

For information on the energy needs of pregnant and lactating females, see Reproduction, p.57.

ACTIVE		WORKING	
2–5 kg	210–420 kcal	2–5 kg	295–590 kcal
6–10	480–705	6–10	675–990
11–20	775–1,180	11–20	1,065–1,665
21–30	1,225–1,600	21–30	1,725–2,255
31–40	1,640–1,990	31–40	2,310–2,800
41–50	2,025–2,350	41–50	2,850–3,310

INACTIVE		SENIOR	
2–5 kg	185–370 kcal	2–5 kg	150–300 kcal
6–10	420–620	6–10	345–505
11–20	665–1040	11–20	545–850
21–30	1,080–1,410	21–30	885–1,155
31–40	1,445–1,750	31–40	1,180–1,430
41–50	1,780–2,070	41–50	1,460–1,690

DIET AND HEALTH

From early in life, offer your dog a fresh, tasty and nutritious diet. As time moves on, modify that diet according to your dog's unique demands. Provide more nutrients when they are obviously needed; for example, as the weather gets colder. Like us, each dog (especially the little ones) has its own preferences for odours, textures and flavours – but bear in mind that finicky eaters are made, not born. Do not turn your kitchen into a canine restaurant with your customer choosing from a varied menu!

Weigh your dog routinely. Steady weight is just about the best simple sign of good health. Weight increases or losses indicate that the natural balance has been upset. Almost certainly something is wrong, and central to resolving the problem may be changing nutrition.

FEEDING A CONVALESCENT DOG

Energy requirements increase during convalescence. At the same time, a dog's desire to eat may be impaired. Unless your veterinary surgeon advises you not to, increase dietary fat as well as protein.
• Feed an easily digested, well-balanced diet – if possible, one that is specifically formulated to help your dog through its illness. Your vet can provide you with a diet formulated for convalescing dogs. These tasty, high energy foods can be eaten from the bowl or gently syringed into the mouth if needed.

• Feed small amounts frequently.
• Warm food to just below body temperature. This enhances aroma and taste and is easy to do in a microwave.
• If feeding dry food, add a little animal fat to enhance the smell. This makes the food more appealing. Alternatively, add water at body temperature.
• Carefully monitor food and water intake, reporting any increases or decreases to your vet.

PREVENTING AND TREATING OBESITY

As with us, fat runs in families. A dog's body condition is influenced by what you feed but also by genetic factors. According to surveys carried out at veterinary schools, certain breeds are more prone to obesity than others; these breeds include the American Cocker Spaniel, Basset Hound, Beagle, Cairn Terrier, Cavalier King Charles Spaniel, Dachshund, Labrador Retriever, Norwegian Elkhound, Rough Collie, and Shetland Sheepdog. If you have a dog belonging to one of these breeds, be extra vigilant about the amount that you feed your dog and about any treats and snacks offered by members of your family.

A dog's appetite is initially stimulated by the scent of food. The need to eat is controlled by the part of the brain called the hypothalamus; after a meal, sugar in the bloodstream travels to the brain, activating the "satiety" centre in the hypothalamus and turning off the need to eat. Low-fat, good-quality carbohydrates such as barley and sorghum can help to control your dog's appetite because they release energy into the bloodstream more gradually than other carbohydrates such as rice, and are better at controlling surges in blood sugar. Fibre or water adds bulk to food, thus "diluting" the calories in it. Added nutrients such as L-carnitine may help to burn body fat.

To combat obesity, keep a record of everything that your dog eats, including all the titbits. This makes you more conscious of all the extras it receives. Ideally, cut out titbits, but if this is not possible replace them with bits of fruit and vegetable. Feed and exercise your dog frequently to help accelerate its basic metabolic rate. Avoid crash diets; as well as upsetting your dog, such diets will only drive its metabolism to be more efficient at fat-storing in the future.

VET'S ADVICE

All of us take pictures of our dogs. Intentionally take side and top photos in the same location and compare your dog's present size with previous images. This is not as accurate as routine weighing but it is very useful for having a technicolour target of the condition you want your dog to return to.

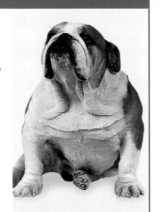

You may need help in sticking to a healthy dog's diet as much as your dog does. If you are being laser-beamed by mournfully melting brown eyes, consult your veterinary staff – they make fine, understanding, tough counsellors. Your vet can provide your dog with a special weight-loss diet. Such products are available as dry or wet foods. While they contain excellent levels of micronutrients, they also contain satisfying bulk. One consequence is that dogs on weight-loss may pass more faeces.

FOOD ALLERGIES AND FOOD INTOLERANCE

A food allergy occurs when a dog's immune system is abnormally sensitive to a component of its food. The allergy usually causes a skin reaction, often itching; it may also affect the gastrointestinal tract and cause vomiting, diarrhoea, or both. Food intolerance is a reaction that does not involve the immune system but may cause vomiting, diarrhoea, or other clinical signs. Any dog at any age may develop a food intolerance.

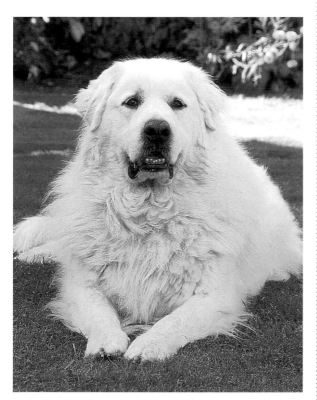

THE HEALTH RISKS OF OBESITY
Overweight dogs are at risk of various health problems. Their ability to exercise is reduced and the work of the heart increased. They also run a very high risk of tearing the cruciate ligaments, in the knees.

BODY SHAPE

A modern urban lifestyle is not what dogs were made for. It can be tedious and dull. Just about the most exciting event is feeding time. Deep down, most dog owners understand this. We know we aren't providing our dogs with the type of physical exercise they really want.

While many owners of obese dogs know they are living with unhealthy companions, some people do not recognize when a dog is simply overweight. Use this chart to assess your dog's body condition.

EMACIATED

- Ribs showing, no fat cover
- Severe abdominal tuck
- Bones at base of tail obvious with nothing between skin and bone.
- No fat palpable in the abdomen

THIN

- Ribs easily felt with minimal fat cover
- Waist very obvious behind ribs
- Bones at base of tail raised with only minimal tissue between skin and bone.
- Minimal abdominal fat

IDEAL

- Ribs palpable through slight fat cover
- Waist visible behind ribs
- Bones at base of tail covered in thin layer of fat
- Minimal abdominal fat

OVERWEIGHT

- Ribs not found easily because of moderate fat cover
- Waist hardly discernible
- Bones at base of tail covered by moderate fat
- Moderate abdominal fat

OBESE

- Ribs disappeared under thick fat cover
- No waist, distended abdomen
- Bones at base of tail difficult to feel through fat
- Extensive abdominal fat

VETERINARY DIETS

With the variety of special veterinary diets now available for dogs, it is easier for vets and owners to ensure a balanced "medical" or "life-stage" diet. There are puppy diets (including special puppy diets for large breeds); high-energy foods for working dogs; reduced-calorie diets for overweight dogs; diets designed for dogs with particular medical conditions; diets for dogs recovering from illness or surgery; and many more.

The top dog food manufacturers provide a wide range of these diets, available through veterinary surgeries. The choice is excellent and ever-increasing, and includes:

- Low-calorie for weight loss

- Low-phosphorus and fibre-enriched for kidney disease

- Low-protein for advanced kidney disease

- Low-sodium for heart disease

- Low-allergen for dogs with food allergies

- Low-mineral or low-protein to prevent bladder stones

- Balanced-fibre for bowel disorders

- High-energy/high-calorie for convalescence or weight gain

- High-fibre for diabetic dogs

- High-fat, low-carbohydrate for slowing cancers

- Predigested for allergy diagnosis and treatment

- Diets with balanced fatty acids to relieve inflammatory skin conditions

- Easily digestible foods for elderly dogs and those with digestive disorders

- Extra nutrients for liver disorders

- Foods with increased crunchiness for dogs with dental conditions.

A dog develops an allergy to a specific ingredient in the diet called an antigen. The most common types of antigens that cause canine food allergies are proteins. Some textbooks implicate beef and dairy proteins as the most likely to cause allergies, but this is not so; allergies are most likely to develop to the most common proteins that a dog eats. In the United States, where beef is the most common protein in dog food, it accounts for about 60 per cent of diagnosed cases. In Britain, where other protein sources such as lamb and chicken are commonly used in dog food, beef and dairy are relatively minor causes of food allergies. The procedures used to make commercial dog food may somehow increase the levels of antigens (substances involved in provoking allergic reactions). As a result, processed food may trigger an allergic response while fresh food using the same ingredients does not. Some vets feel that early weaning or early gastrointestinal infection may also be contributing factors to the development of food allergy later in life.

All dogs, purebred or of mixed breeding, can develop food allergies, but certain breeds are particularly susceptible. These include the Cocker Spaniel, Dalmatian, English Springer Spaniel, Labrador Retriever, Lhasa Apso, Miniature Schnauzer, Shar Pei, Soft-coated Wheaten Terrier, and West Highland White Terrier.

A food allergy is diagnosed by feeding a diet that the dog has not eaten before, for at least a month (and preferably for six weeks to three months). If the allergic reaction clears up, then returns when the former food is fed, this confirms true food allergy. Feed a home-cooked or commercial diet consisting of nutrients known not to cause allergy. Your vet can provide you with an "exclusion diet" formulated from foods your dog is unlikely to have eaten previously, such as capelin (a deep sea fish), tapioca, potato, and duck. Some dog food manufacturers produce hypoallergenic foods with altered antigen size, which lessen the risk of further allergic reactions; such foods may be available from your vet.

NUTRITIONALLY RESPONSIVE SKIN DISEASES

The health of a dog's skin and hair can be affected by imbalances or deficiencies in protein, vitamin A, vitamin E, the essential fatty acids, and zinc. Such deficiencies may be due to poor-quality food, or more probably to poor storage of commercial dog food.

These skin problems, as well as certain others not necessarily due to deficiencies (such as seborrhoea – greasy, flaking skin), can be relieved by vitamin or zinc supplements. (*See also Skin disorders, pp.180–201. For details on vitamins and minerals, see p.89 and p.90.*)

PANCREATITIS

There are many causes of pancreas inflammation including diet. This unpredictable and painful condition can be associated with a low-protein, high-fat diet. If a dog has an episode of pancreatitis, high-fat foods should be avoided in the future (*see also Pancreas and liver, p.292*).

INHERITED DISORDERS OF NUTRIENT METABOLISM

These are rare disorders in which the body cannot absorb or break down a specific nutrient. Recognized conditions include B12 malabsorption in Giant Schnauzers; copper-storage disease in Bedlington Terriers; purine metabolism defect in Dalmatians, which causes them to develop stones in the bladder or urethra (*see Urinary tract, p.298*); and hyperlipidaemia in Miniature Schnauzers, which results in abnormally high blood levels of fats such as cholesterol.

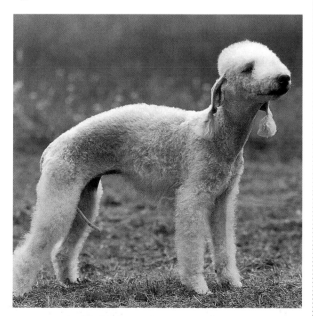

BEDLINGTON TERRIER
Dogs belonging to this breed may suffer from an inherited inability to regulate the amount of copper that they store in the liver. They need a special diet to prevent them from developing copper poisoning.

Q **I'VE READ THAT CHOCOLATE IS TOXIC FOR DOGS, BUT MY PET SHOP SELLS CHOCOLATE DROPS AS DOG TREATS. WHO IS RIGHT?**

A Chocolate in excess is harmful to dogs. It contains a toxin called theobromine; the darker the chocolate, the higher the content of theobromine. Baking chocolate is most dangerous, and white chocolate is least. Just 100 g (4 oz) of baking chocolate can potentially kill a dog under 4 kg (9 lb). Dog "chocolate" is low in theobromine, or in many cases is not chocolate at all but chocolate-flavoured candy.

Q **DOES GARLIC OR ANY OTHER FOOD REPEL FLEAS?**

A Although they are all recommended, neither garlic, onions, nor brewer's yeast repels fleas. Garlic and brewer's yeast are both harmless. Onions, however, may cause anaemia if fed in excessive amounts.

Q **DO DOGS EAT THEIR OWN OR OTHER ANIMAL DROPPINGS BECAUSE OF A DIETARY DEFICIENCY?**

A No, they do not, although even some veterinary textbooks suggest that they do. Dogs eat droppings because they are evolutionary food scavengers. In parts of Asia, pariah dogs are part of the human ecosystem, acting as local sanitation engineers, living off human excrement. Herbivore droppings, for example from rabbits and deer, may be a source of vitamins. In pet dogs, eating animal droppings (coprophagy) is a behaviour of young dogs that, without training intervention, is perpetuated into adulthood.

Q **CAN I FEED CAT FOOD TO MY DOG?**

A If you have a cat and a small dog, chances are your dog will try to convince you that it will die unless it eats cat food. This food is rich in tasty protein, because cats need more protein in their diets than dogs do. While you should never feed dog food to a cat, because a cat's nutrient requirements are unique, a healthy dog can easily convert the extra protein in cat food into energy. Cat food is safe for healthy dogs, but it should be avoided if your dog needs a protein-restricted diet.

DIAGNOSING ILLNESS
asking the right questions

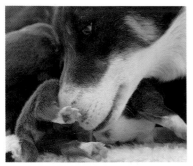

Inherited genes can carry problems

The 20th century saw a huge expansion in scientific knowledge, together with the most spectacular advances ever in the diagnosis and treatment of canine illness and disease. The art of veterinary medicine is to use such knowledge in the best possible way for your dog. To help dogs overcome injury, illness, and disease, owners and vets must make a proper diagnosis of a problem and then give the appropriate treatment and care. We must first ask the right questions, in order to achieve these aims.

Even though medical knowledge has increased, and the ways in which we apply that knowledge have grown more complex, an old-fashioned use of the senses is still at the heart of diagnostics. A vet will observe your dog, using the senses of sight, touch, and smell, and will also want to listen to all you have to say about your dog's condition. From these observations and the clues you give, a vet can then formulate the questions that will permit a correct diagnosis.

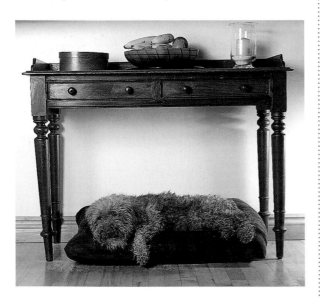

THE IMPORTANCE OF ENVIRONMENT TO HEALTH
Rather than suppressing symptoms, you can help your dog towards recovery by providing a comfortable environment at home; this, along with a good diet and your care, will help its body repair itself.

STEPS TO DIAGNOSIS

Most medical problems seen in veterinary practice can be identified by simply examining the animal, taking its temperature, listening to its heart and breathing with a stethoscope, and talking to you, the dog's owner. Before employing any additional aids, a vet will also consider other possible contributory factors, such as genetic or environmental conditions.

GENETIC CONDITIONS

When we modify dog design through breeding, we increase the risk that some dogs will suffer from medical problems. Genetic defects can occur in any breed and can affect any system in the body. For example, dogs with long backs and short legs, such as Dachshunds, are more susceptible to slipped discs, and dogs with flattened faces, such as Bulldogs and some toy breeds, are more prone to nasal problems.

Responsible breeders know that the best way to avoid inherited disease is through selective breeding of dogs known not to carry the gene for that disease. Although genetic testing is still in its infancy, its influence through selective breeding will be far greater in veterinary medicine than in human medicine.

ENVIRONMENTAL CONDITIONS

The demands of our environment are sometimes at odds with the dog's evolutionary defences. The risk of catching an airborne infectious disease, for example, is low in nature, because dogs would only meet unrelated

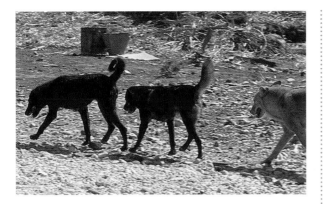

LIVING IN PACKS REDUCES INFECTION
Feral or semi-wild dogs live in closed communities as wolves do, meeting dogs outside the pack only to fight or mate. This reduces the opportunities for infectious diseases to spread. Pet dogs, especially those in towns and cities, meet a far wider range of dogs and face a higher risk from infectious disease unless immunized.

dogs in territory disputes. This risk increases when unrelated dogs are brought together in man-made environments, such as in kennels. The fact that the most common form of upper respiratory tract infection is called "kennel cough" highlights this link between man-made situations and disease. We can enhance a dog's defences by avoiding these risk situations and by vaccinating against transmissible infectious diseases.

UNDERSTANDING CLINICAL SIGNS

Dog owners usually talk about a dog's "symptoms" because that is the term we properly use when telling our doctors about an illness. Dogs experience many of the sensations that we do, but they cannot tell us how they feel. A vet may, for example, see a dog's pale gums and tongue, feel tension in its abdominal wall, and see that it is lethargic. These are, technically speaking, "clinical signs", rather than symptoms: observations made by seeing, hearing, smelling, or feeling. That term is used throughout this chapter, both because it is correct and as a reminder that correct diagnosis of a canine problem depends on lucid observation.

Some of the common problems that vets are asked to treat, such as vomiting, diarrhoea, coughing, and limping, are not diseases but clinical signs. They are your dog's defences against attack, triggered when its body is confronted with something that upsets its equilibrium. A common mistake is to try to suppress the body's natural defences rather than working with

them to fight the threat to homeostasis. Your vet must judge what part of the condition is a manifestation of the problem itself, and what part is the dog's natural defence against the problem. Vomiting, for example, is the most efficient way to rid the stomach of any matter that might be harmful if it travelled further down the digestive tract. Dogs vomit more readily than many other animals because they are natural scavengers and may easily ingest a toxic substance. Diarrhoea serves the same purpose, removing toxins from the intestines as quickly as possible. When expelled, an intestinal irritant may be covered in mucus, and this is a good clue that the large intestine is reacting defensively.

A dog with an infection might develop a fever and associated loss of appetite. These are also clinical signs – defensive measures that reduce the germ's ability to multiply. We should not eliminate them but just ensure that they are not excessive.

Sensible intervention means working with rather than against your dog's inherent ability to heal itself. It means knowing when to operate, when to use drugs (and the effects of those drugs), and what type of hospital or home care is best.

PREDISPOSITION TO PROBLEMS

According to pet health insurance statistics, there are breed differences in susceptibility to illness. Below is a list of the breeds commonly associated with problems in particular body systems.

SYSTEM	BREEDS PRONE TO PROBLEMS
Skin	Doberman
	Boxer
Gastrointestinal	Welsh Terrier
	Doberman
Respiratory	Irish Wolfhound
	Great Dane
Skeletal	Dachshund
	Irish Wolfhound
Cardiovascular	Cavalier King Charles Spaniel
	Irish Wolfhound

DIAGNOSTIC AIDS

A health disorder is an attack on the body by an often invisible enemy. The most successful way to confront and overcome such an attack is to understand the enemy's strategy – how it tries to destroy or bypass natural defences. In the real world of veterinary medicine it is often necessary to deal with health problems without a clear understanding of what the enemy is, let alone what its tactics are.

Your dog's well-being depends first on your noticing when something is wrong and describing to your vet what you have seen, felt, smelt, or heard (*see pp.402–427*). Your vet will then look for clinical signs by performing a physical examination. If this is not enough to make a diagnosis, many simple tests can be carried out at veterinary clinics, using a microscope. In these tests, the vet may examine skin scrapings or samples of body cells or fluids, often on a "while-you-wait" basis. The vet can arrange for further tests on samples to be performed in a laboratory. Vets can also make use of imaging techniques such as X-rays and ultrasound, as well as more sophisticated, and expensive, body scanning. Many diagnostic procedures can be carried out on a conscious dog with minimal restraint, but in some circumstances sedation or short-acting anaesthesia is needed.

LABORATORY TESTS

The range of reliable laboratory tests on blood, urine, faeces, and tissue samples (biopsies) is ever-expanding and comprehensive compared with what was available only a generation ago. As good as these tests are today, this is an area of diagnostics where even greater advances will occur. Most clinical laboratory work is relatively non-invasive (in other words, it does not involve operations such as large incisions). The tests usually require only a blood sample, although some types of tissue have to be removed by aspiration (withdrawal through a hollow needle inserted into the target organ). These samples are used to check cells or the chemical constituents of body fluids in order to diagnose a problem or assess the function of an organ.

X-RAYS

X-ray images (radiographs) are made by passing X-rays (electromagnetic radiation with an extremely short wavelength) through the body and on to photographic plates or fluorescent screens. The X-rays are absorbed to differing degrees by different types of tissue, which therefore show as lighter or darker areas on the images.

X-rays are the best aid for visualizing hard tissue such as bone or stones in the bladder. They are also an excellent diagnostic tool for examining tissues that show up in sharp contrast, such as air-filled lung tissue; for example, in dogs with bronchitis the thickening tissue of chronically inflamed air passages contrasts well with the surrounding air-filled lungs.

The images are less useful, however, if the contrasts are less dramatic. If a dog has swallowed a plastic bag, for example, the bag will not show up in a plain X-ray of the stomach. In cases like this, the dog is fed some "contrast material", such as barium, that absorbs X-rays and appears white on images. An X-ray is taken

Intestine   Intestinal wall

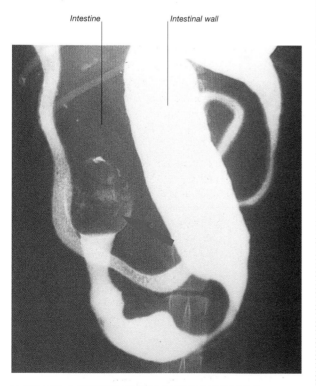

X-RAY OF A FOREIGN BODY IN THE INTESTINES
Dogs sometimes swallow foreign bodies. Some items, such as peach stones or the walnut seen here, pass through the body in stops and starts, making clinical diagnosis difficult and dependent on X-ray.

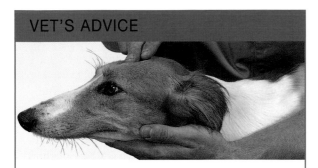
after most of the barium has left the stomach; the bag will trap some of the barium and will then be visible.

ULTRASOUND

Ultrasound uses sound waves of extremely high frequency, far beyond the range of human hearing, to produce images of the interior of the body. It shows areas that are not visible on X-rays, and body parts can be seen moving. Ultrasound revolutionized diagnosis in areas such as heart disease, where the heart valves can be watched as they open and close. Defects are easily seen, and blood flow is readily measured. Whereas with an X-ray it is difficult to differentiate between the wall of the heart and blood inside the heart, with ultrasound the thickness of the wall of the heart can be accurately measured to the millimetre. Ultrasound is a superb aid for examining other organs, such as the adrenal glands, the male's prostate gland, and, of course, the uterus in the pregnant female.

MRI AND CT BODY SCANS

Body scans have enabled ground-breaking advances in diagnostics for brain and joint conditions and for determining the exact size and shape of tumours anywhere in the body. These scans have, for example, revealed that brain tumours are more common than was once realised. Although far more expensive than X-rays, they are extraordinarily accurate in showing exactly what type of problem is occurring almost anywhere in the body.

Computerized tomography (CT) scanning is a specialized form of X-ray, in which the X-ray source and detector rotate around the patient and a computer turns the information into cross-sectional images. In magnetic resonance imaging (MRI), low-frequency radiation is passed through the body in the presence of a strong magnetic field, which causes temporary realignment of atoms within the tissues. Measuring the effects of this realignment gives valuable information about particular body structures. MRI can produce cross-sectional images, like CT scans but with greater contrast, and it can show soft tissue even if it is obscured by bone, unlike CT scanning.

CT and MRI scanners, at one time only available for human medical use, are now available at many veterinary schools and through specialists in most urban areas. The cost of MRI equipment is falling dramatically. In the coming decade, body scanners will become a standard part of the diagnostic armoury in efficient multi-veterinary practices.

THE LIMITS OF KNOWLEDGE

Your vet is looking for information that fits recognized patterns so that he or she can accurately identify your dog's problem. When a disease is diagnosed there may be a specific treatment, but some diseases are difficult to identify even though they produce definite signs. Such conditions are known as "undiagnosed illness". In these cases, a vet may buy time, through good intervention, allowing your dog's natural defences to overcome the condition and effect a recovery.

Q ONCE MY VET HAS MADE A DIAGNOSIS, WHAT CAN I DO TO HELP MY DOG?

A • Follow your vet's instructions and make sure that your dog takes all the medicine prescribed.
• Create a comfortable, secure environment that will be conducive to recovery. Minimize possible physical and psychological stress by giving your pet a quiet place in which to rest when required.
• Integrate the positive values of conventional and complementary therapies. Do not let personal medical judgments interfere with good canine care.
• Remember that time is a great healer. Trust your nurturing instincts: they are often right.

MEDICAL INTERVENTION
the benefits and risks of treatment

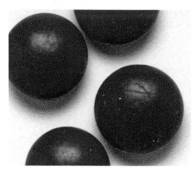

Many drugs are licensed for dog use

Thanks to modern medicines, the prevention and treatment of disease are more successful than ever before. The range of drugs now available includes medicines that will suppress pain; kill infectious organisms; correct hormone imbalances; improve mood; make breathing, digestion, or walking easier; and even delay the wear and tear of old age. Modern drugs help to combat illness by reducing demands on the body systems, thereby giving the body time to use its own resources to defend or repair itself.

In this age of drug therapy we may think that drugs alone are responsible for recoveries from illness. For example, when a wound abscess is treated with antibiotics and the abscess disappears, we credit the antibiotic therapy with the recovery. Antibiotics are powerful and important drugs, but they only ever reduce the number of bacteria. By doing so, they give the immune system time to prepare its counterattack, and to deploy natural killer cells, macrophages, and other components of the natural defence system. The real source of the cure is the immune system.

SIDE EFFECTS OF MODERN MEDICINES
Modern drugs were one of the great successes of 20th-century medicine, and many are licensed for use on dogs. All new drugs must be thoroughly tested for safety and effectiveness before they can be marketed, but they may still have unwanted side effects. This is especially true if they are given in excessive doses or for the wrong reason.

Antibiotics (*see pp.106-7*) destroy bacteria and fungi, giving the natural defences time to coordinate and attack these invaders, but they may also destroy good microbes. Vaccines (*see pp.106-7*) stimulate a dog's immune system to build protection against potentially lethal infectious diseases, but in rare cases they may also cause adverse reactions. Painkillers (*see pp.108-9*) reduce the stress of pain, allowing repair to begin as soon as possible, but they can damage the stomach if incorrectly given. Anaesthetics (*see pp.108-9*) obliterate all sensation, including pain, allowing the

VET'S ADVICE

Hippocrates' first rule of medicine, "Primum non nocere", meaning "first, do no harm", holds true today, and must be the basis for all treatment. Your dog's body wants to be healthy, to maintain homeostasis. Its powers of self-diagnosis, repair, and regeneration are the ultimate success story of evolution. The body has magnificent ways of repairing itself, so give them a chance. Help your dog to deal with health disorders by minimizing environmental risks and augmenting the dog's natural defences through proper care.

vet to carry out tests and perform surgical repairs; however, accidents involving anaesthetics do happen, with potentially life-threatening consequences. Hormones (*see p.328*) stimulate or suppress body functions, but the wrong dose may cause side effects.

DRUG TOXICITY AND ALLERGY
Drugs can be toxic to more than one body system. Problems resulting from drug toxicity include brain or nerve damage (such as blindness or deafness); liver or kidney damage or failure; and bone marrow suppression. A drug may act as a poison and be toxic if too much is given, if it is administered for too long, or if it is not eliminated safely from the body. In other circumstances the dog's body may consider a drug to be "foreign" and mount an immune response to it. That immune response may itself cause problems.

Antibiotics and vaccines are the medicines most likely to provoke the immune system into allergic responses varying from mild to life-threatening. Mild allergic reactions to drugs include itching and scratching, facial swelling, rash or hives, and watery eyes. Moderate allergic reactions include vomiting, diarrhoea, and joint inflammation, while severe reactions include difficulty breathing, collapse, and in some even death (*see p.423*).

You and your vet should be aware of any potential adverse reactions. Drugs are almost always prescribed according to body weight, although dosages may be lower for growing pups than for mature dogs. Exact dosing can be critical, especially in small dogs, and some drugs have very narrow margins of safety. Never assume that what is safe for humans is also safe for dogs (*see pp.112–13*).

Traditional or modern herbal medicines are not necessarily safer than conventional drugs. They may be contaminated with other substances, vary in potency, and have side effects as threatening as those of modern medicines.

DRUG INTERACTIONS

It is always safest to use a single drug or the smallest number of drugs to treat any condition. One drug may affect the absorption of another, or alter the way in which the liver metabolizes another (*see p.292-297*). Drug interactions may reduce the value of a medication or create toxic concentrations. Never give your dog an additional medication without checking first with your veterinary surgeon.

Q **IF THERE ARE RISKS WITH DRUGS, IS IT ALWAYS BEST TO AVOID DRUG TREATMENTS?**

A Absolutely not. Any vet who has practised clinical veterinary medicine for the last 30 years will tell you that, with the help of modern drugs, dogs are now more comfortable and get better faster than ever before. What should be avoided is the use of drugs as an easy but unnecessary option. Some dog owners feel that they are not getting value for money unless their vet dispenses a medicine for a particular condition. Drugs can bring about life-enhancing changes, but take care that they are used properly and judiciously.

Q **ARE WE AT RISK FROM THE DRUGS THAT WE GIVE TO OUR DOGS?**

A Some drugs, such as those given as part of chemotherapy, are dangerous if we absorb them. Ask your vet whether you should wear disposable plastic gloves when handling any medication for your dog.

Q **WHAT DOES "OFF-LABEL" USE OF A DRUG MEAN, AND IS IT SAFE?**

A Drugs are licensed for specific uses. If a drug is found to have additional uses that have not been included in the drug company's initial research, it is used "off label". Off-label uses are usually safe and effective, but drug companies discourage them because adding a new use to existing ones is frequently not in the companies' financial interest. Your vet should discuss any "off-label" use with you and secure your informed consent.

DRUGS DURING PREGNANCY

If your dog is pregnant, always ask your vet before giving it any prescription or non-prescription medication. Anything your bitch consumes during pregnancy may cross the placenta and affect the developing pups. Very few drugs have been tested on dogs during pregnancy to determine whether or not they pose a danger to developing foetuses. As a general rule it is best not to give drugs to a pregnant bitch, especially during the first three weeks of pregnancy.

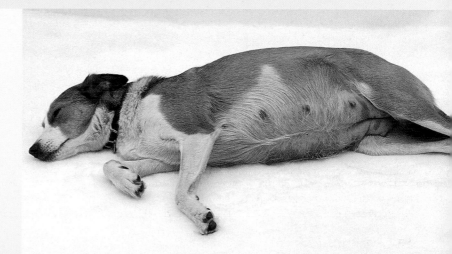

VACCINES AND ANTIBIOTICS

A vaccine harnesses the body's natural ability to defend itself. Vaccination (or immunization) stimulates an immune response that will protect a dog from the natural form of a disease. Antibiotics prevent bacteria and fungi from multiplying (bacteriostatic antibiotics) or destroy them (bactericidal antibiotics).

VACCINES

Vaccination can be a highly effective way of preventing many killer diseases. Until a few decades ago, serious viral illnesses such as canine hepatitis and the highly contagious canine distemper were feared, but now they are rare wherever efficient vaccination programmes have been routinely used. Most vaccines are given by injection, but some, such as Bordetella vaccine to prevent kennel cough, are given by aerosol in the nose.

The effectiveness of vaccines varies: some give lifelong immunity, while others give only partial protection against a particular disease. This is because some viruses (such as human flu viruses) can modify their form, and a vaccine is effective against one form but not another. The form of the canine parvovirus changes in this way, although not as dramatically. The best vaccine manufacturers keep pace with changes in viruses, but some companies, and some vaccines, are more efficient than others.

Vaccines can sometimes fail. A high level of maternal antibodies in pups may "neutralize" a vaccine. A dog may be already infected with the disease but not yet showing clinical signs, or may have a faulty immune system. Vaccines may also be ineffective if they have been handled, stored, or administered incorrectly.

HOW VACCINES DEFEND THE BODY

Vaccines work by sensitizing the immune system to a particular disease-causing bacterium, bacterial toxin, or virus. Most vaccines contain the organism or toxin against which protection is sought; however, this organism has been killed, genetically modified, or weakened so that it does not cause illness but still stimulates the body to produce antibodies against it. If the vaccinated dog later encounters the disease, it remains healthy because it already has the antibodies to destroy the disease-producing agent.

THE ANTIBODY RESPONSE
To infect a cell, a virus must insert its own genes (or DNA) into it. The virus does this by first binding its surface proteins to receptors on the cell surface. In an immune response to the vaccine, antibodies are produced and stick to these viral proteins, preventing them from binding to the cell.

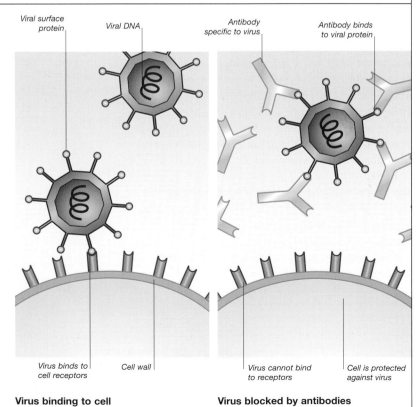

Viral surface protein · Viral DNA · Antibody specific to virus · Antibody binds to viral protein

Virus binds to cell receptors | Cell wall | Virus cannot bind to receptors | Cell is protected against virus

Virus binding to cell　　　　**Virus blocked by antibodies**

HOW ANTIBIOTICS WORK

Antibiotic drugs are either bactericidal (killing bacteria) or bacteriostatic (halting bacterial growth, allowing the immune system to cope with the infection). Once made from moulds but now produced synthetically, penicillin drugs belong to the bactericidal group, and work by disrupting bacterial cell walls.

THE ACTION OF PENICILLIN
Penicillin kills bacteria by causing the walls of bacterial cells to disintegrate so that the cell takes in water, expands, and bursts.

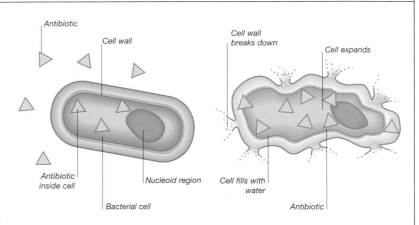

Antibiotic · Cell wall · Antibiotic inside cell · Bacterial cell · Nucleoid region · Cell wall breaks down · Cell expands · Cell fills with water · Antibiotic

Antibiotic invades cell

Cell expands and bursts

ANTIBIOTICS

This group of drugs is used to treat infections caused by bacteria and sometimes fungi. Antibiotics are not effective against viruses.

Most bacteria are susceptible to antibiotics, the most effective of which kill them rather than halting their growth. The antibiotic chosen depends on the type of bacteria and the site of infection. Your vet will often choose a "broad-spectrum" antibiotic – one that is effective against a wide variety of bacteria or fungi – or may arrange for the germ to be cultured in a laboratory in order to match it to the best antibiotic.

Bacteria and fungi commonly live on and in your dog's body, and many types are beneficial. While an antibiotic may kill bacteria causing, say, pneumonia, it may also kill beneficial bacteria in the digestive tract, causing loose stools or diarrhoea.

An antibiotic may fail if it is ineffective against the specific disease-causing germ. It may be given at too low a dose or not for long enough to eliminate the germ. Sometimes the route of administration (by mouth or by injection, for example) does not allow enough of the drug to reach the infection site, perhaps because it is in an abscess or surrounded by dead tissue. Some organisms develop resistance to a previously effective antibiotic. For these reasons you should use antibiotics with restraint, as directed by the vet, and only when there is a clear need for them.

SAMPLE VACCINATION SCHEDULE

Your vet will recommend a vaccination schedule for your area and your dog. Strains of virus differ from one locale to another, and some vaccines offer better protection than others. The example given below is a vaccination schedule used in an urban area where the incidence of rat-transmitted disease is high and vaccine quality is excellent.

AGE	PROTECTION AGAINST THESE DISEASES
8 weeks	Parvovirus, leptospirosis
10 weeks	Parvovirus, leptospirosis, distemper, hepatitis
15 months	Parvovirus, leptospirosis, distemper, hepatitis
1 year later	Leptospirosis for dogs that swim or hunt rodents
Every 3 years	Parvovirus and distemper
For travel	Rabies at three months, repeated every two years

Do not vaccinate if your dog is:

- under eight weeks old
- within 30 days of oestrus or in oestrus
- pregnant or lactating
- undergoing or within 30 days of corticosteroid treatment
- injured, ill, or under any severe stress.

PAINKILLERS AND ANAESTHETICS

Dogs feel pain just as we do (*see p.84*). Painkillers, or analgesics, are drugs that relieve or reduce pain. The two main types of painkiller are narcotic and non-narcotic.

Anaesthetics block all sensation, including pain. General anaesthetics induce unconsciousness; they are used during surgery or for some diagnostic or treatment procedures. Local anaesthetics numb a small area of the body, and are used when your vet wants to carry out a simple procedure on a conscious dog, such as removing a foreign body or stitching a small wound.

NARCOTIC PAINKILLERS

Narcotic painkillers include morphine, pethidine, buprenorphine, and codeine. These mimic endorphins by blocking pain impulses at specific sites. Narcotics are used for severe pain associated with trauma, major surgery, and some forms of cancer. They are controlled drugs and their use is restricted by government regulation. Your veterinary surgeon must keep a register of their use. Codeine is less strong than other narcotics and is often given in combination with non-narcotics such as aspirin.

HOW PAINKILLERS WORK

When tissue is damaged, for example, by injury or infection, it releases prostaglandins. These hormone-like substances produce inflammation and trigger the transmission of pain signals to the brain.

Non-steroidal anti-inflammatory drugs (NSAIDs), such as aspirin, work by preventing prostaglandin production. This reduces inflammation and stimulation of the nerve endings, so fewer pain signals pass to the brain. Paracetamol blocks the pain impulses in the brain itself, preventing the perception of pain.

Narcotic analgesics work by combining with opiate receptors (specific sites in the brain and spinal cord) to prevent pain signals from being transmitted. They act in a similar way to endorphins, substances produced by the body to relieve pain.

THE ACTION OF NSAIDs

These painkillers limit the body's production of prostaglandins, chemicals that trigger inflammation, swelling, and pain. This action prevents the stimulation of nerve endings with pain signals, as well as reducing inflammation and swelling.

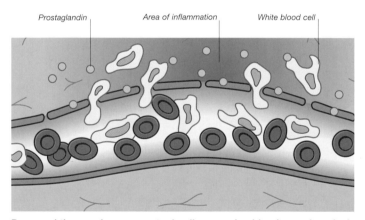

Prostaglandin *Area of inflammation* *White blood cell*

Damaged tissue releases prostaglandins, causing blood vessels to leak.

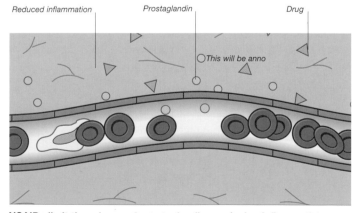

Reduced inflammation *Prostaglandin* *Drug*

This will be anno

NSAIDs limit the release of prostaglandins, reducing inflammation.

NON-NARCOTIC PAINKILLERS

Non-narcotic drugs are commonly used for mild to moderate pain and fever. This drug group includes corticosteroids (*see p.110*), which act by reducing inflammation, and flunixin meglumine, which also fights bacterial toxins. Non-narcotic painkillers also include non-steroidal anti-inflammatory drugs (NSAIDs) and paracetamol.

The NSAIDs, which include ibuprofen and aspirin, work by inhibiting the body's production of prostaglandins, chemicals that trigger pain signals to the brain. Paracetamol blocks pain impulses in the brain itself.

Aspirin has been available for more than a century, and is still widely used for controlling muscle and joint pain in dogs. It is highly effective, but prolonged use may damage the lining of the stomach, causing vomiting and eventually gastric or duodenal ulcers. When giving aspirin, always use a buffered form, pulverized and mixed into a full meal. Your vet can give your dog a drug to accompany the aspirin, which will reduce its toxic effect on the stomach.

Unlike aspirin, paracetamol does not irritate the stomach, but neither does it have an anti-inflammatory effect. This makes it less valuable as a treatment for injury to soft tissues such as muscles and ligaments.

A more recent advance in pain control has been the development of a variety of highly successful and safer non-steroidal anti-inflammatories, such as carprofen (Rimadyl) and meloxicam (Metacam). Studies show these drugs to be better than narcotic painkillers alone for controlling post-surgical pain and chronic bone and joint discomfort. Although these new NSAIDs are tolerated better than aspirin, they may also irritate the stomach lining, causing retching or discomfort.

ANAESTHETICS

General anaesthetic drugs (*see also pp.118*) may be injected or inhaled or both. In some cases, your dog will be given a short-acting anaesthetic intravenously. For longer procedures, anaesthetic gas mixed with oxygen is inhaled, so that when the injected anaesthetic wears off the gas takes over.

Local anaesthetics are applied to a specific area, such as the eye or surface tissue (or around regional nerves). They are usually given by injection but may also be given as eye drops, spray, or ointment. Xylocaine is the most common local anaesthetic used for dogs.

PAINKILLERS CAN BE DANGEROUS

All painkillers are potentially dangerous, especially when used for prolonged periods. The amount of an analgesic should be carefully calibrated according to your dog's body weight. The list below gives the possible side effects of various analgesics, all of which should be administered only on the advice of your veterinary surgeon. One type of painkiller may trigger problems while another, closely related one does not.

DRUG	POSSIBLE ADVERSE EFFECTS
Aspirin	Gastrointestinal irritation and ulceration, eventual damage to joint cartilage
Ibuprofen	Severe gastrointestinal damage
Paracetamol	Severe gastrointestinal damage
Phenylbutazone	Bone marrow suppression, damage to joint cartilage
Flunixin meglumine	Gastrointestinal toxicity
Carprofen (Rimadyl)	Gastrointestinal, kidney, and liver damage
Meloxicam (Metacam)	Gastrointestinal, kidney, and liver damage
Ketoprofen (Ketofen)	Gastrointestinal, kidney, and liver damage

VET'S ADVICE

Use all drugs, even those bought over the counter, only under close veterinary supervision. When giving your dog a painkiller at home, you need to be extremely accurate with the dosage. Overdosing can be critical and lead to serious illness.

Never use two different types of painkiller, such as a corticosteroid and an NSAID, simultaneously. Their toxic side effects can be cumulative. In addition, never use your dog's painkiller for a cat: with some drugs, even a single tablet can be fatal.

HORMONAL AND OTHER DRUGS

Hormones are chemicals that occur naturally in the body and which are released into the bloodstream by a particular gland or tissue and act on tissues elsewhere in the body. They regulate numerous bodily functions, including growth and responses to stress and illness.

Hormonal drugs are similar to natural hormones and have a wide variety of uses. This group of drugs includes corticosteroids, anabolic steroids, sex hormones, and thyroid hormones. The most frequently used, and most misunderstood, are corticosteroids.

CORTICOSTEROIDS

Natural corticosteroids are life-sustaining hormones produced in the adrenal glands. Corticosteroid drugs are often incorrectly called "steroids" and mistaken for anabolic (body-building) steroids, also often called "steroids" (see below).

Corticosteroids are anti-inflammatory agents, and for this reason they are used as anti-inflammatory and antipruritic drugs. They may be applied topically, as part of treatment for a variety of itchy skin conditions, and may also be injected into a specific area, such as a joint or tendon, to reduce inflammation in that area. Taken orally, these drugs treat respiratory disorders by reducing or preventing inflammation of the airways. In addition, corticosteroids can save a dog's life if the animal is in clinical shock (*see p.388*).

There are many different corticosteroid drugs but one simple rule for their use. The drug of choice should be the least potent, given at the lowest dosage that yields clinical improvement. Almost invariably, the drug used is prednisone, prednisolone, or methylprednisolone. All corticosteroids are absorbed into the bloodstream just as fast by mouth as they are by intramuscular injection.

RISKS AND SIDE EFFECTS

Side effects of corticosteroids are less common in dogs than in people, and depend on the dosage and duration of treatment. Common possible adverse effects with some types include excessive thirst, urination, and panting, and increased appetite. There may be short-term personality changes, usually for the worse, such as heightened irritability. Some older dogs, females in particular, become temporarily incontinent. In the longer term, weakness and weight gain may occur.

Corticosteroid withdrawal is not as problematic for dogs as it is for humans. After prolonged use (over one month), the dose should be tapered off over a period of seven to ten days.

Daily therapeutic doses of corticosteroid given for longer than a month suppress the activity of the adrenal glands; therefore, the only safe long-term therapy is administration on alternate days. At higher doses, corticosteroids suppress the immune system.

ANABOLIC STEROIDS

These steroids mimic the anabolic (protein-building) effect of the male hormone testosterone, but their use is not associated with the development of secondary sex characteristics. Anabolic steroids are used in geriatric medicine to build tissue and enhance muscle mass. They promote muscle recovery following injury, and help strengthen bones. This group of steroids has been widely abused by human athletes to build strength and stamina, with serious risks to their health,

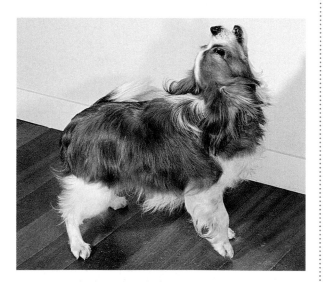

USING MOOD-ALTERING DRUGS
Certain mood-altering drugs, used in conjunction with behaviour retraining, are effective for overcoming behaviour problems. They can, for example, reduce the symptoms of anxiety in your dog, such as howling or excessive barking.

but if you administer them as prescribed for your dog, there are only minimal side effects.

SEX AND THYROID HORMONES

The male hormone (testosterone) is sometimes used to treat hormone-related skin disorders. Female hormones (oestrogen and progesterone) are used for a variety of physical and behavioural conditions. All sex hormones may produce unanticipated behavioural side effects. Thyroid hormone in the form of L-thyroxine is used therapeutically to treat hypothyroidism (*see p.331*).

OTHER DRUGS

A wide variety of other drugs is also available to treat your dog. Those listed below are among the most commonly prescribed.

MOOD-ALTERING DRUGS

In the 1990s a number of mood-altering drugs, originally licensed only for human use, were licensed for veterinary use. These include clomipramine and amitriptyline. Mood-altering drugs are only used in conjunction with behaviour retraining (*see pp.30-39*). By themselves, however, they are not effective at overcoming behavioural problems such as anxiety or destructiveness.

ANTHELMINTICS

This group of drugs is used specifically against parasitic worm infestations. Some types kill or paralyse intestinal worms, which then pass out of the body in the faeces, while others kill worms in other parts of the body. The text on internal parasites (*see pp.166–75*) has a fuller description of anthelmintics.

COMPLEMENTARY THERAPIES

The complementary therapies that may be used for dogs include homeopathic remedies, herbal remedies (*see box, right*), and the physical and other pain relief therapies described on pp.114–15.

If you wish to use complementary treatments for your dog, seek the services of a veterinary surgeon trained in complementary therapies or an individual who has been recommended by a qualified vet. Make sure that you tell your vet what complementary treatments you have given your dog.

HERBAL MEDICINES

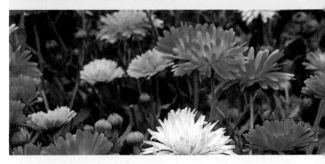

Plants and herbs are an important source of many modern conventional medicines, and for many people around the world they remain in themselves a major part of the medical treatment available for both people and animals. Many herbs are sold as pills or tinctures (extracts in alcohol), but the traditional way of taking them is by drinking an infusion. This medicine is made by pouring boiling water over the flowers or leaves of a plant, then leaving the mixture to steep to release its active ingredients. When the infusion has cooled, it is ready for your dog to drink.

Exercise caution when considering herbal medicine for your dog. Herbal remedies contain constituents that can be harmful in excess. Conventional medicines undergo extensive research and testing to calculate what their toxic doses are, but for most herbs the toxic doses for dogs have not been calculated.

Q ARE ALL DRUGS USED FOR HUMANS ALSO SUITABLE FOR DOGS?

A Not necessarily. Your vet will advise you whether or not a drug is suitable for your dog. Some drugs developed for humans may not be licensed for veterinary use but have proved to be of value. For example, several that act on the stomach lining (sucralfate, misoprostol, ranitidine, cimetidine) can be very effective for a variety of bowel disorders. The choice of drug depends on the medical condition and your vet's experience with the drug.

Q WON'T TRADITIONAL MEDICINES BE SAFER FOR MY DOG?

A Traditional, or complementary, medicines are not necessarily safer. Tea tree oil, for example, has excellent anti-fungal properties but can be toxic in its concentrated form; it may also be topically irritating to dogs with skin sensitivity. Use all medications cautiously, and tell your vet if you give your dog traditional medicines.

OVER-THE-COUNTER MEDICINES

Many medicines are available to humans without a doctor's prescription, or "over the counter" (OTC), although the drugs that are available in this way vary from one country to another. While some of these medicines can be used to treat minor complaints in dogs, a drug that is safe for us will not necessarily be safe for dogs. Conversely, do not assume that a drug that may cause adverse effects in people will do so in dogs. As an example, humans tolerate the painkiller ibuprofen (also sold as Nurofen in the United Kingdom and as Advil, Motrin, and Nuprin in the United States) better than dogs do, while dogs tolerate corticosteroids (such as prednisone and prednisolone) better than we do. Outlined below is a range of over-the-counter drugs that can be used on dogs.

ANTIDIARRHOEALS

Diarrhoea is not itself a disorder but a sign of an underlying problem. It is often the result of ingesting a toxic substance, but in some cases may indicate a serious intestinal condition. Consult your vet if your dog has chronic diarrhoea.

Bismuth subsalicylate (Pepto-Bismol) is safe and effective for acute diarrhoea. Give .25 ml/kg (.125 ml/lb) by mouth every four hours. Loperamide (Imodium) may also control diarrhoea at a dose of .08mg/kg (.04 mg/lb) every six hours, but take care. This is a narcotic drug and it may cause neurological side effects in small dogs and in collie and part-collie breeds.

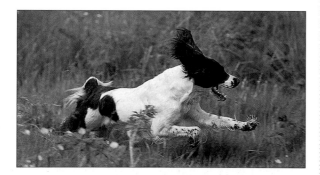

TREATING MINOR AILMENTS AND ALLERGIES
Over-the-counter medicines are useful to treat minor ailments in your dog. Antihistamines, for example, are effective for dogs that are allergic to substances that commonly cause hay fever in humans, such as dust, mould, or pollen and other plant substances.

ANTIHISTAMINES

This group of drugs blocks the effects of histamine, a natural body chemical that is released during allergic reactions such as rashes, itching, and irritation (for example, from insect bites or stings). Antihistamines such as diphenhydramine (Benadryl) are safe, and control seasonal allergic itch in some dogs when given at a dose of 2–4 mg/kg (1–2 mg/lb) every eight to 12 hours. This drug has a sedative effect, which is useful if the itching disturbs your dog's sleep.

COUGH MEDICINES

A persistent cough requires investigation by your vet. Cough medicines with antihistamines are effective only for allergic coughs. Avoid cough medicines containing pseudoephedrine, because this drug may cause toxic side effects. The safest and most effective OTC cough medicines for dogs contain only dextromethorphan. This is effective when given at a dose of 1–2 mg/kg (0.5–1 mg/lb) every eight hours.

EMETICS AND ANTIEMETICS

The most common emetic, syrup of ipecacuanha, is a safe and efficient method of inducing vomiting in dogs, at a dose of 1–2 mg/kg (0.5–1 mg/lb).

Dimenhydrinate (Dramamine) and other similar OTC motion sickness medications are sometimes used for dogs. These are safe for dogs of all sizes when given at a dose of 25–50 mg.

EYE MEDICINES

Artificial tears and irrigating solutions sold for our eyes are also safe for dogs. To apply them, first gently pull the lower lid away from the eye by using a fingertip to draw down the skin below the eye, then allow the drops to fall behind the lid.

GASTRIC ACID-REDUCING DRUGS

At one time, drugs to reduce gastric acid such as ranitidine (Zantac) and cimetidine (Tagamet) were only available by prescription. Because these "H2-receptor blocking drugs" have a wide margin of safety, they are now available over the counter. Cimetidine is safe at 5–10 mg/kg (2.5–5 mg/lb) every 12 hours and ranitidine at 1–2 mg/kg (0.5–1 mg/lb) daily.

LAXATIVES AND ENEMAS

Soluble psyllium fibre prevents constipation by
increasing the bulk of the dog's stools, while emollient
laxatives soften the stools in acute constipation. Avoid
phosphate enemas in small dogs because the level of
phosphate is potentially toxic.

TOPICAL MEDICINES

Locally applied, or topical, medicines are used on the
surface of the body to treat skin disorders. Some types
contain low doses of hydrocortisone; these medicines
are soothing but may increase the risk of bacterial skin
infection. OTC antifungal ointments and creams
containing miconazole or clotrimazole are excellent
and effective against a variety of fungi, including forms
of ringworm, *Malassezia* yeasts, and *Aspergillus*. Take
care when using any topical ointment containing the
local anaesthetic benzocaine, because it may cause
haemolytic anaemia (*see p.257*) in small dogs if the
affected area is licked excessively.

COMPLEMENTARY THERAPIES

Medicines such as herbal, homeopathic, biochemic
tissue salt, and flower remedies are all OTC products.
Common herbal remedies include echinacea for the
immune system, comfrey for wounds, lavender as an
antiseptic, marigold for inflamed skin, and garlic for
digestive disorders. All of these are safe for dogs, but
the therapeutic value of a herbal product varies
considerably according to its method of preparation.
Homeopathic and biochemic tissue salt products are so
diluted that they are invariably safe for dogs, although
some animals are allergic to the lactose in lactose-
based tissue salts. Flower remedies are also harmless.

If you wish to try these therapies, talk to your
veterinary surgeon. Many practices now dispense
complementary remedies from reliable sources.

Some remedies are classed as nutritional supplements.
These medicines may be extracts, such as evening
primrose, flax, or fish oils, or more complex herbal
preparations. High levels of omega-3 fatty acids, as are
found in coldwater-fish oil and linseed oil, may have
an anti-inflammatory effect. Supplements of fish oil
concentrate are thought to reduce discomfort from
chronic skin or joint inflammation and from irritable
bowels. These treatments, and products such as
glucosamine and chondroitin sulphate for joints, are
safe for dogs if given in moderate amounts.

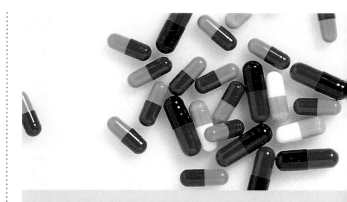

Q **WHERE SHOULD I BUY OVER-THE-COUNTER
MEDICINES FOR MY DOG?**

A Buy from a source that is genuinely knowledgeable
about the products it stocks. This usually means a
pharmacy or a veterinary practice. Pet shops and pet
superstores often have a wide variety of over-the-counter
products, but many of them are of questionable value. You
need to be especially cautious when buying concentrated
herbs or mixes of herbs. When analysed, it is common to
find that herbal preparations, particularly those originating
from China, are contaminated with other herbs, some of
which are toxic to dogs.

Q **DO I NEED TO WORRY ABOUT INTERACTIONS WHEN
USING OVER-THE-COUNTER MEDICINES?**

A Yes, you do. Never give your dog two or more
products, whether over-the-counter or by
prescription, without first discussing what you are doing
with a knowledgeable pharmacist or a vet.

NUTRITIONAL SUPPLEMENTS

Complementary therapies are
not a substitute for professional
veterinary advice. Some remedies,
however, can be useful nutritional
supplements for dogs. Evening
primrose oil, for example, is often
given to reduce itching in certain
skin conditions. So, too, is flax oil
and marine fish oil. All of these
supplements contain fatty acids
thought to be beneficial in
controlling or reducing the
inflammatory response.

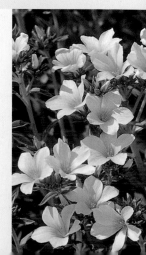

COMPLEMENTARY PAIN THERAPIES

To alleviate short-term pain, veterinary surgeons use a variety of medications (*see pp.108–9*). Chronic pain, however, does not always respond well to conventional therapies. As a result, many dog owners have tried complementary therapies for their dogs; some of these medicines have proved to be beneficial for certain individuals.

ACUPUNCTURE

Acupuncture is thought to work by stimulating the body to release endorphins (natural painkillers) and prostaglandin-suppressing cortisone (which reduces pain and inflammation). Both the American Veterinary Medical Association and the World Health Organization recognize acupuncture as a treatment for joint-related pain. While studies in humans show that acupuncture is effective in relieving back pain, studies in dogs are complicated and difficult to perform (although dogs do not appear to resent the insertion of needles). Veterinary acupuncturists say that the more chronic the pain, the more treatments may be necessary before pain relief is observed.

MANIPULATION THERAPIES

Chiropractors and osteopaths with knowledge of canine anatomy can ease acute pain in dogs by manipulating spinal joints and muscle tissues. This type of treatment is especially useful in breeds such as Dachshunds. Trigger-point therapy is a form of acupressure in which pressure on specific points – so-called trigger points – in muscles is claimed to relieve severe pain associated with nerve inflammation, as well as muscle and joint pain. Veterinary clinicians at Murdoch University in Perth, Australia, say that when pressure is correctly applied, dogs may initially wince or yelp, but after therapy the animals have more mobility and fewer signs of discomfort. They say that trigger-point therapy has been particularly effective in relieving neurological pain not responsive to conventional therapies.

HYDROTHERAPY

Hydrotherapy involves a wide range of techniques to treat pain using water. Ice packs applied to the affected area can reduce pain caused by inflammation, while cold compresses probably dull pain-sensing nerve receptors in the skin and underlying tissue.

Swimming exercise, especially in a heated pool, is one of the best forms of physical therapy. It appears to improve the circulation and reduce the severity of muscle and joint pain. The opportunity to swim may also have a positive psychological effect on a dog that is a natural swimmer: this effect could stimulate the production of natural endorphins and prostaglandin-diminishing corticosteroids.

PHYSICAL THERAPIES

Transcutaneous electrical nerve stimulation (TENS) and other forms of physical therapy, such as pulsating electromagnetic field (PEMF) therapy, may be effective treatments for reducing chronic joint or soft tissue pain in dogs, although they are difficult to apply.

TENS works by transmitting pulses of low-voltage electricity into the body tissues. A small, portable

---

Q MY DOG IS ILL BUT IS BEHAVING NORMALLY – DOES THIS MEAN IT IS NOT IN PAIN?

A Dogs wince or yelp only when they are in severe pain. In all other circumstances most dogs are more stoical than most of us, puttng up with quite severe discomfort unflinchingly. In any situation that we know causes pain in us, from a broken nail to bladder stones, we should always assume that a dog feels pain.

Q IF THE PAIN IS NOT ENOUGH TO MAKE MY DOG COMPLAIN, IS ANY TREATMENT NEEDED?

A Dogs are natural stoics, but the fact that they do not complain does not mean that their pain is only mild. If you think your dog may be experiencing pain, have your vet examine it. Although pain is a sign that the body is working to defend itself, it is also an early warning signal of many underlying health disorders.

Q WHAT CAN I DO TO HELP MY DOG FEEL LESS PAIN?

A Like humans, dogs feel an increased sense of physical well-being through being touched. Stroking your dog is a form of massage, which can be therapeutic in cases of mild to moderate pain (see facing page). Talking to dogs soothingly will also help them feel better.

battery-operated unit sends the current through electrodes attached to the skin. The pulses prevent the passage of pain messages to the brain; their strength and frequency can be adjusted.

PEMF works on the theory that pulsating magnetic fields can improve the oxygen utilization in diseased or damaged body tissues, thereby promoting healing and reducing pain.

British studies suggest that electro-stimulation is as effective as some pharmaceutical painkillers. However, laser therapy units do not appear to offer any benefits.

HERBALISM AND AROMATHERAPY

While a number of herbs are used as topical therapies for pain in people, these remedies are not practical in dogs that tend to lick themselves.

Eucalyptus and tea tree oil are said to stimulate the endorphin system when massaged on the body, but studies found the effect to be no greater than that of massage alone. Natural pheromones, especially sex pheromones, work by distracting a dog from its pain and concentrating its mind on more intriguing matters.

NUTRITIONAL THERAPY

Some nutritional supplements (see p.91) have an anti-inflammatory effect; these medicines reduce the pain of certain inflammatory conditions, such as arthritis.

COMPARING TREATMENTS: A STUDY

In the 1990s, vets at the Ontario Veterinary College, University of Guelph in Canada, dispensed to ten veterinary clinics in southwestern Ontario four different but identical-looking treatments for dogs suffering from developmental joint diseases (see p.366). All the treatments were contained in gelatin capsules. One substance was a placebo consisting only of rice flour. Others consisted of rice flour together with a North American native herbal formula for arthritic pain, traditional Chinese herbs for arthritic pain, or aspirin. Neither the vets nor the owners knew what was in the capsules.

When the vets and owners assessed responses, 40 per cent reported improvements on the placebo alone. A similar number reported improvements on the North American native herbs, while a greater number saw improvements on the Chinese herbs. The greatest improvement was reported for the dogs given aspirin.

TOUCH, MASSAGE, AND RELAXATION

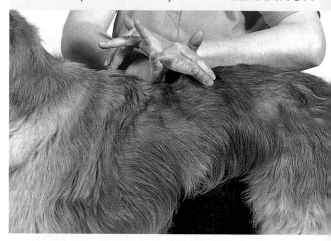

● The use of touch to promote physical and psychological well-being is one of the oldest natural therapies. Touch appears to have powerful benefits for all sociable species, and this is especially true for dogs raised in our homes from puppyhood. Throughout a dog's life, touch is comforting and rewarding. Most of us intuitively understand it is beneficial because we are ourselves rewarded when we touch our dogs. Therapies such as acupuncture, acupressure, shiatsu, Tellington Touch, chiropractic, osteopathy, and massage all involve touch. Even the gentle touch of an acupuncturist inserting needles can be physiologically rewarding, reducing pain and promoting healing.

● For most dogs, human contact when they are unwell is beneficial. Massage has a possibly calming effect on a dog, and can also reduce pain by stimulating or relaxing the muscles and improving circulation. Active touch from an owner may have even more beneficial psychological effects that diminish pain sensation (see p.85). Simply stroking your dog can be a form of massage; the dog will appreciate this kind of attention even more than usual if in discomfort.

● According to Professor Karen Overall, clinical veterinary behaviourist at the University of Pennsylvania's veterinary school, conditioning dogs to relax seems to be an effective way to reduce post-surgical pain. Relaxation techniques are relatively simple to use. A dog is rewarded when it appears calm: its ears are relaxed, there is no intense expression in the eyes, and its breathing is steady. This procedure conditions the dog to find relaxation itself rewarding. The benefits are decreased levels of adrenaline (epinephrine) and blood sugar, lowered blood pressure, and improved digestion, alertness, and immune activity.

SURGERY AND AFTERCARE

Surgery is undertaken either to diagnose or to treat a condition. Diagnostic surgery is usually called "exploratory" surgery. If your dog has pale gums and a swelling abdomen, for example, the vet may do an "exploratory laparotomy" – an operation to open the abdomen – not knowing exactly what he or she will discover. If a problem is found, the vet may perform an operation to correct it, such as a splenectomy (removal of the spleen) to treat internal bleeding from a torn spleen. While surgery is the best form of treatment for tumours, and is usually the fastest way to repair most injuries, it may be difficult to decide whether to operate or simply to allow the body to repair itself.

SURGICAL TERMS

Some of the main surgical terms sound rather similar but have different medical meanings. Adding "ectomy" to the end of a word means "to remove", as in a tonsillectomy – an operation to remove the tonsils. The term "otomy" means "to open and close". A tracheotomy, for example, is a procedure to open the trachea (windpipe), remove something, then close up the opening made in it. Another term, "ostomy", means "to open and leave open". Your vet will carry out a tracheostomy when a dog needs a permanent new opening in the trachea through which to breathe.

GENERAL ANAESTHESIA

If your dog needs surgery under general anaesthesia, you must withhold food for 12 hours before the anaesthetic. This reduces the risk that the dog will vomit food (and choke on it) during or immediately after the operation. Withhold water for the same period unless your vet is worried about your dog's hydration and tells you to leave water for a few hours more.

In most circumstances, the general anaesthesia is induced by giving the dog a short-acting anaesthetic intravenously. The dose is calculated according to a dog's weight, but also according to its health and what other drugs it has had. Lean breeds, such as Whippets and Border Collies, need less anaesthetic than other breeds of similar weight. The dog falls asleep as the drug is injected and remains unconscious for a variable length of time, depending on the drug used.

HOW ANAESTHESIA IS ADMINISTERED

To anaesthetize a dog, the vet first injects a short-acting anaesthetic into a vein. The dog will fall asleep within seconds. The vet then inserts a tube into the windpipe and inflates it. A vaporized mixture of anaesthetic gas and oxgen is now administered via the tube. As the injected anaesthetic wears off, the gas continues to keep the dog unconscious until the surgery is complete.

INTUBATION
Supplying a mixture of oxygen and anaesthetic vapour is the safest method of general anaesthesia. This Golden Retriever has a tube placed in its windpipe that feeds in the gas mixture.

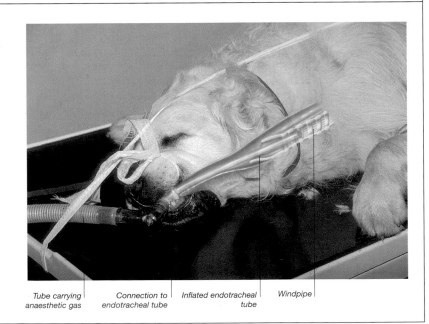

Tube carrying anaesthetic gas — *Connection to endotracheal tube* — *Inflated endotracheal tube* — *Windpipe*

WHAT HAPPENS DURING AN OPERATION

As soon as the dog has become unconscious, a tube (endotracheal tube) is inserted over its tongue into its windpipe and inflated. This keeps its airway clear and is attached to a source of oxygen.

Quick procedures – such as taking an X-ray or removing a foreign body from the ear – often require only the intravenous anaesthetic. For longer surgical procedures, such as routine operations, oxygen is mixed in a vaporizer with an anaesthetic gas. During the operation, the injected anaesthetic wears off while the vaporized gas mixture continues to keep the dog unconscious. At the end of the procedure, the anaesthetic is stopped and only fresh oxygen given until the dog wakes up.

RECOVERY FROM ANAESTHETIC

The time the dog takes to recover depends not only on the injected and inhaled anaesthetics used but also on the painkillers and tranquillizers given before and during surgery. Some anaesthetics, such as intravenous propofol and inhaled isoflurane, are very fast-acting. An anaesthetized dog will be awake minutes after the anaesthetic is stopped. These are very safe drugs but expensive, especially when used on medium to giant breeds. Other anaesthetics, such as intravenous barbiturate and inhaled halothane, are as safe and less costly, but recovery from these drugs takes longer. Further anaesthetics are "reversible", meaning that after a procedure has been completed another drug is given to counteract the effect of the anaesthetic.

Tranquillizers, sedatives, and narcotic painkillers (but not NSAID painkillers) prolong the recovery time. Anaesthetics are removed from the body by the lungs, liver, or kidneys; poor function of any of these organs prolongs recovery and increases the risk from the anaesthetic. Before an anaesthetic is given, a full set of blood tests will reveal any potential problems.

POST-SURGICAL CARE

Licking wounds is a natural behaviour, and from your dog's perspective a surgical incision is simply a wound. Your vet may give you an "Elizabethan collar" or a plastic neck brace that prevents your dog from licking the surgical site. Both you and your dog may initially object to this restriction, but removing it may lead to excess licking. This may, in turn, pull out the stitches, and they would then have to be replaced.

POST SURGERY

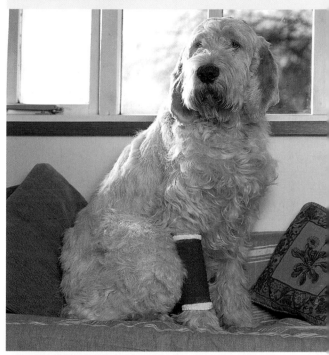

Studies of human patients admitted to hospital for gall bladder surgery showed that those who had windows with views of the surrounding countryside recovered faster and needed fewer painkillers than those people whose rooms overlooked other parts of the hospital. Although little is published in the area, logic and common sense suggest that a pleasant post-surgical environment is as vital for dogs as it is for us. Dogs probably get better faster in their own homes than they do when they are separated from their human families. As soon as it is safe to do so, arrange for your hospitalized dog to return to its own home.

Q **IS IT WORTH THE RISK TO ANAESTHETIZE MY DOG FOR A ROUTINE DENTAL SCALE AND POLISH?**

A Any medical procedure involves risk, but the advances that have been made in the types of anaesthetic now available – and also in the monitors that measure blood oxygen, heart function, and breathing during anaesthesia – are such that the health benefit of a medical procedure almost always outweighs the minimal risk. You and your vet should discuss perceived risks and necessary aftercare before any procedure is undertaken.

IMMUNE SYSTEM
defences against germs and cancer

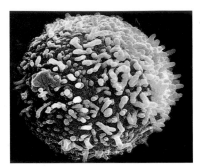

White blood cell

A dog's health depends on an efficient immune system. This system recognizes and destroys any foreign or damaging object inside the body (*see pp.82–83*), including rogue body cells. The system can be activated by physical or psychological causes, and should turn on and off as necessary. If it does not turn on properly, a dog has a poor immune response and is said to be "immunosuppressed". If, on the other hand, the system is oversensitive and will not switch off, allergy or autoimmune disease may ensue.

A healthy immune system recognizes and destroys both external disease-causing microbes, such as viruses and bacteria, and internal dangers such as cancer cells. It is constantly vigilant and occupied with these tasks.

MATERNAL IMMUNITY

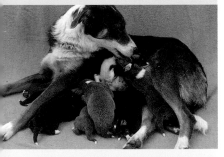

Antibodies conferring immunity to infectious organisms are passed from a mother to her young in the first milk, called colostrum. At birth, the pup's intestines are permeable enough to absorb these antibodies into the blood; after a few days any remaining antibodies remain on the tonsils and lining of the intestines. Maternal antibodies drop to low levels after about 10 to 12 weeks of age. Pups should be fully inoculated against major diseases between 8 and 12 weeks (*see p69*).

HOW THE SYSTEM WORKS
White blood cells are the "soldiers" that guard and protect the body. There are different types, which function in different ways. One type, known as B-lymphocytes, produce molecules called antibodies that attach themselves to microbes; the presence of the antibodies alerts other immune system cells that the microbes are to be killed. The B-lymphocytes are prompted to make antibodies by immune system cells called "helper" T-cells, and to stop antibody production when the job is done by "suppressor" T-cells.

Other lymphocytes, known as "memory" T-cells, patrol the body, recognizing microbes that they have enountered before and mobilizing attack teams. Appropriately named "killer" T-cells attack and destroy virus-infected cells and tumour cells. White cells called macrophages ("big eaters") clean up the affected area by devouring microbes and debris.

A HEALTHY BALANCE
A natural balance exists within the immune system between "helper" and "suppressor" T-cells. In good health, antibodies are produced only when needed and the immune system turns itself on and off. In certain situations, however, such as an overactive adrenal gland, the suppressor cells become dominant and the immune system becomes weakened. In this condition (an "immunosuppressed" state), a dog is susceptible to secondary infections.

AUTOIMMUNE DISEASE
The opposite condition is equally harmful: if helper T-cells dominate, the immune system becomes over-active and loses the ability to differentiate between normal body cells and invaders. Consequently, the immune system begins to attack the body's own tissues, resulting in autoimmune disease. Most dogs with an underactive thyroid gland (*see p.331*), for example, are suffering from an autoimmune disorder in which excess helper cells attack and destroy the dog's thyroid gland. Evidence is mounting that a variety of other conditions in dogs, including certain forms of heart disease in breeds such as the Doberman, are autoimmune in nature.

ALLERGIES
Finally, the imune system may become oversensitive, reacting to harmless substances such as flea saliva, dust mite droppings, plant pollens, or food. This is how allergic disorders develop.

STRUCTURES OF THE IMMUNE SYSTEM

An efficiently functioning immune system is essential to the health of all living beings. In mammals, the system works through almost every part of the body, from the surface of the skin (its largest internal and external component) right into the marrow of the bones. A network of bean-shaped nodes (glands) and connecting vessels, called the lymphatic system, collects fluid (lymph) from body tissues and returns it to the blood, thus maintaining the fluid balance within the body. As lymph filters through the lymph nodes it is enriched with white blood cells called lymphocytes, which are produced in the lymph nodes as well as in the bone marrow, spleen, and thymus. These cells are vital in the fight against infection.

THE IMMUNE NETWORK
The immune system essentially functions through the action of white blood cells circulating in the blood. These cells, in turn, depend on an intricate and finely tuned network of organs, nodes (glands) and vessels throughout the body.

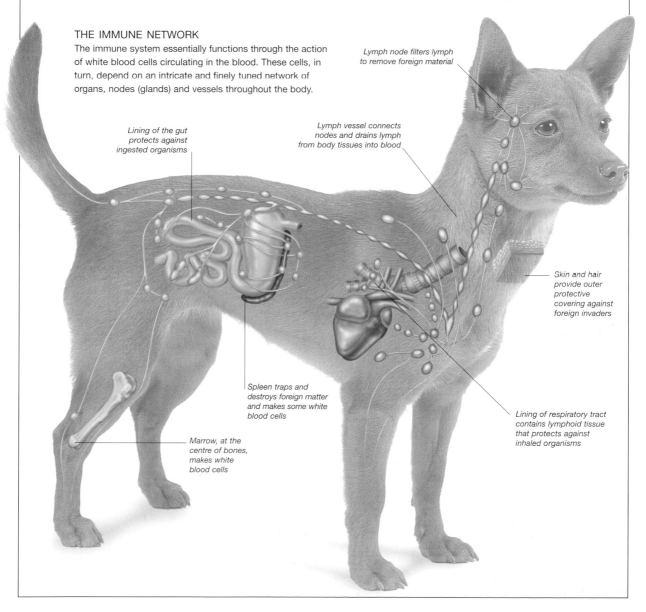

Lymph node filters lymph to remove foreign material

Lining of the gut protects against ingested organisms

Lymph vessel connects nodes and drains lymph from body tissues into blood

Skin and hair provide outer protective covering against foreign invaders

Spleen traps and destroys foreign matter and makes some white blood cells

Lining of respiratory tract contains lymphoid tissue that protects against inhaled organisms

Marrow, at the centre of bones, makes white blood cells

INFLUENCES ON IMMUNE RESPONSE

The ability of the immune system to respond to a challenge is influenced by a number of factors.

THE INFECTIOUS AGENT Various factors connected with the infectious agent (germ or microbe) are important. First is its virulence: some strains of microbe are more likely than others to overwhelm the immune system. The dose also plays a part. Generally, the higher the number of microbe particles to which a dog is exposed, the more likely it is that the immune system will be overwhelmed. Finally, the route by which the microbe enters the body can be significant. Some viruses, for example, can produce illness only if they invade the body via the mucous membranes that line the eyes and nose.

THE HOST In the dog as a whole, age plays an important part. Some organisms are much more dangerous to young pups than to adults, in whom the immune system response is more mature and vigorous. Antibodies that are passed to a pup in the first milk from its mother do, however, provide considerable protection (*see p.69*).

Inherited factors are also important in influencing outcome in a high proportion of cases. As a result, there are some slight variations between breeds in susceptibility to infections.

ENVIRONMENT The conditions in a dog's environment also have an effect. Changes in temperature and humidity somehow affect the immune system's efficiency. So, too, does social stress, although the exact way in which it does so is one of the great remaining questions in immunology.

INFLUENCE OF MEDICAL CONDITIONS

The presence of illness can reduce the vigour of the immune system. Some infections, such as distemper, suppress the immune system; any co-existing illness or infection drains the body of

essential nutrients, ties up parts of the immune system, and reduces its ability to respond efficiently.

Certain diseases can suppress the production of essential immune system components. These diseases include leukaemia, cancers of the lymph tissue, and bone marrow disease.

While both humans and cats can be affected by viral diseases that suppress the immune response (human immunodeficiency virus or HIV in humans, FIV and FeLV in cats), as yet there are no known equivalent causes of immunosuppression in dogs.

INFLUENCE OF SPLEEN REMOVAL

The spleen is the largest organ in the immune system. It functions as a filter, capturing foreign material but also recycling the contents of dying or dead red blood cells. It is home to certain

types of white blood cell belonging to the immune system and a major site for the manufacture of these cells.

Dogs sometimes need to have their spleens removed, either because of a traumatic injury or the development of a tumour. A dog can live comfortably without its spleen, but it will have a reduced resistance to certain types of bacterial infection.

MEDICAL INFLUENCES

Veterinary medicine is used to affect the immune system in two different ways. Inoculation – using a vaccine to introduce dead or modified germs into the dog's body – stimulates the immune system to produce natural antibodies to them, thereby "immunizing" the dog against the dangerous variety of that specific germ (*see p.106*). In dogs that have been inoculated, the antibodies neutralize specific invaders,

VET'S ADVICE

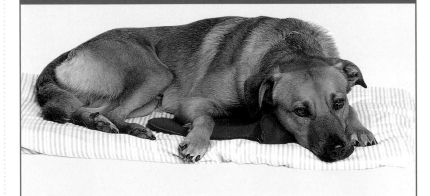

Just like humans, dogs that are ill should be kept in a comfortable, soothing environment and given plenty of love and care to help them recover. As far as possible, maintain an even temperature and quiet surroundings. Provide your dog with a lukewarm, covered hot-water bottle if the temperature might drop and your vet recommends it. Keep a constant supply of fresh water in a clean bowl within easy reach. When your dog's immune system is occupied in fighting an infection, the dog does not need excitement, boisterous activity, or long periods outside in fresh (but cold) air.

or attract killer T-cells to do the work for them. Inoculation also arms healthy body cells with natural chemicals called interferons that are used to fight certain infections. Diseases against which dogs can be inoculated include canine distemper, rabies, infectious canine hepatitis, and parvovirus.

Vets are also able to suppress the immune system whenever it becomes overactive, as it does in allergic reactions or autoimmune conditions. Corticosteroid drugs (*see p.110*) are usually used for this purpose, but in certain circumstances other, more powerful immunosuppressant drugs are more effective.

NUTRITIONAL INFLUENCES

Poor nutrition can impair the immune system, but good nutrition supplies substances that are essential to it. High-quality food provides amino acids, which build all proteins, including antibodies. Food is also a source of antioxidants, which neutralize excess "free radicals" – chemicals that can damage cell membranes. Studies in people show that substances acting as antioxidants also improve the immune response. Antioxidants include the minerals selenium and zinc; vitamins A (as beta-carotene), C, and E; and bioflavonoids. Beta-carotene is thought to improve skin and mucous membrane defences. Vitamin C, which humans must consume in food but dogs can manufacture themselves, increases antibody levels. Vitamin E protects body cells, tissues, and organs.

Some nutritionists believe that vitamin D, the B complex of vitamins, iron, calcium, magnesium, and manganese also have roles to play in maintaining the immune system.

Be sensible with any nutritional supplement; do not give your dog too much. Selenium, for example, is toxic in large doses, but standard vitamin and mineral tablets for dogs, which contain slightly more than the recommended daily amounts, are safe.

NATURAL IMMUNE STIMULANTS

The purple coneflower, *Echinacea purpurea* (*see right*), is a wildflower once used by Native Americans to treat various infections. The Dakota tribe treated diseases in their horses with coneflowers. This is the most popular herb thought to stimulate the immune system, with over 350 scientific studies published on it. The coneflower is said to stimulate macrophages (a type of white blood cell), especially in their action against yeast cells. Herbalists also recommend a number of other plants to treat animals, and more are being studied. According to published research, barberry (*Berberis*) is said to stimulate the immune system in dogs, while aloe (*Aloe vera*), which looks like a cactus but is in fact a member of the lily family (related to onions and garlic), is said to stimulate an immune response in horses.

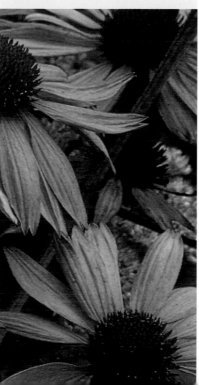

Q WHAT ARE ANTIBODIES AND HOW MANY TYPES EXIST?

A Antibodies, which are also called immunoglobulins or "Ig", are "markers" used for identifying cells to be destroyed by other cells in the immune system. They are proteins, which appear in many different forms. IgM, found in the bloodstream, is the first antibody produced after exposure to an antigen. IgG, the most common type of antibody, is also carried in the bloodstream. IgA is found wherever there is mucus: on the lining of the respiratory, digestive, and urogenital tracts. IgE exists in minute quantities on the surface of a class of immune system cells called mast cells. It plays a role in protection against parasites, and is also a key element in allergic responses.

Q WHAT IS ANAPHYLACTIC SHOCK?

A This condition is a potentially catastrophic IgE-triggered response. It is much more extreme than allergy, the typical response triggered by IgE. Substances released from mast cells and other types of white cell called basophils can constrict the airways and blood vessels inside the lungs, causing sudden respiratory distress. Muscles in the walls of the digestive system and bladder may contract, causing vomiting and involuntary passage of urine. An affected dog may drool saliva; become intensely itchy, especially on the face; lose physical coordination; and collapse. Anaphylaxis occurs more frequently in cats than in dogs. It may be triggered by insect bites and stings, medications such as penicillin, or vaccines. An affected dog needs immediate treatment with adrenaline (epinephrine) and corticosteroids.

IMMUNE SYSTEM DISORDERS

For unknown reasons, vets are diagnosing ever more disorders of the immune system. These disorders fall into two main categories: allergies and autoimmune disorders. (Some autoimmune disorders are described as "immune-mediated" rather than "autoimmune", but the distinction between these two terms is vague.)

Some specific immune system disorders are covered in detail under the body systems where they occur, but because they are so important, a general outline is also provided here.

ALLERGIES In an allergy, the immune system produces an exaggerated, inappropriate, and unnecessary response to a non-infectious substance.

AUTOIMMUNE DISEASE In autoimmune disease, the immune system wrongly turns its destructive firepower on a normal part of the body ("self") rather than on an invader. In these disorders, the immune system damages or destroys essential tissues such as red blood cells, skin cells, and thyroid gland cells. In some "immune-mediated" conditions, antigens (substances or particles of organisms that come from outside the body) circulate in the body with antibodies attached, and lodge in places where they should not be, such as blood vessel walls. The presence of these compounds (antibody-antigen complexes, or immune complexes) can cause inflammation and tissue damage.

ALLERGIES

Allergic reactions, especially to certain foods, drugs, and chemicals, were scarcely known or recognized before the 20th century. The word "allergy", in fact, was only coined in 1906, by a Viennese paediatrician, Baron Clemens von Pirquet. Hay fever, the most common form of allergy occurring in humans, was not mentioned in medical literature until the early 1800s. In 1950 it was still uncommon in both humans and dogs. Among Japanese people, for example, less than 1 per cent suffered from hay fever. Today, however, over ten per cent of the population suffer from it. In Australia today, over one third of the human population have allergies. As the incidence of allergies has increased in people, there has been a similar increase in allergies in dogs.

Allergic reactions may occur on a dog's skin, causing itchiness; on the lining of the airways, causing sneezing, coughing, and difficulty breathing; or on the lining of the gastrointestinal (digestive) tract, causing vomiting or diarrhoea. Chemicals in insect bites (as in flea saliva), certain foods, drugs, plants, dust mites, plant pollens, fungal spores, and even our own shed skin cells (human dander) can set off an allergic reaction in a dog.

THE ALLERGIC RESPONSE

Infectious agents, such as viruses, normally stimulate the immune system to produce protective antibodies. Allergens, usually harmless substances that are inhaled or swallowed, or that come into contact with the skin or eyes, provoke the immune system mistakenly to produce an antibody called immunoglobulin E (IgE).

In allergy-prone dogs (about 15 per cent of the total dog population) a set sequence follows (*see p.126*). First, IgE binds to receptor sites on specialized immune system cells called mast cells. These cells are like primed mines, filled with ten different chemicals. Mast cells exist in the skin and the lining of the stomach, lungs, and upper airways. (They may originally have developed to attack internal parasites such as intestinal worms or lungworms.)

When the dog is exposed to the same allergen again, the substance binds to IgE, already bound to mast cells. This reaction causes mast cells

POLLEN

Though dogs are not as commonly allergic to pollens as are humans, the types of pollens to which dogs and humans develop allergies to are broadly the same. They include the following:

• tree pollens (for example, cedar, oak, ash)

• grass pollens

• weed pollens (such as ragweed).

An assortment of pollen grains from various species of tree, grass, and weeds, magnified 600 times.

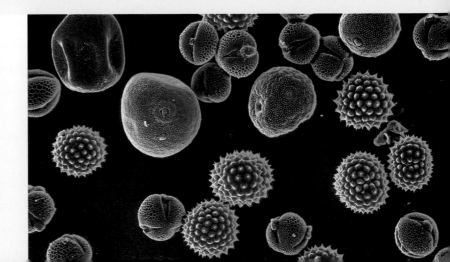

either to release some of their chemical contents or to explode, releasing inflammatory substances such as histamine and prostaglandin.

Dogs and people have mast cells distributed in different regions. While people have lots of these cells in their noses and eyes, and so commonly suffer hay fever, dogs have most of theirs in the skin, and suffer itchiness. Allergies may also affect one or more regions of the gastrointestinal tract.

MODERN CAUSES OF ALLERGIES

The house dust mite, flea saliva, and human dander are common causes of allergy in dogs. By selective breeding, humans have increased the genetic predisposition to allergies in some dogs, and by altering their natural environment we have also increased dogs' exposure to potential allergens.

The following points are some helpful questions to ask when trying to decide if a sick dog has an allergy. Has the problem occurred before? Does it occur at a specific time or season? Does it occur in a particular environment? Are the ears involved? Is there any history of allergies in the dog's breed or immediate family? If the answer to many of these questions is "yes", then an allergic cause is probable.

Q **WHAT IS THE DIFFERENCE BETWEEN ALLERGY AND ATOPY?**

A Allergy occurs when usually innocuous substances (allergens), such as flakes of skin (dander), pollen, mould spores, or house-dust mites, attach themselves to immunoglobulin E (IgE)-tagged mast cells, causing them to release their irritating chemical contents. In some individuals and some breeds, the likelihood of being allergic is inherited. This tendency is called "atopy"; an affected dog is "atopic".

ALLERGIC INHALANT DERMATITIS

Inflammation can be triggered by allergens that are absorbed through the skin, but more frequently by allergens that are inhaled into the respiratory system. In such cases, only some dogs develop respiratory problems. Many others exhibit their allergic response through itchy skin inflammation, especially on the face, feet, and ears.

ALLERGIC CONTACT DERMATITIS

In this condition, the allergic reaction occurs only on parts of the body in direct contact with the allergen. Grass sap, for example, causes a dermatitis (skin inflammation) on the relatively hairless underside of the dog's body.

HIVES (URTICARIA)

This condition, a form of localized and often itchy swelling, is most likely to be triggered by biting or stinging insects, food allergies, and drug reactions.

HAY FEVER

While common in people, hay fever (or allergic rhinitis) is quite uncommon in dogs, for whom inhaled allergens are more likely to trigger itchy skin than sneezing and drippy noses. When hay fever does occur, the allergens are the same as for humans: notably dust, dander, pollen, mould spores, and cigarette smoke.

ALLERGIC BRONCHITIS

Inhaled allergens rarely cause an allergic response in the nose; they are more likely to do so in the air passages (trachea and bronchi) and the lungs. Allergic bronchitis causes a dry, honking cough, similar to that associated with kennel, or canine, cough (*see p.240*).

ALLERGIC PNEUMONITIS

If the smallest air passages in the lungs are involved in an allergic reaction, an affected dog shows signs of pneumonia (*see p.242*). Blood samples show excess

ALLERGY-PRONE BREEDS

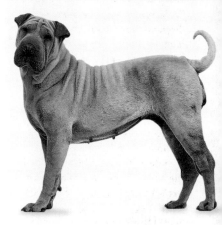

Just as allergies tends to runs in human families, there is also a breed predisposition in dogs. The Shar Pei (above) and Japanese Akita (below) seem particularly susceptible to allergies. Several breeds with predominantly white coats, such as West Highland White Terriers,

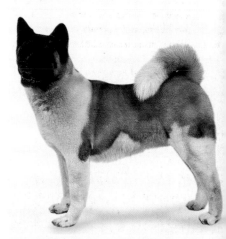

Bull Terriers, and English Setters, are predisposed to produce excessive IgE (immunoglobulin E) and have a higher than normal incidence of skin allergies. Golden Retrievers and West Highland White Terriers have a higher incidence of gastrointestinal allergies. Acquired sensitivities may develop later in life.

numbers of white blood cells called eosinophils; samples of fluid washed out of the dog's trachea (windpipe) may also contain these white cells. The condition is sometimes called PIE (pulmonary infiltrate with eosinophils). Recovery takes several weeks.

ALLERGIC GASTROINTESTINAL CONDITIONS

Allergy is a common cause of a group of disorders called inflammatory bowel disease or IBD. Each affected dog experiences a unique form of IBD, and any of the following conditions may occur. (*See also pp.284–86.*)

ALLERGIC GASTRITIS A food allergy may cause a dog periodically to vomit bile-tinged mucus, usually some hours after eating, or rhythmically, at certain times of day. Affected dogs continue to look well and behave normally.

ALLERGIC ENTERITIS Food allergy causes loose, watery, smelly diarrhoea, sometimes associated with bile-tinged vomiting. The frequency of bowel movements remains normal.

EOSINOPHILIC ENTERITIS This form of allergy often produces stools with the consistency of cow manure. Blood samples show increased numbers of eosinophils (a type of white cell). The dog may be thin, with a dull coat.

ALLERGIC COLITIS When the colon (large intestine) is affected, dogs pass bloody diarrhoea. There are many causes of colitis in dogs. Food allergy, or allergic colitis, is only one of them. Surprisingly, food allergies may cause no gastrointestinal problems but may trigger an allergic response in the skin, sometimes confined to the face or ears.

DIAGNOSIS AND TREATMENT OF ALLERGIES

Vets usually recommend avoidance as the best treatment for allergies. Finding the cause of an allergy has to be done through taking the history and by a process of trial and error, using skin tests or blood samples, special diets, and sometimes temporary removal of the dog from its normal environment. Determining the specific causes can be frustratingly difficult.

For immediate relief from allergy, vets try to "turn off" the allergic reaction at its source. Although many different chemicals are released when mast cells explode, only one of them, histamine, can be effectively controlled; drugs called antihistamines are used for this purpose. More recently, an "anti" for another chemical, a leukotriene, has been licensed for use in people suffering from allergies and asthma.

To relieve skin allergies, frequent shampoos are recommended. A terrier's rough coat, for example, is ideal for "capturing" mould spores and pollen, but washing can remove them. In addition, vets increasingly recommend high-dose essential fatty acid (EFA) supplements. EFAs are thought to affect prostaglandin synthesis, diminishing the intensity of mast cell explosions.

HUMAN ALLERGY TO DOGS

Every dog carries a protein called Can F-1 on flakes of its skin and perhaps in its saliva. This protein can cause allergic people to sneeze and wheeze. (If you have one parent with allergies you have an almost 50 per cent risk of developing allergies. If both your parents are allergic your risk increases to about 70 per cent.) Contrary to popular belief, there are no dog breeds that pose a lower risk of allergy than

CONTACT AND INHALED ALLERGENS

A common unwanted immune response, causing problems such as skin itchiness, involves a type of antibody called immunoglobulin E (IgE). It occurs in response to foreign substances (allergens) when they come into contact with the skin, or are inhaled or ingested.

MECHANISM

The body produces IgE on first exposure to the allergen. The IgE "primes" immune system cells called mast cells by attaching itself to them. On subsequent exposure, the binding of allergen to IgE causes the mast cells to release inflammatory substances such as histamine.

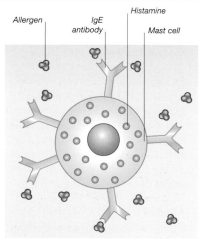

Allergen | IgE antibody | Histamine | Mast cell

Mast cell primed with IgE antibodies

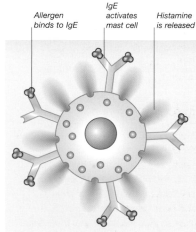

Allergen binds to IgE | IgE activates mast cell | Histamine is released

Response on subsequent exposure

INGESTED ALLERGENS

Some food substances can cause an allergic response in the gut lining. This response involves mast cells to which IgE antibodies have attached themselves. The mast cells release chemicals such as histamine, which can have effects on the muscle in the intestinal wall and on blood vessels in the gut lining, and lead to vomiting and diarrhoea. Allergens may also enter the bloodstream through the gut and spread to produce symptoms in other body areas, such as hives on the skin.

MECHANISM

The allergen penetrates the gut lining. In the submucosal layer of the gut wall, it causes "primed" mast cells to release histamine. This chemical stimulates the smooth muscle to contract and blood vessel walls to swell, leading to bowel upsets. The allergen also diffuses into the bloodstream.

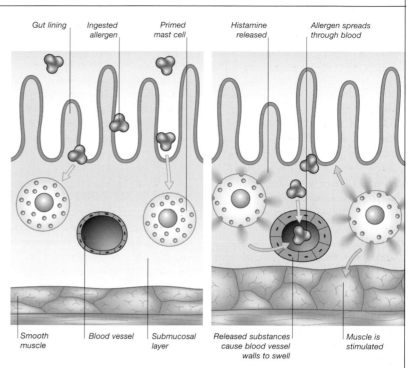

Gut lining | Ingested allergen | Primed mast cell

Histamine released | Allergen spreads through blood

Smooth muscle | Blood vessel | Submucosal layer

Released substances cause blood vessel walls to swell | Muscle is stimulated

Allergen penetrating gut wall

Allergic response in submucosal layer

---

others. All breeds, including non-moulters such as Poodles and hairless ones such as the Chinese Crested, produce Can F-1. We are less likely to be allergic to dogs that are routinely bathed and clipped; these activities reduce the concentration of Can F-1. Dry, flaky, or oily skin conditions increase levels of Can F-1.

AUTOIMMUNE DISORDERS

The disorders in this group result from the inability to differentiate between "self" and "not-self". They lead the body to produce an auto-antibody – in effect, an antibody against the body's own tissues. Some of the disorders known as "immune-mediated" occur due to the development of antibody-antigen complexes (see p.124). Autoimmune disease can be triggered

by bacteria and viruses or even by drugs, tumours, and possibly vaccines. Although conditions such as immune-mediated haemolytic anaemia (see below), systemic lupus erythematosus (see p.200), and hypothyroidism (see p.331) are still relatively rare, there has been an increased incidence of diagnosis of autoimmune disorders since the 1960s. This increase may be because of better diagnostic abilities in this field, but many vets feel that both the incidence of disease and diagnostic ability have increased.

IMMUNE-MEDIATED HAEMOLYTIC ANAEMIA (IMHA)

In this condition, the immune system attacks and destroys red blood cells. IMHA is the most common of all canine immune system diseases. The condition

may be triggered by viruses, but also by drugs, perhaps vaccines, and even by cancer. It may occur devastatingly quickly or develop more gradually. The more overwhelming and rapid the destruction of red blood cells, the graver the outlook is.

In peracute (sudden) instances, an affected dog is lethargic and may have a fever for one to three days, after which its breathing rate increases and its gums become pale. The dog passes dark urine. It may have difficulty walking. Dogs with subacute (more gradual) IMHA develop the same signs but over a longer period, while those with chronic IMHA experience intermittent flare-ups of the illness.

DIAGNOSIS AND TREATMENT The diagnosis of IMHA is based on clinical signs and blood tests. Rapid and vigorous treatment with corticosteroid drugs or other, more powerful immunosuppressant drugs is vital. The use of blood transfusions is controversial; they may actually make the condition worse, because the overactive immune system attacks the fresh red blood cells. There are rare circumstances, however, in which a blood transfusion is the only way to sustain the dog's life.

IMMUNE-MEDIATED THROMBOCYTOPENIA (IMT)

The term "thrombocytopenia" means a reduced number of small cells called platelets, or thrombocytes, in the blood. Platelets play an important part in blood clotting; a lack of them can cause unexpected bleeding and bruising.

IMT occurs most frequently in females, whether spayed or not, and especially in Poodles, after an oestrous cycle. It may occur after an infection, and may also be an immune response to certain drugs. The first sign may be unexpected bruising seen on the relatively hairless parts of the body. An affected dog's stools may be tarry and black from bleeding into the gastrointestinal system, and there may be signs of blood in the urine. Some dogs suffer from nosebleeds.

DIAGNOSIS AND TREATMENT Your vet needs to differentiate IMT from IMHA and from other bleeding disorders. An accurate blood platelet count is vital. Corticosteroid drugs are the usual treatment. Transfusions of blood and platelets, combined with the use of powerful immunosuppressant drugs, are sometimes necessary. As with IMHA, some dogs develop a chronic form of the disease and need long-term treatment with immunosuppressants.

AUTOIMMUNE NEUTROPENIA

Neutropenia is a deficiency of neutrophils (a type of white blood cell). Certain drugs, such as sulphas (used to treat forms of colitis) and some anti-seizure medications, may trigger the immune system to suppress neutrophil production. This reponse increases the risk of bacterial infection. The condition is usually transient and responds to treatment with corticosteroid drugs.

IMMUNE-MEDIATED ARTHRITIS

This form of arthritis is a disease caused by the formation of antigen-antibody complexes (immune complexes; *see p.124*). It occurs in many forms, and may be associated with muscle inflammation (polymyositis) or with nerve inflammation (polyneuritis). All forms of immune-mediated arthritis are treated with corticosteroid drugs and other immunosuppressant drugs. Some dogs with rheumatoid arthritis benefit from having an affected joint surgically fused and stabilized.

IMMUNE-MEDIATED MENINGITIS

This rare condition, an inflammation of arteries in the meninges (membranes that line the brain), is also associated with the development of immune complexes. It has been seen in young Akitas, Beagles, Bernese Mountain Dogs, Boxers, and German Short-haired Pointers. Affected dogs suffer from intermittent apparent neck pain, rigidity, and a reluctance to move. Episodes last for about a week. The use of corticosteroid drugs reduces the signs of the illness.

NASAL SOLAR DERMATITIS

Some autoimmune diseases affect skin cells. Nasal solar dermatitis, also called discoid lupus erythematosus, is the most common and occurs most frequently in certain breeds living in sunny climates. It is commonly known as collie nose, because the breeds most at risk include Rough and Smooth Collies and the Shetland Sheepdog. White German Shepherd Dogs and Siberian Huskies are also at risk.

DIAGNOSIS AND TREATMENT The condition is diagnosed by visual examination, and treated with topical corticosteroid drugs and sunscreen.

OTHER AUTOIMMUNE SKIN DISEASES

These conditions are uncommon. The most common, pemphigus foliaceus, initially mimics an allergic dermatitis with a secondary bacterial infection affecting the muzzle, nose, ears, and the skin around the eyes. Systemic lupus erythematosus (SLE) may cause

IMMUNE-MEDIATED HAEMOLYTIC ANAEMIA

This condition typically affects middle-age females. It is life-threatening and there are frequent complications. While some individuals experience only one episode, in many others the disease recurs. Life-long drug therapy may be needed; however, this treatment, in turn, leads to further complications associated with chronic use of corticosteroids and other immunosuppressant drugs.

TYPE	MOST AFFECTED	FREQUENCY	OUTLOOK
Peracute	German Shepherd Dogs 2–6 years old	10–20 per cent of all cases	Fatal in over 50 per cent of cases
Subacute	Females, especially Cocker Spaniels	70–80 per cent of all cases	Fair to good
Chronic	Small breeds	under 5 per cent	Unpredictable

ANTIGEN-ANTIBODY COMPLEXES AND THEIR ACTION

In some forms of skin and joint disease, immune complexes form and become deposited in the skin, or in the synovial membrane lining a joint. They trigger the release of destructive chemicals from different types of cells. These chemicals cause erosion to the surfaces of the joints, leading to chronic arthritic changes.

MECHANISM
An antigen (often nuclear material from other cells that has been ingested by a macrophage) is later "presented" on the macrophage surface and combines with an antibody, making an immune complex. It may trigger other cells to release destructive chemicals called cytotoxins.

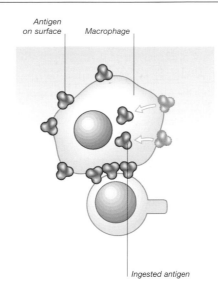

Antigen on surface   *Macrophage*

Ingested antigen

Antigen ingested by macrophage and presented on its surface

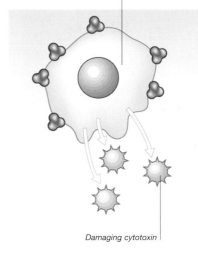

Macrophage

Damaging cytotoxin

Release of tissue-damaging factors

---

similar skin problems and also affect internal organs. All forms of pemphigus and SLE are serious and need vigorous treatment with immunosuppressant drugs. Other autoimmune skin disorders include erythema multiforme, topical epidermal necrolysis, and familial dermatomyositis. (*See also pp.200–01.*)

IMMUNODEFICIENCY CONDITIONS

These disorders are extremely rare. Canine Granulocytopathy Syndrome, found in Irish Setters, is one such problem. It causes white cells called granulocytes to increase in number but function inefficiently or not at all, permitting life-threatening bacterial infection. Cyclic Haematopoiesis of Gray Collies (and of Irish Wolfhounds) is a condition in which production of white blood cells (neutrophils) in the bone marrow intermittently shuts down, allowing bacterial infection to take hold.

IMMUNE-MEDIATED ARTHRITIS

The most common form of immune-mediated arthritis is idiopathic polyarthritis ("idiopathic" means "of unknown cause"). This condition does not cause erosion (destruction of tissue surfaces) within the joint, but does produce inflammation and other features such as loss of appetite and an intermittent fever. Signs of lameness come and go, and affect one or more joints. Erosive or rheumatoid polyarthritis eventually causes chronic pain with visible swelling, often in the smaller joints. A unique form of erosive polyarthritis affects some Greyhounds.

TYPE	AFFECTED BREEDS	AFFECTED JOINTS	DIAGNOSIS
Rheumatoid polyarthritis	Young to middle-aged toy breeds	Joints near end of limbs (digits)	Early X-rays
Plasmacytic synovitis	Large breeds	Knee	Examination of joint fluid
Idiopathic polyarthritis	Gun dogs Toy breeds 2–4 years old Guarding breeds (German Shepherd Dog, Doberman)	Some but not all joints	Examination of fluid from several joints

TUMOURS
cancer and other abnormal growths

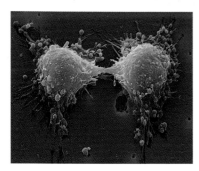

Cancerous cells dividing

A tumour is an abnormal mass of tissue that forms when cells in a specific area of the body reproduce at an increased rate. Tumours are divided into two broad categories: malignant (cancerous) and benign (noncancerous). Malignant tumours invade surrounding tissues and may also spread via the bloodstream or lymphatic fluid to other organs in the body. Benign tumours usually grow slowly and do not spread. In dogs, tumours occur most commonly in the skin, mammary tissue, bones, lymphatic system, spleen, and liver.

Tumours are relatively common in dogs. Most are benign. Malignant tumours may cause concern – the word "cancer" is highly charged and its associations very frightening – but some cancerous tumours can be treated successfully.

WHAT CAUSES TUMOURS?

While benign tumours have a variety of possible causes, from viral infection to injury or genetic predisposition, all cancers arise from the same basic mechanism: damage to genes. A cell may become cancerous when certain genes that control vital processes such as cell division become damaged. These faulty genes may be inherited. Some dogs have specific cancer-producing genes. For example, three in five Bernese Mountain Dogs die as a result of tumours that have a direct genetic cause. In other individuals or breeds, the genetic link is more complicated.

Whatever the genetic predisposition, cancer formation is usually triggered by environmental factors. Some, such as sunlight, are known to be capable of damaging genes directly; these factors are called carcinogens. Others, such as diet or stress, may have an indirect effect on cancer development.

The immune system is normally very efficient at destroying abnormal cells, but cancer cells trick the natural killer cells of the immune system into regarding them as "self" and therefore not destroying them. Having eluded the body's natural defences, cancer cells multiply rapidly to form a tumour, and may then spread around the body.

DESCRIBING TUMOURS

The medical names of most tumours end in "-oma". For example, lipoma and adenoma are types of benign tumour. Malignant tumours are classified according to where they originate. Carcinomas arise from the tissues that line the surfaces of a dog's organs; sarcomas form in tissues such as muscles, blood vessels, and bones; and lymphomas develop in the tissues of the lymphatic system.

BREED PREDISPOSITION TO FATAL CANCER

According to actuarial statistics from Britain's largest pet insurer, the breeds most at risk of dying from cancer are:

- Irish Wolfhound
- Rottweiler
- Afghan Hound
- Standard Poodle
- Weimaraner
- Staffordshire Bull Terrier

- Boxer
- Cairn Terrier
- Old English Sheepdog
- Golden Retriever
- Flat-coated Retriever

Breeds with an average risk include:

- Doberman Pinscher
- English Springer Spaniel

- Labrador Retriever
- Great Dane

The breeds least at risk include:

- Border Collie
- Random-breds
- West Highland White Terrier
- Yorkshire Terrier

- Cocker Spaniel
- German Shepherd Dog
- Shetland Sheepdog

CANCEROUS TUMOUR

Cancer occurs when body cells divide and grow in an uncontrolled manner. Cancer cells are irregular in shape and size, and often bear little resemblance to the cells from which they arose; this characteristic irregular appearance is often used to help diagnose cancer. A cancerous tumour is a collection of these abnormal cells. Such tumours infiltrate neighbouring tissues by forcing their way between normal cells. They may also spread to more distant parts of the body through the bloodstream or lymphatic system. The cells in a cancerous tumour obtain oxygen and nutrients from surrounding blood vessels so, as the tumour enlarges, it may invade existing blood vessels or stimulate new blood vessels to form within it.

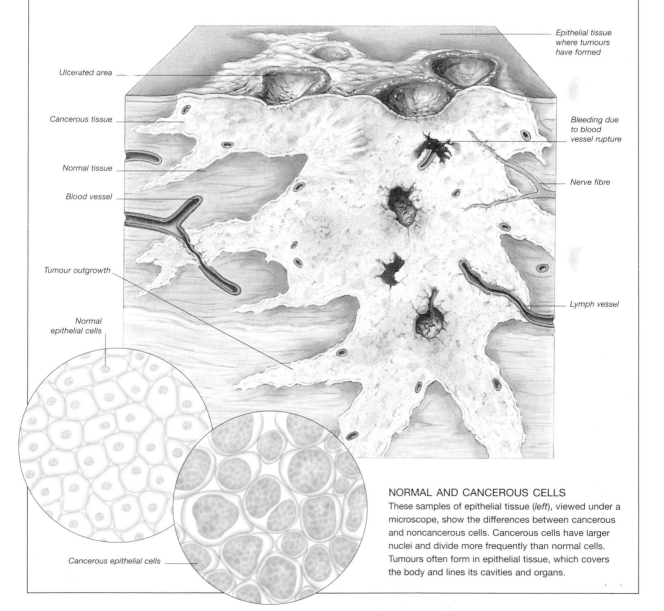

Epithelial tissue where tumours have formed

Ulcerated area

Cancerous tissue

Normal tissue

Blood vessel

Tumour outgrowth

Normal epithelial cells

Bleeding due to blood vessel rupture

Nerve fibre

Lymph vessel

Cancerous epithelial cells

NORMAL AND CANCEROUS CELLS

These samples of epithelial tissue (*left*), viewed under a microscope, show the differences between cancerous and noncancerous cells. Cancerous cells have larger nuclei and divide more frequently than normal cells. Tumours often form in epithelial tissue, which covers the body and lines its cavities and organs.

INVESTIGATION AND TREATMENT

DIAGNOSING TUMOURS

Many tumours, such as those in the lymph nodes, are visible on or under the skin. The appearance or "feel" of these tumours may suggest a diagnosis to your vet. Other tumours may be discovered when your vet carries out a routine physical examination or may be suspected from your dog's symptoms. When making a diagnosis, your vet will consider your dog's age, medical history, and breed, and he or she may perform some of the following tests.

IMAGING TECHNIQUES

X-rays and ultrasound scanning are often used to detect tumours in internal organs. Magnetic resonance imaging (MRI) scans give detailed information about tumours, but they are costly to perform. If a tumour is detected using imaging techniques, tissue sampling or exploratory surgery may then be necessary to confirm the diagnosis.

TAKING SAMPLES

It is often difficult for a vet to make a diagnosis without examining some of the tissue from the tumour under a microscope. Small tumours may be removed completely, while for larger ones your vet may either remove a small piece of abnormal tissue (known as taking a biopsy) or use a needle and syringe to withdraw a sample of cells from the tissue (fine-needle aspiration). For some types of tumour, such as those of the liver or spleen, blood tests may be necessary for diagnosis.

ASSESSING THE DANGERS OF TUMOURS

The main question your vet wants to answer when diagnosing a tumour is whether it is malignant or benign. This determines how dangerous the tumour is to your dog's health.

BENIGN TUMOURS

These tumours are usually harmless. Some, however, grow very large and compress surrounding tissues, which can cause pain and impair the function of nearby organs. In addition, certain types, such as Sertoli cell tumours (*see p.137*), produce hormones and can cause symptoms by disturbing the dog's hormonal balance.

THE MOST COMMON SIGNS OF CANCER

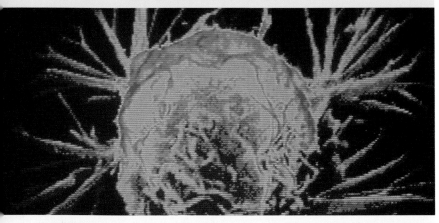

Magnified cancer cell

It is important to be vigilant for changes in your dog's health, especially for older dogs, in which cancer is more common. Some cancers, such as those affecting the skin, are visible and may be discovered during grooming or a routine examination. Cancers of the internal organs are often more difficult to detect, and an owner may first suspect that a dog is ill because of a change in its behaviour or appearance. If you notice any of the signs listed on the right, contact your vet as soon as possible. The earlier cancer is detected, the more promising the outcome.

The most common signs of cancer, reported by the American Veterinary Cancer Society, are:

- abnormal swelling that persists or continues to grow
- loss of appetite
- bleeding or discharge from any opening
- persistent lameness or stiffness
- reluctance to exercise or lack of stamina

- sores that do not heal
- weight loss
- offensive odour
- difficulty eating or swallowing
- difficulty in breathing
- straining to urinate or defaecate.

Q HOW DO CANCEROUS TUMOURS SPREAD?

A The defining feature of a cancer is its ability to spread not only locally but also to distant sites in the body by a process called metastasis. In metastasis, a cancer cell detaches from a tumour and travels in the bloodstream or the lymphatic fluid to a new location, where it multiplies to form a new, or secondary, tumour. To do this, the migrating cancer cell must survive attack from the immune system and stimulate the growth of blood vessels to provide oxygen and nutrients.

MALIGNANT TUMOURS

Malignant tumours are always harmful. How immediate a threat a malignant tumour poses depends on its location, its rate of growth, and whether it has spread to other organs. The World Health Organization has established a staging and grading system for malignant tumours. Many cancer specialists use this method to classify the seriousness of a tumour. "Staging" describes the extent of a tumour, while "grading" gives an impression of its malignancy at the cellular level.

TREATING TUMOURS

If a tumour is found to be benign and is not causing symptoms, it may not require any treatment at all. Your vet may simply want to monitor the tumour at regular intervals to check that it does not become cancerous or grow too large. Large tumours may need to be surgically removed to reduce pressure on nearby organs. Hormone-secreting tumours are also usually removed.

If a cancer is discovered, your vet will discuss with you whether it can be cured or whether the realistic aim of treatment is control, or palliation. In either case, there are four possible treatments: surgery, radiotherapy (irradiating a tumour with X-rays), chemotherapy (using drugs), and immunotherapy (stimulating a dog's immune system to attack the tumour). Treatment may include one or more of these possibilities.

While these are the medical treatments, there are also the uniquely veterinary treatments – simple pain control or euthanasia. This is an emotion-laden topic filled with ethical dilemmas. Ultimately, you and your vet must decide what is best for your dog.

SURGERY

Overwhelmingly, the most effective treatment for any bothersome tumour is surgery. Whenever possible, your vet will want to remove the tumour

together with a band of the healthy tissue around it. If there is a likelihood of spread, as there is with cancerous mammary tumours, your vet may want to remove the tumour, its surrounding tissue, and the local lymph nodes that serve that part of the body.

RADIOTHERAPY

This treatment is used on localized, radiation-sensitive tumours when it has not been possible to remove the mass completely or if the mass is inoperable. Radiotherapy is particularly useful for soft tissue sarcomas, squamous cell carcinomas, mouth and nasal cavity tumours, and mast cell tumours. Since the equipment is costly and potentially dangerous, radiotherapy is carried out at specialist veterinary centres.

CHEMOTHERAPY

In this treatment, anticancer drugs kill fast-multiplying cells. Certain types of lymphoma and leukaemia respond well to it, especially in small dogs, and transmissible venereal tumours may also be treated with drugs. For all other types of cancer, chemotherapy may improve quality of life but is unlikely to increase life expectancy. The drugs may cause unpleasant side effects.

IMMUNOTHERAPY

The corticosteroid drug prednisolone has been used for years to enhance quality of life and prolong survival time in dogs with certain forms of cancer, including lymphoma. More recently, research has concentrated on ways of stimulating the immune system to attack a cancer. Although immunotherapy is still not widely available, results are promising, especially for aggressive lymphosarcomas and mast cell tumours.

PALLIATIVE THERAPY

A significant difference between the therapies used for dogs and those for people is one of ethics. Most vets feel it is not acceptable for a dog to suffer during treatment. The consequence is that chemotherapy and radiotherapy are used less aggressively in dogs than in people. The objective is minimal or no side effects. When this goal cannot be attained, we should consider a dog's emotional and physical well-being. Sometimes the best course of action is not to attempt to cure the cancer but rather to preserve the dog's quality of life, even if this means a shorter life expectancy. This is the aim of palliative therapy. Pain relief is an important part of palliative care.

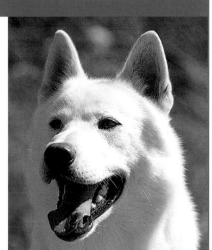

VET'S ADVICE

Certain risk factors for cancer in dogs, such as genetic predisposition and old age, cannot be controlled, but other factors can. Feed your dog a balanced diet to support the immune system, avoiding additives known to be carcinogenic. Keep your dog fit; excess body fat promotes certain cancers, including mammary cancer. Light-coated dogs should not be allowed outside in direct sunlight for long periods of time. Examine your dog regularly. Routine veterinary check-ups are especially important for dogs over seven years old.

SKIN TUMOURS

Because of their location, skin tumours are the most commonly diagnosed tumours in dogs, accounting for half of all tumours that vets see. The majority of skin tumours can be identified fairly accurately just by visual examination, but for some tumours procedures such as biopsy, blood sampling, and X-ray or ultrasound scanning may be needed to make an accurate diagnosis.

For more information about noncancerous skin conditions and their treatment, refer to Skin and Hair (*see pp.176–201*).

PAPILLOMA

This is a benign wart caused by infection with a virus. Papillomas occur most commonly in young dogs. They tend to appear as small, pink, cauliflower-like masses. Those dogs that develop papillomas typically have whole crops of them at the same time.
DIAGNOSIS AND TREATMENT Diagnosis is usually by visual examination. Papillomas may look unsightly, but they need to be removed only if they bleed, become infected, or otherwise cause problems. In time, papillomas disappear without treatment.

LIPOMA

A lipoma is a benign tumour of fat cells, common in older, overweight female dogs. Lipomas are painless. They form under the skin and may develop anywhere on the body. The tumours feel like smooth oblong masses. They usually grow slowly but can become extremely large.
DIAGNOSIS AND TREATMENT Diagnosis is by visual examination and usually also biopsy. Surgical removal is warranted if a lipoma is interfering with movement, is growing quickly, or is very unsightly. In rare circumstances, what appears to be a lipoma is in fact a malignant variety called a liposarcoma. To give some idea of how rare this condition is, I see lipomas in dogs on a daily basis but have only seen one liposarcoma in over 30 years of veterinary practice.

ADENOMA

This is a benign tumour. Adenomas in the skin and around the eyes arise from oil-producing sebaceous glands and are called sebaceous adenomas. In unneutered mature male dogs, another type, perianal adenoma, may develop from the glandular tissue around the anus (*see below*).

Sebaceous adenomas are almost always hairless, lobulated growths less than 2cm (¾in) in diameter. In rare cases, what appears to be a benign adenoma may actually prove to be a malignant adenocarcinoma, which has the potential to spread to other organs, such as the lungs.
DIAGNOSIS AND TREATMENT Diagnosis is by visual examination and biopsy. Removal is not necessary unless a growth ulcerates, grows quickly, or is larger than 2cm (¾in); all of these signs indicate that it may be a malignant adenocarcinoma.

PERIANAL ADENOMA

This type of adenoma needs the male hormone testosterone in order to grow. Perianal adenomas most commonly occur in male dogs over seven years of age. They look and feel like round, hard masses in the tissue around the anus. In many cases, the adenoma ruptures through the skin and may be noticed by an owner because the dog licks the anal area more intensively.
DIAGNOSIS AND TREATMENT Diagnosis is by visual examination. The adenoma will need to be surgically removed. Neutering, which removes hormonal nourishment from these tumours and consequently slows their growth dramatically, should be carried out at the same time as removal of the perianal adenoma in order to prevent recurrence of the condition.

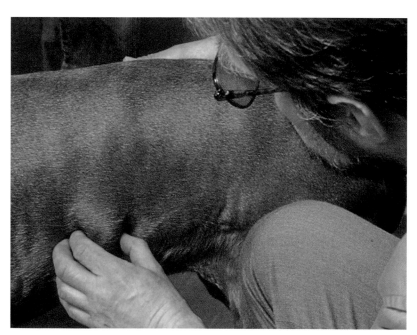

LIPOMA UNDER A DOG'S SKIN
This dog has an unusually large lipoma, a type of benign tumour consisting of fat cells. As shown, a lipoma can be felt under the dog's skin during a physical examination. It is usually diagnosed visually and by taking a sample of cells from the tumour for analysis.

NONCANCEROUS TUMOURS

A noncancerous tumour has a fibrous outer capsule that separates it from surrounding normal tissue. The surrounding tissue may become distorted as the tumour grows, but it is not breached by the tumour. The cells of a benign tumour are regular and resemble normal cells.

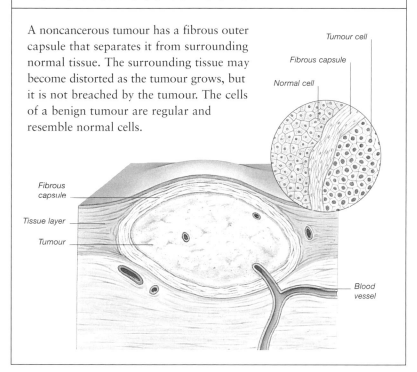

Tumour cell
Fibrous capsule
Normal cell

Fibrous capsule
Tissue layer
Tumour
Blood vessel

BREEDS AT RISK

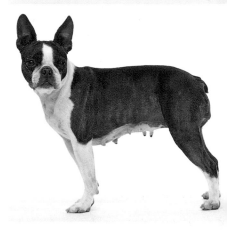

Breeds prone to mast cell tumours include:

- Boxer
- Bernese Mountain Dog
- Boston Terrier (above)
- Bulldog
- Golden Retriever (below)
- Labrador Retriever

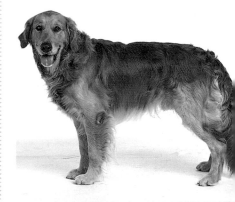

Breeds prone to melanomas include:

- Boxer
- Boston Terrier
- Scottish Terrier

Breeds prone to histiocytosis include:

- Bernese Mountain Dog

HISTIOCYTOMA

This is a benign skin tumour with a round, raised, hairless, often red appearance. Histiocytomas most often occur in young dogs between one and three years old.

DIAGNOSIS AND TREATMENT Diagnosis is by visual examination and biopsy. Some histiocytomas will shrink and eventually disappear following topical treatment with corticosteroid drugs. Most, however, need surgical removal for accurate diagnosis to differentiate them from more troublesome mast cell tumours (*see p.136*).

HISTIOCYTOSIS

Certain breeds, such as the Bernese Mountain Dog, are particularly prone to a malignant skin condition called histiocytosis. This condition occurs most commonly in dogs between three and eight years of age. An affected individual develops skin nodules; the dog also loses weight, is lethargic, and appears generally unwell.

DIAGNOSIS AND TREATMENT Diagnosis is by visual examination and biopsy. Unfortunately, histiocytosis does not respond well to chemotherapy, and the condition is usually fatal.

BASAL CELL TUMOUR

Most common around the head or neck of dogs over seven years old, these hard, raised nodules are usually benign. Some basal cell tumours, however, are malignant.

DIAGNOSIS AND TREATMENT Diagnosis is by visual examination and tissue sampling. In most cases, the entire tumour, along with a good margin of surrounding normal tissue, is removed for analysis by a pathologist. This prevents the need for further surgery should the tumour be found to be cancerous. If the tumour is difficult to remove completely, a biopsy is taken.

MAST CELL TUMOUR

While half of all mast cell tumours are benign, the rest are malignant. Frustratingly, they all look the same on the skin. These tumours usually occur in dogs over eight years old, but they may also affect younger individuals of certain breeds, notably Boxers, Labrador Retrievers, and Golden Retrievers. Mast cell tumours vary enormously in appearance. Most commonly, they look like histiocytomas (*see p.135*), being raised, red, sometimes ulcerated masses on the skin. The tumours may grow slowly or quickly.

Mast cell tumours (just like normal mast cells) produce chemicals causing inflammation, such as histamine. This may lead to symptoms such as swelling and redness, and also to more remote problems, such as stomach ulcers.

DIAGNOSIS AND TREATMENT Diagnosis is by visual examination and tissue sampling. The mast cell tumour will be surgically removed and examined by a pathologist. If it is cancerous, further treatments may include chemotherapy or immunotherapy.

Q WHY ARE OLDER DOGS MORE LIKELY TO GET CANCER?

A Dogs over seven years old are at greater risk of most types of cancer. This is in part because their cells have had more time to develop genetic damage, and in part because a dog's natural defences against cancer, particularly the cells and chemicals of the immune system, gradually become less efficient with increasing age.

Q HOW FAST DO CANCEROUS TUMOURS GROW?

A Tumour growth rates are measured by the time it takes for the number of cells to double (the "doubling time"). The doubling time of a tumour varies from about one month to two years.

SQUAMOUS CELL CARCINOMA

Squamous cell carcinomas vary enormously in appearance, from hard and flat to red and cauliflower-like. This type of tumour is malignant and is more likely to occur on lightly pigmented areas of the body, including the nail beds, nose, and lips. Squamous cell carcinomas aggressively invade surrounding tissue. Some tumours may spread to regional lymph nodes, and eventually to the lungs. Others are "low grade", or less malignant.

DIAGNOSIS AND TREATMENT Diagnosis is by visual examination and analysis of the tissue. Squamous cell carcinomas have to be surgically removed together with a large area of the surrounding normal tissue, because they have a tendency to spread. In addition to removing the tumour, the vet may take a sample of tissue from local lymph nodes in order to check for cancer cell migration. Radiotherapy at the site of removal may also be necessary.

MELANOMA

Melanomas appear as black or brown nodules and sometimes have a crusted surface. They may occur anywhere on the skin, on the lips, or in the mouth. While skin melanomas (except those around the nail beds) are usually benign, those that develop inside the mouth are more likely to be malignant. Malignant melanoma is a serious form of skin cancer that often grows rapidly and spreads both locally and to other organs in the body.

DIAGNOSIS AND TREATMENT Diagnosis is by visual examination and analysis of the tumour tissue. As for squamous cell carcinoma, surgical removal of the melanoma together with a wide area of surrounding tissue is the usual treatment. Following removal of a malignant melanoma, radiotherapy may be given at the surgical site, and at any sites to which the cancer has spread, to ensure that all the abnormal cells have been destroyed.

SKIN GROWTHS THAT RESEMBLE TUMOURS

Some skin growths look or feel like tumours but are actually distinct types of skin disorder. Veterinary surgeons can distinguish between these relatively harmless conditions and potentially dangerous skin tumours by visual examination and tissue sampling.

SEBACEOUS CYST

When a hair follicle becomes blocked, the sebaceous gland connected to that follicle cannot secrete sebum (the oily substance that these glands produce to lubricate the skin). The sebum then accumulates within the follicle rather than running out to cover the skin surface. The hair follicle becomes dry, developing a texture like cottage cheese, and grows into a dome-shaped swelling called a cyst. These cysts are common in mature Pekingese and Cocker Spaniels, among other breeds. Sebaceous cysts may become infected.

DIAGNOSIS AND TREATMENT Diagnosis is by visual examination and by viewing a sample of fluid from the cyst under a microscope. Sebaceous cysts that are causing pain or that restrict movement require surgical removal.

HAEMATOMA

A physical injury may cause a blood blister (haematoma) under the skin, and this can be mistaken for a tumour. Haematomas most commonly occur on the ear flaps, especially in Labradors and Golden Retrievers (*see p.228*).

DIAGNOSIS AND TREATMENT Large haematomas are usually drained. Some ear haematomas require surgery.

TUMOURS OF THE MALE REPRODUCTIVE SYSTEM

Tumours of the reproductive organs in male dogs are common. Testicular tumours are among the most common, and fortunately most benign, of male canine tumours.

TESTICULAR TUMOURS

These tumours are common in male dogs over seven years old, typically occurring around ten years of age. They are a particular hazard for dogs that have one or both testicles undescended (*see p.317*); such animals have almost a 50 per cent likelihood of developing a testicular tumour.

The tumours may develop in one or both testicles. There are three kinds: seminomas, interstitial cell tumours, and Sertoli cell tumours. Seminomas and interstitial cell tumours (also called Leydig cell tumours) may cause enlargement of the affected testicle or just produce a developing hardness in the testicle. Sertoli cell tumours produce the female hormone oestrogen. In addition to an enlarged or irregular testicle, dogs with these tumours may show symmetrical hair loss, mammary gland enlargement with sore teats, and a pendulous, floppy prepuce (foreskin).

Most testicular tumours are benign, but some seminomas and Sertoli cell tumours are malignant.

DIAGNOSIS AND TREATMENT Diagnosis is by physical examination of the testicles and sometimes also biopsy. Because the testicles hang from the body, surgical removal of a tumour is simple and effective, unless the testicle has not descended but has remained within the abdominal cavity. Surgery is still effective in these cases, but it has to be more invasive.

PROSTATE TUMOURS

Hypertrophy (enlargement) of the prostate gland is a common condition in unneutered male dogs over six years of age, but prostate tumours are rare in these dogs, especially in comparison to their incidence in human males. An enlarged prostate gland in a neutered (desexed) dog is, however, very likely to be due to a tumour rather than hypertrophy. Prostate gland tumours may be either benign or malignant.

DIAGNOSIS AND TREATMENT Diagnosis is by physical examination and sometimes also by imaging. Surgical removal of the prostate gland is the only treatment for tumours, and analysis of the tumour tissue is carried out afterwards to assess the degree of malignancy. Because of the location and form of the prostate, however, complete surgical removal of the gland is difficult and is associated with a known risk of subsequent urinary incontinence.

TUMOURS OF THE FEMALE REPRODUCTIVE SYSTEM

Tumours of the reproductive organs occur relatively frequently in female dogs, and mammary tumours are the most common type.

MAMMARY TUMOURS

Mammary tumours most commonly develop in females over six years old. They are often multiple, occurring near one or more of the bitch's ten or twelve teats. About half are malignant. Most mammary tumours, whether benign or malignant, are painless, mobile masses. Some bitches, however, develop an invasive, painful inflammatory form of breast cancer, often in the glands that are closest to the groin. This form of cancer is very difficult to differentiate from an acute bacterial infection (*see p.325*). Malignant breast cancer tends to spread locally to nearby lymph nodes, and sometimes also more widely, especially to the lungs.

DIAGNOSIS AND TREATMENT Mammary tumours can usually be felt under the skin. If you feel a lump in your dog's breast tissue, do not delay. See your veterinary surgeon as soon as you can.

RISK FACTORS INFLUENCING MAMMARY TUMOURS

Spaying is the single most important factor influencing the risk of a bitch developing mammary tumours. An unspayed female has a one in four chance of developing a mammary tumour. This risk is eliminated if a bitch is spayed before her first season. Even spaying after one season reduces the risk of mammary tumours by over 90 per cent.

Breeds prone to mammary tumours include:

- Dachshund
- Poodles
- Boston Terrier
- Spaniels
- Retrievers

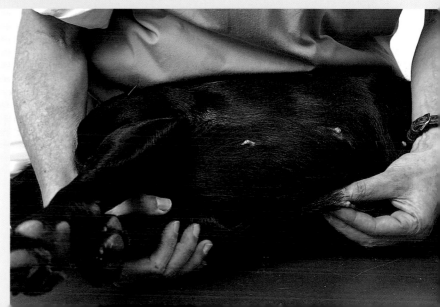

Breast lumps, together with some surrounding normal tissue, are always surgically removed and examined by a pathologist. Because breast cancer spreads, chest X-rays are taken before breast surgery to determine the extent of the cancer. Surgery offers a high cure rate for benign tumours, a moderate rate for malignant tumours less than 2cm (¾in) in diameter, but a poor rate for large or inflammatory forms of breast cancer. When surgery is not practical due to poor health of the dog or the extent of cancer spread, chemotherapy or immunotherapy may enhance an individual's quality of life as part of palliative care.

The best prevention for mammary tumours is spaying (see p.137). If a bitch has not been spayed at the time

of surgery to remove a mammary tumour, this procedure should also be done to prevent recurrence, although spaying at this stage will not increase the likelihood of a cure if the tumour is found to be malignant.

VAGINAL TUMOURS

Vaginal tumours are uncommon in bitches, but are most likely to occur in unspayed individuals over ten years old. Most are benign, being lipomas (see p.134) or leiomyomas (tumours arising from smooth muscle tissue), but some may be malignant: these include leiomyosarcomas, mast cell tumours, and squamous cell carcinomas (see p.136). Vaginal bleeding or discharge, excessive licking of the vulval area, or a visible mass inside the vulva are signs of a tumour.

DIAGNOSIS AND TREATMENT Diagnosis of vaginal tumours is by physical examination and sometimes also biopsy. Surgical removal is the usual treatment and is successful in most cases.

OVARIAN TUMOURS

Ovarian tumours are rare in bitches. Most cause no signs.

DIAGNOSIS AND TREATMENT Most ovarian tumours are diagnosed during routine ovariohysterectomy operations (see p.316) in older animals. More common are ovarian cysts, which may also be detected at the time of surgery.

TRANSMISSIBLE VENEREAL TUMOUR

This rare type of tumour is transmitted during mating. Cauliflower-like growths may develop on the penis or in the vagina or vulva.

DIAGNOSIS AND TREATMENT Diagnosis is by physical examination. Weekly treatment for up to six weeks with the chemotherapeutic drug vincristine sulphate usually produces a cure. Radiotherapy is another possible and effective form of treatment.

BONE TUMOURS

The most common bone tumours are malignant, quickly spreading from the affected bone to the lungs. Malignant bone cancer is very rare in small dogs. It is more common in moderate-sized breeds such as Boxers, and the risk increases further in larger breeds.

OSTEOSARCOMAS

Osteosarcomas most commonly occur in the long bones of the legs; less frequently, they arise in the jaw or in the ribs. These tumours, which cause the dog pain when pressed, are often diagnosed in mature dogs that develop lameness with no history of an injury to the affected leg.

DIAGNOSIS AND TREATMENT A simple X-ray usually enables a diagnosis. The most common treatment is amputation one joint above the affected bone. This may be done if the lungs are free of cancer, and if you and your vet have determined that your dog will not have too much difficulty walking on three legs. In general, the younger the dog and the smaller the breed, the better the chance that the dog will recover mobility after amputation surgery. Although limb-sparing surgical techniques to treat osteosarcoma have been developed, these are not routinely available at present.

CHRONDROSARCOMAS

These malignant tumours are relatively painless swellings involving cartilage tissue. Chondrosarcomas occur most commonly in the nose, ribs, and hips, although they may also develop in the cartilage of the limbs.

DIAGNOSIS AND TREATMENT Diagnosis is by X-ray of the affected area and biopsy of the tumour. Surgical removal is the preferred treatment, but may not be possible, depending on the location of the chrondrosarcoma. In these cases, radiotherapy may prolong life, but it does not provide a cure.

Q **CAN A DOG LEARN TO WALK AGAIN AFTER AMPUTATION OF A LIMB TO REMOVE A TUMOUR?**

A Watch any lightweight dog with a severe lameness and it will be obvious that it gets around well on three legs. Mobility problems are more likely to occur in heavy or older individuals.

Dogs normally carry more weight on their front legs than on their hind legs. All but the very largest individuals easily cope with the loss of a hind leg due to a tumour or an accident. Healthy, well-muscled dogs often regain excellent mobility even if they lose a front leg to amputation. Unfortunately, however, tumours such as osteosarcomas are most common in the forelegs of older individuals belonging to the giant breeds. Before amputation surgery is undertaken, you should take into consideration the chance of recovery of mobility after the amputation and the long-term welfare of your dog. Your vet will be able to advise you of the best course of action.

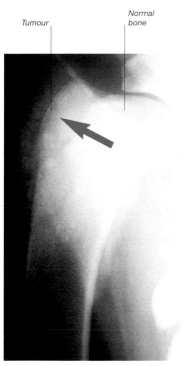

Tumour / Normal bone

X-RAY OF AN OSTEOSARCOMA
This X-ray of the top of the humerus shows proliferation of calcified tissue outside the normal contour of the bone.

OSTEOCHONDROMAS AND OSTEOMAS

Osteomas and osteochondromas are both types of benign tumour that form as hard masses in bone tissue. These tumours are uncommon, and most often occur in younger dogs.

DIAGNOSIS AND TREATMENT These tumours are diagnosed by X-ray or bone biopsy. Surgery is necessary only if the mass is causing pain or is restricting mobility.

SOFT TISSUE TUMOURS

There is an unpleasant variety of tumours that may occur anywhere in any soft tissue of the body, such as organs, blood vessels, and lymphatic tissue. These tumours may be benign or malignant. Malignant soft tissue tumours are called sarcomas.

WIDESPREAD SOFT TISSUE TUMOURS

These tumours are classified according to the type of soft tissue from which they arise. Benign fibromas develop from fibrous connective tissue, as do malignant fibrosarcomas (which are more common in dogs than fibromas). Benign haemangiomas develop from the lining of blood vessels and occur most frequently in the spleen, while malignant haemangiosarcomas may occur in the spleen, heart, liver, and skin. Other types of sarcoma include haemangiopericytomas, arising from the tissue that surrounds blood vessels, and Schwannomas, arising from cells in the sheaths covering nerve fibres. Lymphomas and lymphosarcomas, which are both cancerous, develop from lymphatic tissue.

Certain forms of cancerous soft tissue tumour, including some types of lymphoma, are highly malignant. Cells from these tumours spread rapidly to other organs of the body, most frequently to the lungs or the liver.

DIAGNOSIS AND TREATMENT Soft tissue tumours are diagnosed by physical examination, biopsy, and sometimes also imaging techniques. Surgical removal is always the treatment of choice. This is curative when the tumour is benign, as in the case of a haemangioma of the spleen. Malignant soft tissue tumours are usually treated with a combination of surgery, radiotherapy, and chemotherapy.

The prognosis depends upon the location of the tumour and the stage the tumour has reached. The outlook is poor for dogs with cancer that has spread around the body, but palliative therapy can provide pain relief in these circumstances.

TUMOURS IN THE LUNGS

Primary lung cancer (lung cancer that originates in the lungs) is rare in dogs, especially as compared to its incidence in humans. The most obvious reason for this is that dogs do not smoke!

BREEDS AT RISK

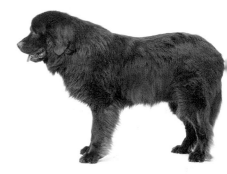

Giant breeds are most at risk of developing malignant bone cancer. Genetic factors are thought to play a part in this breed predisposition, but the exact mechanism of genetic susceptibility is not known. Tumours most often develop in the bones of the front legs, and, as with many other cancers, older individuals are most commonly affected.

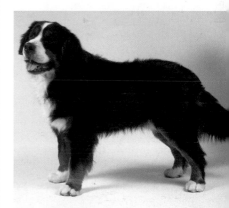

Breeds with a high incidence include:

- Rottweiler
- Bernese Mountain Dog (above)
- Pyrenean Mountain Dog
- Newfoundland (top)
- Great Dane
- Irish Wolfhound

Unfortunately, secondary lung cancer, spreading either from bone tumours (*see p.138*) or from other soft tissue, is relatively common.

DIAGNOSIS AND TREATMENT X-rays of the chest sometimes enable diagnosis, although exploratory surgery may also be necessary. Whenever a malignant tumour is discovered elsewhere in the body, the chest is usually X-rayed as well, to determine whether the cancer has spread to affect either the lungs or the lymph nodes in the chest.

If the cancer has spread to the lungs, the outlook is poor; there is no curative treatment for lung cancer in dogs. Palliative therapies may be helpful in improving the animal's quality of life, but it is likely that the vet will suggest euthanasia in these circumstances.

TUMOURS IN THE HEART

Tumours developing in the heart tissue are uncommon and occur mostly in middle-aged and older dogs. They may be either benign or malignant.

Depending on its location in the heart, the tumour may cause a build-up of fluid in the chest cavity, and thus interfere with breathing (*see p.243*), or it may interrupt the blood supply from the liver to the heart (*see p.292*), causing the liver to enlarge and eventually leading to a fluid build-up in the abdominal cavity. Both of these conditions are life-threatening and often present a greater immediate threat to health than the potential malignancy of the tumour.

DIAGNOSIS AND TREATMENT X-rays of the chest are sometimes diagnostic, although exploratory surgery may also be necessary. Surgical removal of a heart tumour is often effective.

TUMOURS IN THE SPLEEN AND LIVER

Tumours may develop in any of the organs within the abdomen, such as the spleen and the liver. Spleen tumours are more common in large breeds, especially the German Shepherd and the retrievers. These tumours tend to be symptomless in the early stages. As a result, they may reach a large size before being diagnosed, and they are often discovered only when affected dogs become depressed and lethargic as the tumours start to bleed.

Tumours may arise in the liver (primary liver tumours), but this organ is also a common site for secondary tumours, which spread from a cancer originating elsewhere in the body.

DIAGNOSIS AND TREATMENT Diagnosis is by physical examination, analysis of blood samples, X-rays, and ultrasound scanning. Removing the spleen cures benign tumours (haemangiomas), but malignant ones (haemangiosarcomas) may already have spread by the time of diagnosis, most commonly to the liver. Tumours affecting only one lobe of the liver may be surgically removed; more extensive liver tumours have a graver prognosis.

TUMOURS IN THE DIGESTIVE TRACT

The most common types of digestive tract tumour are adenocarcinomas, lymphomas, and lymphosarcomas. The typical signs of such tumours include loss of appetite, vomiting, diarrhoea, and straining to defaecate.

DIAGNOSIS AND TREATMENT Imaging techniques are used in diagnosis, but exploratory surgery may also be necessary. The affected section of the digestive tract, and its associated lymph nodes, are surgically removed. Chemotherapy prolongs remission.

NUTRITIONAL THERAPY FOR SOFT TISSUE CANCERS

Nutritional therapy may be of value in combatting certain cancers, particularly lymphomas and lymphosarcomas (*see p.141*). Dogs suffering from cancer need plenty of vitamins and minerals, which should be obtained in the diet or in some cases through nutritional supplements. The use of antioxidants, such as vitamins A, C, and E and the mineral selenium, is slightly problematic, however. No doubt antioxidants help to keep body cells healthy, but their nourishing value may help to keep cancer cells healthy as well. Discuss the value of nutritional supplements with your veterinary surgeon or cancer specialist.

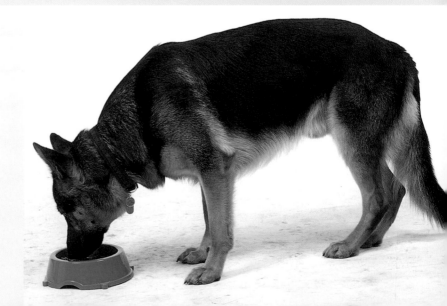

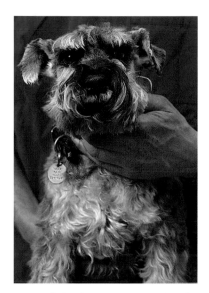

FEELING SWOLLEN LYMPH NODES
This dog has enlarged lymph nodes in the neck. The vet is gently feeling the neck, trying to ascertain whether the swelling is caused by a tumour.

TUMOURS IN THE URINARY TRACT

Within the urinary system, tumours at the neck of the bladder are more common than kidney tumours. All types of urinary tract tumour occur most frequently in older dogs. The first sign of a tumour is often blood-tinged urine. Bladder tumours may cause straining to urinate.

DIAGNOSIS AND TREATMENT Diagnosis is by imaging and sometimes also exploratory surgery. While an affected kidney may be surgically removed, surgical correction for bladder cancer is more problematic.

LYMPHATIC TUMOURS

Lymphoma and lymphosarcoma are cancers that develop from lymphatic tissue. This tissue is mainly located in the lymph nodes, but is also present in certain organs and other body structures, including the bone marrow, liver, spleen, intestines, and skin.

Lymphatic tumours most often occur in dogs over seven years old. The first sign of illness is often a swelling at a single lymph node located in the neck, armpit, groin, or hind leg. Involvement of lymph nodes in the chest leads to breathing difficulties. Intestinal involvement causes loss of appetite and gastrointestinal symptoms. Skin lymphoma mimics a variety of less severe skin diseases.

DIAGNOSIS AND TREATMENT A diagnosis is made by examining a sample of fluid collected from the tumour. While only one lymph node may be enlarged, in most dogs the disease has become more widespread by the time of diagnosis.

The affected lymph node is surgically removed. Blood counts and bone marrow biopsy indicate whether the tumour has spread. Chemotherapy may produce a prolonged, sometimes even permanent, remission in small individuals, but this treatment is less effective in larger dogs.

There is evidence that some cancer cells, particularly those in lymphomas and lymphosarcomas, thrive on carbohydrates. Some nutritionists advise avoiding a carbohydrate-rich diet and recommend a high-fat diet instead. This type of diet is both tasty and energy-dense. Fed on a long-term basis, it may "starve" certain cancer cells that cannot use fats for energy.

LEUKAEMIA

Leukaemia is a broad name for any cancer in which there is a disorganized proliferation of white blood cells. All forms of leukaemia are rare in dogs. When the disorder does occur, the signs are non-specific, such as weight loss, lethargy, and anaemia (*see p.256*).

DIAGNOSIS AND TREATMENT Diagnosis is made from blood or bone marrow samples. Chemotherapy usually results in at least a temporary remission.

Q **ARE COMPLEMENTARY THERAPIES EFFECTIVE IN CANCER TREATMENT?**

A No known complementary therapy cures any form of cancer. It does no harm, however, and may be beneficial for some dogs if, through diet and physical contact therapies, you can improve nutrition and your dog's sense of well-being.

Q **DOES A DOG'S EMOTIONAL STATE INFLUENCE RECOVERY?**

A There is now fascinating evidence that for people with cancer, a positive feeling or a feeling of well-being prolongs survival time. In one study, churchgoers survived longer than non-churchgoers of the same age and social and economic status, and with the same forms of cancer. Some may attribute this to divine intervention. Others will say that prolonged survival is a result of belief or contentment. In any social species, including dogs, touch has a powerful effect. If your dog has any form of cancer and enjoys physical contact with you and your family, indulge it. In some as yet undefined way you may be helping your dog's body fight the cancer.

Q **IS CANCER TREATMENT PAINFUL FOR A DOG?**

A Surgery is normally carried out using some form of anaesthesia to prevent pain. Other treatments, such as radiotherapy, may cause some pain, and chemotherapy may produce side effects. Your vet will administer drugs to help control any pain or side effects. In some cases, however, it may be best not to put your dog through painful treatments in the hope of a cure for the cancer, but rather to make the most of the time for which it can live comfortably.

INFECTIOUS DISEASES
viruses, bacteria, and fungi

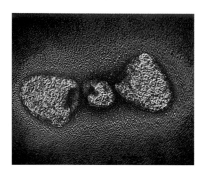

Rabies virus particles

A variety of infectious agents, such as viruses, bacteria, and fungi, cause illnesses in dogs; these tiny organisms are commonly called microbes or germs. A healthy dog's natural physical defences may be able to destroy harmful organisms, but a very young or old dog, or one that is already ill, may be at greater risk of disease. Some infectious diseases can be prevented simply with good hygiene, or by avoiding areas in which diseases are known to occur. Others, however, require veterinary aid to prevent or treat them.

Viruses are nature's smallest and most efficient parasites. They cannot survive for long, or multiply, outside living cells; a virus has to invade a cell and take over that cell's genetic apparatus before it can multiply. Some types of virus cause little damage to their "host" cells, but others are powerfully destructive, wiping out the cells in which they multiply.

Q ARE THERE TREATMENTS FOR VIRAL INFECTIONS?

A In human medicine there are drugs for HIV and human herpesviruses. For dogs, however, there are drugs to kill bacteria and fungi, but none to kill viruses.

Q CAN DOGS CONTRACT MAD COW DISEASE?

A Probably not. Mad Cow Disease (BSE) is caused by a malformed protein called a prion. Eating infected beef has led to "new variant" Creutzfeldt–Jakob Disease (nvCJD) in some people and Feline Spongiform Encephalopathy (FSE) in some cats, but there are no reported cases of prion disease in dogs or other canines.

Like all living cells, a bacterium consists of genetic material and a cell wall. Most bacteria multiply simply by dividing in two once they reach a certain size. A unique type of extremely small bacteria are called rickettsiae; unlike all other bacteria, these germs can only multiply inside living cells.

Fungi are involved in decomposing the remains of other organisms. They usually exist as multi-celled, thread-like mould, but can also live in a single-celled yeast form. Yeasts multiply by forming bud-like spores. Under certain conditions, some yeast-like fungi are pathogenic (able to cause disease).

Most canine bacterial and fungal infections respond to antibiotic drugs, but there are no drugs to treat viral infections; an infected dog's recovery depends on its body's ability to contain or destroy the germ. Most serious viral infections can, however, be prevented with vaccines. Certain vaccines are also available to prevent or alleviate some common bacterial infections.

HOW A VACCINE WORKS

A vaccine harnesses the body's natural ability to defend itself. Vaccination, or immunization, stimulates an immune response that will protect a dog from the natural form of a disease.

Vaccine manufacturers use three types of material: dead pathogens; living ones that have been modified so that they do not cause clinical illness; or harmless bacteria that are genetically engineered to manufacture bits of virus particle and thereby stimulate the body to produce antibodies against a virus. These modified microbes, or parts of microbes, are introduced into the body as a vaccine. Most are given by injection; some, such as the Bordetella vaccine to prevent kennel cough, are given by aerosol in the nose.

EFFECTIVE VACCINATIONS

Vaccinations against viral diseases are usually effective. Canine hepatitis virus and canine distemper, for example, were once both killers but are now rare wherever efficient vaccination programmes have been routinely used.

Vaccination is effective if a virus exists in a single "form". Some viruses, however, such as those causing human flu and canine parvovirus, can modify their form by changing the structure of their protein coat. A vaccine may be effective against one form but not another. Not all vaccines are equally effective. Neither is every vaccine against a specific virus similar; some offer longer-term protection than others.

GERMS THAT INFECT DOGS

Germs are microorganisms that cause disease. There are three principal types. Bacteria are single-celled organisms that can exploit all kinds of environment. Most live in harmonious co-existence with their hosts, but some, called pathogenic bacteria, cause disease. Fungi usually exist in the environment as multi-celled moulds, but may also live in the body as single-celled yeasts. Viruses are the smallest infectious agents; a virus is basically no more than a package of genetic material (either DNA or RNA) encapsulated in a protective protein coat. The six types of microscopic pathogens that may infect dogs are shown below.

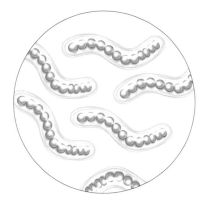

STREPTOCOCCI

Some of these bacteria cause pus-forming infections and, in humans, are responsible for diseases such as tonsillitis, scarlet fever and "strep throat". Other streptococci form part of the normal flora on a dog's skin and superficial mucous membranes.

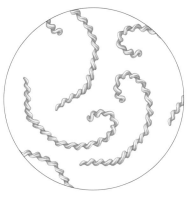

LEPTOSPIRA

These bacteria are spirochetes; they are shaped like spiral threads. Leptospira often contaminate water found near livestock and areas where wild rodents live. In dogs, they cause a disease called leptospirosis (*see p.151*) that affects the kidneys.

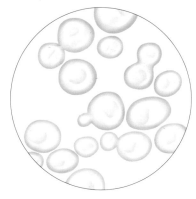

BLASTOMYCES

The spores of this fungus are found in parts of the United States, where they cause blastomycosis (*see p.157*) in dogs. They are often found associated with soil that is not exposed to direct sunlight and is rich in rotting debris and bird droppings.

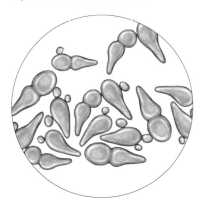

MYCOPLASMA

These organisms are an unusual type of bacteria that form part of the normal flora of a dog's body. When conditions permit, they occasionally become pathogenic, causing an infection resembling pneumonia or an infection of the urinary tract.

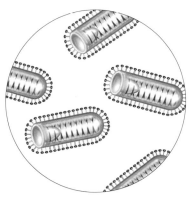

RHABDOVIRUS

These germs are bullet-shaped viruses, one of which is responsible for causing rabies (*see p.144*) in dogs. They contain RNA and have an outer coat of protein, which makes them vulnerable to many detergents, soaps, and solutions of disinfectant.

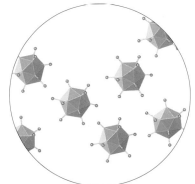

ADENOVIRUS

Adenoviruses are 20-sided particles. One type causes infectious canine hepatitis. They contain DNA but are not coated with protein; as a result, they are resistant to soaps and detergents. They are, however, vulnerable to iodine and bleach.

VIRAL DISEASES

Viruses are inert when existing in the environment, but they need to invade living things in order to reproduce and multiply. Most viral infections do not create symptoms in the host animal because they are easily destroyed by the host's immune system, but some kill the cells that they invade and produce a disease or illness that manifests as clinical symptoms. Antibiotics have no effect on viruses, but vaccination prior to infection by a virus will stimulate the immune system to defend the host successfully against the disease.

RABIES

This is an invariably fatal viral disease of carnivores and bats, and exists on every continent except Antarctica and Australia. Vaccinations have reduced the incidence in many developed countries, but rabies remains prevalent in many developing nations, where dogs are important carriers.

Specific wild carnivores in different parts of the world play a primary role as transmitters of rabies and reservoirs of the disease: foxes in Europe, skunks and raccoons in the United States, and the mongoose in southern Africa. Bats do the same in Latin America.

Rabies is caused by a rhabdovirus (*see p.143*). This microorganism is transmitted in contaminated saliva, usually through bites but sometimes through licking. The saliva of a rabid dog is teeming with viruses – it is often turned into a froth because of the dog's increased rate of respiration.

The rabies virus follows a cycle (*see left*), working its way from the entry site through the nervous system to the spinal cord and finally to the brain. From here the virus moves on, via the nervous system, to the salivary glands in particular, but also to the digestive system and the lungs. The time that elapses between a bite and the first manifestation of the disease can be as little as a week or as long as a year, depending on how long the virus remains in the muscle where the bite has occurred. One of the worrying aspects of rabies is that the saliva may be infected with the virus for as long as two weeks before the animal shows any signs of infection.

Rabies may initially cause little more than a limp. More commonly, the first signs are mild changes in the dog's behaviour. Usually affectionate animals may become irritable and reclusive, while nervous dogs may become more outgoing.

Rabies manifests itself in two forms, with most individuals having mixed clinical signs of both. In the paralytic, or "dumb", form of the disease, an affected dog finds it difficult to move. In addition, paralysis of the throat muscles prevents swallowing, leading to drooling saliva.

In the more excitable form, known as "furious" rabies, a dog becomes irrationally aggressive, showing no fear. An excessive sensitivity to light is fairly common. (Dogs do not seem to experience a fear of water, from which humans with rabies commonly suffer.) The furious stage may last for up to a week. It usually gives way to a final paralytic stage, which lasts for a couple of days, followed by death.

THE RABIES CYCLE

Rabies virus travels from the site of the wound via the nerves to the brain, where it causes inflammation (encephalitis). The journey may take two to eight weeks, or even longer when the bite is in an area distant from the brain. The virus then travels via the nerves to the salivary glands, where it concentrates, ready to spread through bites to other animals. Clinical signs of rabies may develop within a week of exposure, but in some individuals it has taken a year after a bite before changes in behaviour have occurred.

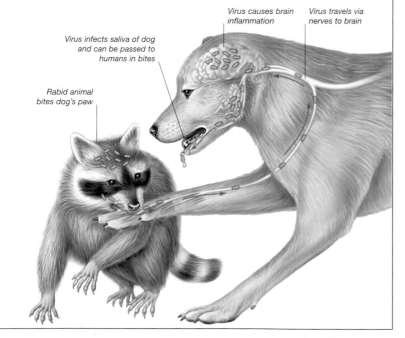

Virus causes brain inflammation

Virus travels via nerves to brain

Virus infects saliva of dog and can be passed to humans in bites

Rabid animal bites dog's paw

DIAGNOSIS Clinical signs may suggest rabies, but a conclusive diagnosis of the disease depends entirely on microscopic examination of the brain tissue. Accurate diagnosis is essential because of the hazard to people in contact with a potentially rabid dog.

TREATMENT There is no effective means of treating an infected dog. A human being who has been exposed to, or bitten by, a suspected or known rabid dog needs immediate attention. Flush and clean the bite wound with soap and water or disinfectant – this measure can kill some of the viruses and gain valuable time before the (now painless) rabies antiserum can be administered.

PREVENTION All dogs (and cats and ferrets) living in regions where rabies is endemic should be routinely vaccinated against the disease. Dogs should be given booster vaccinations according to the manufacturer's recommendations (usually every two to three years) or to comply with local laws.

ADVICE If your dog has been bitten by an animal that you either know or suspect is rabid, then take the following precautions.

If your dog has been vaccinated, put on rubber gloves, then thoroughly and immediately clean the bite wound with soap and water. Your vet will administer a booster vaccination. Keep your dog under close observation at home for at least 45 days, reporting any suspicious symptoms to your vet.

If your dog (or cat or ferret) has never been vaccinated against rabies, contact your local health department and arrange quarantine kennelling for six months. Your pet will be vaccinated one month before release. If a six-month period of quarantine is not a practical option, euthanasia is the recommended alternative.

PSEUDORABIES

This very rare disease is caused by a herpesvirus. It produces clinical signs similar to rabies – hence its name. It is also called Aujesky's disease or, more colloquially, mad itch. Humans are not susceptible to this infection but all of our domesticated species are possible hosts. Pigs are the main reservoir for the virus, but they rarely show any symptoms or die from the disease.

Dogs contract pseudorabies by eating raw pork that has been infected with the herpesvirus. As with rabies, the virus travels along the nerves to the brain – in this case, from the mouth and tonsils. Infected dogs suffer an intense itching of the head and madly scratch themselves in their search for relief. Death invariably occurs within a few days of infection.

DIAGNOSIS AND TREATMENT Clinical signs and history are the best basis for diagnosis. After death, the virus can be identified from brain and tonsil tissue. There is no effective treatment.

PREVENTION Never feed raw butcher's pork waste to your dog. This is the best way of avoiding the disease and preventing its spread.

PARVOVIRUS

Parvovirus was first recognized in North America, Europe, and Australia in 1978, after an outbreak of gastrointestinal haemorrhaging occurred in domestic dogs. No canine blood sample prior to 1976 has antibodies to the virus; this fact suggests that 1976 is the year when the disease first appeared. Current research at Cornell University suggests that canine parvovirus arose as a mutation either of feline parvovirus or of a related form of parvovirus occurring in foxes.

Known as canine parvovirus type 2 (CPV-2), the virus is extremely tough, capable of surviving outside a dog for almost six months. It is resistant to soaps, detergents, and disinfectants, but not to chlorine bleaches.

The virus is spread in contaminated faeces. It enters its victim via the mouth, when the animal does something as simple as licking its foot pads. Young pups, under 16 weeks of age, are prone to the most serious forms of parvovirus infection.

TAKING DOGS TO RABIES-FREE COUNTRIES

Historically, dogs entering rabies-free countries such as Australia, New Zealand, Japan, the United Kingdom, Ireland, Norway, Sweden, and the State of Hawaii had to go into quarantine, usually for 4 to 12 months, to prevent rabies from entering the country and infecting wildlife. In 1996, Sweden and Norway replaced quarantine for some dogs by microchip identification, vaccination, and a follow-up blood sample to confirm a high level of protection. In 2000, the UK set up a Pet Travel Scheme (PETS); this scheme now includes other countries, including Australia.

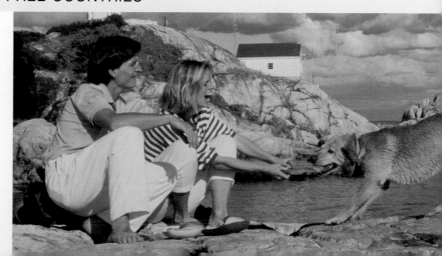

The virus penetrates the tonsils. It then progresses, via the lymph system and the bloodstream, to the lining of the intestines, as well as the bone marrow, lymph nodes, and thymus gland – areas where the body cells multiply rapidly. In severe cases, the results include abdominal pain; lethargy; occasionally fever; vomiting; and diarrhoea, which is sometimes bloody. Clinical shock induced by viral damage can cause death if a dog is not treated efficiently. Other individuals have milder signs, such as loose, bulky stools. When the disease first appeared many pups died suddenly of heart failure, but this occurrence is now extremely rare.

GAINING IMMUNITY

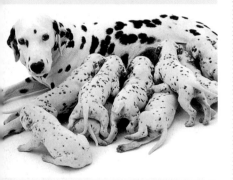

Young pups are most at risk from any infection, but they do inherit immunity against diseases to which their mother has been exposed (see pp.120–29). This immunity comes in the form of maternal antibodies, which are passed in the first milk that is suckled. Such acquired protection gradually fades and disappears almost completely by, at the latest, 12 weeks of age. Eventually, a dog will generate its own protection when its white blood cells learn how to produce antibodies. They do so when exposed to specific infectious agents – whether a virus, bacterium, or fungus. They also do so when exposed to the modified infectious agents used in vaccines.

DIAGNOSIS A diagnosis is based on history and symptoms, and confirmed by identifying virus particles or virus antigens in a stool sample analysed at a local laboratory. There is a simple antibody blood test that your vet can perform, but false negative results are common due to maternal antibodies or antibodies from vaccination. Depressed white blood cell counts occur in about one-third of affected individuals.

TREATMENT Shock control is vital, as are pain control and the prevention of dehydration (caused by the massive fluid loss during diarrhoea). Antibiotics are often used to prevent a secondary bacterial infection entering the bloodstream from the damaged intestines.

PREVENTION With effective veterinary intervention, most dogs should survive a parvovirus infection. They will then have lifelong immunity to the disease. New strains of parvovirus, however, are constantly evolving.

Vaccination gives very good but not necessarily full protection against the disease; the level of protection depends on the virus strains that are used by the vaccine manufacturer. In addition, the antibodies that young pups inherit from their mothers are particularly troublesome in preventing effective parvovirus vaccination. With early types of vaccine, the maternal antibodies would destroy the virus in the vaccine. Further inoculations were necessary until the pups reached over 16 weeks of age, or sometimes for longer, until the maternal antibodies disappeared and the vaccine could become effective. Recent types of vaccine, in contrast, are efficient at combating maternal antibodies. One European manufacturer, Intervet, produces a vaccine that gives full protection with a final inoculation at 10 weeks of age.

If it is left alone, parvovirus can contaminate an environment for some months. The virus can, however, be killed by cleaning. It is resistant to many household cleaners but not to bleach. If your dog has had a parvovirus

infection, clean any areas contaminated by its faeces with a solution of one part bleach to 16 parts hot water. Apply the solution to the area for 15 minutes, then rinse with clean water.

CORONAVIRUS ENTERITIS

This is a gastrointestinal infection caused by canine coronavirus (CCV). The virus was discovered, almost by accident, when canine parvovirus spread worldwide in the late 1970s.

Dogs of all ages and breeds can pick up the infection from other animals or their faeces. In most cases the infection is "subclinical", causing no signs of illness. Young dogs are more likely to develop the clinical disease; the signs include vomiting, diarrhoea, and lethargy lasting for a week to ten days.

DIAGNOSIS A diagnosis is usually based on clinical signs; in addition, the virus can be identified by microscopic examination of stool samples.

TREATMENT Supportive treatment with electrolyte fluids to combat fluid loss is usually all that is necessary. A vaccine is available in the US, but its cost and limited value may not justify its use.

ROTAVIRUS ENTERITIS

Rotaviruses cause diarrhoeal infections in many animal species, including dogs, cats, humans, pigs, cows, and horses. Canine rotavirus infections, like those of the canine coronavirus, are usually subclinical. They cause symptoms of mild gastroenteritis, such as diarrhoea and dehydration, in some pups under two weeks old.

DIAGNOSIS AND TREATMENT No reliable techniques have been discovered for diagnosing canine rotavirus. Supportive treatment with electrolyte fluids is usually all that is necessary.

FADING PUPPY SYNDROME

Pups under four weeks "fade" or die suddenly. These "faders" show several clinical signs: they stop feeding, cry, are lethargic, show discomfort when touched, and may have a nasal

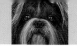

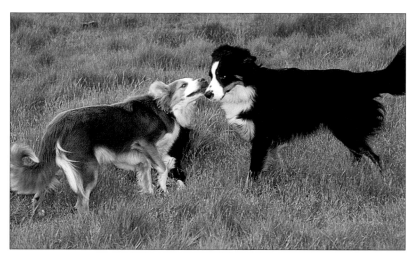

FROM ONE DOG TO ANOTHER
Dogs are naturally inquisitive. They like to explore sounds and smells and, with a great deal of licking and sniffing, to check out other dogs. These harmless investigations provide an opportunity for pathogens to be transmitted from one dog to another.

discharge. In contrast, infections at five weeks of age or older cause, at most, a mild nasal inflammation (rhinitis). Of the many causes of "fading puppy syndrome", canine herpesvirus (CHV) is perhaps the most important. Studies of CHV antibodies reveal that the infection is common in many countries.

DIAGNOSIS AND TREATMENT Fading Puppy Syndrome is confirmed either by isolating the herpesvirus or by post-mortem findings. At present there is little that can be done either to treat infected pups or to prevent infection.

PREVENTION Experimental vaccines have not been completely effective. Herpesviruses (such as the human cold sore herpesvirus) remain dormant in carriers and are activated by stresses such as pregnancy. This virus should be considered whenever there are multiple deaths in young litters.

DISTEMPER
This disease is under control in most of North America, Western Europe, and Australia, but is still a leading cause of death in dogs worldwide.

Clinical signs vary, but they often develop from an initial fever, lethargy, and runny eyes and nose to vomiting, diarrhoea, dehydration, coughing, and a sticky yellow eye and nose discharge. With antibiotics many affected dogs improve, but then several weeks later encephalitis (brain inflammation) occurs, causing convulsions, confusion, and irrational behaviour such as constant chewing. Some dogs go blind.

Pups that survive distemper infection develop mottled adult teeth. Some survivors may also have intermittent, painful, spasmic muscle jerks known as myoclonus; this jerking may initially happen while the dog is sleeping or relaxing, but later it may occur at any time. Affected dogs often whimper or cry. Although the muscle spasms may occur throughout life, they become less severe with time.

Hardpad is another name for distemper. The virus attacks the skin on the nose and footpads, causing thickening and cracking. Although this form of distemper was common until the early 1970s, it is rarely seen today in North America or Western Europe.

DIAGNOSIS A diagnosis is usually based on clinical signs. Sometimes, analysis of spinal fluid is also carried out.

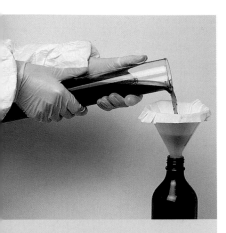

Q DO HOMEOPATHIC NOSODES OFFER ANY PROTECTION AGAINST VIRUSES?

A Nosodes are homeopathic medicines containing disease organisms. The evidence is that nosodes offer no protection. In one study, carried out by Professor Ronald Shultz at the University of Wisconsin's School of Veterinary Medicine, dogs were given nosodes for parvovirus prepared by a well-known homeopathic pharmacy. The nosodes were produced using diarrhoea from dogs with clinical parvovirus. When the treated dogs were later exposed to parvovirus, all of them contracted serious disease.

Q DO VIRUSES CAUSE LYMPHOID CANCERS IN DOGS AS THEY DO IN CATS?

A Lymphomas in cats, and in cattle, are caused by a group of viruses called retroviruses. Although particles that look like retroviruses have been seen in tissue from dogs, there is still no evidence that canine lymphomas, lymphosarcomas, or leukaemias are caused by a virus infection.

TREATMENT A range of treatments are usually necessary to counteract various elements of distemper. Antibiotics are used to control opportunist bacteria or prevent them from causing secondary infection. Fluid therapy is given to control the dehydration, and anti-nausea drugs are administered to stop vomiting. Anticonvulsants, sedatives, and painkillers are needed for dogs that develop neurological signs.

The success of the treatment will depend on how effectively the dog (usually a pup) mounts its own immune system response. This factor, in turn, is influenced by the general health and nourishment of the individual.

PREVENTION Breeding females should be vaccinated against canine distemper virus two weeks before mating, to ensure that they can provide high levels of protective maternal antibodies for their pups. The pups should be vaccinated one or more times between eight and 12 weeks of age, depending on the local risk of infection.

To protect the home, household detergents and disinfectants are usually enough to deactivate the virus and decontaminate areas that have been occupied by an infected dog.

INFECTIOUS CANINE HEPATITIS

This now rare disease was formerly often confused with canine distemper. It is caused by an adenovirus called canine adenovirus type 1 (CAV-1). This virus occurs worldwide and is a close relative of CAV-2, one of the viral causes of kennel cough (*see below*).

Infectious canine hepatitis occurs most frequently in unvaccinated dogs under one year of age. Many dogs develop CAV-1 antibodies by the age of two years, and subsequently the disease is rarely fatal.

The virus is transmitted by contact between dogs and enters the lymphatic system – and eventually the blood – through the tonsils. It targets the liver, the kidneys, the inner lining of the

blood vessels, and the eyes. Within a week, the dog's antibodies have done their work and the virus remains only in the eye and in the kidneys, from where it is excreted in the urine.

Many, if not most dogs, experience an infection with only a one-day fever. Young pups under six weeks old may suffer acute abdominal pain and die of shock within a day. Death is so rapid that owners sometimes think their pups have been poisoned. Older dogs have a high fever and abdominal pain, and produce bloody vomit and diarrhoea. Some become overly sensitive to light.

Dogs that recover from the infection often develop clouding of the cornea, causing so-called "blue eye", which takes a few weeks to clear.

DIAGNOSIS The diagnosis depends on symptoms and a medical history of no vaccination. Occasionally, serology (analysis of the fluid in blood) or biopsy (examination of a tissue sample) is carried out to confirm the diagnosis.

TREATMENT In the absence of a cure, effective treatment for the hepatitis depends on the quick and efficient control of pain and shock. Fluid replacement is vital. Antibiotics may be used to prevent bacteria from causing a secondary infection.

PREVENTION The first vaccines, based on CAV-1, protected against the virus but occasionally caused "blue eye". At present, all modified-live hepatitis vaccines are produced from CAV-2. They cross-protect against infectious canine hepatitis and kennel cough without initiating "blue eye".

The virus is resistant to common household detergents and disinfectants. It may, however, be deactivated with solutions of iodine or chlorine bleach, diluted 1:32 in water.

KENNEL COUGH COMPLEX

"Kennel cough", also known as canine infectious tracheobronchitis or canine cough, is a contagious disease of the respiratory system that is caused by a variety of viruses and bacteria. Each of these germs initiates similar signs, including a typical dry, non-productive cough with a distinctive honking sound.

The coughing occurs because the pathogens temporarily destroy the tiny hair-like projections, or cilia, that line the larynx, trachea, and bronchi in the upper respiratory tract. (Normally, the cilia protect the airways by creating rhythmic movements, which remove irritants by wafting them up and out of the respiratory system.) In addition, the pathogenic microorganisms have a chance to move deeper into the lungs.

The most important cause of kennel cough is *Bordetella bronchiseptica* (*see p.152*), a relative of the bacteria that cause whooping cough in humans. The most common viral causes are canine parainfluenza virus (CPIV) and canine adenovirus-2 (CAV-2), a close relative of canine hepatitis virus (CAV-1). Kennels and other places where dogs are kept together are prime sites for the transmission of the disease. Stress, poor ventilation, and the proximity of dogs that may be harbouring one of the causative pathogens are all contributory factors.

Around five days after airborne exposure to one of the pathogens, an affected individual develops the high-pitched, honking cough. While some dogs recover within a couple of days, others suffer from a more unpleasant and longer-lasting condition called tracheobronchitis, due to complications brought on by opportunist bacteria and fungi. These pathogens cause various symptoms, such as lethargy, fever, eye or nose discharges, loss of appetite, and sticky saliva at the corners of the mouth. In addition, the affected dog may have paroxysms of coughing accompanied by retching. In some circumstances, a complicated case of kennel cough can appear similar to the respiratory phase of canine distemper infection.

DIAGNOSIS Clinical signs and recent medical history are used to diagnose the disease. Washes of fluid from the trachea are sometimes taken to isolate the exact cause of a cough.

TREATMENT Cough suppressants reduce paroxysms of dry coughing and make a dog more comfortable. Antibiotics are used on individuals at risk from a secondary infection, or on those with affected lungs. Bronchodilators are beneficial for dogs with narrowed air passages. Medication to break down mucus is also sometimes used. In certain circumstances, a corticosteroid is needed to suppress coughing and reduce inflammation.

Supportive therapy is also necessary. This treatment includes rest and the avoidance of stressful situations that trigger a coughing attack.

PREVENTION Environments in which kennel cough has occurred should be cleaned with a half-hour exposure to chlorine bleach, diluted 1:32 in water. Bordetella vaccine given intranasally stimulates local immunity within the respiratory tract, but this protection only lasts from two to nine months. Injections of vaccines against CAV-2 and parainfluenza reduce but do not eliminate the risk of kennel cough.

VET'S ADVICE

Kennel, or canine, cough is not the only cause of coughing. A dog may chew on a rough object that damages its throat; the resulting cough sounds very similar to a hacking kennel cough. A more serious cause is a "heart cough". A heart inefficiency can cause fluid to collect in the lungs, and this build-up, in turn, triggers non-productive coughing. It is easy to confuse the early stages of a heart cough with a mild kennel cough. If your dog starts to cough, contact your vet.

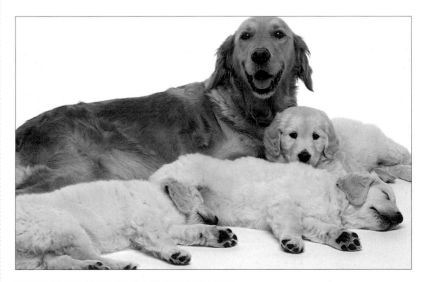

PASSING ON ANTIBIOTICS THROUGH MILK
A mother's milk contains protection against infectious diseases, but it may also carry other substances, including drugs. These substances can have an effect on the pups; for example, antibiotics can affect the digestive microflora developing in a pup's intestines.

BACTERIAL INFECTIONS

Bacteria are single-celled organisms that, unlike viruses, do not need other living cells in order to multiply. They are very versatile, self-contained, and able to grow almost anywhere – from the crevices and mucous membranes of an animal's mouth to the deepest and most inhospitable regions of the planet. Most bacteria belong to what is called the "normal flora" and are beneficial, helping to maintain the environment in which they live.

In dogs, some types of bacteria live on the skin and the hair, while other types thrive inside the body – for example, in the large intestine and the reproductive tract. The beneficial effects of intestinal bacteria include aiding digestion and even contributing to the manufacture of vitamins.

Certain types of bacteria, however, will cause disease if they are given the opportunity – for example, in an animal suffering from a viral disease or a young pup with an immune system that is not yet strong enough to cope with a virulent pathogen. Not usually part of the normal flora of the body, these pathogens are the ones that concern us and our dogs.

ANTIBIOTICS

Most bacteria are susceptible to antibiotics, which either prevent them from multiplying or actively kill them. Antibiotics are chemically synthesized drugs, yet virtually all of them are copies of natural substances made by microorganisms for their own defence and protection. Antibiotics that are commonly used by veterinary surgeons include amoxicillin, cephalosporins, doxycycline, enrofloxacin, and clindamycin.

As bacteria find ways of resisting the powerful effects of antibiotics, pharmaceutical companies constantly search for new substances that microorganisms produce to protect themselves. (*See also pp.106–07.*)

GASTROINTESTINAL INFECTIONS

Four pathogenic bacteria – *Salmonella*, *Campylobacter*, *Escherichia coli* and possibly *Helicobacter* – cause such symptoms as acute vomiting, acute infectious diarrhoea, cramp, and fever. Pups, young dogs, and dogs that are weakened by viruses or poor nutrition are especially prone to these infections. An illness can last from four to ten days, with chronic diarrhoea often continuing for another 30 or more days. The dehydration that results from acute diarrhoea is a considerable concern in small dogs and pups.

Salmonella, *Campylobacter*, and pathogenic *E. coli* are contracted by eating contaminated food, drinking contaminated water, or contact with infected animal droppings, or from surfaces contaminated by diarrhoea from an affected individual.

Salmonella is a hardy bacterium that can stay alive in soil and manure for years. *Campylobacter* can live for more than a month in unpasteurized milk or in water. Some strains of *E. coli* form part of the normal flora of the gut, but a viral disease of the intestine can trigger other strains of *E. coli* to become dangerously pathogenic.

DIAGNOSIS *Salmonella* is found in stool samples. *Campylobacter* is identified by the history; it is more common in pups than in adults. Pathogenic *E. coli* is revealed by culture and sensitivity tests. *Helicobacter*, a bacterium that may cause stomach inflammation, can be diagnosed only by endoscopic biopsy.

TREATMENT Signs of the illness, such as pain and vomiting, need to be controlled. Fluids are administered intravenously to control dehydration. Antibiotics are rarely effective; they are seldom used to treat *Salmonella* or *E. coli* but are more commonly used to treat *Campylobacter*. *Helicobacter* infection is treated with a combination of antibiotics and bismuth subsalicylate.

ADVICE *Salmonella* and *Campylobacter* may cause a zoonotic infection (*see pp.434–35*). People at increased risk, such as those who are elderly, ill, and HIV–positive, should not handle pups with these infections.

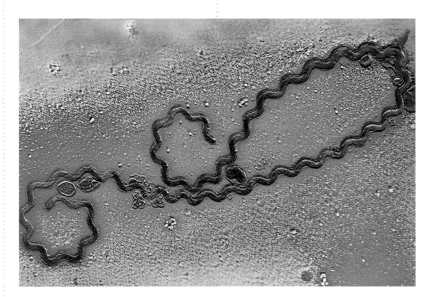

LEPTOSPIRAL BACTERIUM
The bacteria that cause leptospirosis are long, thin, and shaped like a spiral. One of the most common culprits for leptospirosis in dogs is *Leptospira canicola*, which causes the kidneys to become inflamed but does not usually produce any lasting damage.

LEPTOSPIROSIS

This disease is caused by spirochete bacteria, including *Leptospira canicola*. Many dogs can develop the infection without showing clinical signs. They become carriers, spreading the disease to others.

When illness does occur, it may cause kidney inflammation (nephritis) or a more generalized disease involving the liver and often accompanied by blood in the urine. Clinical signs, which appear between four and 12 days after infection, include lethargy, fever, vomiting, and redness of the mucous membranes and conjunctiva of the eyes. In severe cases, there may be jaundice and a yellowing of the mucous membranes.

DIAGNOSIS Blood tests may reveal increased numbers of white blood cells, a reduced platelet count, and kidney involvement. Serum samples show an increasing level of antibodies. Sometimes the leptospiral bacteria may be seen under the microscope in urine or tissue samples.

TREATMENT Support therapy including intravenous fluids is given according to the signs. Appropriate antibiotics are given for at least three weeks, or often for longer periods.

PREVENTION Leptospiral bacteria are spread in the urine of carrier animals such as rodents and skunks, and can contaminate water and soil in places where these animals congregate. In areas where leptospirosis is a potential problem, dogs should be routinely vaccinated. Leptospirosis vaccine does not guarantee protection, however; rather, it protects some individuals and reduces the seriousness of any infection in others. Present vaccines provide immunity lasting for up to 18 months. Routine booster inoculations may be necessary for some dogs.

ADVICE Leptospirosis is a zoonotic disease, transmissible to humans (*see pp.434–35*). If your dog develops this infection, ensure strict hygiene during the treatment phase.

DOGS AS CARRIERS OF HUMAN DISEASES

Dogs can not only contract bacterial diseases such as tuberculosis from humans but, in a more troublesome way, can also be carriers of human infections. They can, for example, pick up and carry our streptococcal infections without showing signs of illness. If a member of your family is suffering from "strep throat", scarlet fever, rheumatic fever, tonsillitis, or pneumococcal pneumonia and is given antibiotics, your dog should be treated with the same or another appropriate antibiotic.

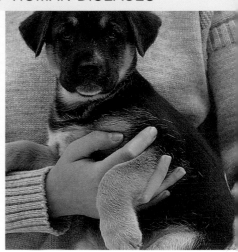

BRUCELLOSIS

This is a worldwide infection, first identified in the 1960s and caused by *Brucella canis*. Geographically, there is considerable variation in its incidence. In some parts of North America up to five per cent of stray dogs are infected, while in Great Britain and Australia the incidence is much less than one per cent. Brucellosis is usually most prevalent among dogs that are kept in kennels.

In acute cases, individuals show enlarged lymph nodes in the groin area, and in some cases the nodes beneath the jaw are also enlarged. Many infected individuals, however, show no clinical signs of illness. The bacteria may remain in an infected individual for as long as two years, during which time the dog develops immunity.

The optimum time for the spread of *Brucella* bacteria is during breeding. The bacteria are transmitted through infected urine, or through the semen of male dogs and the vaginal discharges of females. Infected male dogs may become infertile, or they may have an inflammatory condition affecting the testicles (orchitis) or the prostate gland (prostatitis). Pregnant females who are infected often abort their foetuses at six to eight weeks of gestation. If the pups are born alive, they usually fade and die within a few days.

DIAGNOSIS AND TREATMENT A positive blood culture, to detect the bacteria, is the most definitive method of diagnosis. A test for antibodies is more practical when larger numbers of dogs need to be screened. A negative test is a true negative, but false positives are not uncommon. If a dog tests positive, more specific (and more expensive) antibody tests are available.

In breeding kennels a test-and-remove policy is the most practical option. Affected dogs can remain *Brucella* carriers for years. Antibiotics clear bacteria for as long as they are used, but are not always effective in eliminating the disease.

PREVENTION All dogs used for breeding should be blood-tested. A negative test essentially confirms that a dog is free from the disease.

ADVICE *Brucella canis* is theoretically a zoonosis (*see pp.434–35*); human beings can catch the disease, although cases of human infection are very rare. The risks of catching it can be reduced by wearing rubber gloves and taking sensible hygienic precautions when handling aborted pups, tissue, or fluids from infected animals.

TETANUS

Almost all warm-blooded animals can contract this non-contagious infection, which is caused by *Clostridium tetani*. The bacterium thrives without causing disease in the horse's intestinal tract, and is found in soil contaminated by horse or cow manure.

Clostridium usually enters the body through a deep, penetrating wound in the skin. Once inside the wound, in conditions where oxygen is lacking and the body's tissue is decaying, the bacteria produce a poisonous chemical, or toxin, which upsets the infected animal's nervous system.

Symptoms may appear within a few days but usually show up some weeks after the injury. The leg muscles of the affected dog may contract violently in random spasms. The limbs may extend in a rigid manner, and the jaws become locked – hence the common name for tetanus, which is lockjaw.

The mouth becomes difficult to open, and there is a characteristic "smile" caused by muscular retraction of the lips and eyes. The forehead muscles contract, making the ears stand up, and the third eyelids may be more apparent. Death results from a combination of dehydration, breathing problems, and general exhaustion.

VET'S ADVICE

Many bacterial diseases are active across species. As well as acting as carriers for some human diseases, dogs can also pick up infections that are harmful to them, some of which are quite surprising. One of my patients was a German Shepherd Dog that contracted TB by licking the sweat from the face of her HIV–positive owner, who did not know at the time that he had TB.

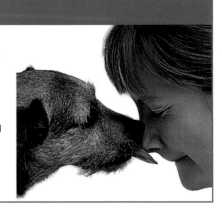

DIAGNOSIS It is important to spot the clinical signs early and to eliminate the possibility of strychnine poisoning, which causes similar symptoms.

TREATMENT If your dog has been injured, always make sure that any wound is cleaned and disinfected thoroughly and promptly to stop the infection spreading. Early intervention by a vet can avoid death.

Tetanus antitoxin, together with antibiotics, such as penicillin, and sedatives are used. Intravenous fluids are often given to combat dehydration. Complete recovery from tetanus may take several weeks, so follow-up supportive care is essential.

PREVENTION Unlike human beings, dogs have a naturally high resistance to *Clostridium*, so routine vaccination is not undertaken.

INFECTIOUS TRACHEOBRONCHITIS

Bordetella bronchiseptica is the most important and the most common cause of infectious tracheobronchitis in dogs. Other viral causes are covered in Kennel Cough Complex (*see p.148*).

This disease is an inflammation of the upper respiratory tract including the larynx, the trachea, and the bronchi (airways leading to the lungs). Affected dogs suffer from a distinctive, dry, hacking cough sometimes accompanied by a clear discharge from the nose and eyes. When the disease is complicated by a secondary bacterial infection, the cough may be accompanied by fever, lethargy, and a purulent (pus-filled) discharge from the nose.

DIAGNOSIS A wash of fluid taken from the dog's trachea, or a culture grown from a nasal swab, will confirm the presence of *Bordetella*.

TREATMENT Keep your dog in a warm, draught-free environment. Humidify the air in the room to reduce coughing. Antibiotics by mouth or injection are not particularly effective for *Bordetella*, because the bacteria stick like glue to the lining of the windpipe. (A nebulizer, which delivers drugs in droplets of

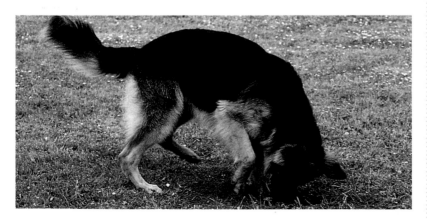

BACTERIA IN THE SOIL
Some disease-causing bacteria inhabit the soil. *Clostridium tetani*, for example, is common in soil contaminated by cows and horses, and even in well-rotted manures. When the spores of *Clostridium* enter a wound, they germinate and then produce the toxin that causes tetanus.

vapour, is perhaps the best route of antibiotic administration, but is impractical for most dogs.)

PREVENTION Use *Bordetella* vaccine, which is effective for two to nine months, when your dog is visiting a high-risk environment or if *Bordetella* infection occurs with high frequency in your locality.

TUBERCULOSIS

Dogs usually contract tuberculosis by inhaling *Mycobacterium tuberculosis* or by catching it from the respiratory secretions of people suffering from TB. Frequently, the lung infection does not cause any clinical signs because the dog's immune system can deal with the bacteria. When the mycobacterial disease does materialize, the dog suffers from coughing, lethargy, loss of condition, and laboured breathing.

DIAGNOSIS Chest X-rays will reveal tubercular lesions in the lungs. Bacteria in samples of sputum (mucus from the airways) or in tracheal washes may be seen under the microscope. Intradermal skin tests (*see pp.180–81*) are available but are seldom used for screening dogs.

TREATMENT The obvious health risk to people makes treatment a dilemma, and euthanasia becomes the best choice. In circumstances where treatment is an option, virtually permanent antibiotic therapy may be effective. Vaccination against TB is not available.

PREVENTION Tuberculosis is increasing in the human population, particularly amongst people from hygienically and economically poor regions of the world and amongst people who are HIV–positive. Any dog living in a household where human tuberculosis has been diagnosed is at risk.

STAPHYLOCOCCUS SKIN INFECTION

Staphylococci are among the most common bacteria existing on the skin. Most are part of the skin's natural flora but, if given the opportunity, the organisms can become pathogenic,

causing either superficial or deep skin infection. Some strains of staphylococci are more virulent than others.

The most common sign of disease is a local, pus-producing skin infection following a scratch or a skin puncture. There may also be inflammation of the hair follicles, or folliculitis (*see p.196*). Deeper infection can lead to the development of pus-filled boils or, in more severe cases, carbuncles. The latter, when they rupture, can seed the bacteria into the bloodstream, spreading disease to other tissues and causing septicaemia. Staphylococci may also be associated with infections of the ears and the urinary tract.

DIAGNOSIS AND TREATMENT A diagnosis is based on the clinical history, signs, and a bacterial culture. Antibiotics from the cephalosporin group are the treatment of choice.

ACTINOMYCOSIS AND NOCARDIOSIS

Actinomyces bacteria are part of the mouth's normal flora, while *Nocardia* bacteria live predominantly in the soil. These thread-like bacteria usually gain entry through skin wounds, causing visible abscesses.

Both actinomycosis and nocardiosis are uncommon diseases, in which the lymph nodes become swollen in the region around the wound site. When infection moves deeper – for example, if it is carried deeper into body tissues on a foreign body such as a migrating grass seed – the infection may break into the chest or the abdomen, causing pus to accumulate there.

DIAGNOSIS AND TREATMENT Clinical signs will be confirmed by a laboratory bacterial culture, which will identify the organism responsible.

Simple abscesses are lanced and then flushed with antiseptic. Deeper infection, however, requires more aggressive treatment, which includes daily flushing and cleansing of the area with disinfectant, accompanied by antibiotics for at least a month.

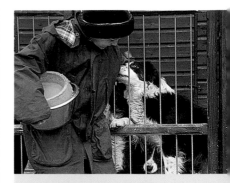

Q SHOULD ALL PUPPIES BE ISOLATED UNTIL THEY COMPLETE THEIR INITIAL VACCINATIONS?

A Exposure to an infectious disease before a pup has produced protective antibodies against that disease is medically risky. On the other hand, isolation from other dogs, people, and animals until two weeks after a final primary inoculation is socially and behaviourally risky. Where I practise, most people have their dogs fully vaccinated. As a consequence, when I assess risk, the risk of poor social development if a pup is kept isolated is greater than the potential medical risk if it meets other dogs before it has completed its primary inoculation. Talk to your vet about the pros and cons of early canine socializing where you live.

Q ARE DOG SHOWS, KENNELS, CANINE GROOMERS, AND VETERINARY CLINICS SOURCES OF INFECTIOUS DISEASE?

A Vets usually destroy all known canine infections with disinfectants. Dog shows and quality kennels usually demand up-to-date vaccination records. If you take your dog to a groomer, ensure that they carry out efficient vaccination checks and disinfection.

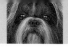
RICKETTSIAL DISEASES

These newly identified diseases are due to an exceptional group of bacteria called rickettsiae. These germs behave, in some ways, more like viruses than like bacteria. They are as small as virus particles and need to invade living cells in order to multiply. Most are passed on through the bites of external parasites such as ticks, fleas, lice, and mites.

LYME DISEASE

This is the most common of the tick-borne diseases. Lyme disease is caused by the spirochete bacterium *Borrelia burgdorferi*. It is named after Old Lyme, Connecticut, US; it was first recognized in the 1970s, when doctors in this area noticed that children, in particular, were suffering from unusual recurrent diseases of the joints. The infection (Borreliosis) has since been identified throughout the United States, predominantly in the northeast and the mid-Atlantic regions but also in the midwest and the Pacific northwest. In addition, it is found in most parts of Europe, Northern Australia, and other regions of the world where ticks exist.

Lyme disease occurs during the tick season (from May to August in the northern hemisphere) in woodland areas. Different species of tick are carriers and transmitters of *Borrelia burgdorferi*, and different mammals act as the main reservoirs of the bacterium. In the American northeast, for example, the main reservoir population is the white-footed mouse. The tick bites the mouse, picks up the disease, and then bites a dog or human, transmitting the bacteria in its saliva. The ticks keep the disease in the reservoir when they bite previously uninfected mice.

Up to half of all free-roaming dogs in endemic areas have antibodies to *Borrelia* but show no signs of illness. The most common sign of Lyme disease in dogs is lameness, which is sometimes accompanied by fever, lethargy, and weight loss.

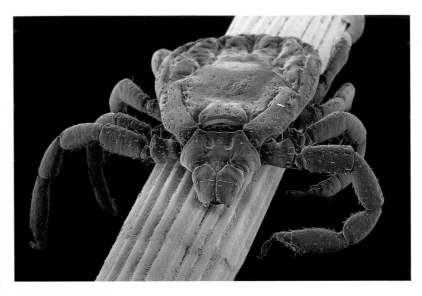

BROWN DOG TICK
The brown dog tick is responsible for transmitting the bacteria which cause canine ehrlichiosis and hemobartonellosis. It may also be responsible for transmitting infectious cyclic thrombocytopenia.

DIAGNOSIS Blood tests showing rising antibody levels to *Borrelia burgdorferi* indicate exposure. Vaccinated dogs, however, can have a positive result. In addition, the test results can remain negative during the initial weeks after exposure to the bacterium.

TREATMENT Antibiotics from the tetracycline group (such as doxycycline) or those from the penicillin group (such as amoxycillin) are very effective.

PREVENTION During the tick season, dogs should be protected against ticks with specially developed products and collars. A vaccine that gives protection for six months is available for dogs that are at high risk, although the need for it is questionable because of the fact that so many cases are subclinical and almost all are self-limiting.

ADVICE There is no hard evidence that dogs diagnosed with Lyme disease pose a risk to their owners or other people. In other words, it is not a zoonosis as such. If your dog shows a positive test, though, then you may well have been exposed to the same tick population and should therefore be tested.

ROCKY MOUNTAIN SPOTTED FEVER

This disease is misleadingly named: in fact, most cases occur in forest regions of the American southeast, far from the Rocky Mountains. It is caused by *Rickettsia rickettsii* and occurs during the tick season. It causes a high fever, lethargy, loss of appetite, coughing, inflammation of the eyes, and general

VET'S ADVICE

Lyme disease is currently an important subject because it affects humans as well as dogs. Although ticks are the most common means of transmission of this bacterial infection, it can also be spread by fleas and other biting insects. Effective use of specially developed products such as fipronil, which gives protection against both ticks and fleas, is an excellent way to control Lyme disease.

muscle and joint pain. There may be bleeding problems, such as nosebleeds or blood in the urine or stools.

DIAGNOSIS A reduction in platelets (thrombocytopenia) is often seen on a blood smear, and a rapidly increasing antibody count is usually diagnostic.

TREATMENT An antibiotic from the tetracycline group given for 14 days is effective. A positive response is seen within a few days. Corticosteroids may also be used to counter inflammation.

PREVENTION Minimize tick exposure and use a specially developed anti-tick product or collar.

EHRLICHIOSIS (TROPICAL CANINE PANCYTOPENIA)

This tick-borne disease was first diagnosed in the United States among military dogs during the Vietnam War. It occurs mostly in the southern United States and in Mediterranean Europe, including all of Spain. It is caused by *Ehrlichia canis* and transmitted in bites from infected brown dog ticks (*Rhipicephalus sanguineus*).

Affected dogs have enlarged lymph nodes and a fever for up to a week. They are often lethargic, appear stiff, and lose their appetite. There may be bleeding problems such as nosebleeds or blood in the urine or stools. Some dogs develop vague neurological signs, for example, stupor, lameness, and vagueness. Untreated dogs appear to recover after two to four weeks. Some authorities think that certain breeds, such as German Shepherds are more susceptible to the disease than others.

DIAGNOSIS Blood counts early in the disease show reduced platelets (thrombocytopenia). In chronic illness, both red and white blood cell numbers also drop (pancytopenia). *Ehrlichia canis* may be identified in blood cells. A positive test for *Ehrlichia canis* antibodies confirms the diagnosis.

TREATMENT Early treatment with an antibiotic from the tetracycline group (such as doxycycline) is very effective. When the disease has become chronic

and bone marrow production is suppressed, antibiotic therapy must continue for months; even then, the outlook is uncertain.

PREVENTION Minimize tick exposure and use a specially developed anti-tick product or collar.

INFECTIOUS CYCLIC THROMBOCYTOPENIA

This disease is caused by *Ehrlichia platys* and was first detected in Florida in the 1970s. It occurs from Texas to the Atlantic seaboard. There may be bleeding problems, such as nosebleeds or blood in the urine or stools.

DIAGNOSIS AND TREATMENT A cyclical drop in blood platelets occurs but there are few signs of illness. Platelet numbers drop and then rapidly return to normal. Affected dogs seldom need treatment, but if necessary tetracycline antibiotics are given.

SALMON DISEASE

This disease is caused by rickettsia bacteria (*Neorickettsia helminthoeca* and the Elokomin fluke fever agent) that infect salmon in the waters of the Pacific Northwest of America, from San Francisco to Alaska.

Five to seven days after eating infected raw fish, dogs vomit and then rapidly develop explosive watery to bloody diarrhoea. The dogs become weak and lethargic, and may have enlarged lymph nodes as well as eye and nose discharges.

DIAGNOSIS The clinical signs are similar to those of parvovirus (*see p.145*). Diagnosis is confirmed by a history of eating raw fish and by identification of rickettsia or associated liver flukes in a sample of faeces.

TREATMENT Both pain control and rehydration are essential. In addition, an antibiotic drug from the tetracycline group (such as doxycycline) is usually given to combat the infection.

PREVENTION Do not feed raw salmon to dogs. Freezing or smoking salmon will lower the risk.

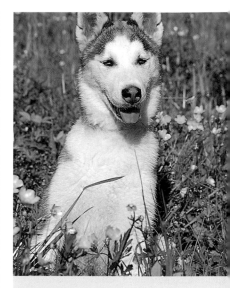

Q WHAT SHOULD I DO IF I SEE A TICK ON MY DOG ?

A In some regions of the world, such as Great Britain, ticks are rarely more than a disgusting nuisance. In other areas, including continental Europe, North America, and Australia, they carry a variety of infectious diseases such as the rickettsial diseases described on these pages.

If you see a tick, spray it with insecticide to kill it. Alternatively, cover it in vaseline to smother it. A few hours later, using either a commercially produced tick remover (available from your vet) or tweezers, grasp it as close to the skin as possible and, with a gentle rotation, disengage it from the skin. Gentle removal is imperative; forced removal may leave its mouthparts embedded in the skin, causing soreness and inflammation. More seriously, squeezing the tick increases the risk of infectious agents or toxins entering the dog's circulation. Dispose of a tick by placing it in a jar with some alcohol. Screw on the lid tightly.

FUNGAL INFECTIONS

Fungi are primarily responsible for the decomposition of organic material. They include yeasts and moulds (and mushrooms, smuts, and rusts, but these forms do not cause infections in animals). In certain circumstances, usually associated with an underlying malfunction of an animal's immune system, certain fungi can cause illness. Their spores can enter the body via the respiratory tract, or through a cut or a puncture of the skin.

Fungal diseases are divided into two categories: the common skin and mucous membrane conditions, such as ringworm, thrush, aspergillosis, and malassezia; and much more rare systemic fungal infections that affect various organs of the body, including the lungs and the liver.

RINGWORM

Dermatophytosis, or ringworm, is overwhelmingly the most common fungal infection to afflict dogs. In otherwise healthy individuals with efficient immune systems, antibodies eventually overcome the infection. Medical treatment remains necessary because of the high risk of spread to other animals and to humans during

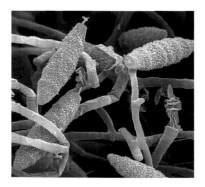

RINGWORM
The fungi that cause ringworm are called dermatophytes. They infest the outer layers of the skin, hair, and nails, where they thrive on the shed skin cells and feed on keratin, a protein that is rich in sulphur.

the weeks that it takes for the immune system to respond.

Several different types of fungi (dermatophytes) cause ringworm. The fungi thrive on keratin, a protein found in dead skin cells that have been shed. The infections produce a variety of hair and skin lesions.

Ringworm is discussed in more detail in Skin Problems (*see p.184*), because this is a skin infection and resembles other skin problems.

DIAGNOSIS Ringworm is diagnosed by clinical signs and fungal culture. The most common form of the infection (*Microsporum canis*) is detected by fluorescence under ultraviolet light.

TREATMENT The condition is treated effectively with antifungal drugs from the topical imidazole group (such as miconozole and ketoconazole) and oral antibiotics (such as griseofulvin), given for at least one month.

CANDIDIASIS

This yeast infection of the skin and mucous membranes, commonly known as thrush, is more common in young or elderly people than in dogs. It is most likely to occur in dogs with chronic illness or those on long-term antibiotics or drugs that suppress the immune system.

Candida infection usually causes a moist skin inflammation. When the mucous membrane of the genital tract is involved, there is a creamy white discharge. Systemic infection, though possible, is extremely rare.

DIAGNOSIS AND TREATMENT Diagnosis is made by microscopic identification or culture. Antifungals from the imidazole group are the treatment of choice. All known causes of immune suppression should, when possible, be removed prior to treatment.

ASPERGILLOSIS

Aspergilla fungi live in hay, straw, and animal feed. Given the opportunity, they may invade the tissues of a dog's respiratory tract, causing infection.

An affected dog, often one with a long nose (such as a collie) initially has a watery nasal discharge and sneezing; the sneezing is eventually accompanied by bleeding from the nose.

DIAGNOSIS X-rays of the nose show bone destruction caused by the fungus. Culture from swabs or nasal flushing reveals *Aspergilla*. Blood sampling may reveal antibodies to the fungus.

TREATMENT Treatment is difficult. One method involves placing temporary drains into the sinuses and nasal passages, allowing twice-daily flushing for one to two months with antifungal medication. Oral antifungal drugs may also be used. Radical surgery is rarely successful.

MALASSEZIA

The yeast *Malassezia pachydermatis* is an opportunist fungus implicated in a disease of the ear called otitis externa (*see p.226*). It is also involved in producing crusting diseases of the skin (*see pp.196–97*).

SYSTEMIC FUNGAL INFECTIONS

Internal (systemic) fungal infections are limited to specific regions of North America (*see right*). They do not exist in Great Britain, continental Europe, or Australia. Many dogs are exposed to the fungi that cause these infections, but most exposures cause the dog to develop strong immunity rather than illness. Systemic fungal infection is uncommon, occurring most frequently in dogs that are poorly nourished and living in sub-standard hygiene or in dogs suffering from chronic infections.

Prolonged use of corticosteroids or broad-spectrum antibiotics can affect a dog's ability to resist disease organisms, and so may also predispose the animal to systemic fungal infection. These diseases become part of a differential diagnosis for systemically ill dogs that do not respond to conventional antibiotic therapy.

HISTOPLASMOSIS

Most instances of histoplasmosis, which is caused by *Histoplasma capsulatum*, produce no clinical signs. Where signs are present, they may include fever, weight loss, and muscle wasting, coughing, vomiting, or diarrhoea.

DIAGNOSIS AND TREATMENT Chest X-rays, blood profiles, and both culture and cytology (cell analysis) studies are used for diagnosis.

Mild infections are treated with a long course of an antifungal drug such as ketoconazole or itraconazole.

PREVENTION Keep your dog away from chickens, bats, and all areas that are contaminated by their droppings.

COCCIDIOIDOMYCOSIS

Most cases of coccidioidomycosis (also called San Joaquin Valley fever) exhibit no symptoms. The disease is caused by the fungus *Coccidioides immitis*. When symptoms appear, they may include pneumonia or, commonly, infection of the long bones and the gut. The condition is often life-threatening.

Coccidioidomycosis sounds similar to a disease called coccidiosis, but the two are totally different – coccidiosis is a protozoal disease of the intestines.

DIAGNOSIS AND TREATMENT The disease is diagnosed by identifying the fungus in biopsy or culture specimens. Antifungal drugs are used for long-term treatment, often for a year or more.

CRYPTOCOCCOSIS

Cryptococcus fungi usually affect the brain, causing behaviour changes, head pressing, blindness, loss of balance, or seizures. Rarely, cryptococcosis, which is caused by *Cryptococcus neoformans*, is a localized infection, causing skin nodules that ulcerate and drain.

DIAGNOSIS AND TREATMENT The fungus is identified from a biopsy or culture specimens. Antifungal drugs are not particularly effective in treating this condition because of the involvement of the central nervous system.

BLASTOMYCOSIS

The clinical signs of this disease, which is caused by *Blastomyces dermatitidis*, are most commonly those of bronchitis and pneumonia. Some dogs develop skin lesions that ulcerate and drain.

DIAGNOSIS AND TREATMENT The fungal organism is revealed by microscopic examination of tracheal washes, biopsy, or culture. An antifungal from the imidazole group, together with amphotericin B, is used in prolonged treatment. Amphotericin B is, however, a potentially dangerous antibiotic that is toxic to the kidneys.

SPOROTRICHOSIS

This fungal disease, which is caused by *Sporothrix schenckii*, appears as nodules at the site of skin punctures. Further nodules may develop in the lymph nodes nearby. It is rarely systemic (in other words, it hardly ever spreads throughout the body), but in some circumstances the disease affects the lungs and liver.

DIAGNOSIS AND TREATMENT The fungus is revealed by microscopic examination of a nodule biopsy.

Wounds infected with the fungus are cleaned with potassium iodide, and antifungals from the imidazole group are given orally.

ADVICE Humans may contract this infection from cleaning the wounds of a dog. Always wear gloves when cleaning and draining wounds.

SYSTEMIC FUNGAL INFECTION RISK AREAS

The organisms that cause many of the systemic fungal infections are confined to certain geographical regions of North America. Some inhabit particular ecological habitats. For example, the fungus *Histoplasma capsulatum*, which causes histoplasmosis, inhabits soil that is rich in nitrogen.

FUNGAL DISEASE	LOCATION	SOURCE
Histoplasmosis	Texas and up the Missippippi and Ohio River Valleys to the Great Lakes, into Ontario and Quebec, and over to the Appalachian Mountains	Inhaled spores from soil
Coccidioidomycosis	Dry Southwestern region, including California and northern Mexico	Inhaled spores from dust in cactus country
Cryptococcosis	Wherever pigeons are common	Inhaled spores from dry pigeon droppings
Blastomycosis	Similar to range for histoplasmosis but including the whole Eastern Seaboard	Inhaled spores from dry bird droppings in shaded organic debris
Sporotrichosis	North and central United States, spreading into the Maritime Provinces, Quebec, and Ontario	Spores that enter small puncture wounds, especially in hunting dogs

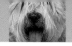
EXTERNAL PARASITES
fleas, lice, ticks, and mites

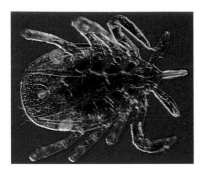

Nymph stage of a tick

Parasites are organisms that live on or in animals, but offer no benefits or may even be detrimental, drawing nourishment by feeding on their "hosts". Parasites on or in the skin are called external parasites or ectoparasites. They range in importance from harmless, barely noticeable beasts to a range of more problematic creatures that can be highly irritating or even life-threatening for your dog. Fortunately, most external parasite infestations are relatively easy to diagnose and will respond to existing therapies.

The most common external parasites affecting dogs are fleas. Furthermore, although they prefer dog's blood, fleas are quite happy feeding off humans too – and the presence of fleas causing bites around the ankles is certainly not a popular feature in the home. These ubiquitous little creatures are without doubt the single most common cause of medical skin conditions in dogs, and canine skin problems account for more visits to the vet than any other single condition. Other external parasites, such as ticks, are not as common, but are potentially more worrying. In many regions of the world, ticks transmit potentially life-threatening rickettsial and protozoal diseases, such as Lyme disease and Rocky Mountain spotted fever.

HOW PARASITES ARE TRANSMITTED

Some external parasites (dog lice, for example) are transmitted to pet dogs through direct contact with other dogs. Others may be picked up through contact with other animals such as foxes. Demodex mites are passed on by mothers to their pups soon after birth and become a problem only if a dog's immune system fails. Ticks and harvest mites are picked up directly from areas of grass and other vegetation, where the parasites lie in wait for a suitable host. Flea problems often start when a dog first arrives in a home where a flea-affected pet lived previously; immature forms of the insect can survive for many months in places such as carpets or bedding, waiting for new hosts to turn up.

Q DO DOG PARASITES ONLY AFFECT DOGS?

A Some parasites are highly host-specific in their habits — they will live in or on, and feed from, only one host species. Dog lice, for example, only affect dogs and never spread to people. Other parasites show a preference for one species but are happy to feed on others. For example, the most common flea affecting dogs will also feed on people and cats (in fact it is primarily a cat flea). Another example, the dog scabies mite, can temporarily affect a person who comes into contact with an affected dog.

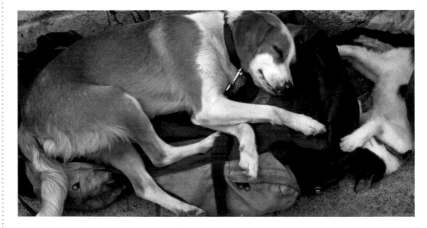

TREAT ALL ANIMALS FOR INFESTATIONS
Most external parasites are contagious to other dogs. Many also pass to and from other species such as cats or rabbits. If one of your pets has parasites, assume that they all do.

SOME EXTERNAL PARASITES OF DOGS

The common external parasites of dogs are either insects (six-legged creatures such as fleas and lice) or arachnids (eight-legged creatures related to insects, such as ticks and mites). The four different parasites depicted here are not shown to scale – the flea and tick are shown about 20 times life size, while the two types of mite are drawn over 100 times life size. Other important external parasites include lice, which can cause anaemia as well as irritation, harvest mites, ear mites, and Cheyletiella mites.

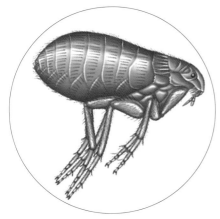

FLEA

An adult flea is brown, about 2.5 mm in length, and can be seen with the naked eye. It typically causes itching on a dog's back, in its groin, and around its hindquarters. Fleas can move quickly through a dog's hair and are difficult to catch.

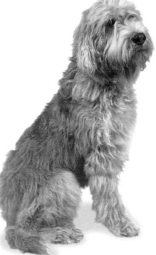

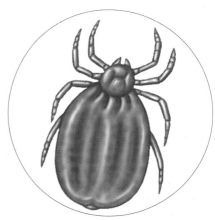

DEMODEX MITE

Demodex mites are cigar-shaped, about 0.2 to 0.4 mm in length (invisible to the naked eye), and have eight tiny legs. They occur normally in dog skin, but the presence of large numbers can cause hair loss or more serious problems.

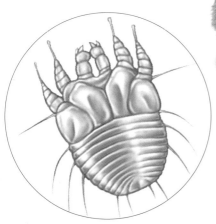

SCABIES MITE

An adult scabies mite is about 0.4 mm in length (hard to see with the naked eye), roughly oval in shape, and pale-coloured. It tunnels in the skin, causing severe itching and inflammation around the dog's ear tips, elbows, chest, and face.

TICK

Ticks are about 2–5 mm in length, have eight legs, and may swell to many times their normal size when engorged with blood. They may attach to any part of a dog, but are commonly found around the ears or between the toes.

DIAGNOSIS AND TREATMENT

All dogs are likely to suffer from external parasites at some time, so it is best to check your dog's coat and skin every few weeks and treat preventatively on a regular basis.

DIAGNOSIS

The signs of a possible external parasite infestation in a dog include scratching, skin inflammation (especially in areas such as the ears, face, chest, elbows, and between the toes), red bumps on the skin, hair loss, or dandruff from the neck down to the tail (in the case of one type of mite infestation). Some external parasites (such as fleas and ticks) are large enough to be visible to the naked eye, while lice leave tell-tale eggs glued to their host's hair. Mites, however, can only be seen when your vet examines skin scrapings from an affected dog under a microscope.

TREATMENTS

Since the 1980s, pharmaceutical companies have developed many new chemical treatments for controlling or preventing fleas and other external parasites. These medications are much more effective than the old flea collars. The treatments are summarized in the table on p.161 *(opposite)*. When using any treatment, you should always follow the manufacturer's or your vet's instructions.

INSECT GROWTH REGULATORS

Insect growth regulators (IGRs), which include the compounds methoprene and pyriproxyfen, mimic natural insect hormones and work by interfering with the development of flea eggs and larvae so that they cannot grow into adults. They do not kill adult fleas, and will not affect other insects or any

mammals. Some IGRs are applied to the dog in the form of collars and sprays, while others are applied to the environment. These treatments are ideal to use in homes with young children or people who are sensitive to other insecticides. As well as being used in the house, modern forms can be used in the garden. The original IGRs broke down rapidly in sunlight, a problem when trying to rid the whole environment of fleas. More recent formulations do not have this problem.

INSECT DEVELOPMENT INHIBITORS

Insect development inhibitors (IDIs) interfere with insect growth. The most widely available, lufenuron (Program), inhibits the formation of chitin, which provides the external skeleton of insects. Lufenuron is used for flea control in dogs but does not kill adult fleas and does not control ticks. It is given orally or as a spot-on application and enters the dog's bloodstream. When a female flea bites the dog it ingests the chemical, and the eggs it lays will never hatch as they cannot develop into other stages.

It can take 12 to 16 weeks' use of an IDI on its own to reduce a flea population to a minimal level.

NEUROTRANSMITTER INHIBITORS

Neurotransmitter inhibitors interfere with parasites' nervous systems, paralysing their breathing apparatus. Selamectin (Stronghold, Revolution) is absorbed through the dog's skin and spread via the blood, concentrating in the dog's sebaceous glands, where it comes out in the hair follicles and is soon present in skin all over the body. It kills fleas, scabies mites, and ear mites, and stops flea eggs developing. It is also active against heartworms and some intestinal worms.

Fipronil (Frontline) is an extremely powerful disruptor of the insect central nervous system. It is applied as a spray or "spot-on" treatment to the dog's skin (not fur) and within 24 hours spreads via natural oils to all areas of the body. It can be used to control fleas, Cheyletiella mites, and harvest mites and is also toxic to ticks.

Imidacloprid (Advantage) is applied as a spot-on treatment and works in a similar way to fipronil. It is not active against ticks, however.

NATURAL NEUROTOXINS

Pyrethrins are natural products that are derived from chrysanthemums. They also affect parasites' nervous

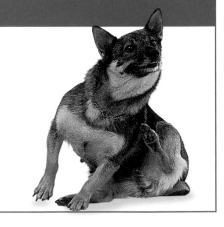

VET'S ADVICE

Most of us rightly assume that peristent scratching is usually due to irritation from fleas. If your itchy dog lives where fleas are active, use of a product that kills fleas is a logical first treatment. Scratching, however, may lead to a secondary bacterial infection, which requires antibiotics. Fleas are not the only cause of scratching – allergy may be a possibility, and requires bathing and antihistamines.

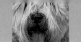

systems (causing convulsions and paralysis) but have the disadvantage of being toxic at high concentrations to humans, dogs, and cats, as well as to fleas, lice, and mites. They may also cause dermatitis (skin inflammation) on contact with the skin. Micro-encapsulated pyrethrins cause fewer adverse side effects than natural form pyrethrins. Permethrins are synthetic pyrethrins that are less likely to cause dermatitis but are highly toxic to cats.

MONOAMINE OXIDASE INHIBITOR

Amitraz (Preventic) is used in dogs to interfere with ticks' metabolism, causing the ticks to detach and die. It works within hours of application, spreading through the oils on the dog's hair to cover the entire coat. The collars on the market are designed to release the chemical consistently over a period of time, preventing new ticks from attaching for up to three months.

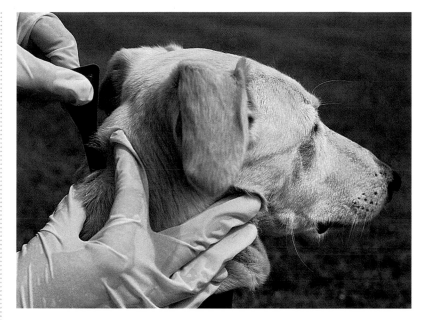

MODERN PARASITE TREATMENTS
Unlike the older treatments that were dusted, sprayed, or shampooed over the whole coat, many modern treatments can be applied as a "spot-on" treatment to the back of the neck. They spread to give effective protection to the whole body.

EXTERNAL PARASITE PREVENTION AND CONTROL

MECHANISM OF ACTION	CHEMICAL (AND TRADE) NAME	FORMULATION	TREATS
Insect growth regulator (IGR)	methoprene	spray, collar, fogger	fleas
Insect growth regulator (IGR)	pyriproxyfen	spray, spot-on, fogger	fleas
Insect development inhibitor (IDI)	lufenuron (Program) (lufenuron with milbemycin) (Sentinel)	pill, oral liquid	fleas (Sentinel also protects against some worms)
Neurotransmitter inhibitor	selamectin (Stronghold, Revolution)	spot-on roundworms, ticks	fleas, ear mites, scabies mites, lice, heartworms,
Neurotransmitter inhibitor	fipronil (Frontline)	spot-on, spray	fleas, ticks, Cheyletiella and harvest mites
Neurotransmitter inhibitor	imidacloprid (Advantage)	spot-on	fleas
Naturally occurring neurotoxin	permethrins/pyrethrins	spot-on, spray, shampoo	fleas, lice, Cheyletiella mites, mosquitoes (repellent)
Monoamine oxidase inhibitor (MAOI)	amitraz (Preventic)	collar	ticks
Cell growth inhibitor	selenium sulphide (Seleen)	shampoo	Cheyletiella mites

INSECT PARASITES

The main insect parasites of dogs are fleas and lice. Mosquitoes can also be a problem, although they do not actually live on dogs.

FLEAS

Fleas are wingless, blood-sucking insects, with flattened bodies and three pairs of powerful jointed legs, which they use for jumping. Fleas thrive whenever and wherever humidity is above 50 per cent and the temperature is over 20°C (68°F). Although there is a specific dog flea, *Ctenocephalides canis*, it is rare. Most dog infestations are with the cat flea *Ctenocephalides felis*. Human fleas, *Pulex irritans*, are also sometimes found on dogs.

Under ideal conditions, a flea can complete its life cycle in just over two weeks, but when food is scarce the cycle can be as long as 21 months. That is why flea problems may return to an infested house even when it has been uninhabited by pets for well over

a year. It is important to realise that for every flea on your dog, there are likely to be 100 more in the local environment at different stages in their life cycle. These include flea larvae in the dog's bedding, in the garden, in your car, and anywhere else where the dog rests. The larvae live off organic debris including flea dirt (dried droppings left by adult fleas) and human skin scales. Fleas in the pupal stage will also be present, often deep in carpets or amongst organic material in the garden. Adult fleas start hatching from pupae in response to triggers indicating the presence of a possible host – these include heat, motion, vibration, or an increase in carbon dioxide levels. Once an adult flea has hatched, it jumps onto the first available source of nourishment (dog, cat, or other mammal).

SIGNS OF INFESTATION A dog troubled by fleas will scratch the affected area. A flea infestation can be diagnosed by finding fleas on the dog or seeing white and black ("salt and pepper")

grains, about the size of sand grains, in the dog's coat. These particles are flea eggs (white) and faeces (black). Fleas can carry disease, but flea allergy dermatitis (FAD), a sensitivity to flea saliva, is by far the most common skin problem in dogs (*see p.191*). Flea bites can also trigger bacterial skin infections (*see p.196*). Very heavy flea infestations in a small dog or pup can cause anaemia (reduced numbers of red cells in the blood).

TREATING THE DOG AND ENVIRONMENT
If a flea problem exists in your home, it is pointless to treat just the dog. The whole environment (including the car and garden), as well as any contact animals, must be treated to remove fleas in all stages of the life cycle. When planning treatment, do not forget any pet cats. If cats go outdoors they get reinfested with fleas, bringing them back into the treated environment.

Ideally, treatment should start before the flea season begins in your area (generally in the spring). Several different anti-flea treatments are

---

FLEA LIFE CYCLE

Adult fleas feed every few days via bites through a dog's skin. These blood meals are needed before sexual activity can take place. A fertilized female lays up to 50 eggs a day. Most are dislodged by scratching and drop to the floor or ground. The life cycle proceeds via larval and pupal stages to hatching of new adults.

LENGTH OF STAGES
Only a small part of a flea's life cycle is spent feeding on a dog; most is spent in the dog's environment. The adult fleas can live for 6 to 12 months, but much of this time is spent "off" the dog. The pupal or cocoon stage can last from a few days to a year or more.

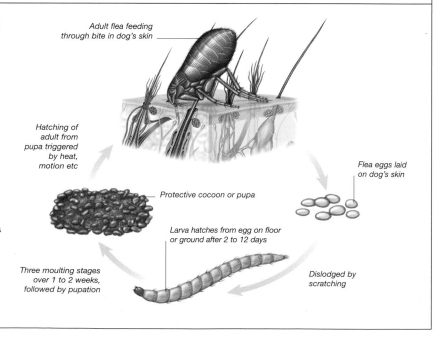

Adult flea feeding through bite in dog's skin

Hatching of adult from pupa triggered by heat, motion etc

Protective cocoon or pupa

Flea eggs laid on dog's skin

Larva hatches from egg on floor or ground after 2 to 12 days

Three moulting stages over 1 to 2 weeks, followed by pupation

Dislodged by scratching

available (*see p.161*). These include insect growth regulators (IGRs), insect development inhibitors (IDIs), neurotransmitter inhibitors, natural neurotoxins, and others.

TREATMENT PRECAUTIONS IGRs and IDIs such as methoprene, pyriproxyfen, and lufenuron (Program) should be used only when the dog has no flea allergy dermatitis (FAD). If fleas are irritating your dog, use a topical product such as fipronil (Frontline), imidacloprid (Advantage), or selamectin (Stronghold, Revolution). Never treat cats with products that are licensed only for use on dogs.

CARPET TREATMENT Professional carpet treatment with sodium polyborate, sodium tetraborate, or sodium borate can be highly effective for preventing flea eggs and larvae from maturing. Many treatments come with one-year guarantees. Do not treat your carpets yourself with laundry-grade borax. The National Animal Poison Control Center (in the United States) reports increasing cases of serious eye, respiratory, and kidney problems in small dogs (and cats) when laundry-grade borax powder has been used for this purpose.

INEFFECTIVE TREATMENTS Some devices and remedies that should not be relied upon for dealing with fleas include ultrasonic flea collars, Brewer's yeast, tea tree oil, garlic, and cedar. None of these effectively controls fleas.

MOSQUITOES

Mosquitoes can be as great a nuisance to your dog as they are to you, and in some parts of the world (including Australia and parts of North America) they transmit heartworm disease to dogs (*see pp.254–56*). Keep dogs indoors at twilight when mosquitoes are most active. Try permethrin or pyrethrin-based mosquito repellents, but do not use DEET, a chemical often used to repel mosquitoes from people. DEET can be toxic if consumed, and dogs commonly lick themselves.

LICE

Lice are wingless insects that come in two varieties: biting lice, which feed on skin, and sucking lice, which feed on blood. An overwhelming infestation of sucking lice can lead to severe anaemia (reduced numbers of red cells in the blood) resulting in lethargy.

The species of lice that affect dogs are different from those that affect people. But like human lice, they leave their eggs (called nits) glued to hair. These are usually more noticeable than the 2–3 millimetre-long lice themselves.

DIAGNOSIS AND TREATMENT The presence of nits proves that a dog is, or has been, affected by lice. Nits can be mistaken for flakes of dandruff, but their egg-like appearance becomes obvious under a magnifying glass. An affected dog should be shampooed weekly for four weeks with a pyrethrin or permethrin shampoo. In addition, treat the dog's grooming equipment, and its bedding and sleeping quarters, with an insecticidal spray. Anaemic dogs should be given nutritional supplements with iron and vitamins and a balanced diet.

ARACHNID PARASITES

Arachnids are eight-legged animals that are distinct from, though related to, insects. (Both insects and arachnids belong to a larger animal group, the arthropods.) The main arachnid parasites of dogs are ticks and mites.

TICKS

Ticks are a group of blood-sucking arachnid parasites. They live at ground level, and are stimulated into activity by triggers such as heat, motion, vibration, or shadow, which indicate that a potential host is nearby. Once it has climbed onto a host, a tick inserts its head through the skin and feeds, gorging itself with blood.

Dogs are attractive to the brown dog tick, *Rhipicephalus sanguineus*, found worldwide. Two other tick species pose

---

Q **WHERE CAN ONE GO IN THE WORLD TO ESCAPE FLEAS?**

A If you want to ensure minimal flea problems, move to an area that is more than 1,500 metres (5,000 feet) above sea level. That could include some places in the Alps and Pyrenees in Europe, and large areas of the western United States. Fleas do not like high altitudes. They also do not thrive in very hot, cold, dry, or humid conditions, but these tend to be uncomfortable for dogs and humans, too.

Q **CAN VACUUMING ALONE GET RID OF FLEAS?**

A Thorough vacuuming of the home is a necessary part of dealing with fleas, but it will not remove all fleas, in all stages of the life cycle, from the dog's environment. Vacuuming and then applying insecticides is a fast way of getting rid of fleas. Vacuuming sucks up different stages of the flea life cycle and also straightens the carpet pile, allowing subsequent insecticidal sprays to penetrate deeper. The heat and vibration from vacuuming also encourage adult fleas to emerge from pupae. You should dispose of the contents of the vacuum cleaner carefully, because it contains fleas in varying stages of their life cycle.

Q **ARE SHAMPOOS, SPRAYS, OR DIPS BEST FOR REMOVING FLEAS FROM MY DOG?**

A Shampoos are not as effective as sprays or dips (also called rinses), because shampoos leave little residual insecticide on your dog. Dogs are not as frightened by pump sprays as by aerosols. Always wear rubber gloves when using dips or sprays.

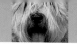

LIFE CYCLE OF A HARD TICK

Hard ticks have a four-stage life cycle. These stages are egg, six-legged larva (not shown), eight-legged nymph, and adult. Usually, each of the last three stages has to feed on a host such as a dog to proceed to the next stage. Much of a tick's life is spent sitting on a blade of grass or leaf, waiting for a suitable host to pass by.

FROM EGG TO ADULT
A female tick lays thousands of eggs, and then dies. Larvae hatch from the eggs a few weeks later, feed (if they can find a host), and grow into nymphs over a period of 2 to 3 weeks. The same pattern is repeated for transformation from nymph to adult.

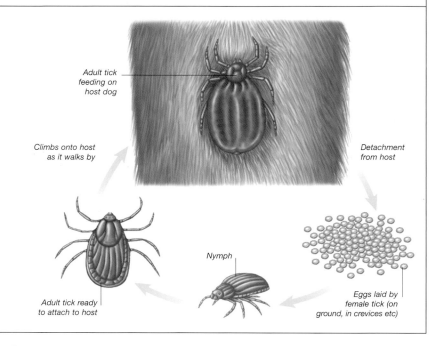

Adult tick feeding on host dog

Climbs onto host as it walks by

Detachment from host

Nymph

Adult tick ready to attach to host

Eggs laid by female tick (on ground, in crevices etc)

---

particular hazards: *Dermacentor variabilis* in North America, and the paralysis tick, *Ixodes holocyclus*, in eastern Australia. Various other species affect dogs in different parts of the world. A heavy tick infestation can lead to anaemia through blood loss. Ticks are also responsible for skin problems, caused by their irritating saliva, or paralysis, due to a poison (neurotoxin) in their saliva. They can also trigger bacterial skin infections (see p.196).

Ticks transmit a variety of infectious diseases including Lyme disease (see p.154), Rocky Mountain spotted fever (see p.154), and Babesia (see p.175). These diseases are not passed on until a tick has been attached and feeding for several hours. Ticks and tick-borne diseases are a problem during spring and summer in temperate climates, year round in warmer regions.

DIAGNOSIS AND TREATMENT A tick infestation is diagnosed by finding one or more ticks on the dog's skin. To remove a tick, use tweezers to grasp it as close as possible to the dog's skin, then pull it slowly out. Be sure to wear gloves for this task, because a tick's blood may contain organisms that are dangerous to humans. After the tick has been removed, clean the bite area with an antiseptic. If it is possible that the tick was feeding on the dog for several hours, watch out for signs of possible tick-borne disease in the dog.

PREVENTION Ticks can be prevented from attaching to a dog with the use of collars such as those containing amitraz (Preventic). Note that some tick-prevention drugs are effective only against certain varieties of tick. Always examine your dog thoroughly after a walk through tick-infested areas.

SARCOPTIC MANGE

Sarcoptic mange is the most intensely irritating parasite-induced skin disease of dogs. It is caused by the scabies mite, which is microscopic in size and highly contagious. The mite provokes the dog to chew, lick, and scratch the affected area, further damaging the skin. The elbows and ear tips are often inflamed and lose hair. The chest and face may also be affected. Affected dogs scratch intensely. Tickling the dog's ear tip triggers a reflex foot-thumping response from the hind leg on the same side.

DIAGNOSIS AND TREATMENT Skin scrapings of affected areas reveal mites that have burrowed a few millimetres into the skin to lay their eggs. It is often difficult to find mites on skin scrapings. A blood test for antibodies to the scabies mite is available. Scabies infestation can be suspected if a dog has classically intense itchiness, has recently been in contact with other dogs (or foxes or wombats), or been in a region with carrier animals, and responds to anti-mite treatment.

The best treatment is selamectin (Stronghold, Revolution), which is applied as a spot-on and repeated two weeks later. Anti-inflammatory corticosteroids may also be used.

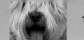
Amitraz dips repeated weekly for six weeks may be used if there is a reason not to use selamectin. All dogs that have been in contact with the affected one should also be treated.

WARNING Ivermectin (Ivomec) by injection has been used successfully to treat sarcoptic mange infection in dogs. It is not licensed for this use, however, and it is known to have adverse effects on the brain in certain collie breeds, including the Rough and Smooth Collie, Shetland Sheepdog, Old English Sheepdog, Australian Shepherd, and crosses of these breeds.

CHEYLETIELLA MANGE

These large, transparent, highly contagious mites are most common in commercial kennels, catteries, and breeding establishments with poor hygiene. Affected pups develop moderate to thick dandruff from the neck down the back to the tail. The ears are sometimes affected. Some pups (or kittens) are itchy but many if not most are not. (An older name for Cheyletiella is "Walking Dandruff".)

DIAGNOSIS AND TREATMENT In an affected dog, mites can be seen on microscopic examination of coat brushings or skin samples taken by sticky tape application or scraping. Treatment is by spraying the dog with fipronil (Frontline) every two weeks for six weeks. Alternatively, the dog can be treated with a lime-sulphur dip. The use of pyrethrin or permethrin shampoos is also effective.

PREVENTION Good environmental hygiene and the use of flea control products such as fipronil (Frontline) prevents this uncommon parasite.

RISK TO HUMAN HEALTH Cheyletiella can affect humans, causing an itchy pimply rash, especially on the arms. Mites can live for up to ten days off a dog. If a person is affected, the rash clears soon after all dogs are treated.

DEMODECTIC MITES

Demodex mites are natural cigar-shaped inhabitants of hair follicles in most animals. Unlike other external parasites, they are not contagious. Mothers pass these mites to their pups within a few days of birth. The mites cause problems when the skin's normal immune protection fails. In the juvenile form of disease, affected dogs suffer from relatively mild and local hair loss. In the more severe and uncommon adult form, disease expands from local to generalized and may be life-threatening. Because demodectic mange is more than a simple reaction to a parasite, it is discussed in more detail under Skin problems (*see p.183*).

EAR MITES

The ear mite, *Otodectes cynotis*, is still only too common in dogs and cats. Prevention and treatment are simple and effective and are discussed under Ear problems (*see pp.222-31*).

CHIGGERS

Chiggers, or harvest mites, live in decaying vegetation. Their larvae, which can be seen with a magnifying glass, are parasitic, sucking on a dog's skin. Dogs come in contact with these larvae, especially on the feet, when exercising in grassland during late summer and early autumn. The mites cause itchy inflammation between the toes, but also on the ears and around the mouth, especially on dogs with short coats such as the Doberman Pinscher.

DIAGNOSIS AND TREATMENT Mite larvae can be seen under magnification in skin scrapings from affected areas. Fipronil (Frontline) spray is the best treatment. Pyrethrin or permethrin shampoo are also effective treatments. The use of corticosteroid drugs and antihistamines may be beneficial to reduce intensive itchiness and self-mutilation. Use thiabendazole drops if the dog's ear canals are affected.

PREVENTION To avoid an infestation keep your dog out of long grass during chigger season.

SCABIES TRANSMISSION TO HUMANS

Dog scabies is caused by a different mite from the one that causes human scabies, but the dog scabies mite can still affect humans, causing itchiness that may last for up to three weeks. The majority of human cases involve a person's forearms or hands (between the fingers) that have come in contact with an affected dog. A dog scabies infection in a person usually clears up quickly once the dog has been successfully treated. This photograph shows a scabies mite, magnified approximately 100 times.

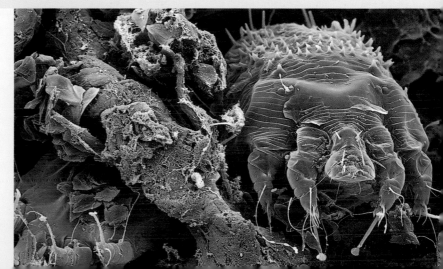

INTERNAL PARASITES
causes, treatment, and prevention

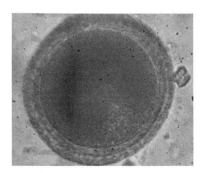

Roundworm egg

Many organisms live inside other animals, causing no problems, even producing benefits for their "hosts". The digestive tracts of dogs and other mammals contain bacteria that help break down food and provide an example of a productive, mutually beneficial relationship. Internal parasites, or endoparasites, are organisms that live in animals but offer no benefits and may be detrimental, drawing nourishment from their hosts. Different parasites can live in organs such as the intestines, heart, lungs, liver, and kidneys.

Internal parasites vary in size from large but often relatively innocuous tapeworms, to microscopic but potentially deadly single-celled animals called protozoa. Parasites have evolved to live on or in all mammals. In return, our immune systems have developed strategies to cope with them.

WORMS
In dogs, the most common internal parasites are worms, which fall into two main groups, nematodes and cestodes. Nematodes are cylindrical, cream-coloured worms. They include roundworms, hookworms, whipworms and threadworms, which all live (as adults) in the intestines, and some other nematodes that live in the heart, lungs, or other organs. Cestodes, or tapeworms, are flattened worms that consist of several joined segments. These live in the small intestine.

Some nematodes, such as roundworms and hookworms, have life cycles involving migration of tiny larvae through the host's body. When this happens, the host's immune system develops immune defences, such as the production of antibodies. As a result, these parasites are usually a problem only with young pups, who have not yet produced antibodies, or animals with failed immune systems. Worms that only live in the intestines, such as tapeworms, do not provoke an immune response, so a dog can get re-infested each time it consumes a tapeworm egg.

PROTOZOA
Protozoa are microscopic single-celled animals. Many different types live freely in the environment and cause no harm. Only a few are important parasites of mammals. Some of these spend part of their life cycles in intermediate hosts such as insects. Others are capable of developing into forms called cysts that can survive for long periods in the environment. When protozoal parasites invade a mammal, they often provoke an immune response and never cause recognizable illness. But they can be dangerous when they trick the immune system by living within white blood cells or when they infect individuals with immune system weakness or failure.

PUBLIC HEALTH RISKS

Many internal parasites of dogs produce eggs that are passed in the dog's faeces. These eggs can survive for long periods in the environment and if swallowed by another dog will produce a new infection. If a person accidentally consumes roundworm eggs (a child licking fingers that have contacted faecally-contaminated soil, for example), this can also produce some potentially serious health problems. These problems can be combatted by cleaning up after your dog in parks and gardens.

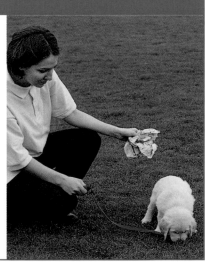

THE RANGE OF INTERNAL PARASITES IN DOGS

A variety of internal parasites that can affect dogs are shown here. The majority live in the intestinal tract, where they have a ready source of nutrients and can largely escape the dog's immune defences. Some have suckers or an arrangement of hooks on their surfaces that they use to attach themselves to the dog's intestinal walls. Often they cause few problems, but they can cause disease if they use up essential nutrients or feed on the host's blood, block the intestinal tract, or damage its walls. The only parasites shown here that do not live in the intestines are the heartworms and the *Leishmania* protozoa. The latter are introduced via sandfly bites into blood, where they immediately affect white blood cells.

SIZE RANGE

The parasites shown here are not to scale. An adult dog tapeworm can be up to 50 to 75 centimetres in length. Adult roundworms and heartworms are smaller (several centimetres in length). The two types of protozoa shown (*Giardia* and *Leishmania*) are microscopic (less than 0.001 mm in length).

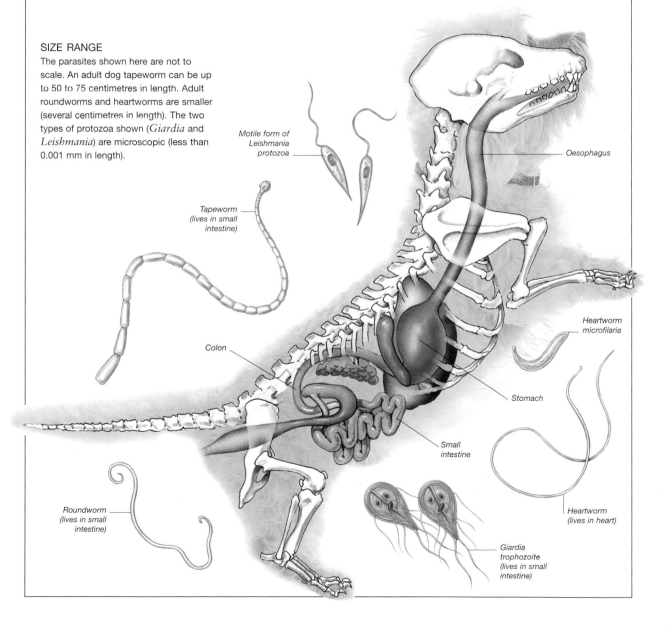

Motile form of
Leishmania
protozoa

Tapeworm
(lives in small
intestine)

Oesophagus

Heartworm
microfilaria

Colon

Stomach

Small
intestine

Roundworm
(lives in small
intestine)

Heartworm
(lives in heart)

Giardia
trophozoite
(lives in small
intestine)

INTESTINAL WORMS

The main intestinal worms in dogs are roundworms, hookworms, and whipworms (three different types of nematode), and tapeworms.

ROUNDWORMS

Roundworms are the most common worms in dogs. The most important species is *Toxocara canis*. An infestation with this worm is known as toxocariasis. Roundworms may cause mild vomiting and diarrhoea in pups. Occasionally, pups or adults pass spaghetti-like worms in their stools. Rarely, a severe worm load may cause a pot-bellied appearance, abdominal pain, dehydration, even death.

TRANSMISSION Pups get *Toxocara* from their mothers while in the womb or from milk. Later they can contract worms from contaminated soil or living conditions.

DIAGNOSIS AND TREATMENT An infestation is diagnosed from finding worm eggs in the dog's faeces on microscopic examination. Treatment with deworming agents such as selamectin (Stronghold, Revolution) is highly effective.

PREVENTION A pregnant bitch should be treated with a deworming agent recommended by your vet during the last weeks of pregnancy to reduce puppy infection and environmental contamination. Pups should be dewormed every two weeks starting at two weeks of age until 12 weeks old. Over six months of age, healthy male dogs should be dewormed yearly. Females should be dewormed after each oestrus cycle. All dogs should be dewormed after treatment with corticosteroid drugs (which weaken the immune system) and whenever they have been stressed by illness. It is often most practical to deworm dogs routinely, twice yearly.

RISK TO PUBLIC HEALTH *Toxocara canis* can cause a condition in humans known as visceral larva migrans, or human toxocariasis. This can occur when a person, usually a child, accidentally consumes a *Toxocara* egg from faecally-contaminated soil. The egg evolves into a larva, but because it is in the wrong host it fails to complete its natural life cycle. Instead, it moves to the lungs, liver, even the eyes where it forms into a cyst and provokes an inflammatory response. This can cause anything from coughing or wheezing to blurred vision or even loss of vision. Routine use of effective wormers and cleaning up after your dog are the two most effective ways to reduce the incidence of toxocariasis in both dogs and humans. Human toxocariasis should not be confused with a completely different disease, toxoplasmosis, which is sometimes transmitted to humans from cats and other animals. Toxoplasmosis is an occasional cause of blindness in children. Toxocariasis can also sometimes cause blindness in humans, but this is extraordinarily rare.

ROUNDWORM LIFE CYCLE

An adult roundworm lives in a dog's intestine and produces eggs which pass out in its faeces. When a dog swallows an egg it hatches into a larva. Hatched larvae encyst in tissues or (in young pups) move via the lungs to the intestine and grow into adult worms. In pregnant and lactating bitches, encysted larvae reactivate and can infect the pup; they also grow into adults in the mother.

PUP INFECTION
Most pups are infected by their mothers in the womb or from her milk. They can also become infected by ingesting worm eggs.

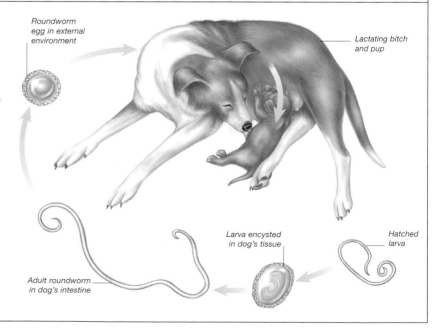

Roundworm egg in external environment

Lactating bitch and pup

Larva encysted in dog's tissue

Hatched larva

Adult roundworm in dog's intestine

HOOKWORMS

Hookworms are tiny parasites that latch onto the lining of their host's intestines and suck blood. This can cause anaemia (low red blood cell count) and symptoms such as diarrhoea (sometimes containing blood), poor appetite, weakness, and weight loss. The most important hookworm species in dogs is called *Ancylostoma caninum*. Although only one half to one centimetre (one quarter to one half inch) in length, this worm, common in areas with hot humid climates such as many parts of Australia and the southern United States, can cause severe disease. Another species, *Uncinaria stenocephala*, can survive in colder climates but causes less serious illness.

TRANSMISSION Adult hookworms produce eggs that pass out of the body in faeces and hatch into larvae on moist ground. The larvae can infect new hosts by several different routes. Pups usually acquire the disease as a result of larvae infecting the mother and passing to the pup in her milk or across the placenta while the pup is still in the womb. Pups and adult dogs can also become infected by accidentally ingesting hookworm larvae in the soil or on grass or by direct penetration of larvae through the pads on the feet or skin on the belly. Finally, pets can become infected by eating the meat of another animal that contains the parasite. Once inside a new host, most larvae eventually move to the host's intestines, but some become encysted in muscle, or in a pregnant bitch may migrate to the mammary glands or uterus.

DIAGNOSIS AND TREATMENT An infestation is diagnosed by finding hookworm eggs in a sample of the dog's faeces, but signs of disease may develop before eggs are seen. Pups often deteriorate quickly from massive blood loss, passing dark or bloody red diarrhoea. Rehydration (restoring the pup's water balance) and treatment for

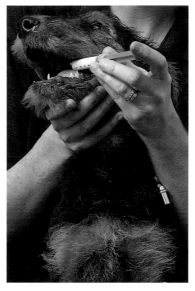

ADMINISTERING MEDICINE
Deworming medicines are available as tablets, granules, or liquids. Granules and liquids are best for giving precise dosages to growing pups.

shock is essential. Some adult dogs carry hookworms and pass their eggs but are free of signs of disease. Others develop serious signs of illness similar to those seen in pups. Worming with a drug such as fenbendazole (Panacur) or pyrantel (contained in Canex and Drontal) eliminates adult worms but not all encysted ones. Repeat worming every two weeks for eight weeks is recommended.

PREVENTION Dogs that have recovered from illness are often hookworm carriers, reinfesting the environment. Good environmental hygiene and preventative worming of pregnant bitches reduce risks from hookworm.

RISK TO PUBLIC HEALTH Hookworm larvae living in soil can penetrate human skin and cause an itchy, bumpy skin condition known as creeping eruption or "cutaneous larva migrans". The use of antihistamine cream is beneficial in relieving the itchiness, although the condition clears without any specific treatment.

WHIPWORMS

Whipworms are thread-like parasites, 5–7 centimetres (2 – 3 inches) in length. They inhabit the colon and small intestine and are blood suckers causing dogs with heavy infestations to develop bloody diarrhoea and weight loss.

TRANSMISSION The worms produce eggs, which pass out in the dog's faeces. A new host can become infected only by ingesting the eggs.

DIAGNOSIS AND TREATMENT Unlike hookworms and roundworms, whipworms do not produce many eggs. This makes diagnosis by examining the dog's faeces for eggs more difficult. Treatment is with a deworming drug and has to be repeated monthly for at least three months.

PREVENTION Whipworm eggs are very stable, surviving for years in the environment. Good park and garden hygiene (stoop and scoop) is the key to reducing environmental contamination.

Q **DO DOGS CARRY HUMAN THREADWORMS?**

A No. Human threadworms cannot be acquired or passed on by dogs.

Q **ARE THERE ANY DRUGS THAT ELIMINATE ALL WORMS?**

A No, but almost. Selamectin (Stronghold, Revolution) is effective for roundworms and heartworms but not tapeworms.

Q **ARE THERE ANY EFFECTIVE COMPLEMENTARY THERAPIES FOR INTERNAL PARASITES?**

A Western-trained vets working in poor regions of the world have observed the effective use of some herbal remedies for worm infestations. However, these cause some discomfort to the dog.

TAPEWORM LIFE CYCLE

The most common tapeworm in dogs is *Dipylidium caninum*. The adult worm lives in the dog's small intestine, with its scolex (head) attached to the intestinal wall. It has many segments. As new segments grow at the worm's head, older ones are pushed towards its tail. These drop off at the tail and are excreted in the dog's faeces or crawl out of its anus. An excreted segment consists of a sac of worm eggs. The eggs are released, and some are eaten by flea larvae in the dog's bedding. The flea larvae grow into adult fleas, which contain young tapeworms. If a dog accidentally ingests one of these fleas, the tapeworm grows into an adult, completing the life cycle.

TAPEWORM SEGMENTS
A freshly excreted tapeworm segment is up to one centimetre (0.4 inch) in length, white, quite flat, and capable of movement. It may resemble a grain of white rice. As it dries, it may look more like a sesame seed. Segments may be seen in an infected dog's faeces or around its anus. Sometimes a string of segments is passed.

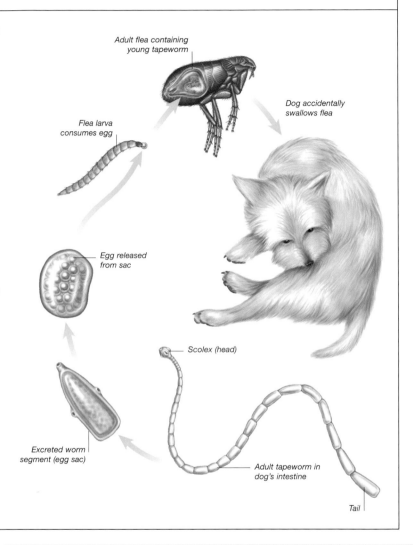

Adult flea containing young tapeworm

Dog accidentally swallows flea

Flea larva consumes egg

Egg released from sac

Scolex (head)

Excreted worm segment (egg sac)

Adult tapeworm in dog's intestine

Tail

TAPEWORMS
Several different types of tapeworm affect dogs. In many species, the tapeworm spends part of its life cycle in an animal other than the dog (the other infected animal is called the "intermediate host"). For the most common dog tapeworm, *Dipylidium caninum*, fleas are the intermediate hosts. This tapeworm can be expected in any dog (or cat) that has had a heavy flea infestation. *Taenia* species of tapeworm occur in dogs that hunt or

TYPES OF TAPEWORM

NAME	INTERMEDIATE HOST
Dipylidium caninum	Fleas and lice
Taenia species	Rats, mice and rodents, rabbits
Diphyllobothrium latum	Freshwater fish
Echinococcus granulosus	Sheep, goats, cattle, deer
Echinococcus multilocularis	Fox or rodents

scavenge wildlife. *Diphyllobothrium* occurs in areas such as the Arctic and New England in dogs (and people) that eat raw freshwater fish. *Echinococcus* species occur in many parts of the world including continental Europe and Australia and are a serious hazard to human health.

DIAGNOSIS AND TREATMENT Tapeworms rarely cause illness in dogs, but it can be upsetting (for the owner) to see tapeworm segments in a dog's faeces or around its anus. Treatment with praziquantel (Droncit, Drontal) is effective against all tapeworms.

RISK TO PUBLIC HEALTH *Echinococcus* species, while causing few problems in dogs, can cause a fatal infection known as hydatid disease in people. Affected dogs or foxes (and dingoes in Australia) pass eggs that are consumed by sheep and other grazing animals. The infected animals develop fluid-filled structures in their tissues called hydatid cysts; these contain forms of the worm that can reinfect dogs. Humans can also act as intermediate hosts for this tapeworm, developing cysts that cannot be destroyed by drugs. Because hydatid disease is so serious, dogs living with sheep should be treated preventatively with praziquantel (Droncit, Drontal) every two months. As part of their Pet Passport Schemes, countries such as Norway, Sweden, Australia, New Zealand, and the UK require that all dogs and cats entering their countries are treated with praziquantel. This virtually eliminates the risk of a pet bringing *Echinococcus* into these countries.

STRONGYLOIDES

This parasite is sometimes called a threadworm (not to be confused with the human threadworm, *Enterobius vermicularis*). It is an uncommon worm, sometimes found in dog kennels with poor hygiene in humid, subtropical climates. Its life cycle resembles that of roundworms. Affected pups have watery or bloody diarrhoea and may develop pneumonia if many worms migrate at the same time through the lungs.

DIAGNOSIS AND TREATMENT An infection is diagnosed by finding worm eggs or larvae in faecal specimens. An anti-worm agent is given for five days and a repeat course given a month later.

RISK TO PUBLIC HEALTH Humans can infect dogs and they can infect us with *Strongyloides*. Infected individuals should be isolated during treatment.

OTHER WORMS

A few worm parasites reside in organs other than the intestines.

HEARTWORMS

The worm *Dirofilaria immitis* spreads via mosquito bites and can grow to a considerable size in a dog's heart and pulmonary arteries. It is a particular hazard in Australia. The symptoms and treatment are discussed fully in Cardiovascular system, *pp.254–56*.

LUNGWORMS

Two different types of worm known as lungworms occasionally affect dogs, causing a cough. Infection by *Capillaria aerophila* occurs when the dog eats earthworms containing infectious larvae. *Filaroides osleri* is most often contracted by pups from their mother's saliva. Dogs contract the lung fluke, *Paragonimus kellicotti*, in parts of North America by eating contaminated crayfish. Treatment with deworming agents is effective for lung flukes and *Capillaria*, but eliminating *Filaroides* is more difficult.

RARE WORMS

Other rare worms include *Spirocerca lupi*, which creates nodules in the dog's oesophagus leading to difficulty swallowing. It can be treated with deworming drugs. The giant kidney worm, *Dioctophyma renale*, is a mink parasite that sometimes affects dogs. It can attain enormous size and is treated by removal of the affected kidney.

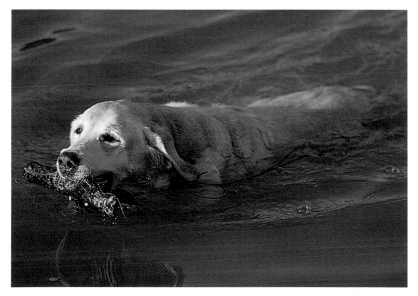

DANGERS OF SCAVENGING
A dog should be discouraged from chasing or killing any other animal, picking up a dead animal in its mouth, or eating its meat. The meat may contain encysted forms of parasites that could be bad for the dog's health. For example, a dog may contract different parasites from eating fish or sheep remains. Also discourage a dog from drinking from ponds and puddles.

PROTOZOAL PARASITES

Some protozoal parasites are relatively inconsequential but others are potentially life-threatening. While some intestinal protozoa are relatively easy to eliminate with safe and simple drugs, others can be frustratingly difficult to overcome.

COCCIDIA

Coccidia are protozoa that infect the intestines and can cause a watery diarrhoea. They primarily cause problems in newborn pups. Coccidia are opportunistic parasites, rarely causing disease unless pups are stressed and living in unsanitary conditions. Affected pups have mild diarrhoea, which may progress to become mucus-covered and tinged with blood, go off their food, and become dehydrated.

DIAGNOSIS AND TREATMENT Coccidia are commonly found in normal pup faeces but they multiply when pups are stressed in some way, for example when they have other internal parasitic conditions such as roundworms. In a pup with coccidiosis, coccidia eggs (oocysts) can usually be detected when faecal samples are examined under a microscope. Treatment includes giving the pup fluids for dehydration when necessary, improving hygiene, eliminating other parasites and the use of antiprotozoal drug therapies such as amprolium. Antibiotics, especially sulpha drugs such as trimethoprim-sulpha, are used to eliminate bacterial infections that follow on from the underlying protozoal cause.

PREVENTION Coccidia parasites are passed in an affected animal's faeces. To prevent spread, it is important to isolate ill animals from other dogs. In a premises where one or more pups have been found to be affected, measures should be taken to dispose of all dog faeces as quickly as possible, preferably by burning. An additional useful measure is to clean the affected pup's environment with a solution that kills coccidia, such as aluminium hydroxide. Good hygiene should be maintained, and young pups subjected to minimal stress.

GIARDIASIS

This increasingly common infection, caused by protozoa belonging to the genus *Giardia*, now occurs in dogs (and cats and people) worldwide. Dogs contract giardiasis by drinking water contaminated with cystic forms of the *Giardia* parasite (oocysts). In most circumstances there are no obvious

GIARDIA LIFE CYCLE

A dog usually acquires a *Giardia* infection by drinking water that has been contaminated with the cyst form of the parasite. In the dog's intestine, the cysts develop into moving, feeding forms called trophozoites, which cause disease symptoms. The trophozoites are capable of dividing and multiplying by binary fission (splitting in two). Some form into cysts, which are passed out in the dog's faeces.

CYSTS AND TROPHOZOITES
The cysts are non-moving cells with a thick wall, which helps them to survive in inhospitable environments. The trophozoites are moving forms of the parasite with tiny suckers on their surfaces. These allow the parasites to attach to the dog's intestinal wall.

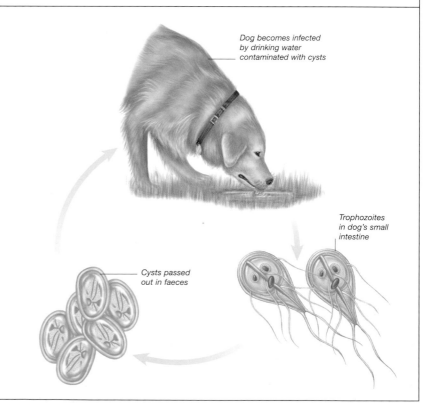

Dog becomes infected by drinking water contaminated with cysts

Trophozoites in dog's small intestine

Cysts passed out in faeces

signs of disease, but some dogs develop persistent, bulky, smelly "cow manure" stools. These unpleasant bowel movements may occur intermittently or become chronic (continue for weeks or months).

DIAGNOSIS AND TREATMENT Oocysts are only shed intermittently by *Giardia* parasites. These are seen on examination of stool samples under a microscope. Because infected dogs are sometimes not producing any detectable oocysts, blood tests are more accurate for establishing whether the disease is present in a particular dog. Giardiasis is relatively simple to treat with either metronidazole (Flagyl) or fenbendazole (Panacur). Metronidazole should not be used in pregnant bitches.

PREVENTION Water contaminated by wildlife is the cause of both human and dog infection. Bottled water and, in developed countries, tap water from the public supply is generally safe. Any other water for human or dog consumption should be filtered, boiled, or treated with sterilizing tablets before it is drunk.

TOXOPLASMOSIS

The causative agent of toxoplasmosis is the protozoal parasite *Toxoplasma gondii*. This parasite rarely causes significant illness in pups. In unusual circumstances it may cause a variety of signs of disease including fever, loss of appetite, breathing difficulties, and a swollen abdomen.

DIAGNOSIS AND TREATMENT
Toxoplasmosis is diagnosed by finding a higher than normal level of antibodies to the parasite in a sample of the infected animal's blood. As with coccidiosis, antibiotics may be used to suppress bacterial infections that develop in consequence of the underlying protozoal disease.

RISK TO PUBLIC HEALTH There is a remote public health hazard from feline toxoplasmosis but not from canine toxoplasmosis. Cat-related

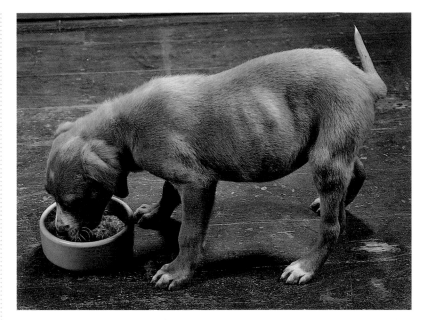

PUPPY WITH SWOLLEN ABDOMEN
A pup's stomach is like a holding tank and typically appears swollen after every meal. This swelling usually diminishes before the next meal. If the stomach remains swollen and the pup looks skinny as this one does, there is a strong possibility it is carrying a heavy worm load.

toxoplasmosis causes hundreds of cases of childhood blindness each year. The cat is the principal host for *Toxoplasma gondii*. For a period of up to four weeks after the first occasion a cat contracts this parasite by eating contaminated wildlife, it passes infectious oocysts in its stool. Livestock accidentally consume infectious cat faeces. The result is that their raw meat contains *Toxoplasma* organisms. Large numbers of people have been exposed to toxoplasmosis, probably (in most cases) through eating undercooked meat, usually without developing any obvious illness. Problems arise if a pregnant woman who has not previously been exposed to toxoplasmosis comes into contact with *Toxoplasma* during the first three months of pregnancy. This can occur if she eats undercooked meat or comes in contact with contaminated cat faeces while gardening or handling cat litter. In these circumstances, her baby may be born blind and have other serious

brain injuries. Pregnant women who test negative for antibodies against *Toxoplasma* should thoroughly cook any meat they eat and wear rubber gloves when handling meat, gardening or cleaning the cat's litter tray. If a woman tests positive for the antibodies, she has had previous exposure to *Toxoplasma* and there is no risk to her foetus.

Pet cats can also be tested for immunity to toxoplasmosis. An immune cat is unlikely to shed infectious oocysts. Dogs, even those with toxoplasmosis, are not a hazard to pregnant women because they do not pass infectious oocysts.

A further complication with the perceived risks of dog faeces is that journalists have sometimes confused toxoplasmosis and toxocariasis, a disease caused by a dog roundworm (*see p. 168*). This has lead to some misleading stories appearing in newspapers about dog faeces blinding children.

LIFE CYCLE OF LEISHMANIA PARASITE

The *Leishmania* parasite spends part of its life in sandflies and part in mammals such as dogs. When a sandfly bites an infected mammal, it ingests macrophages (types of white blood cell) containing a form of the parasite. In the sandfly, the parasite is released and transforms into a motile form (with a whip-like tail). When the sandfly bites another mammal, motile parasites enter the mammal's blood via the wound, are consumed by white blood cells, and revert to the original form.

FOUR-STAGE CYCLE
Some of the main stages in the parasite's life cycle are shown here. Within the dog, infected white blood cells are also continuously bursting and releasing parasites, which then infect new white blood cells.

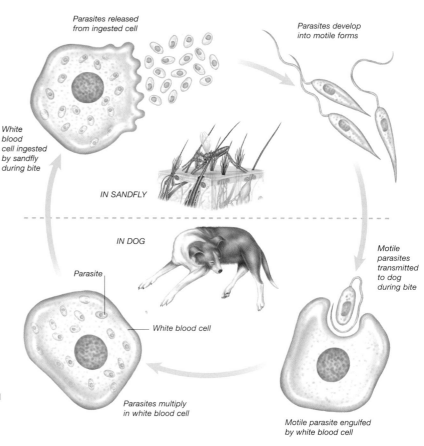

Parasites released from ingested cell

Parasites develop into motile forms

White blood cell ingested by sandfly during bite

IN SANDFLY

IN DOG

Motile parasites transmitted to dog during bite

Parasite

White blood cell

Parasites multiply in white blood cell

Motile parasite engulfed by white blood cell

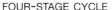

NEOSPORA CANINUM
The illness caused by this protozoal parasite is an "emerging disease" that is not yet fully understood. The causative parasite looks similar under a microscope to *Toxoplasma gondii,* the cause of toxoplasmosis. The complete life cycle of the parasite has yet to be established, but it is known that the infection can be transmitted from mother to pup within the uterus via the placenta. Affected dogs, usually pups between three and six weeks of age, develop muscle and nerve conditions ranging from lameness to sore muscles to muscle wasting and paralysis. Sometimes several pups in the same litter are affected. Some infected dogs, particularly adults, may have no obvious signs of disease.

DIAGNOSIS AND TREATMENT A rising level of antibodies to the parasite, measured in the animal's blood, indicates a recent infection. Effective treatments, based on antiprotozoal drugs, are being developed.

LEISHMANIASIS
This serious protozoal infection, also called kala-azar, is the most common and serious parasitic disease in dogs in southern Europe. It affects up to 40 per cent of dogs throughout Greece, extending halfway up the Adriatic coast of former Yugoslavia and Italy. It is established on the Mediterranean coast of Italy and France and throughout Spain and Portugal. It does not occur in Australia. In North America it was first reported in 2000 among pack hounds in some areas of the southeastern United States.

The disease is usually acquired as a result of sandfly bites. The parasite affects types of white blood cells called macrophages. A sandfly picks up white blood cells infected with *Leishmania* parasites when feeding on an infected dog and transmits the parasites to another dog (or other mammal) when it takes another meal. The recent occurrence of the disease among pack hounds in the United States is perplexing. As there are no sandflies in the affected region, how it arrived in North America and how it is transmitted there remains uncertain.

There are two forms of the disease. In the usually non-fatal cutaneous (skin) form, an affected dog develops crusty, dandruffy areas that may become discoloured, even ulcerated. In the almost always fatal visceral form, there is anaemia (low red blood cell count), sometimes diarrhoea and almost always some damage to the liver and spleen. Affected dogs lose their vigour and may look emaciated.

DIAGNOSIS AND TREATMENT Leishmaniasis is diagnosed by finding organisms in smears taken from lymph nodes or in skin scrapings. Anti-Leishmania drugs are licensed in some countries. Even with treatment the outlook is poor for any dog with the visceral form of leishmaniasis.

PREVENTION Sandflies bite at night. Dogs should be kept indoors from dusk until dawn in localities where sandflies exist.

RISK TO PUBLIC HEALTH Humans can also contract leishmaniasis and there has been some concern that an infected dog is a health hazard to its human family. Evidence from Mediterranean Europe suggests that an infected dog is only a potential hazard to individuals with weakened immune systems, such as those who are HIV-positive.

BABESIOSIS

Babesia parasites affect red blood cells and are transmitted by ticks between mammals such as dogs, cattle, sheep, and occasionally humans. These parasites occur in many regions of the world including parts of Europe, Asia, Africa, and some northern parts of Australia. They are unusual in North America, although found in some dogs in the southeastern United States ranging up to Massachusetts. Affected dogs are listless from severe anaemia (low red blood cell count) and may pass dark-coloured urine.

DIAGNOSIS AND TREATMENT *Babesia* may be seen in blood samples from affected animals. Antibody tests are also used for detection. As with leishmaniasis, anti-Babesia drugs are licensed in some (European) countries.

PREVENTION Dogs in regions of Europe, Asia, Africa, and Australasia where this parasite lives should be routinely treated with tick prevention measures such as the use of fipronil (Frontline) spray or the wearing of an amitraz (Preventic) collar.

AMERICAN TRYPANOSOMIASIS

The protozoal parasite *Trypanosoma cruzi* is common in Central and South America but fortunately rare in North America and does not occur in Australasia. It is transmitted when certain blood-sucking insects called "assassin bugs" or "kissing bugs" take a meal from a dog, or from humans. While feeding, the bug defaecates, passing the protozoa in its faeces. The dog or person scratches the bite and the protozoa, called trypanosomes, enter the bloodstream, where they invade white blood cells. As with all parasites, pups are more susceptible than adults. Signs of the disease (which is also known as Chagas' disease) may include enlarged lymph nodes, fever, and incoordination. The heart and muscles may be affected.

DIAGNOSIS AND TREATMENT The disease is diagnosed by the finding of trypanosome parasites in blood samples during acute stages of the disease. Tests for antibodies to the parasite are also used. There are at present no effective treatments for American trypanosomiasis.

PREVENTION Transmission of the disease can be reduced by the use of insecticide to eliminate the blood-sucking assassin bugs from homes in regions where they exist.

IMMUNE BENEFITS?

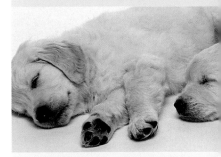

Recent evidence suggests that contact with parasites early in life may be beneficial. Researchers at Cambridge University noted that most African people show evidence of past or present parasitic infestations but suffer only low levels of autoimmune disorders such as diabetes or rheumatoid arthritis. In Europe, Japan, and North America, the incidence of parasites is low but the incidence of autoimmune disease is significant and increasing.

These relationships could be explained by simple coincidence but for an intriguing discovery. Animal studies have shown that diabetes, an autoimmune disease, is usually triggered by special immune cells called TH1 cells. Parasitic infestations stimulate a similar but slightly different cell called TH2. High TH2 levels seem to inhibit TH1 manufacture and activity, and the lower the TH1 activity the lower the risk of autoimmune disease.

The increase in the incidence of autoimmune disease in dogs has coincided with more effective worming of young pups. At present there is no evidence to prove a link between these two seemingly unrelated facts, but the possibility that there is a real causal link is being actively investigated by veterinary immunologists.

SKIN AND HAIR
the dog's first line of defence

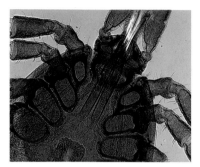

Microscopic view of a tick

Skin disease accounts for about two out of five of dogs' visits to the vet. The reason is obvious. It is easier to see when something is wrong with the skin than it is for any other body system. A dog's skin may be affected by parasites, most commonly fleas, and by bacterial and fungal infections. Skin problems may also result from a response of the immune system, as occurs in allergies, or from a variety of hormonal and hereditary disorders. In addition, some diseases affect the condition of a dog's coat and may even cause hair loss.

Skin is durable, elastic, and capable of excellent self-repair when damaged. A layer of fat beneath the dermis (lower layer of skin) offers insulation and further physical protection.

FUNCTIONS OF THE SKIN

The dog's skin and hair are its first line of defence against physical damage and microbial invasion. The skin forms a protective barrier between the harsh environment of the outside world and the internal organs. Some of the surface skin cells produce a pigment called melanin that gives colour to the skin and hair, and protects the skin from ultraviolet radiation in sunlight.

The skin is the body's largest sensory organ, infiltrated with millions of nerve endings that monitor the environment. These nerve endings influence body temperature and also, through pain sensitivity, how a dog responds to potential dangers.

The skin is also an important organ of the immune system. It contains immune cells that multiply when the skin is injured, causing inflammation, which is necessary for repair. Other immune system cells, such as mast cells, explode when irritated, releasing chemicals that provoke scratching and rubbing. Sometimes the skin thickens

as a defensive response, forming areas such as elbow calluses, to reduce the likelihood of the skin breaking and pathogens getting through.

THE DOG'S COAT

Hair provides physical protection for the skin, including protection from ultraviolet radiation in sunlight, and also offers insulation.

In most dogs, the coat is made up of two kinds of hair: coarse, protective "guard" hair, and finer, insulating "down" hair. In breeds such as the German Shepherd Dog, guard hair naturally predominates. Selective breeding has eliminated the downy coat from some breeds; for example, Yorkshire Terriers have only about 100 hairs per square centimetre compared to the 500 hairs per square centimetre of most Nordic breeds. Other breeds, such as the Boxer, have no downy hair and only short guard hair. These dogs have diminished physical insulation.

Hair grows from pits called follicles in the skin. Growth occurs in cycles, in which a rapid growth phase (anagen phase) is followed by a long resting stage (catagen phase). Inevitably for most dogs, shedding (telogen phase) then occurs. In this stage, hair detaches from its anchor in the follicle. Licking,

rubbing, rolling, or grooming help to remove loosened hair. The growth cycle is affected partly by the environmental temperature, but more strongly by increasing or decreasing daylight. Hormones, nutrition, stress, and genetic factors also influence the cycle.

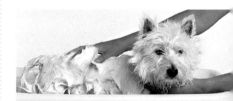

Q IS BATHING MY DOG GOOD FOR ITS SKIN?

A Bathing your dog about once a month helps to keep its skin clean and healthy. It is a fallacy that shampooing dries the skin and makes hair brittle. Provided you use a mild shampoo, the opposite is true.

Q DOES BATHING REMOVE FLEAS?

A Bathing does not get rid of fleas. If fleas are a problem, use an effective flea-control product on your dog and in its environment.

CROSS SECTION OF SKIN AND HAIR

The skin consists of two main layers: the epidermis, the thin outer layer; and the dermis, the thick inner layer; the epidermis comprises sheets of tough, flat cells, which are shed as dander through natural wear and tear. Skin derives its strength from the protein keratin, which also makes up the hair and nails. The dermis is made of strong, elastic tissue. It contains nerve endings that respond to heat, pressure, and pain; blood vessels; sebaceous glands, which release an oily fluid to moisten and waterproof the skin; and sweat glands in the foot that are involved in temperature regulation. Beneath the dermis is a layer of fat that provides insulation. Hair grows from hair follicles – modified regions of epidermis that reach into the dermis.

TYPES OF HAIR

Most dogs have a mixture of coarse, protective hair, and fine, insulating down. Arrector pili muscles, attached to each coarse hair, tense to pull the hair upright when the dog is cold or frightened.

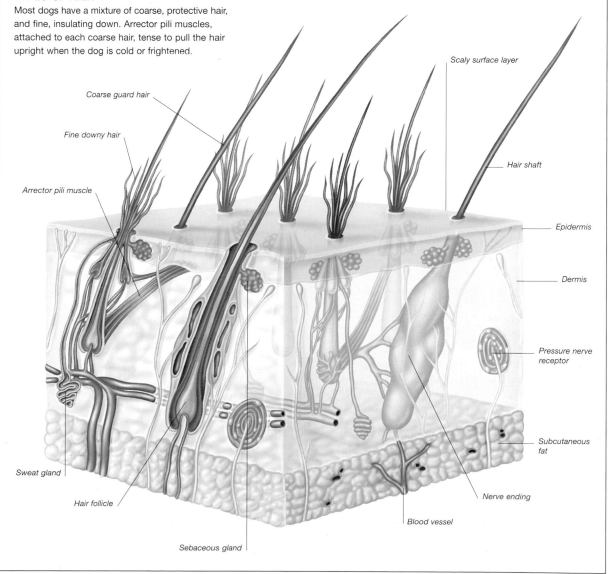

Coarse guard hair

Fine downy hair

Arrector pili muscle

Sweat gland

Hair follicle

Sebaceous gland

Scaly surface layer

Hair shaft

Epidermis

Dermis

Pressure nerve receptor

Subcutaneous fat

Nerve ending

Blood vessel

CARE OF THE SKIN AND HAIR

Dogs keep their hair and skin in good condition by licking, scratching, dry bathing (rolling in dust), or simply by getting wet. Saliva contains natural antiseptics, and licking and scratching are normal activities that are beneficial in moderation. Rolling and rubbing are ways in which a dog massages its skin, removes debris from areas that it cannot reach with its tongue or paws, and activates its sebaceous glands. A primary function of the sebaceous glands is to secrete oil (sebum), which waterproofs the skin and hair and enables dirt and debris to be washed out of the coat whenever it gets wet. The sebaceous gland secretions also have antimicrobial properties.

You can also help your dog to keep its skin and hair healthy by regular

KEEPING CLEAN

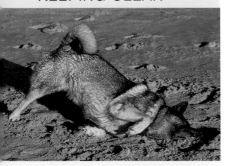

Rolling in dust or sand is a natural way in which dogs look after their skin and coat. Rolling has a massaging effect on the dog's skin, which, apart from feeling good to the dog, has the following benefits:
• the dog dislodges stubborn debris that it cannot remove by grooming with its tongue and paws;
• the sebaceous glands in the skin are stimulated. These glands produce an oily substance called sebum that waterproofs the skin and makes the coat look sleek. Sebum also contains chemicals that prevent infection.

bathing and grooming. There is a wide range of grooming items designed for different coats, including slicker brushes for fine or short hair; pin brushes for longer hair; and thinning scissors and stripping combs for thinning dense coats. See opposite for specific advice on dealing with different hair types.

Grooming and bathing are ideal opportunities to examine your dog for signs of skin and hair problems. The following areas can easily be checked.

THE EARS

Check your dog's ears routinely for odour, inflammation, or wax build-up. Do not worry about a little ear wax; the wax is a natural form of protection. Only remove the wax if there is a great deal of it. Use a proprietary ear wax remover, available from your veterinary surgeon, or simply wipe the inside of the ear with a cotton ball moistened with mineral oil. If wax builds up again within the week, take your dog to the vet for a checkup.

Floppy-eared dogs, such as Cocker Spaniels, Labrador Retrievers, and Basset Hounds, are more prone to ear problems because the inside of their ears is damp and warm, encouraging the growth of yeasts, mites, and bacteria.

Hair growing down the ear canal is a considerable nuisance in particular breeds. All naturally wire-haired breeds have ear hair, as do Poodles, Shih Tzus, Lhasa Apsos, and many Yorkshire Terriers. This hair needs to be removed weekly or even daily. Fingernails or tweezers work well. Grasp a few hairs at a time and pull them out. This task is usually quite easy and not upsetting to your dog. Always give a treat after plucking ear hair.

THE EYES

Some breeds, of which the Yorkshire Terrier is a classic example, develop "sleep" in the corners of their eyes.

This is simply mucus, a natural protective secretion that keeps the eyes clean. Overnight, it often forms a small, hard, crusty ball that catches in the hair at the corners of the eyes. It is often easy to pick off the "sleep" with your fingernails, but if the mucus is stuck, first soften it with a cotton ball dipped in lukewarm water. If left unattended, the dried mucus provides a haven for bacteria, which may cause a skin infection to develop in the corners of the eyes.

HAIRY FEET

Some breeds, including all the spaniels, grow an abundance of hair, top and bottom, between their toes. This hair acts like a magnet for dirt, debris, and grass seeds (sometimes called foxtails) that, once caught in the hair, can easily penetrate the skin. This problem may lead to the formation of a swelling called an interdigital cyst (see p.186). Using blunt-tipped scissors, carefully cut away excess hair on the feet. A professional groomer or veterinary nurse can show you how to do this.

ANAL SACS

Certain breeds, including Dachshunds, retrievers, and spaniels, are especially susceptible to problems with the scent sacs around the anus (see p.290). There is a scent sac under the skin on either side of the anus, at the "four and eight o'clock" positions. The sacs contain a malodourous discharge that is disgusting to us, but is enormously attractive to other dogs.

Avoid conditions such as painful abscesses in this region by checking the sacs before bathing your dog. They normally empty naturally, but should be drained if they are full. (Sacs that are full feel like hard grapes.) Your veterinary surgeon can empty blocked anal sacs; alternatively, you can learn how to do it yourself (see p.290).

DIFFERENT COAT TYPES AND HOW TO GROOM THEM

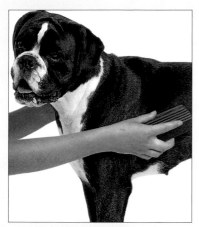

SMOOTH COATS

Dogs such as Boxers that have smooth, thin coats need brushing about once a week. Use a hound glove or rubber brush, as shown above, and brush gently with the lie of the coat. This action removes loose hair and stimulates the skin's oil glands to make the coat look healthy and sleek. Stubborn debris in the coat may be removed by applying cooking oil to soften it.

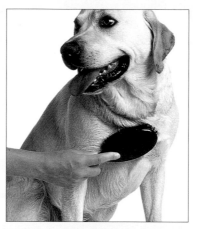

SHORT, THICK COATS

In dogs such as Labrador Retrievers, the undercoat needs the most attention. Use a slicker brush with the lie of the coat to clear tangles, then against the lie to remove loose hair. Use a bristle brush to get rid of any remaining debris. Finish with a fine-toothed comb; pay special attention to the thickest hair, on the neck and tail. Brush once weekly, or twice weekly during moults.

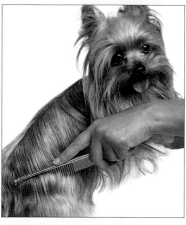

SILKY HAIR

Some long-haired breeds, such as the Maltese and the Yorkshire Terrier, have no protective undercoat and thin skin that is susceptible to laceration. This makes them sensitive to irritation from rough grooming. First, tease out tangles with a slicker brush, then use a bristle brush to position the hair. Follow by combing. Brush daily, trimming untidy ends at least once a month.

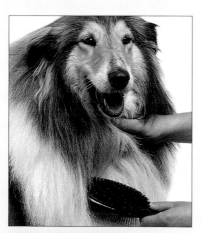

LONG, DENSE COATS

For dogs such as Rough Collies, remove tangles with a slicker brush, then use a pin brush to penetrate through the density of the coat. After thorough pin-brushing, use a wide-toothed comb throughout the coat, paying particular attention to the feathers on the legs, chest, hindquarters, and tail. Brush daily and trim excess hair monthly.

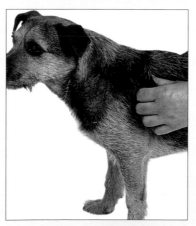

WIRY COATS

Dogs such as Border Terriers, with wiry coats, should be brushed twice weekly in the same way as for other short, thick coats (*see above*). They also need their coats stripped. Once a month, thin any overgrown hair on the back by running a stripping comb through it. Wiry coats should be stripped professionally every three to four months.

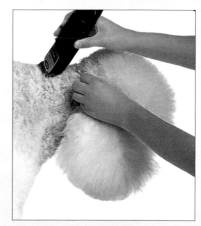

NON-MOULTING COATS

Clipping is necessary every six to eight weeks in breeds such as Poodles or the Bichon Frise, whose coats simply keep growing. Daily brushing is important, and clipping should be done as necessary after grooming and bathing. It is often best to leave clipping to a professional groomer, especially if you want a particular style.

DIAGNOSING SKIN DISEASES

CLASSIFYING SKIN PROBLEMS

There are several ways of approaching the description and classification of skin conditions. Classification is important for diagnosis and treatment.

PRIMARY OR SECONDARY?

Most skin problems are primary; that is, involving only the skin. Others are secondary problems – manifestations on the skin of more complicated internal conditions. Sunburn (*see p.197*), for example, is a primary skin condition, whereas ulcers that develop due to a disease of the immune system (*see p.200*) are described as secondary, a symptom of a more general problem.

CAUSES OR SIGNS?

Veterinary surgeons often classify skin diseases according to their causes, as shown in the box on the opposite page. For dog owners, however, it may be more useful to start by identifying any abnormalities on their dog's skin. In the following pages, rather than following a traditional classification, skin diseases are presented according to clinical signs that you are likely to see. The information starts with a discussion of conditions that cause hair loss; these conditions are followed by problems causing "lumps and bumps", skin pigment changes, itchiness, pimples, scaling and crusting, and finally erosions and ulcers.

This descriptive classification has some practical advantages, but it is important to bear in mind that skin diseases are rarely discrete problems causing just one type of clinical sign. Virtually all of them cause a whole range of signs, and in some cases these signs vary during the course of the disease. As an example, parasites, particularly fleas, are responsible for causing the majority of irritating skin conditions. A single insect can cause inflammation, scaling, bleeding, and crusting, erosions, ulcerations, lumps, and hair loss. Therefore, there is bound to be some overlap between classifications according to signs. Conditions are listed on these pages according to the symptoms that they most commonly produce.

GENERALIZED OR LOCALIZED?

When looking at skin diseases in terms of signs, it can be useful to note which parts of the body are affected. Many skin disorders, such as allergic dermatitis (*see pp.190–93*), can affect several or all areas of the body surface at once. Localized skin conditions are those, such as tumours (*see p.188*) or injection reaction (*see p.186*), that affect only one particular part of the body surface or are restricted to a small area of the skin.

DIAGNOSTIC METHODS

If you are concerned about the condition of your dog's skin or hair, arrange a veterinary check-up. Your vet will carry out a thorough physical examination and use one or more of the following techniques to help diagnose the cause of the problem.

RESPONSE TO TREATMENT

Most often, the vet examines your dog, makes a diagnosis, then dispenses a treatment, such as parasite control or antibiotics. A complete response is not only a cure; it is also diagnostic. The problem is what the vet expected.

SKIN SCRAPINGS

The vet gently scrapes the surface of the affected skin and looks at the scrapings under a microscope. This test may be done to identify causes of itchiness such as scabies (*see p.197*) or Demodex mites (*see p.183*).

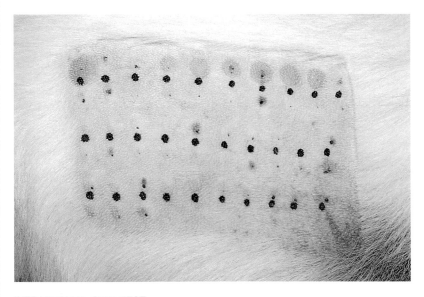

INTRADERMAL SKIN TEST

An intradermal skin test relies on varying skin reactions to potential allergens, to reveal the cause of allergic skin disease. In the test above, various potential allergens have been introduced into the skin and different levels of inflammatory reaction have been provoked.

SKIN SMEAR

The vet applies adhesive tape firmly to itchy areas, then peels it off the skin and examines the resulting smear under a microscope. Skin smears can detect Malassezia yeast (*see p.196*), Cheyletiella mites (*see p.196*), bacteria, and inflammatory cells.

SKIN BIOPSY

A skin biopsy reveals what is happening to skin cells. This is a particularly useful procedure, especially for skin conditions that are difficult to diagnose. A biopsy, or sample of skin cells, is usually taken with a small tool called a biopsy punch and then examined under a microscope.

BACTERIAL OR FUNGAL CULTURE

A sterile swab of an affected area of skin may be taken for bacterial culture. This enables the vet to identify the infectious agent. Hair may be removed for a fungal culture to determine if ringworm (*see p.184*) is present.

ULTRAVIOLET EXAMINATION

A hair sample is placed under ultraviolet light in a dark room. Hair infected with the most common type of ringworm (*Microsporum canis*) will fluoresce.

INTRADERMAL SKIN TESTING

To help diagnose specific causes of allergic itchiness, small amounts of potential irritants, such as pollens, dust mite, human dander, and flea saliva, are injected into the skin. The injection sites are monitored for inflammation and itchiness. This procedure is best performed by an experienced veterinary dermatologist.

ELISA TESTING

To avoid the inconvenience of testing a dog itself, ELISA tests for allergies are done in test tubes. The reliability of these tests has improved, making it possible for general practice vets to make accurate diagnoses of the causes of canine allergic itchiness.

PATCH TESTING

Patch testing is used to diagnose allergic contact dermatitis (*see p.193*). Suspected causes of allergies are applied under a patch to the skin, and the skin is later checked for inflammation.

BLOOD TESTS

Hormonal imbalances cause a variety of skin changes. Blood tests are used to monitor hormone levels. Autoimmune conditions (*see p.200*) are diagnosed by immunological blood tests.

DIET CHANGE

Food, and specifically the protein in food, can cause itchy skin disease. Feeding an "exclusion diet" (a unique protein and unique carbohydrate that a dog has never had before) for at least four to six weeks can be diagnostic of food allergy if itchiness diminishes on the diet (*see pp.97–98*).

ENVIRONMENT CHANGE

Itchy skin allergies can be triggered by human dander, house dust mites, and even contact with freshly cut grass. Your vet may suggest an environment change (if it is practical) to help make

CLASSIFICATION

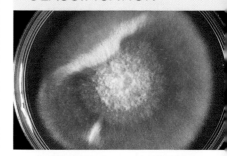

Skin diseases are often classified by cause, as in the following examples:

PARASITES

Flea or tick infestation (*pp.162–64*), Demodex mite disease (*p.183*)

INFECTION

Abscess (*p.188*), General bacterial skin infection (*p.196*), Furunculosis (*p.200*), Ringworm (*p.184*)

HORMONAL

Hair loss due to underactive thyroid gland (*p.182*)

IMMUNE-MEDIATED

Allergic dermatitis (*pp.190–93*), Autoimmune conditions (*pp.200–01*)

NUTRITIONAL

Zinc-responsive dermatosis (*p.195*)

TUMOURS

Lipoma (*p.188*), Melanoma (*p.188*), Histiocytoma (*p.188*)

HEREDITARY

Sebaceous adenitis (*p.195*), Hereditary seborrhoea (*p.194*), Colour dilution alopecia (*p.187*)

ANATOMICAL

Skin fold infection (*p.198*)

ENVIRONMENTAL

Interdigital cysts (*p.186*), Sunburn (*p.197*), Acute moist dermatitis (*p.198*)

commonly an overactive adrenal gland
(*see p.335*), an underactive thyroid
gland (*see p.331*), diabetes mellitus
(*see p.336*), a tumour, or failure of the
immune system.

DIAGNOSIS AND TREATMENT In pups
affected by localized Demodex mite
disease, 9 out of 10 cases clear up
spontaneously over a period of two
months. More generalized disease is a
potentially serious disorder demanding
rigorous treatment.

The aim of treatment is to find the
underlying cause of Demodex mite
proliferation and eliminate or control
the primary problem. At the same
time, the skin is treated with a benzoyl
peroxide shampoo to remove scale and
with amitraz to kill mites. (Follow
your veterinary surgeon's instructions
carefully when using amitraz; it kills
mites but can be toxic to your dog and
to you.) Antibiotics may be given to
control secondary bacterial infection.
Corticosteroids have, controversially,
been used in the past to suppress
itchiness in Demodex mite disease,
but this is no longer considered a
suitable treatment.

RINGWORM

Ringworm is a fungal infection of the
hair and hair follicles. It may affect any
part of the body but often develops
on the face and ears. It occurs more
frequently in pups than in adult dogs.
The most common cause of ringworm
is *Microsporum canis*, but other types
of fungi (*Microsporum gypseum* and
Trichophyton mentagrophytes) can
also cause the disease.

Affected individuals typically show
skin irritation resembling an allergic
reaction, and a circular loss of hair,
where infection occurs; however, not
all dogs respond typically. The less
common ringworm-producing fungi
(*M. gypseum* and *T. mentagrophytes*)
often cause more inflamed and
irregular areas of hair loss. Affected
hair can easily be pulled from the skin.
Ringworm does not usually cause
itchiness, but secondary bacterial
infection may occur, producing crusts
that cause the dog to lick and scratch
itself excessively.

DIAGNOSIS AND TREATMENT Ringworm
infection can mimic a variety of other
skin conditions, and conversely many

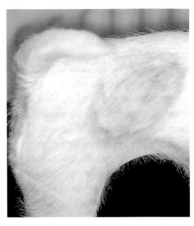

RINGWORM HAIR LOSS
This roughly circular patch of hair loss,
with accompanying skin inflammation and
redness, is typical of infection with the
fungi that produce ringworm.

problems that look like ringworm turn
out to be something else. Diagnosis is
therefore by signs along with specific
tests. Hairs infected with *M. canis*
fluoresce under ultraviolet light, while
hairs infected with other causes of
ringworm do not. A fungal culture
confirms diagnosis, but because culture
can take a week or more treatment
often begins before culture reveals the
type of fungus involved.

Mild cases of ringworm in healthy
dogs are usually overwhelmed by the
immune system and improve without
treatment. Pups, and individuals with
more severe infections or compromised
immune systems, are less capable of
caring for themselves. Even if only a
small area is visibly infected, such dogs
should be completely bathed in an
antifungal shampoo. Small areas of
infection are then treated topically
with an antifungal cream or lotion
(usually miconazole or ketoconazole).
Treatment continues until at least two
weeks after all of the signs have
disappeared, or two weeks after fungal
culture is negative. In severe cases,
your vet may give oral antibiotics –
usually griseofulvin, which should be
given for at least four weeks.

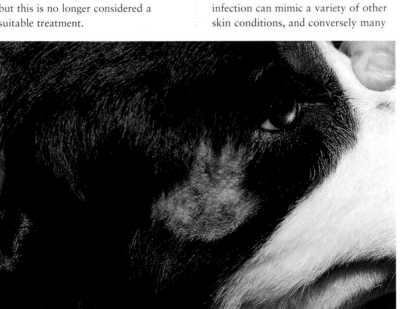

HAIR LOSS DUE TO DEMODEX MITE DISEASE
The bald patch in this dog's coat has been caused by infestation with the Demodex
mite. This condition also causes the skin to become oily and thickened.

EXCESSIVE LICKING

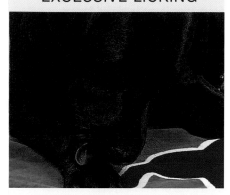

Many veterinary dermatologists and behaviourists think that excessive licking, to the point where a dog causes damage to its own skin, is a condition that has psychological or emotional causes. It is a so-called "psychogenic" disease.

Breeds most often affected include:

- Doberman
- German Shepherd Dog
- Great Dane
- Irish Setter
- Labrador Retriever (above)

BEHAVIOURAL CAUSES OF HAIR LOSS

Persistent licking or scratching can cause localized hair loss and also injure the underlying skin.

LICK DERMATITIS

This common condition is also known as lick granuloma or acral dermatitis; the variety of names is a clue to its complexity. The essential sign is licking, usually on the forelegs, leading to localized thickening of the skin and associated hair loss. The skin becomes pinkish-red, shiny, and sore, and the surrounding hair is stained a mahogany colour from saliva. Continued licking may lead to ulceration of the skin. Lick dermatitis is most common among mature male dogs.

DIAGNOSIS AND TREATMENT Diagnosis is based upon the dog's medical history and elimination of other possible causes of hair loss. Treatment involves prevention of further licking and the elimination of secondary bacterial infections. An Elizabethan collar prevents licking while healing of the skin occurs. In some instances, damage is so severe that conventional surgery, cryosurgery (freezing), or local steroid injection is necessary. There has been some reported success using anti-anxiety drugs such as amitriptyline and clomipramine to reduce licking behaviour, although it is not known whether these drugs reduce "anxiety" or simply lessen the tingling pain sensation. Boredom is thought to play an important role in this condition, so any treatment programme involves a re-evaluation of the dog's lifestyle.

ENVIRONMENTAL CAUSES OF HAIR LOSS

In some cases, hair loss is triggered by particular factors encountered in the environment, such as plant seeds, or by grooming practices such as clipping.

PRESSURE SORES AND ELBOW CALLUSES

Heavyweight dogs put extraordinary pressure on their elbow skin when they lie down. The skin responds by thickening its surface, producing adherent scale, or "callus". Eventually, the hair is lost and the callus comes into direct contact with the ground. In particularly heavy dogs, calluses may also develop over the bony prominences of the hips or the hocks. The calluses may crack, bleed, and become infected by bacteria.

DIAGNOSIS AND TREATMENT Calluses occur in middle-aged or older heavy dogs. Secondary infection is treated with antibiotics. Severely cracked skin may need surgical repair. Dry calluses are lubricated with petroleum jelly or humectants (moisturisers). Heavy dogs

Q ARE SOME BREEDS MORE PRONE TO HAIR PROBLEMS?

A Certain breeds are prone to alterations in the quantity and quality of their hair. The Boxer, English Bulldog, French Bulldog, and Miniature Schnauzer can develop a cyclical hair loss followed by regrowth. Airedales have a similar condition that causes a saddle-like loss of hair. Other breeds, including the Siberian Husky, Irish Water Spaniel, Portuguese Water Dog, and Curly-coated Retriever, can develop woolly, rust-coloured coats. All of these uncommon conditions appear to be genetic in origin. They may be seasonal or permanent.

Q HOW SAFE ARE TREATMENTS FOR RINGWORM?

A Commonly prescribed drugs for ringworm are safe and effective for most dogs. Griseofulvin and ketoconazole, however, can cause birth defects; they should not be given to pregnant dogs or handled by pregnant women.

Q HOW CONTAGIOUS IS RINGWORM?

A Ringworm spreads as easily among dogs as athlete's foot spreads among us. As with athlete's foot, there need not be direct contact with the carrier. Ringworm can be left in the environment by a carrier, then picked up by another dog. If your dog has ringworm, isolate it from other pets until your vet gives the all-clear. Cover its bedding or any furniture that it lies on with a sheet, and wash the sheet every two days using a mild bleach solution to kill ringworm spores. Give your home a thorough vacuuming. Dip all of your dog's grooming implements in a solution of one part bleach and 32 parts water.

SKIN LUMPS AND BUMPS

There is a wide range of conditions that produce lumps and bumps on the skin surface. Cancer is one of them, but such disorders also include many relatively harmless forms of skin tumour and growth. See Tumours (*pp.130–41*) for more detailed coverage of this group of skin conditions.

CYST

A cyst is a sac-like cavity. A skin cyst (epidermoid cyst) is a round, firm, discrete, painless swelling that develops within a hair follicle. Epidermoid cysts often contain a cheese-like substance. These cysts are often wrongly referred to as sebaceous cysts.

DIAGNOSIS AND TREATMENT   Cysts are diagnosed by examination and biopsy if necessary. They are treated by draining. Do not squeeze cysts; this only causes local inflammation and heightens the risk of infection.

ABSCESS

An abscess is a deep infection that is walled off in a pocket of tissue under the skin. Bacteria are deposited by an object such as a tooth or claw that

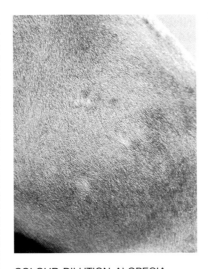

COLOUR DILUTION ALOPECIA
In this blue Weimaraner, patches of blue-coloured hair have become brittle and dull, and the hair in these places has begun to fall out, leaving bare, dry skin.

penetrates the skin. White blood cells attack the invaders, while the body walls off the "battlefield" to prevent the skirmish from spreading elsewhere. Abscesses may feel hot, and the surrounding skin may be reddened. An abscess is a common form of foreign body reaction (*see p.186*).

DIAGNOSIS AND TREATMENT   Abscesses are diagnosed by examination and, if necessary, biopsy. They are treated by draining and antibiotics.

HAEMATOMA

A haematoma is an accumulation of blood under the skin as a result of injury. Vigorous shaking of the head can also cause haematoma on the ear flaps. Haematomas may be hot and reddened, but are rarely painful.

GRANULOMA

A granuloma is a connective tissue response to any object that penetrates the epidermis (outer layer of the skin). Granulomas tend to be raised, firm swellings that lack discrete margins. A granuloma is a common response of the skin to a "sterile" foreign body,

such as to a needle in an injection reaction (*see p.186*).

DIAGNOSIS AND TREATMENT
Granulomas often spontaneously diminish in size. Any lump that does not shrink should be examined by a vet.

PAPILLOMA

This is a cauliflower-like growth protruding from the skin. Affected dogs frequently have crops of such growths at the same time. Papillomas may be pink and are painless. They do not usually need to be treated unless they become injured or infected.

LIPOMA

A lipoma is the name for a tumour of fat cells. Lipomas may occur anywhere on the body and are most common in older individuals. They are usually painless and can be felt under the skin as soft, round growths. They are treated by surgical removal.

PERIANAL ADENOMA

This condition is a discrete swelling in the tissue around the anus, in older male dogs. It often causes the dog to lick the anal area excessively. The tumour is treated by surgical removal.

HISTIOCYTOMA

This tumour is a button-like, raised lump that may be red and inflamed and can form anywhere on the body. It is most common in young dogs.

SKIN CANCERS

A variety of cancerous skin tumours, including melanomas, basal cell tumours, squamous cell carcinomas, and mast cell tumours, may cause lumps and bumps on the skin. Most of these conditions are more common in older dogs. All of these tumours are potentially dangerous; they are treated by surgical removal of the growth together with a wide margin of the surrounding healthy tissue. Cancer is confirmed by an examination of the tissue removed from the tumour.

VET'S ADVICE

Those of us who live close to our dogs and groom them regularly find lumps and bumps earlier than ever before. I am happy to say that year by year I am asked to comment on ever-smaller skin masses. This is marvellous because the earlier a condition is seen, the easier it is to treat. While many dog owners are concerned they have found a cancer when they come across a lump, more often than not the lump is something much less serious.

PIGMENT CHANGES

Some skin conditions produce loss of skin pigment, while others cause increased pigmentation. Many causes of pigment changes are of no medical consequence, but some are good clues to the presence of other conditions.

HYPOPIGMENTATION

Pigment can be lost after virtually any form of skin damage. In addition, some individuals inherit a condition called vitiligo, in which some parts of the body spontaneously lose pigment. Other dogs lose pigment, either seasonally or permanently, only from their nose leather (*see right*). Immune-mediated diseases such as pemphigus and lupus erythematosus (*see pp.200–01*) may also cause pigment loss, especially in Collies and German Shepherd Dogs from one to three years old.

DIAGNOSIS AND TREATMENT A skin biopsy is necessary to enable accurate diagnosis of pigmentation loss. Autoimmune conditions are treated with immune-suppressing drugs. For vitiligo, all you can do is protect the skin by keeping the dog out of bright sunlight and using sunblocks. There are no known treatments or dietary supplements that promote the return of skin pigmentation. Tattooing has sometimes been used medically to protect hypopigmented ear skin from sunburn, but tattooing itself may cause an allergic or irritant skin reaction.

HYPERPIGMENTATION

Exposure to sunlight, and almost any form of chronic skin irritation or inflammation, may trigger changes in the skin that can lead to increased pigmentation, or hyperpigmentation. Chronic allergies (*see pp.124–27*) is a common cause of hyperpigmentation. Other causes include infections such as malassezia (*see p.196*); parasitic infestations (*see p.190*); and hormonal imbalances such as an underactive thyroid gland (*see p.331*) or overactive adrenal glands (*see p.335*). This condition is often accompanied by thickening of the skin.

DIAGNOSIS AND TREATMENT A skin biopsy may be diagnostic. Blood tests may also be performed to identify underlying causes such as hormonal fluctuations. Hyperpigmentation often clears up when the underlying cause is controlled or eliminated.

ACANTHOSIS NIGRICANS IN DACHSHUNDS

The Dachshund uniquely suffers from a hyperpigmentation condition of its armpits called acanthosis nigricans. Although the exact cause is poorly understood, the skin darkens as a consequence of chronic inflammation.

DIAGNOSIS AND TREATMENT Diagnosis is by signs, breed, and elimination of other causes. Topical corticosteroid cream is sometimes used to relieve the inflammation.

NASAL PIGMENT CHANGES

Some individuals of certain breeds are born with black noses that eventually fade to brown, freckled, or pink. These breeds include the Afghan Hound, Doberman, German Shepherd Dog, Irish Setter, English Pointer, Poodle, and Samoyed. Breeders have a curious name for this: "Dudley nose".

In other breeds, the nose leather fades from black to milk-chocolate in winter, then darkens again in summer. Affected breeds include the Bernese Mountain Dog, Golden Retriever, Labrador Retriever, and Siberian Husky. Breeders call this form of pigment change "snow nose".

In still other breeds, it is not only black nasal leather pigment that is lost; the black pigment on the lips and eyelids also fades and then disappears. This occurrence is a sign of the skin condition vitiligo (see above).

All of these conditions are aesthetic rather than medical problems and do not require treatment. They are thought to be hereditary in nature.

BREEDS AT RISK

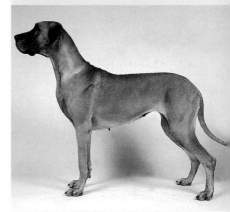

Breeds most likely to suffer from vitiligo include:

- Collie
- Doberman
- Labrador Retriever
- Newfoundland
- Rottweiler
- Tervueren (Belgian Shepherd)

Breeds at increased risk of loss of pigment in the nose leather include:

- German Shepherd Dog
- Golden Retriever
- Labrador Retriever
- Poodle
- Samoyed
- Siberian Husky

Breeds most susceptible to hyperpigmentation include.

- Beagle
- Boston Terrier
- Boxer
- Cocker Spaniel
- Dachshund
- Doberman
- Great Dane (above)
- Irish Setter
- Old English Sheepdog
- Scottish Terrier
- Shar Pei
- Weimaraner
- West Highland White Terrier

ITCHY SKIN OR PRURITUS

A dog's environment today, like ours, is radically different from that in which it evolved. In the United States and Canada, for example, the majority of humans spend 95 per cent of their time either indoors or in transport. So do our dogs! Modern houses are relatively airtight with higher humidity and temperature than ever; these conditions are ideal for enabling dust mites to multiply. For increasing numbers of dogs, exposure to dust mites triggers immune system cells in the skin to release their chemical contents, many of which are irritating and cause itchiness.

Diagnosing the cause of itchiness can sometimes be difficult because there need not be any inflammation (or secondary infection) associated with itchiness. Responding to itchiness is the most common way in which dogs can tell their owners that there is something wrong with their skin. Dogs react to itching by licking, nibbling or chewing, scratching, biting, rubbing, or rolling. These responses can cause the formation of scales and crusts, which are an ideal environment for secondary skin infection. Persistently itchy skin may also lead to adverse personality changes, including loss of tolerance, irritability, and aggression.

Allergies are an obvious cause of itching. Possible allergic conditions include flea allergy dermatitis (*see below*), atopic dermatitis (*see p.192*), food allergy dermatitis (*see p.192*), allergic contact dermatitis (*see p.193*), and allergic staphylococcal dermatitis (*see p.193*).

PARASITES

Specific causes of itching include parasites such as scabies mites, harvest mites, ear mites, fleas, lice, ticks, Cheyletiella mites, and maggots. (*See also pp.158–65.*)

DIAGNOSIS AND TREATMENT Parasites are seen on the skin or found on skin scrapes or smears. Treatment is aimed at eliminating the cause and any secondary conditions. Antihistamines and corticosteroid drugs are often given to relieve itching and to prevent further skin damage from licking and scratching. Frequent shampooing removes scales and crusts.

BACTERIAL AND FUNGAL INFECTIONS

Bacterial infections (*see pp.150–53*) and fungal infections (*see pp.156–57*) can also cause itchiness.

DIAGNOSIS AND TREATMENT Bacteria or fungi will be found on skin smears or cultures. Treatment is designed to eliminate the cause and address any secondary conditions. Antihistamines and corticosteroids are often used to relieve itching, thus preventing further skin damage from licking and scratching. Frequent shampooing removes scales and crusts and thus prevents secondary infection.

ALLERGIES

An allergy is an abnormal reaction of the immune system to a foreign substance. In most individuals, the substance produces no symptoms, but in a susceptible individual, it triggers an allergic reaction (*see pp.124–27*).

Substances that can produce an allergic response (allergens) include pollens, grass sap, certain infectious agents and parasites, and certain foods.

If you or I suffer from an allergy, we are likely to have itchy eyes and a runny nose or, worse, lung congestion. When dogs have allergic reactions, they develop itchy skin. The skin may become so itchy that dogs damage themselves by increased scratching, licking, and chewing, and may develop a whole range of additional secondary complications, such as bacterial or fungal infections. Itchy skin disease in dogs has become more common over the last few years, and allergy has become one of the most important causes of itchy skin.

DIAGNOSIS AND TREATMENT Allergies are diagnosed by intradermal skin tests or ELISA tests, exclusion diets, or environmental control. Treatment aims at eliminating the cause and clearing up any secondary conditions. For allergies this is not always possible, simply because determining the exact causes of allergies is a frustratingly

SEARCHING FOR FLEAS

It is not always easy or necessary to find a flea. Finding flea droppings is just as diagnostic as discovering the culprits themselves. Droppings are shiny and black, like specks of coal dust. They are easy to see on the skin of white- or tan-haired dogs but more difficult to find amongst dark hair. Simplify the search by sitting your dog on a white surface. In the picture on the right, the dog has been placed on some paper. With your hand, vigorously brush against the lie of the coat. This action dislodges flea droppings on to the paper. Apply a piece of damp tissue or cotton wool to any black debris. If mahogany to red colour runs from the debris, it is flea dirt, confirming the presence of fleas.

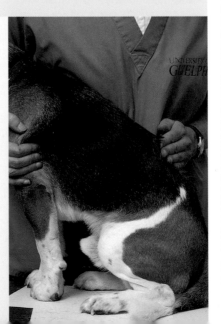

THE PROCESS OF INFLAMMATION

The skin is the largest organ of the immune system. Its tissues contain a variety of "sentinel" white blood cells. When invading microorganisms, or foreign bodies such as shards of glass, penetrate the skin surface, these white blood cells release chemicals that increase the permeability of tiny blood vessels, called capillaries, around the invasion site. The porous capillaries attract other white blood cells, called phagocytes, which are always on patrol in the circulation; the phagocytes then leak out of the capillaries into the affected area. The chemicals that cause this leakage, together with other substances (such as histamine) released by the damaged tissues, cause local, itchy inflammation. The area becomes red and swollen, and may be painful and warm.

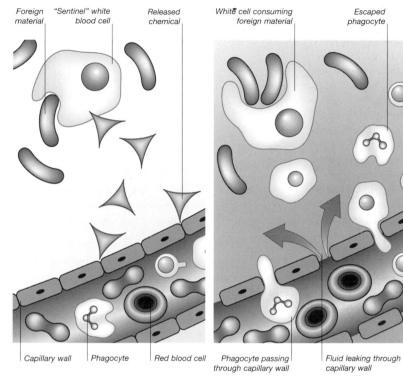

Foreign material   "Sentinel" white blood cell   Released chemical   White cell consuming foreign material   Escaped phagocyte

Capillary wall   Phagocyte   Red blood cell   Phagocyte passing through capillary wall   Fluid leaking through capillary wall

Release of inflammatory chemicals   **Leakage of phagocytes**

time-consuming affair. Antihistamines and corticosteroids are often used to relieve itching and prevent further skin damage from licking and scratching. Frequent shampooing removes allergens, as well as scales and crusts, from the skin surface.

FLEA ALLERGY DERMATITIS

This most common of all dog allergies is triggered by a reaction to substances in flea saliva that are left after a flea has a blood meal. If your dog is scratching but has no signs of skin damage and you know fleas are about, assume that a flea has caused the itch.

Flea allergy dermatitis (FAD) initially causes immediate itching and scratching, followed by red, raised pimples. These pimples are most likely to occur over the rump and in the groin. Eventually, the skin becomes thickened and darker, and may also be dry, sticky, or scaly.

DIAGNOSIS AND TREATMENT An ELISA blood test or intradermal skin test can be used to confirm a flea allergy. Treatment involves eliminating fleas and preventing their return (*see pp.160–63*). Both the dog and its environment are treated.

If your dog suffers from FAD, do not rely on biological flea control products, such as insect growth regulators, that prevent fleas from reproducing. Your objective is to kill fleas as quickly as possible, to prevent them from having further meals and provoking more allergic response. Use insecticides such as selamectin (Stronghold, Revolution)

Q WHY DO FLEAS MAKE DOGS SO ITCHY?

A Flea saliva is injected into the dog's skin as the flea feeds. The saliva contains inflammatory histamine-like chemicals. Eventually, in hypersensitive individuals, a single flea, taking a single meal, triggers a dramatically itchy response.

Q WHAT IS THE BEST WAY TO PREVENT RECURRENCES OF FLEA ALLERGY DERMATITIS?

A Year-round control is required. Routinely treat all pets with insecticides. Protect your home with insect growth regulators, which stop eggs and larvae from hatching.

or imidacloprid (Advantage) on all your dogs (and any cats) as a preventative measure, beginning at least a month before the flea season begins in your area. In warm climates, you have to combat fleas all year round.

ATOPIC DERMATITIS

This intensely itchy condition is the second most common allergic skin disease. Allergens such as dust mite droppings, human dander, or seasonal pollens, are inhaled or settle on the skin, and provoke an excessive antibody immune response (see p.126), triggering inflammation and itchiness. Atopic dermatitis, also called atopy, takes time to develop and typically starts in dogs from six months to three years old. The ears, which are one of the most sensitive parts of the skin, are often the first area to become itchy and inflamed. Licking the paws, groin, or armpits, or licking the paws and then rubbing the face, leads to mahogany staining from saliva, a sign of chronic irritation. Bacterial complication is common, leading to pustules, crusts, erosions, and ulcers (see pp.194–200).

DIAGNOSIS AND TREATMENT Atopic dermatitis is frequently complicated by secondary bacterial or fungal infection. Microscopic skin examination is used to diagnose atopic dermatitis, while fungal and bacterial cultures are used to identify the opportunist microbes. A thorough history-taking and clinical evidence from a full year of changing seasons offers the best information for an accurate diagnosis. Intradermal skin testing and ELISA testing are both useful for finding the specific causes of atopic dermatitis.

Antihistamine drugs reduce itching in some dogs, although only in a minority. Corticosteroids are excellent when used sparingly. If used at a low dose for only a few days, they can relieve the problem before secondary infection develops. Appropriate medicated shampoos and antibiotics control any secondary infection.

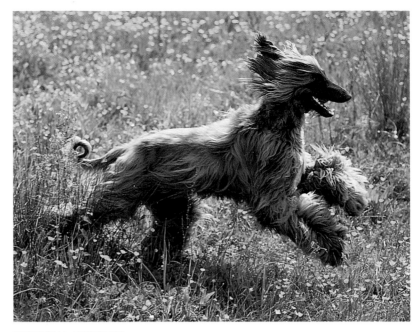

SEASONAL IRRITANTS
Dogs can develop a canine version of hay fever when exposed to pollens during the summer months. Pollens may be inhaled or irritate the skin by direct contact. Dogs that have an allergic reaction to pollens develop extremely itchy skin, which becomes inflamed and may become pustulated and ulcerated. These problems cause excessive licking and scratching.

PREVENTION Avoiding known allergens is the best treatment, but when that is not possible, dietary supplementation with essential fatty acids found in evening primrose oil, marine fish oil, or linseed oil (EPA and DHA fatty acids) may reduce inflammation and itch. Routine bathing and the use of humectants (moisturizers) cleanses the skin of potential allergens and developing scale, in which bacteria and fungi thrive. Desensitizing vaccines, containing the allergens to which the dog is sensitive, are quite effective in about one third of cases of atopy.

FOOD ALLERGY DERMATITIS

This condition is an underestimated cause of itchy skin disease. The immune system's abnormal antibody response is the same as for atopic dermatitis (see left). After a dog has ingested a trigger food, irritating chemicals are released that cause the dog to scratch and lick

its skin. These responses cause papules and then pustules to form; if left untreated, erosion and ulceration occur (see pp.198–200). The resulting rash very often involves the ears and groin, but it can occur anywhere on the body.

DIAGNOSIS AND TREATMENT A presumptive diagnosis of food allergy is made when a new, or hypoallergenic, diet is fed and the condition clears up. A hypoallergenic exclusion diet is one consisting of foods that the dog has never eaten before (see pp.97–98). The hypoallergenic diet must be fed for at least six weeks to enable a confirmed diagnosis of food allergy dermatitis. A definitive diagnosis is made only if itchiness returns when previous foods are reintroduced.

Home-prepared food is best, but may be difficult practically for some people. In addition, it is difficult for owners to ensure that they consistently give the same quantities of certain nutrients each day. A good alternative is to feed your dog a commercially prepared hypoallergenic diet. Ask your vet's advice, however, before choosing any special diet; there are many on the market and not all are exactly what they say they are.

ALLERGIC CONTACT DERMATITIS AND IRRITANT CONTACT DERMATITIS

These itchy skin conditions develop on the least hairy parts of the body – the chin, belly, feet, and scrotum – after either frequent contact with allergens such as grass sap (allergic contact dermatitis) or a single contact with an irritating substance (irritant contact dermatitis). The two conditions cause identical skin reactions: inflammation leading to the formation of pustules (*see p.194*), and general bacterial skin disease (*see p.196*). Contact dermatitis can develop even after exposure to seemingly innocuous items such as plastic or rubber food bowls; flea collars; fabric dyes; leather; and drugs

Q ARE SOME FOODS MORE LIKELY THAN OTHERS TO CAUSE ALLERGIC DERMATITIS?

A No, although early research suggested that beef and dairy products were prime culprits. This finding occurred because the research was done in the USA, where these products are common constituents of dog food. Dogs are most likely to become allergic to foods to which they have been frequently exposed.

Q IS THERE A DIET THAT WILL NOT CAUSE FOOD ALLERGY?

A There is no ideal diet. Some dogs are born with a tendency to develop food allergy. There is evidence, however, that for some affected dogs it is best to feed fresh rather than processed food.

such as neomycin (which is commonly used in ear medicines).

DIAGNOSIS AND TREATMENT A diagnosis is based on the dog's medical history. Treatment of either condition involves removing the cause of the irritation and treating any residual inflammation and secondary infection with anti-inflammatory drugs, antihistamines, and antibiotics as necessary.

ALLERGIC STAPHYLOCOCCAL DERMATITIS

The *Staphylococcus* species of bacteria are common and useful microbial inhabitants of the skin. Some allergic dogs, however, have a hypersensitivity reaction to the presence of these bacteria, developing an intense itch and skin inflammation. Consequent skin damage allows the bacteria to multiply even more and, as a result, exacerbates the condition.

DIAGNOSIS AND TREATMENT Examination of a sample of skin cells, followed by bacterial culture and combined with appropriate allergy testing, confirms the diagnosis of this uncommon problem. Antibiotics are used to treat the condition.

URTICARIA

Also known as hives, urticaria is an intensely itchy allergic condition consisting of raised red areas, often appearing on the face. Insect bites are the most common cause of urticaria, but the condition can also be triggered by oral or injected antibiotic drugs, insecticides, and even soaps. The skin of the eyelids, in particular, becomes puffy and itchy.

DIAGNOSIS AND TREATMENT A diagnosis is based on the time when urticaria occurs, because it usually develops within 30 minutes of exposure to the cause. An antihistamine drug is the most common treatment. If urticaria occurs as a result of a substance applied to the coat, an affected dog should be rinsed thoroughly.

BREEDS AT RISK

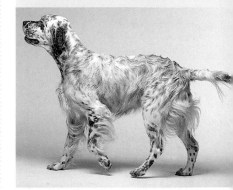

Several breeds with predominantly white coats are predisposed to produce excessive amounts of certain antibodies and have a higher incidence of skin allergies.

Breeds susceptible to atopic dermatitis include:

- Boxer
- Bulldog
- Bull Terrier
- Cairn Terrier
- Dalmatian
- English Setter (above)
- Fox Terrier
- Golden Retriever
- Labrador Retriever
- Lhasa Apso
- Miniature Schnauzer
- Scottish Terrier
- Shar Pei
- Staffordshire Bull Terrier
- West Highland White Terrier

PIMPLES

Small, raised lumps are called pimples. There are two main types of pimple: pustules and papules. A pustule is a small, elevated pimple filled with pus. A papule is a small, elevated pimple filled solidly with inflammatory cells. When they burst, pustules and papules can lead to skin erosion.

PUSTULES AND PAPULES

Pimples result from inflammation. Within the skin, specialized cells called mast cells, part of the immune system, act as "gatekeepers", regulating the skin's response to threats. Mast cells produce chemicals that are very efficient for disease and parasite control but trigger inflammation. Another class of defence cells, called memory T-cells, monitor the skin surface for dangerous microbes that they have met before.

Inflammation is part of natural repair but it leaves the skin prone to infection. Skin infections start as pimples, but within a day these erode and change to scales and crusts, then erosions and skin ulcerations. Bacterial skin disease is, overwhelmingly, the most common cause of pustules and papules. Most bacterial diseases are listed under erosions and ulcerations (*see pp.198–200*).

DIAGNOSIS AND TREATMENT Minor, superficial bacterial or fungal infections are relatively harmless; the affected skin will be lost as cells are constantly sloughed off and replaced by new, healthy cells. The dog will help the sloughing process by licking the skin.

SCALING DISEASES

Scales are bits of the skin surface. They may flake off, as particles of dandruff, or remain on the skin, building up as calluses. Scaling is often associated with increased activity of the oil-producing sebaceous glands; this sign is called seborrhoea. In "dry seborrhoea", there is increased flaky scaling. In "wet seborrhoea", scale is retained in the skin oil, producing an unpleasant, greasy, smelly coat.

HEREDITARY SEBORRHOEA

Excess scale develops on the skin. The scaling leads to either an excessively dandruffy appearance in the coat, often accompanied by itching, or an oily, malodorous skin.

DIAGNOSIS AND TREATMENT Diagnosis is often based on signs alone, although biopsies are conclusive. Treatment is aimed at eliminating opportunist infection and reducing scaling. There is evidence that oral vitamin A therapy

BREEDS AT RISK

Breeds particularly likely to develop seborrhoea include:

- Basset Hound
- Cocker Spaniel
- Doberman
- English Springer Spaniel
- Irish Setter
- Labrador Retriever
- Miniature Schnauzer
- Shar Pei
- West Highland White Terrier

(8,000 to 10,000 IU twice daily) may be useful for some dogs that have hereditary seborrhoea. Antiseborrhoeic shampoos (selenium sulphide, coal tar, sulphur/salicylic acid, or benzoyl peroxide) or anti-malassezia shampoos are used as often as every other day, initially, to reduce scale. Humectant (moisturizing) sprays may be beneficial. Dietary supplements such as evening primrose oil are also useful. Lifelong treatment is necessary.

COMEDO SYNDROME

This is a harmless and fairly common condition of Miniature Schnauzers, in which papules develop over the dog's back. You can feel these "blackheads" when you stroke an affected dog. Bathing the dog with a benzoyl peroxide or other antiseborrhoeic shampoo effectively removes at least some of the blackheads. Antibiotics are necessary only when there is a secondary bacterial infection of the hair follicles.

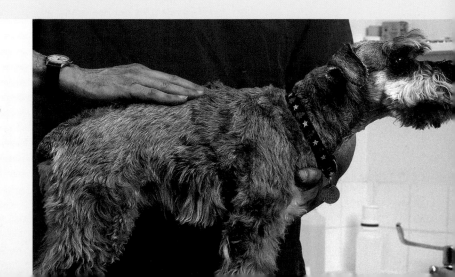

EPIDERMAL DYSPLASIA IN WEST HIGHLAND WHITE TERRIERS

Very young West Highland White Terriers can have a highly unpleasant form of hereditary seborrhoea called epidermal dysplasia. Initially, affected individuals are just itchy, but soon they lose hair from their feet and trunk. The skin becomes scaly and greasy, and the itching increases in intensity. Eventually, the dog's skin becomes thicker (lichenification) and darker (hyperpigmentation). Secondary bacterial infection or malassezia fungal infection (*see p.196*) is very common in dogs with hereditary seborrhoea and especially epidermal dysplasia.

DIAGNOSIS AND TREATMENT These are the same as for hereditary seborrhoea. Westies often need corticosteroids to reduce intense itchiness.

SEBACEOUS ADENITIS

This inherited scaly condition occurs primarily in three- to seven-year-old Standard Poodles, but also in Akitas and Samoyeds. Skin inflammation destroys the local sebaceous glands, leading to adherent yellow scale and hair loss. Secondary bacterial infection is common in this condition.

DIAGNOSIS AND TREATMENT Diagnosis is often based on clinical signs alone but a skin biopsy gives a definitive diagnosis. Treatment is aimed at eliminating opportunist infection and reducing scaling. Antiseborrhoeic shampoos (selenium sulphide, coal tar, sulphur/salicylic acid, or benzoyl peroxide) or anti-malassezia shampoos are used as often as every other day, initially, to reduce scale. Humectant (moisturizing) sprays may also be beneficial, as may dietary essential fatty acid supplements.

ICHTHYOSIS

Some dogs develop an adherent scaling called ichthyosis on their pads. I have seen this inherited scaling condition most frequently in Cavalier King

Charles Spaniels and West Highland White Terriers. The treatment for ichthyosis is the same as for hereditary seborrhoea, although oral retinoids (etretinate or isotretinoin) are also reported to be effective.

ZINC-RESPONSIVE DERMATOSIS

Zinc is required for hair growth and maintenance of the skin. A deficiency in this mineral can lead to a condition called zinc-responsive dermatosis. In some immature fast-growing Nordic breeds, scale develops on the foot pads and nose leather. In mature Siberian Huskies and Alaskan Malamutes, scale develops around the eyes, ears, mouth, prepuce, and vulva. Scaling leads to crust and hair loss. The condition develops at one to three years of age.

DIAGNOSIS AND TREATMENT These conditions are diagnosed by blood testing for zinc levels. Treatment is by dietary zinc supplementation, although older Siberian Huskies do not respond as well as other breeds.

Bull Terrier pups can inherit a lethal disease (acrodermatitis) diagnosed by low blood zinc levels, which does not respond to supplementation and for which there is no effective treatment.

VET'S ADVICE

Regular and frequent shampooing with an antiseborrhoeic product containing selenium sulphide, coal tar, salicylic acid, or benzoyl peroxide is the best way to deal with a persistently oily, greasy coat due to hereditary seborrhoea. Your vet will be able to recommend a suitable type of shampoo. Apply the shampoo all over the coat, then rinse thoroughly. Using a hand-held shower, as shown here, is ideal for removing shampoo, along with skin scales and dandruff.

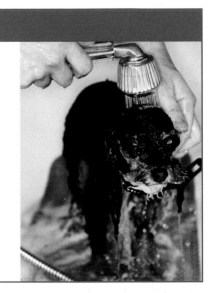

Q IS SEBORRHOEA THE SAME AS DANDRUFF?

A Effectively, yes it is. The sebaceous glands provide the oily waterproofing for a dog's coat. Just enough produces a wonderful shine, but a variety of conditions can cause the glands to be over-active. One consequence is "dry seborrhoea", which produces a flaky deposit like human dandruff. Another form of over-activity causes "oily seborrhoea", making the coat greasy and slightly sticky to touch. Oily seborrhea also results in a "doggy odour", common in breeds such as Cocker Spaniels.

Q IS DANDRUFF NORMAL WHEN A DOG MOULTS?

A It very often is, and increased grooming while a dog is moulting may temporarily increase the problem. Treat severe dandruff with an antiseborrhoeic shampoo recommended by a vet. Medicated tar shampoos are often used. Avoid zinc pyrithione shampoos made for people; they may be unsafe as whole-body shampoos in dogs.

CHEYLETIELLA

This barely visible skin mite causes scaly dandruff over a dog's back. Cheyletiella primarily affects pups, and responds to standard flea control treatment. (*See also p.165.*)

LEISHMANIASIS

The *Leishmania* parasite, transmitted by sandfly bites, causes leishmaniasis. The signs include hair loss, skin inflammation and scaling, and crusting that leads to ulcers, especially on the ears and the lips. (*See also p.174.*)

DIAGNOSIS AND TREATMENT The condition is diagnosed from blood samples or biopsies of skin or lymph nodes. Treatments include injections of antimony compounds (meglumine antimoniate) by mouth.

CRUSTING DISEASES

The surface of a dog's skin (epidermis) is relatively thin. When pustules and papules appear, they remain for only a short time before breaking down to form a crust. These crusts consist of serum and cells from the blood, and inflammatory cells. Your vet is more likely to see crusts rather than their precursors, and will make a differential diagnosis according to the factor that has caused the crusting disease.

CRUSTY NOSE

The nose is normally wet and cool, but it may naturally become dry when the dog is sleeping, has a fever, or is excited. A persistently crusty or scabby nose, however – a condition once known as "hardpad" – is a minor sign of distemper infection (*see p.147*). Some autoimmune conditions, such as pemphigus and lupus (*see pp.200–01*), can also cause the nose to become dry and scabby. In certain breeds, especially flat-faced dogs such as the Pug, Pekingese, and Boxer, the nose leather thickens and crusts with age, becoming like horn. This condition is called nasal callus or hyperkeratosis.

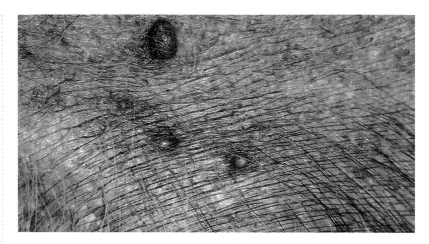

PUSTULES IN GENERAL BACTERIAL SKIN INFECTION
Bacterial infection is the most common cause of pustules on the skin. These small lumps rapidly break down and form crusts on the skin surface. Broken pustules or crusting can allow infection to develop and lead to more serious conditions.

DIAGNOSIS AND TREATMENT Dogs that recover from distemper infection often spontaneously recover from hardpad. The dry nose should be lubricated with antibiotic ointment or petroleum jelly.

GENERAL BACTERIAL SKIN INFECTION

Bacteria are by far the most common cause of crusting skin conditions. In most instances, they multiply because other conditions allow this process to happen; such conditions include allergy (*see pp.124–27*), hormonal skin disease (*see p.182*), seborrhoea (overactivity of the sebaceous glands), scabies (*see below*), and comedo syndrome in Miniature Schnauzers (*see p.194*).

Superficial infection initially causes pimples to form, and the pimples then break to cause crusting. The hair follicles may also become infected, leading to folliculitis (*see below*). Deep infection causes more generalized inflammation, redness, and crusting; this condition is called pyoderma. Oozing sores and other, more dramatic manifestations of skin infection are described below.

DIAGNOSIS AND TREATMENT A diagnosis is made by culturing a sample of skin cells for bacteria or by skin biopsy. A bacterial sensitivity test helps the vet to select the best antibiotic for treatment. Your vet will prescribe drugs according to whether the infection is superficial or deep. In addition, antiseptic shampoos are very effective for controlling superficial skin infection.

FOLLICULITIS

This condition is inflammation of hair follicles. Pustules form within the inflamed follicles; often, the follicles develop into sinuses (widened cavities) that drain on to the surface of the skin. If the infection goes deeper into the skin, it is called furunculosis (*see p.200*). The condition occurs most frequently in the armpits, abdomen, and groin. As with most bacterial infections, it is a complication of other conditions, such as allergy (*see pp.124–27*) and parasite infestations.

DIAGNOSIS AND TREATMENT The underlying primary cause needs to be identified and treated. Antiseptic and antiseborrhoeic shampoos, such as those containing benzoyl peroxide, help to flush out the follicles. Oral antibiotics are often necessary for at least two weeks. Certain antibiotics, specifically erythromycin, clindamycin, tetracycline, and perhaps penicillin drugs, may be used for their anti-inflammatory properties as well as for their antibacterial action.

MALASSEZIA DERMATITIS

The Malassezia yeast, originally called *Pityrosporum*, was once thought to be an almost irrelevant finding in skin disorders but is now considered to be a major cause of itchy skin disease. It causes itchy redness of the skin, often in the region between the toes. If it occurs in the ears, it provokes the production of smelly, yellow ear wax.

Malassezia is usually an opportunist infection; it is common in dogs with allergic skin disease. The skin irritation leads to crusting, which may occur anywhere on the body, including in the ears. Certain breeds appear to be particularly predisposed to developing malassezia dermatitis; they include the Basset Hound, Cocker Spaniel, Dachshund (smooth), Poodle, and West Highland White Terrier.

DIAGNOSIS AND TREATMENT Malassezia can be seen in skin smears examined under the microscope. Sometimes, the yeast may be present without causing disease. A true diagnosis depends on the response to treatment, which may be with a topical antifungal shampoo or, for more serious infections, with oral antifungal medication such as ketoconazole. Infected ears often need individual attention.

SCABIES

Infestation with the scabies mite almost invariably causes intense itchiness. Crusting develops in regions of skin favoured by the mites; these areas include the tips of the ears and the elbows, but also any area where the dog has scratched itself intensively.

DIAGNOSIS AND TREATMENT Scabies is diagnosed by signs and skin scrapings. It is treated with selamectin, and sometimes also with corticosteroids and antibiotics to control itching and secondary infection respectively.

SUNBURN, HEAT BURNS, AND CHEMICAL BURNS

White-coloured individuals exposed to intense sunshine can suffer sunburn from the ultraviolet radiation in the light. Sunburn leads to crusting on the ears and nose. Thermal (heat) burns are most commonly caused by splashes of boiling water or hot oil; such burns may not be noticed until the covering hair falls off several days later, revealing the skin damage. Chemical burns may be caused by a variety of substances (*see pp.412 and 416*).

DIAGNOSIS AND TREATMENT Diagnosis is based on the dog's medical history. Thermal burns often become infected; for this reason, topical and oral antibiotics, together with painkillers, are used to treat them. If your dog has suffered a chemical burn, always examine the inside of the mouth to see if any further injuries have been caused by the dog licking the affected area.

CANCER

Squamous cell carcinoma and, less frequently, basal cell carcinoma may develop and form crusts, especially on areas of sun-damaged skin. White-coated individuals, or dogs that have congenital or acquired hair loss, are most at risk of developing skin cancer. (*See also pp.134–36.*)

DIAGNOSIS AND TREATMENT Initially, skin tumours (especially those that occur on the ear tips) are difficult to differentiate from sunburn. Diagnosis is confirmed by skin biopsy. These types of tumour should be surgically removed, together with a wide margin of surrounding healthy tissue.

PROBLEMS WITH THE NOSE

In intensely sunny climates, ultraviolet light exposure causes sunburn or nasal solar dermatitis, with inflammation and ulceration leading to crusting. It occurs most frequently in Collies (who are particularly prone), Shetland Sheepdogs, and Australian Shepherd Dogs. Affected dogs should be kept out of direct sunlight; if this is not possible, protect them with a minimum 30 SPF sun block. Nasal callus can be picked or rubbed off but the underlying tissue bleeds easily. Lubricate the nose daily with petroleum jelly to prevent excess callus formation.

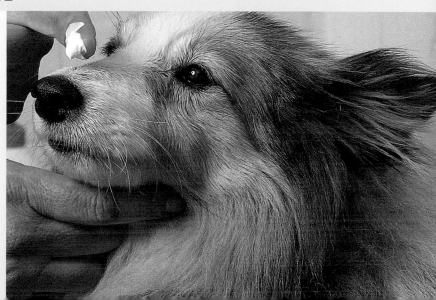

EROSIONS AND ULCERS

These types of skin damage have many causes, but are usually due to bacterial infection. These infections begin as pustules (*see p.194*) on the skin or in hair follicles. The pustules break down, creating crusts and eventually leading to more severe conditions.

Superficial damage to papules and pustules is called erosion. When an erosion breaks through the full skin thickness it is called an ulcer. The progress from pustule to erosion can be very fast; for example, less than a day in acute moist dermatitis (*see below*).

There are several conditions causing erosion and ulceration. A particularly deep and serious type of ulceration is furunculosis, which develops from folliculitis (*see p.196*). In its most severe form, furunculosis occurs in the skin tissue around a dog's anus, causing great discomfort.

ACUTE MOIST DERMATITIS

The first sign of this infection, also called "hot spot" or summer eczema, is often a sticky, sometimes smelly mat of hair that the dog scratches or chews. If this hair is parted, the skin beneath is found to be red, hairless, and oozing serum (fluid from the blood). Whether or not the sore is painful varies from dog to dog. Acute moist dermatitis is most likely to occur in humid weather, and in long-haired dogs that have especially dense coats. The Golden Retriever, in particular, may have a genetic predisposition to the condition.

DIAGNOSIS AND TREATMENT Other possible causes of the symptoms, such as fleas, should first be ruled out. Affected areas are treated by shaving and cleansing with topical antiseptics. Oral antibiotics are often given, together with corticosteroid drugs to reduce discomfort. The dog should wear a protective collar or neck sleeve for a week or more to prevent licking while healing occurs.

SKIN FOLD INFECTION

Where folds of skin rub together, a unique microclimate exists that favours the growth of bacteria. This growth leads to erosion and ulceration, producing a wet, inflamed, and often smelly skin condition. Male dogs may develop infection on the scrotum and adjacent skin; extremely fat females with their vulvas hidden in folds of skin are prone to skin inflammation and erosion within the skin folds. Some breeds are especially vulnerable to facial skin-fold infection (*see below*).

DIAGNOSIS AND TREATMENT The fold is cleaned with an antiseptic shampoo such as benzoyl peroxide. Topical antibiotic and anti-inflammatory medication is often beneficial. The area is then cleaned daily with substances such as benzoyl peroxide gel until the infection has cleared up. You can help to prevent recurrence by cleaning folds daily with mild antiseptic solutions and drying thoroughly. Surgical elimination of a fold ensures a complete cure with no possibility of recurrence.

PUPPY ACNE AND PUPPY IMPETIGO

Both of these conditions, as the names suggest, affect young adolescent dogs. Puppy acne begins as blackheads in the hair follicles on the chin and lips. The spots quickly develop into pimples, then crusts and erosions. If left untreated, large ulcerated areas may develop. Puppy impetigo is a bacterial condition affecting the groin. Pustules develop and then rupture, leaving brown crusts.

DIAGNOSIS AND TREATMENT For puppy acne, cleaning the lips and chin after meals with an antiseptic, such as dilute chlorhexidine or a benzoyl peroxide solution, reduces the frequency and severity. Infection in the hair follicles is treated with an appropriate antibiotic. Benzoyl peroxide is also an effective treatment for puppy impetigo. Both conditions tend to disappear with age.

ANATOMICAL PREDISPOSITION TO LIP-FOLD INFECTION

All dogs have a natural fold of skin on their lower lips, but this fold is particularly exaggerated in the spaniel family and especially in Cocker Spaniels. Affected dogs are able to lick their lips, but they cannot reach their lip folds. If food or other debris accumulates within the fold, bacteria are likely to multiply there, producing a painful and often very smelly infection. The risk of lip fold infection can be dramatically reduced by routine daily cleaning of the dog's lip folds after each meal.

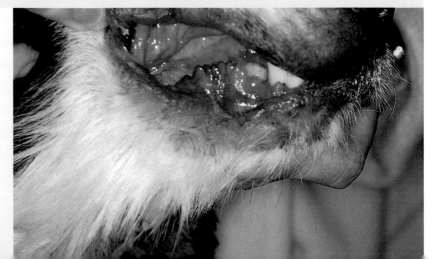

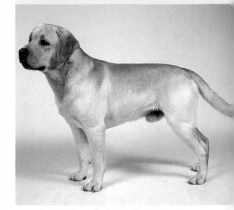

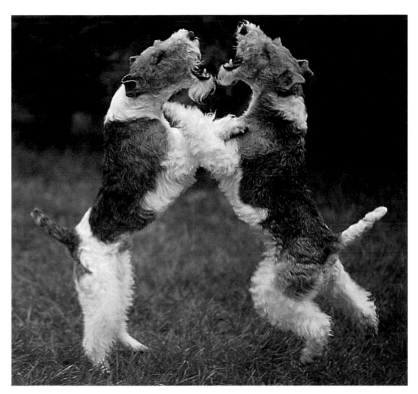

WAR WOUNDS
Injuries inflicted during dog fights often penetrate deep into the tissue. These "war wounds" provide opportunities for bacteria to enter the surface of the skin and infect the underlying tissues. The infection may lead to a condition called cellulitis, in which the skin becomes sore and inflamed, and sometimes severely ulcerated.

PUPPY STRANGLES
This potentially serious skin infection, also called juvenile pyoderma, occurs in pups between one and four months old. Sudden swelling and inflammation develops on the chin, lips, ears, and face. Local lymph nodes become swollen. Pustules, crusts, erosions, and then ulcers rapidly appear on the affected areas of skin. Puppy strangles is thought to be associated with some form of failure of the immune system occurring in young dogs.

DIAGNOSIS AND TREATMENT Antibiotics alone rarely cure puppy strangles. Antibiotics used in conjunction with corticosteroid drugs, however, do usually result in improvement and recovery, which usually takes from two to several weeks.

CELLULITIS
Skin injuries such as dog bites, other skin puncture wounds, and deep scratches or lacerations may cause cellulitis, a bacterial infection of the underlying tissues. The affected area is hotter and redder than normal. Left untreated, cellulitis often breaks through the skin, causing a deep, rough ulcer.

DIAGNOSIS AND TREATMENT If an area of cellulitis has ulcerated, your vet may provide you with a dilute antiseptic solution for flushing the wound twice daily. If it has not ulcerated, antibiotics and painkillers are used. The affected area is also soaked several times a day with warm salt water to bring any underlying abscess or boil to a head. Once it has ripened, the abscess or boil will be drained by lancing.

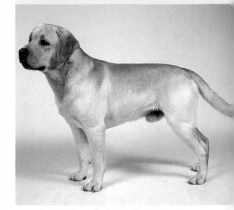
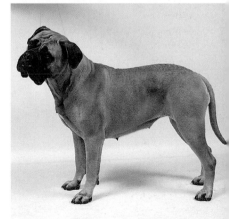

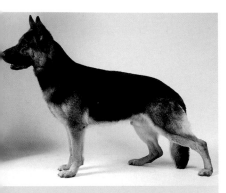

Q **WHY ARE GERMAN SHEPHERD DOGS SO SUSCEPTIBLE TO ANAL FURUNCULOSIS?**

A Some experts believe that breed standards play a role. These standards call for the tail to be carried very low. As a result, a warm, moist microenvironment develops under the tail in the anal region, which is ideal for bacterial multiplication. This occurrence alone would not cause a problem but for the fact that some German Shepherd Dogs also inherit a tendency to weakness of the immune system, the reason for which is not known. The combination of these two factors leads to the high incidence of anal furunculosis in the breed.

Q **ARE AUTOIMMUNE DISEASES IN DOGS INCREASING IN INCIDENCE?**

A These conditions are certainly being diagnosed far more frequently today than ten years ago, but that does not necessarily mean they are becoming more common. Autoimmune diseases are difficult to diagnose. Blood test results are rarely definitive; skin biopsies are more accurate. The increased diagnosis rates may be due to the fact that vets today are more aware of these rare conditions and are more likely to take skin biopsies as part of their assessments.

FURUNCULOSIS AND ANAL FURUNCULOSIS

Furunculosis is a deep form of infection, often occurring together with bacterial folliculitis (*see p.196*). It may occur in any breed of dog, anywhere on hair-covered parts of the body, after Demodex mite infection (*see p.183*), but it most commonly occurs in German Shepherd Dogs, in the hairless skin around the anus.

Anal furunculosis is often first noticed when an affected dog licks its bottom more frequently. The area may be inflamed and is often ulcerated, with variably sized open wounds. The infection penetrates deep into the perianal tissue. Anal furunculosis is very uncomfortable for the dog. The tail may be elevated and the bottom licked or bitten. Some dogs are faecally incontinent; others strain but pass no faeces. The region can be very smelly.

Although this condition occurs primarily in German Shepherd Dogs, it may also occur in German Shepherd crosses and other breeds, usually in dogs between four and seven years of age that have compromised immune systems. These other susceptible breeds include collies and collie crosses, Irish Setters, Jack Russell Terriers, Labrador Retrievers, Leonbergers, and Old English Sheepdogs.

DIAGNOSIS AND TREATMENT Diagnosis is based on the signs. Although bacterial cultures may reveal common infectious microorganisms such as the bacterium *Staphylococcus intermedius*, or opportunist bacteria such as *Proteus*, *Pseudomonas*, or *Escherichia coli*, this condition seldom responds to treatment with antibiotics alone. Antibiotics in conjunction with corticosteroids eventually control furunculosis in many dogs, although treatment is usually necessary for several months. The immunosuppressant drug cyclosporin, given orally, has been successfully used to treat anal furunculosis.

When the ulceration is extensive, surgical repair is necessary. This repair may be carried out using conventional surgery, electrosurgery, cryosurgery (freezing), or laser surgery (which has been particularly successful).

ACTINOMYCOSIS AND NOCARDIOSIS

These infections are rare causes of ulcerating skin disease. They are contracted from soil contaminated by fungi, usually by hunting dogs. They cause systemic disease, affecting the lymph nodes, lungs, and bone.

DIAGNOSIS AND TREATMENT Diagnosis is confirmed by culturing material collected from a draining ulcer. All sites of infection will be surgically opened and drained. Long-term antibiotic therapy is needed.

AUTOIMMUNE DISEASE

A variety of autoimmune conditions, in which the dog's immune system malfunctions and attacks the body's own tissues, cause ulcers on the skin. (*See also pp.127–28.*)

DISCOID LUPUS ERYTHEMATOSUS

This autoimmune skin condition is triggered by exposure to sunlight. It causes crusting, erosion, ulceration, and hair loss on the nose, lips, ears, and around the eyes. These areas often bleed when they are touched.

Discoid lupus erythematosus is more common than was previously realized. "Collie nose" (nasal solar dermatitis; *see p.128*) is, in fact, a form of the condition. Not only collies are affected: white German Shepherd Dogs, Siberian Huskies, and Shetland Sheepdogs can all develop it.

DIAGNOSIS AND TREATMENT Diagnosis is confirmed by skin biopsy. The best treatment for discoid lupus erythematosus is topical corticosteroid cream. The best prevention is to keep the dog out of sunlight. When this is impossible, apply a sunblock (SPF 30) daily to protect the dog's skin.

SYSTEMIC LUPUS ERYTHEMATOSUS

This rare condition is far more serious and far more pervasive than discoid lupus erythermatosus. It causes scaling, crusting, eroded skin lesions, with pigment and hair loss. These lesions, however, are a relatively minor problem. Equally serious structural attacks are taking place within, affecting the blood, kidneys, and other organs.

DIAGNOSIS AND TREATMENT Diagnosis is confirmed by blood tests, including an antibody test. Even with vigorous treatment with corticosteroid drugs and more potent immune-suppressing drugs, the prognosis remains only fair.

BULLOUS PEMPHIGOID

This disorder is extremely rare in dogs, and most often occurs in collies and Dobermans. It causes blisters and ulcers on the skin of the body. The prognosis is poor.

TOXIC EPIDERMAL NECROLYSIS AND ERYTHEMA MULTIFORME

Toxic epidermal necrolysis is a painful ulcerative skin condition affecting the foot pads and the mouth. The disorder may be triggered by factors such as infection, drugs, and cancer. Erythema multiforme is a less severe form of the condition, producing red-rimmed, oval skin eruptions.

BREEDS AT RISK

Breeds at increased risk of systemic lupus erythematosus include:

- Collies
- German Shepherd Dog
- Poodles
- Shetland Sheepdog
- Spitz-type breeds

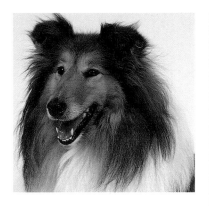

SUSCEPTIBLE BREED
Collies are particularly susceptible to a range of autoimmune disorders, many of which lead to skin problems such as crusting and ulceration.

DIAGNOSIS AND TREATMENT Treatment for toxic epidermal necrolysis includes removing the trigger factor, if possible, and treating with intravenous food and fluids, corticosteroids, painkillers, and antibiotics. Even with treatment, the prognosis is very poor. Most dogs with erythema multiforme, on the other hand, spontaneously recover.

NODULAR PANNICULITIS

This is an autoimmune condition affecting subcutaneous fat. Lumps in the fat layer ulcerate and drain, leaving scars on the skin surface.

DIAGNOSIS AND TREATMENT The lumps in the subcutaneous fat are surgically removed. Medical treatment includes corticosteroids and sometimes also vitamin E supplementation. Unlike other autoimmune skin conditions, this disorder is not potentially fatal.

FAMILIAL DERMATOMYOSITIS

Familial dermatomyositis is a rare inherited condition affecting muscle and skin tissue. The disorder is seen only in collies and Shetland Sheepdogs. Affected dogs experience transient episodes of skin inflammation, leading to crusting, erosion, and ulceration, around the eyes, ears, muzzle, and tail.

The facial muscles may shrink in size. Familial dermatomyositis is not life-threatening, and can be treated with corticosteroid drugs.

PEMPHIGUS CONDITIONS

In these rare conditions, the immune system attacks the walls of skin cells. At least four different types of canine pemphigus have been documented; the following two are the most common.

PEMPHIGUS FOLIACEUS

In this condition, superficial blisters and pustules suddenly develop, usually symmetrically on the face and foot pads. Crusting usually follows around the eyes and on the lips, nose, ears, and feet.

DIAGNOSIS AND TREATMENT Diagnosis is based on physical examination, skin biopsy, and blood tests. Affected dogs are treated with long-term corticosteroid therapy together with more potent immunosuppressant drugs. The prognosis is variable.

PEMPHIGUS VULGARIS

In pemphigus vulgaris, blisters and pustules develop where the skin meets mucous membranes around the lips, nostrils, eyelids, anus, prepuce, and vulva. Mouth lesions are the most common symptom.

DIAGNOSIS AND TREATMENT Biopsy confirms this condition. Treatment is the same as for other autoimmune diseases, but the outlook is poor.

OTHER CAUSES OF EROSION AND ULCERATION

Other conditions causing erosion and ulcers include chronic Demodex mite infestation, especially in older dogs (see p.183); overactive adrenal glands (see p.182); kidney failure (see p.308); skin cancers, especially squamous cell carcinoma (see pp.134–36); and injuries, including burning, freezing, sun damage, scalding from the chemicals in urine, drug reactions, and insect bites.

EYES AND VISION
anatomy and care

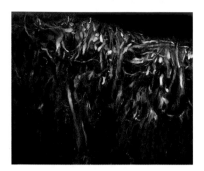

Retinal scar under microscope

Animal behaviourists tell us that all mammals use their eyes not only for seeing but also to communicate their moods and emotions to other animals. We are magnetically drawn to a dog's eyes, and for good reason – they can be very expressive and revealing, and form an important part of the intimate relationship that dogs and humans share. Dogs' eyes naturally evolved to help them track and hunt prey, but humans have now created many new breeds, some with distinctive eyes that require regular care and attention.

Dogs' eyes look similar to human eyes, but they differ from ours in several ways. They are more flattened than human eyes. The lens can change shape and alter the eye's focal length, but not as well as in human eyes. Dogs' eyes may be more sensitive to light and movement than ours – assets that help them to hunt, especially in dim light – but their power to produce a sharp image is poorer than ours. The muscles that change the shape of the lens are weaker than in human eyes, so dogs have poorer near vision; this why a dog has difficulty finding a tennis ball lying right in front of its nose.

On the other hand, dogs have large pupils and more laterally placed eyes than us, which gives better peripheral vision and makes them able to follow moving objects more accurately. A dog's ability to see to the side (peripheral vision) varies according to breed and is usually greater than ours; a Pekingese has 5–10 degrees more peripheral vision than we do, while a typical terrier has 20–30 degrees more.

PROTECTIVE STRUCTURES
The eyeball sits deep in a bony socket. It is cushioned on a layer of fat and supported and protected by the two eyelids. Eyelashes, which grow only on the upper lid, help to prevent foreign objects from coming into contact with the eyeball. A third eyelid, called the nictitating membrane, functions like a windscreen wiper, brushing debris from the cornea (the transparent, tough surface of the eye).

A film of tears constantly bathes the third eyelid and the conjunctiva, the membrane that lines the eyelids. Tears ensure clear vision, prevent the eye from drying out, and fight infection. Excess tears drain via a channel called the nasolacrimal duct into the nose.

DETECTING LIGHT AND COLOUR
The light-sensitive cells of the retina are called rods and cones. In dogs' eyes, the majority of these cells are rods, which are designed to detect even weak light; dogs can, therefore, see better than we do in relative darkness.

To help gather all the available light in dark or dim conditions, dogs have a colourful, reflective layer of cells behind the retina, called the tapetum lucidum. This layer is usually found in the upper portion of the eyeball. It may vary in colour, size, and shape. Beneath the lower part of the retina is the tapetum nigra, a dark layer that protects the retina from the glare of sunlight.

Dogs have poor colour vision; they are thought to see colour in much the same way as people with red–green colour blindness. The few cone cells in the retina enable a dog to distinguish between yellow and blue, but it is the cells' ability to distinguish between shades of grey that is most important to a dog's visual system.

PROMINENT EYES

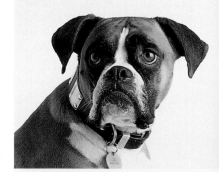

Many humans find large eyes more attractive than smaller ones. One result of this preference is that we selectively bred many dogs, such as the Boxer (*see above*), to have more prominent eyes than their wolf ancestors. This development has increased the risk of eye disease and especially of problems due to trauma.

ANATOMY OF THE EYE

The amount of light entering the eye is controlled by contracting or dilating muscles in the coloured iris. Light passes through the transparent cornea and the fluid-filled anterior chamber, then through the pupil, the round opening in the centre of the iris. The ciliary body and suspensory ligaments adjust the shape of the lens, focusing the light through the jelly-filled posterior chamber on to the retina, at the back of the eye. Light-sensitive cells in the retina translate the energy from the light waves into nerve impulses; these signals are transmitted to the brain along the optic nerve (which begins at the optic disc).

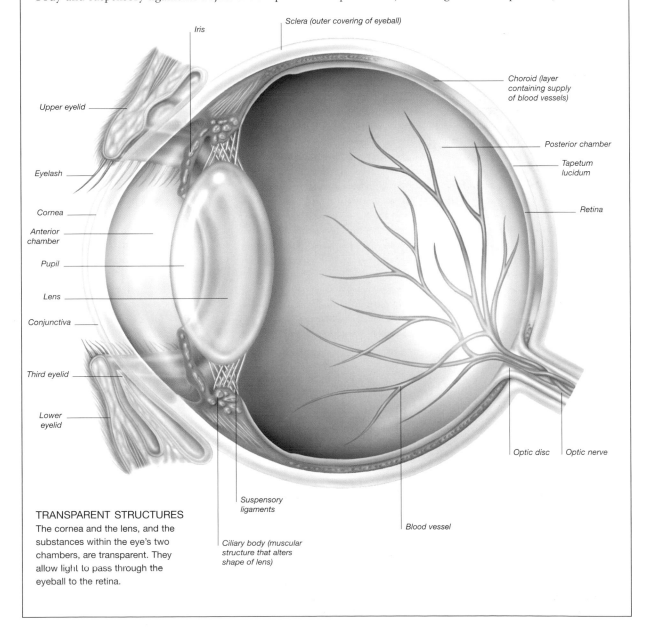

Iris

Sclera (outer covering of eyeball)

Choroid (layer containing supply of blood vessels)

Upper eyelid

Posterior chamber

Tapetum lucidum

Eyelash

Cornea

Anterior chamber

Retina

Pupil

Lens

Conjunctiva

Third eyelid

Lower eyelid

Optic disc

Optic nerve

Suspensory ligaments

Blood vessel

Ciliary body (muscular structure that alters shape of lens)

TRANSPARENT STRUCTURES

The cornea and the lens, and the substances within the eye's two chambers, are transparent. They allow light to pass through the eyeball to the retina.

TAKING CARE OF YOUR DOG'S EYES

A dog's eyes should be bright, shining, and free of debris and discharge. The skin around the eyes should appear healthy and normal.

Remember that the eyes are delicate and sensitive; when you carry out routine grooming, take special care with brushes and combs.

CLEANING THE EYES

Check your dog's eyes every day. At the same time, look for evidence that may warn you of a problem. Keep a watch for any gradual or striking symptoms, such as your dog blinking in an abnormal way, squinting, or pawing at one or both of its eyes.

If mucus from an eye discharges on to the surrounding skin, as commonly happens when the eyes react to dust or some other irritant, remove it gently with damp cotton wool. If the mucus has already dried into a hard crust, however, as frequently occurs with Yorkshire Terriers and some other breeds, first soak the crust with a little water to make it soft, then carefully remove it with your fingers or with a piece of damp cotton wool.

SPECIAL CARE FOR PROMINENT EYES

If your dog is a flat-faced breed with bulging eyes, such as the Pekingese, Boston Terrier, Pug, or Maltese, you need to pay special attention to its eyes.

Check daily that the nasal fold of skin, at the inner corner of each eye, is not touching the eye. Chronic contact with the eye leads to an overflow of tears, and to a pigment deposit in the cornea that reduces vision. If this problem occurs, contact your vet to discuss reducing the size of the fold. Clean the tear overflow at least once a day to reduce the risk of inflammation and infection in the skin fold.

In flat-faced breeds, there is a risk that an eye injury may cause the eyeball to be dislodged from its socket. If this problem has just occurred, quickly clean the eye with water (or saliva, if necessary). Then grasp the upper and lower eyelids and gently massage the eyeball back into the socket. If you take immediate action, you may be able to save your dog's eyesight.

If the injury is older and swelling has occurred, however, do not try to push the eye back in. Instead, cover it with a clean, damp cloth or sponge, keep your dog as quiet as possible, and get immediate veterinary help. Soaking the cloth or sponge in salt water or a supersaturated solution of sugar will help to preserve the eye.

RECOGNIZING SYMPTOMS

Reduced or lost vision may have both inherited and acquired causes. The primary cause may be either in the eye itself or in the brain.

Some conditions may cause clinical signs, such as pain or a deterioration in vision, without any visible changes. Obvious signs of pain include sensitivity to touch and increased irritability; other signs include loss of appetite, over-sensitivity to light, lethargy, and whining. Squinting, or blepharospasm, is also a sign of pain: a squinting dog should be seen by a vet the same day. The most painful eye conditions include glaucoma (*see p.218*), corneal injuries and ulcers (*see p.215*), uveitis (*see p.218*), and keratitis (*see p.215*).

TEAR OVERFLOW AND EYE DISCHARGES

A clear, colourless discharge is simply an excess of tears. Over-production of tears may be a response to an allergy, physical irritants, or wind blowing in the face (*see p.212*). Overflow also occurs when tears do not drain properly from the eyes into the nasal cavity. A yellowish-green discharge usually indicates an infection (*see p.211*).

SIGNS INVOLVING THE EYE SURFACE

The third eyelid protrudes naturally in some breeds, and is often visible when the eye needs protection. It may also protrude because of pain or certain neurological disorders. In some flat-faced breeds, the eyelid may even fold over on itself (*see p.215*).

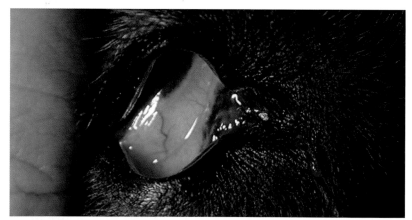

PROTRUDING THIRD EYELID
Normally, the third eyelid remains hidden unless it is cleansing the eye surface. In some breeds, however, such as the Great Dane, Saint Bernard, Basset Hound, and Bulldog, it protrudes and the associated tear gland becomes enlarged.

The conjunctiva (membrane lining the eyelids) and the sclera (white of the eye) may become inflamed for a variety of reasons (*see p.211*). The cornea may become reddened due to bleeding or to the growth of blood vessels in response to previous damage.

A crust or inflammation may develop around the eye because of a problem within the eye socket but also because of a skin condition in the eye area (*see pp.208–10*).

CLOUDY, BULGING, OR SUNKEN EYES

Corneal damage that leads to fluid accumulation, and changes to the lens, can both cause cloudiness of the eyes (*see pp.215–17*). Bulging may occur because the eye has increased in size, or may be due to pressure behind the eye, as in glaucoma (*see p.218*) or eye socket conditions (*see p.221*). The eyeball may appear sunken when there is pain or when it has collapsed.

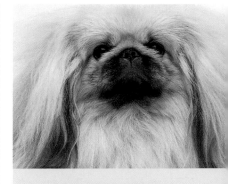

WHAT TO DO WHEN THERE IS A PROBLEM

When you discover a problem in one or both of your dog's eyes, take action right away because it may be a sign of something serious. The condition may appear minor, but it could have serious repercussions if left untreated. The chart below gives you guidance for what to do with certain problems.

EYE PROBLEM	ACTION
Eye hanging out	First aid and see vet immediately
Surface of the eye damaged	First aid and see vet immediately
Bleeding, swelling, severe bruising	First aid and see vet immediately
Foreign body or blood in the eye causing squinting, blinking, tears, rubbing, or oversensitivity to light	First aid and see vet immediately
Eye closed as if in pain	See the vet the same day
Sudden change in the ability to see	See the vet the same day
Pupils irregular	See the vet the same day
Surface of the eyes cloudy or grey	See the vet the same day
Eye intensely bloodshot	See the vet the same day
Green or yellow discharge	See the vet the same day
One or both eyes larger than normal	See the vet the same day
Dog unwilling to open an eye	See the vet the same day
Eyes "ticking" rhythmically in one direction	See the vet the same day
Dilated pupils	Check for shock (*see p.388*) If signs of shock are apparent, see vet immediately
Excess tears	Bathe eyes in tepid salt water
Rubbing of eyes or face	Examine for irritation
Sudden sensitivity to light	Phone vet for advice
Visible third eyelid	Phone vet for advice

Q **CAN MY DOG ACTUALLY WATCH TELEVISION?**

A All dogs are able to watch television, but whether a dog can see a picture depends on the quality of television transmission. Generally speaking, dogs have no difficulty with transmission used for UK or continental Europe. The transmission speed used in North America and elsewhere, however, is more difficult for some dogs to resolve into an image. Videos are a wonderful alternative. Some boredom-relieving videos are available especially for dogs.

Q **WHEN A DOG WITH PROMINENT EYES BUMPS INTO SOMETHING, WHY DOESN'T IT SHUT ITS EYES?**

A There is some anatomical evidence to suggest that some breeds of dog have less "touch-sensitivity" to their eyes than other breeds; in other words, some individuals, often those with prominent eyes, are less concerned when something touches their eyes. As a result, they have a greater risk, and a higher incidence, of corneal damage.

DIAGNOSIS AND TREATMENT

In other areas of the body it is often most practical to discuss problems according to specific diseases and their symptoms; for example, all problems causing hair loss are grouped together (*see pp.182–89*). The eyes are different. Because so much is visible, problems are grouped according to eye anatomy. In the following pages, the information starts with eyelid problems, then covers those of the conjunctiva, the third eyelid, and the surface of the eye. Conditions affecting the (visible) lens and (relatively invisible) retina are then listed, and the section finishes with advice on coping with blindness.

DIAGNOSTIC METHODS AND TOOLS

When you first notice that something is wrong with your dog's eyes, alert your vet. He or she will conduct an examination, not only of the eyes but also of the rest of the body. Your vet knows that, while most eye problems are primary (originating in the eyes), some begin elsewhere and involve other systems; these problems are called

secondary conditions. An example of a sign indicating a secondary condition is a single pupil that is constricted. This sign may show that there is damage to the eyeball, but it can also indicate nerve or brain injury. An example of a secondary condition is an allergy that can cause conjunctivitis but may also involve the dog's skin, respiratory tract, or digestive system.

Your vet will use one or more of the following diagnostic methods to determine the particular cause of your dog's eye condition.

RESPONSE TO TREATMENT

Many conditions, both primary and secondary, are reasonably self-evident to an experienced vet. A diagnosis is confirmed when a dog completely responds to the prescribed treatment.

VISUAL EXAMINATION

The ophthalmoscope is one of the most important diagnostic aids. This hand-held device illuminates and magnifies a part of the eye, enabling your vet to see otherwise invisible damage and disease. It is particularly

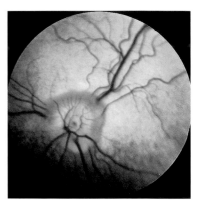

OPHTHALMOSCOPIC VIEW OF EYE
The retina and the blood vessels are clearly visible in this view. Changes to the vessels and to the reflectivity of the retina can indicate progressive retinal atrophy.

useful for examining the eyelids, cornea, iris, lens, and retina. The ophthalmoscope enables the vet to view the texture and blood supply of the dog's retina, and to determine exactly what is happening when there is corneal damage or changes to the lens (such as cataract formation).

FLUORESCENT DYE

Even with an ophthalmoscope, corneal damage may still be invisible. In this situation, a sterile paper strip containing fluorescent dye is applied to the eye. The dye stains the damaged corneal tissue, thereby highlighting the exact region and extent of a corneal injury.

In the event that your dog's eyes are overflowing with tears, your vet may flush fluorescent dye into the tear duct to find out if it is open and operating properly (*see p.206*).

TEAR PRODUCTION MEASUREMENT

Increased or decreased tear production is measured by the Schirmer test, in which a graded strip of sterile paper is applied to the eye to soak up the tears.

VET'S ADVICE

Regular check-ups by your vet will usually include an eye inspection. This check is especially important as dogs grow older. The eyes are vulnerable and susceptible to many problems that may have apparently invisible beginnings. Do not simply assume that your dog's eyes are all right just because you cannot see anything wrong. Your vet's expertise in diagnosis and special equipment will find things that are not visible to the eye of an owner. Any sign of pain without an obvious cause should be investigated.

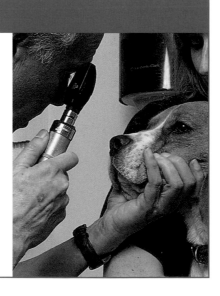

PRESSURE MEASUREMENT

A tonometer is a device that measures intraocular pressure, the pressure in the chambers of the eyeball. It will be used to test for increased pressure, a feature of glaucoma (see p.218).

LABORATORY TESTS

Analysis of discharges, tissue biopsies, and samples of blood and other fluids is performed in the laboratory. If there is a yellow-green discharge from the eye, for example, a bacterial culture and sensitivity test may be performed on a sample of the fluid to determine the best antibiotic to use in treatment. Blood tests can also be carried out to identify the primary cause of conditions such as anterior uveitis (see p.218).

IMAGING TECHNIQUES

Procedures such as taking X-rays and MRI or CT scanning may be carried out when the usual diagnostic methods fail to yield a result or for situations in which an inaccessible part of the eye is involved. These imaging procedures are primarily used to examine the socket region behind the eyeball and to detect the presence of tumours.

If a dog has an advanced cataract in one lens, the vet may be unable to see the retina with an ophthalmoscope because the cataract blocks the view. In this situation, an imaging technique called electroretinography will be used to reveal the health of the retina. This diagnostic procedure is usually carried out by a veterinary ophthalmologist.

TREATMENTS

Your vet may administer or prescribe one of a whole range of drugs, from antibiotic ointments to corticosteroid drops. In certain instances, he or she may recommend surgery.

The following pages (pp.208–21) give relevant details of the treatments for various disorders of the eye.

GIVING EYE MEDICINES

Make sure that a medicine reaches the part of the eye for which it is intended. You may find that a team effort is necessary. While one person holds and reassures the dog, the other instils the medication (see below). Speak calmly to your dog and tell it to sit where it cannot back away – for example, in a corner. If the dog is small, you could lift it up on to a table.

When applying ointment or drops to the eye, make sure that the medicine container does not come into contact with the eye at any time. The container could possibly damage the eye surface; in addition, it may carry dirt or other contamination, which could cause infection. Always praise your dog and give it a food or toy reward after giving eye medicines.

Always follow the instructions on a medicine container. Make sure that you dispose of unused medicine according to the instructions on the packet.

HOW TO APPLY MEDICINE TO A DOG'S EYE

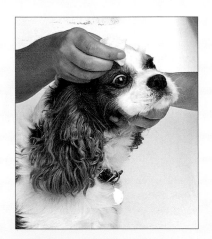

PREPARING THE EYE
Clean away any eye discharge with cotton wool dampened in tepid or warm water. If you are using eye drops, simply tilt the head backwards slightly and, from above, squeeze a drop on the upper part of the eye. If you are using ointment, warm the tube in your hands to help it run smoothly.

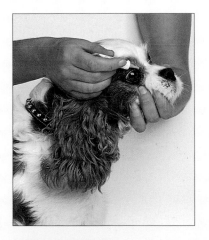

APPLYING OINTMENT
Pull down the lower eyelid to form a pocket for the ointment. Rest the hand holding the tube of ointment against the dog's head, to prevent the ointment container from hitting the eye if the dog moves. Squeeze a line of ointment in the space between the lower eyelid and the eyeball.

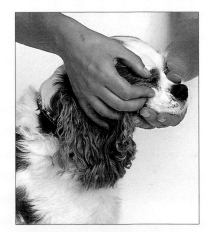

SPREADING OINTMENT
Gently close the eye with your thumb and forefinger for a few seconds, which will spread the ointment evenly over the eye and throughout the socket. Cold ointments often appear grey or white, but body heat will cause them to turn colourless within minutes and the eye will soon clear.

EYE INJURIES

If your dog is pawing at one of its eyes, you need to prevent injury to the area; pawing or rubbing dramatically increases the risk of damaging the cornea and creating a serious problem. You can protect the eye by applying a soft bandage to cover the dewclaws of the forelegs. Even better, improvize an Elizabethan collar (*see p.385*) and secure it to your dog's collar.

CHEMICALS IN THE EYE

If a chemical substance gets into one or both eyes, flush the eyes for at least 10 minutes with plenty of fresh water (*see p.412*). Follow the instructions on the chemical's packaging for a more specific treatment. Protect the eyes to prevent further damage, and take the dog to your vet immediately.

FOREIGN BODIES

Blinking, squinting, avoiding light, and pawing at the eyes may indicate the presence of a foreign body. Using your thumb, pull up the upper eyelid and look closely beneath the lid for any foreign bodies. Pull down the lower lid with your other thumb and carefully look inside that lid as well.

Flush out non-penetrating foreign objects using tepid water. Alternatively, moisten a gauze swab and gently ease the irritant out of the eye. If you cannot remove it, cover the eye with a dressing to prevent further injury, and secure the dressing with a stretchy covering (*see p.395*), then take your dog to the vet immediately.

Do not try to remove a foreign body that has penetrated the eye. Instead, use a bandage or Elizabethan collar to protect the eye and seek immediate veterinary attention. (*See also p.398*.)

EYELID CONDITIONS

Under normal conditions the eyelids efficiently protect the eye, but when their anatomy is faulty they can cause damage. Some dogs are born with abnormal eyelids, while others acquire problems through injury or disease.

ENTROPION

This is a condition in which the eyelids roll inwards. Entropion is inherited in some breeds (*see opposite*), but it may also develop from scarring injuries to the skin around the eyes or after prolonged eyelid infection (blepharitis). Squinting, or blepharospasm, also causes the eyelids to roll inwards, but this problem is temporary. Rolled-in skin irritates the eyes, causing excess tear production and inflammation. There is also increased risk of injury to the cornea and general eye infection.

DIAGNOSIS A vet can tell the difference between entropion and squinting by putting a drop of local anaesthetic on the eyes: the drug relaxes squinting but does not alter true entropion.

TREATMENT Entropion is corrected surgically. A crescent of skin is removed from the eyelid, then the lid is drawn into a more normal position.

ECTROPION

This eyelid defect is the opposite of entropion. The lower eyelids are everted (turn outwards), causing the pink conjunctiva to be visible and more susceptible to inflammation, injury, or contact with debris. Some breeds of dog are born with ectropion of the lower lid (*see opposite*), but the condition may also develop either as a natural part of the aging process or as a result of the skin losing its elasticity.

TREATMENT Mild ectropion is fairly common, particularly in older individuals. If your dog is affected, examine the eyes daily and cleanse the exposed conjunctiva with cotton wool dipped in tepid salt water or with a proprietary eye wash. More severe cases need surgical correction to tighten up the eyelids.

ABNORMAL EYELASHES

In some dogs, eyelashes abnormally grow from the margin of the eyelids, a condition called distichiasis. In others, normal eyelashes turn inwards, rather than away, and make contact with the eye; this condition is called trichiasis. Both of these problems cause constant irritation and heighten the risk of conjunctivitis and corneal damage.

DIAGNOSIS AND TREATMENT You will be able to see the eyelashes lying in the film of tears against the eyeball. Plucking out the lashes with tweezers gives temporary relief, but they usually grow back again. Surgical removal of the hair follicles is usually the most effective treatment, but chemical freezing (known as cryotherapy) and electrolysis are also used.

FACIAL HAIR PROBLEMS

It is not only eyelashes or hair on the eyelids that can irritate a dog's eyes. So, too, can the hair on the nasal fold of flat-faced breeds, and the long facial hair on unclipped Yorkshire Terriers, Old English Sheepdogs, Bearded Collies, Lhasa Apsos, and all other breeds in which hair can overhang the eyes. If you are not planning to show your dog, consider routinely trimming this hair. If you do show it, let it become used to wearing a non-snagging elastic band to hold the hair away from its eyes.

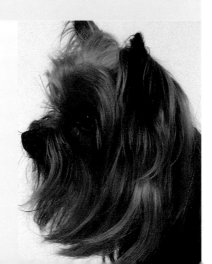

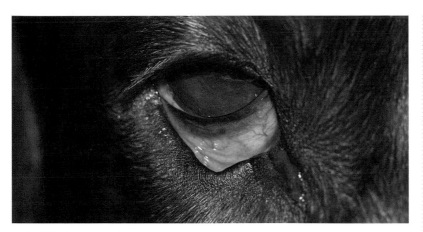

DROOPY LOWER EYELID
Hounds, spaniels, and other breeds with loose facial skin are particularly prone to ectropion, in which their lower eyelids fold outwards and make their eyes look droopy. Hunting dogs, after a hard day's work, may occasionally and temporarily show signs of ectropion.

EYELID INFLAMMATION

Bacterial infection causes the eyelids to thicken and redden, producing mucus and pus. If the crust that builds up on the edges of the lids is not removed, it may "glue" the eyelids together.

This condition, called blepharitis, is most commonly seen in young pups. It is also the most common eye condition associated with canine distemper (*see p.147*). In older dogs, it is almost always associated with an underlying skin disease such as allergy, Demodex mite disease, autoimmune disease, or the effects of an underactive thyroid gland.

DIAGNOSIS AND TREATMENT The vet will arrange a culture and sensitivity test to reveal the bacterial cause and the range of effective antibiotics.

To treat blepharitis, soak off the crusts with a warm, wet flannel. Apply an antibiotic eye ointment following your vet's instructions; oral antibiotics may also be used. The underlying condition must be controlled before blepharitis will disappear.

ACUTE EYELID SWELLING

Your dog may experience an allergic reaction to an insect bite, an injection given by your vet, or even to food, causing the eyelids to swell suddenly.

DIAGNOSIS Affected dogs become very itchy and rub their face and eyes. As with hives (*see p.125*), this reaction usually occurs within 30 minutes of contact with the allergen.

TREATMENT Usually, the only treatment that is necessary is a combination of an oral antihistamine and topical corticosteroid eye drops or ointment, administered over the course of a day.

STYES AND CHALAZIONS

The eyelids are lined with individual oil-producing glands called meibomian glands. If one of these glands becomes infected, a red, tender swelling called a stye develops. If a gland becomes blocked, its contents build up to form a hard, non-tender mass. This swelling creates a firm bulge on the edge of the eyelid, known as a chalazion.

DIAGNOSIS AND TREATMENT Styes and chalazions are diagnosed by a vet. To treat a stye, apply a warm compress (a warm, wet flannel) at least three times a day to bring it to a head. Your vet may then choose to lance the stye using a scalpel or a pin. Topical and sometimes oral antibiotics are used, as are painkillers. A chalazion will be surgically removed, usually from the conjunctival (inner) surface of the lid.

BREEDS AT RISK

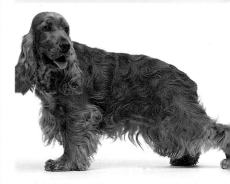

Breeds known to be affected by entropion include:

- Bernese Mountain Dog
- Bloodhound (upper lid)
- Bulldog
- Cocker Spaniel (above)
- Chow Chow
- Golden Retriever
- Great Dane
- Labrador Retriever
- Pyrenean Mountain Dog
- Saint Bernard (upper lid)
- Shar Pei (upper and lower lids)

Breeds prone to ectropion include:

- Hounds
- Spaniels
- Heavyweight giant breeds

Breeds known to suffer from abnormal eyelashes include:

- Bulldog
- Cocker Spaniel (above)
- Dachshund
- Pekingese
- Poodle
- Weimaraner

Q WHAT IS THE MOST COMMON CAUSE OF CONJUNCTIVITIS?

A Physical irritation from dust, debris, or wind is probably the most common cause. The happy dog hanging its head out of the window of a fast-moving car may be revelling in the experience but is also running a high risk of eye injury. (If your dog must hang its head out of the window, let it do so in the driveway.)

Q DO A DOG'S EYES BECOME BLOODSHOT WHEN IT IS TIRED?

A In theory they may do, but if your dog's eyes are bloodshot look for a reason other than its being tired. Bloodshot eyes, sometimes known as pinkeye but more accurately called conjunctivitis, is much more commonly caused by dust, allergy, or infection.

Q WHAT CAN BE USED TO CLEAN INFLAMED EYES?

A Tepid water with cotton wool is fine, but even better is a pH-balanced eye wash. The most readily available are those prepared for human eyes and available from a chemist. More expensive, but even better, are artificial tears, which are also available on the eye care counter at the chemist.

Q ARE THERE ANY EFFECTIVE COMPLEMENTARY THERAPIES FOR CONJUNCTIVITIS?

A The treatment most likely to be effective is eyebright, *Euphrasia officinalis*. This herb has been used for centuries for bathing and brightening sore eyes. Roman chamomile flower, *Chamaemelum nobile*, is also commonly used.

EYELID TUMOURS

Tumours can develop in any part of the eyelid tissue. The most common form of eyelid tumour is a benign adenoma of a meibomian gland. The cells of these glands, which are unique to the eyelids, produce an oil that helps to prevent tears from evaporating from the surface of the eyeball. The tumour produces a proliferation of cauliflower-like tissue attached to, and protruding from, the affected gland. Meibomian gland adenomas may occur as either single or multiple tumours.

Other tumours that may develop on a dog's eyelids include: sebaceous adenomas, which usually appear in older dogs and are commonly benign; melanomas, which are tumours of the pigment-containing skin cells; and papillomas, or warts.

DIAGNOSIS AND TREATMENT Adenomas and other tumours will be diagnosed by your vet. If necessary, tumours will be removed surgically.

ABNORMAL EYELID OPENINGS

The condition microblepharon, in which dogs have small eyelid openings, is uncommon. On rare occasions, pups are born with their eyelids fused (ankyloblepharon). If the pup's eyelids do not open of their own accord in the four to ten days after birth, veterinary intervention is necessary.

Individuals of some breeds, such as the Shetland Sheepdog, may be born with small eyelid openings, which give the dog the appearance of small eyes. When this condition is extreme, a veterinary surgeon may recommend a surgical enlargement of the opening.

Flat-faced breeds commonly have abnormally large eyelid openings (macroblepharon). This makes their eyes attractively prominent but also prone to popping out of their sockets (proptosis). In addition, the eyes are at risk of chronic rubbing from nasal fold skin, which causes corneal pigmentation or other damage (*see p.204*).

HAIR LOSS AROUND THE EYES

Chronic tear overflow may cause loss of hair around the eyes. So, too, can a variety of other parasitic, allergic, and metabolic conditions. For some dogs, aging brings with it a "peri-orbital" hair loss. Others lose hair around the eyes for hormonal reasons. If your dog is losing hair on the eyelids for no apparent reason, see your vet.

CONJUNCTIVAL AND TEAR DUCT CONDITIONS

Conjunctivitis, also known as "red eye", is an inflammation of the eye's protective mucous membrane, the conjunctiva. This membrane lines the inside of the eyelids and the surface of the eyeball as far as the cornea. Conjunctivitis is probably the most common eye disorder that owners see.

The condition often occurs when the conjunctiva is irritated by a hair or a foreign body. If both eyes are inflamed, however, then it may be an indication of more serious problems elsewhere, either within the eyeball itself or in other parts of the body. Allergic conjunctivitis, associated with sneezing (rhinitis), appears to be increasing in dogs. As well as causing local inflammation, conjunctivitis is associated with various discharges that give clues to the cause of the problem. If the eye is infected, for example, the discharge becomes yellowish-green.

Tear production and conjunctivitis are intimately associated. Tears not only keep the surface of the eye moist and glistening but also contain substances that fight infection. Some elements of tears produced in the lacrimal glands – one lying just under the bony ridge at the top of the eye socket, and the other in the nictating membrane. Other components of tears are produced in the meibomian glands, in the eyelids, and by mucus-producing cells in the conjunctiva. Mucus acts like a wetting agent and holds the watery tears to the cornea. The oil from the meibomian glands forms a layer on top of the tears and stops them from evaporating or spilling out of the eye. Excess tears drain from the eye through a large duct, the nasolacrimal duct, into the nasal cavity.

Three tear problems may occur. There can be excess tear production (*see p.212*); blocked tear drainage; and, most serious of all, reduced tear production, or "dry eye" (*see p.213*). Reduced production of tears dries the cornea and increases risk of corneal damage and conjunctival infection.

DISCHARGES

A clear, colourless discharge usually indicates that the eye is suffering from a physical or allergic irritation. Dust, wind blowing in the face, and cold air may all trigger a watery discharge from both eyes. Allergens such as pollens can do the same, but allergy is often accompanied by an itchiness that makes the dog rub its face. Watery discharge from a single eye is usually caused by a foreign body.

A jelly-like discharge of mucus may result from irritation by a foreign body or from an infection. Both of these problems will trigger increased mucus production from the conjunctiva. A yellowish-green discharge is pus, which means that infection is present and must be treated at once.

BACTERIAL AND FUNGAL CONJUNCTIVITIS

Like the skin, the conjunctiva acts as host to many normal bacteria and fungi. Injuries, foreign bodies in the eye, viral infections or, most important of all, a reduction in tear production will allow some of these bacteria and fungi to grow exuberantly. As a result, they cause an infection.

Symptoms of one of these infections include redness, a yellowish-green discharge, and crusting on the eyelids. Dogs may blink, squint slightly, or paw at and rub their eyes. In neonatal

conjunctivitis, a newborn pup may suffer an infection before or after the eyelids have separated, usually between 10 and 14 days. Pups with fused eyelids (ankyloblepharon) are prone to neonatal conjunctivitis. The eyelids bulge or appear swollen, and there may be a discharge. If your pup is affected, you must let your vet know at once in order to prevent more serious disease.

DIAGNOSIS AND TREATMENT It is very important to determine the cause of bacterial or fungal conjunctivitis. The infection itself is diagnosed by culture and sensitivity tests and is treated with the appropriate topical antibiotics. To treat the condition, you can use sterile saline eyewash to flush the eye several times each day. If there is a crust, soak it in warm water, then loosen and remove it with a warm, damp flannel.

VIRAL CONJUNCTIVITIS

The viruses that cause distemper and hepatitis also predispose the eyes to developing bacterial conjunctivitis (*see pp.144–49*). Distemper, in particular, is

associated with reduced tear production and the subsequent development of dry eye (*see p.213*).

DIAGNOSIS AND TREATMENT An early diagnosis of distemper is sometimes made by examining a conjunctival scraping for viral particles. Secondary bacterial infection is treated with appropriate antibiotics. The eyes are kept moist with proprietary saline eye wash and monitored carefully for the possible development of dry eye.

PARASITIC CONJUNCTIVITIS

In the western United States there is a parasitic worm, *Thelazia californiensis*, that can inhabit the space between the eyelids and the eye (the conjunctival sac). The presence of this worm causes conjunctivitis known as thelaziasis.

DIAGNOSIS AND TREATMENT Locating the worm by eye examination confirms thelaziasis. The vet uses a drop of local anaesthetic and removes the worm with forceps. Alternatively, the eye is flushed with an anti-parasitic solution specially prepared for the eye.

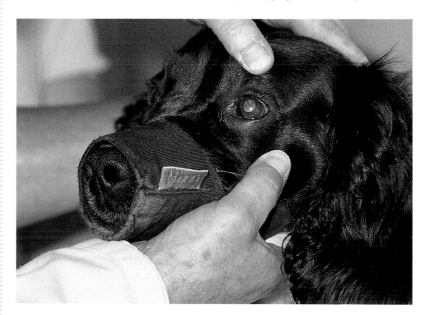

RED EYE
The conjunctiva is the membrane covering the white of the eye and the back of the eyelids. When it is irritated by a physical irritant or an infection, the membrane becomes inflamed and turns red. Conjunctivitis is one of the most common conditions affecting a dog's eye.

TEAR DRAINAGE

Two lacrimal (tear) glands in each eye produce the water in tears. This water forms a middle layer in the tears; the inner, mucous layer comes from the conjunctiva and the outer, oily layer from the eyelids. One tear gland lies above the eye, just below the bony ridge of the eye socket. The other gland forms part of the third eyelid and produces tears in the lower half of the eye. In general, both glands produce a roughly equal amount of tears. In each eye, tears collect in the corner nearest the nose and drain away through two channels (the upper caniculus and lower caniculus) along the nasolacrimal duct and into the nasal cavity.

NASOLACRIMAL DUCT
Tears naturally drain from the eye through the nasolacrimal duct and pass into the nasal cavity. If this duct is blocked or (as happens with some poodles) is poorly formed, tears overflow on to the face.

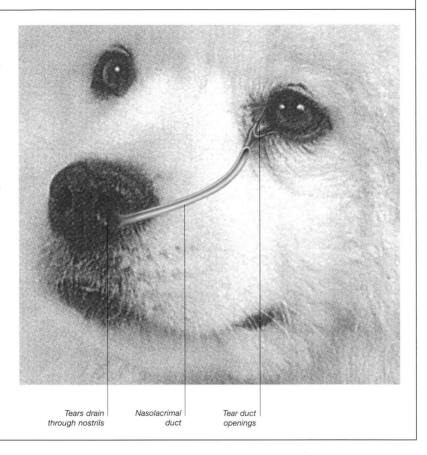

Tears drain through nostrils   Nasolacrimal duct   Tear duct openings

TEAR OVERFLOW (WATERY EYES)

Many conditions produce the symptom of tear overflow, in which an excessive amount of tears fills the eyes. Most of the possible causes are described in this chapter. These problems include: foreign bodies in the eye (*see p.218*); eyelid problems such as entropion or ectropion (*see p.208*); abnormal eyelashes (*see p.208*); facial hair that touches the eye (*see p.208*); blepharitis (*see p.209*); acute allergic swelling of the eyelids (*see p.209*); eyelid tumours (*see p.210*); corneal ulcers (*see p.215*); and conjunctivitis (*see p.211*). Causes that originate within the dog's eyeball include anterior uveitis (*see p.218*) and glaucoma (*see p.218*).

In addition, tear overflow may occur either because the normal drainage system for tears is blocked (*see above*) or because the duct was too narrow or was absent from the nose at birth. This poor drainage is called epiphora. Some breeds have an inherited predisposition to blocked tear ducts (*see opposite*).

The most common reasons for nasolacrimal duct problems are: the duct is swollen because of a bacterial infection; or mucus produced by the conjunctiva either plugs the opening of the duct in the corner of the eye or forms a blockage in the canal.

DIAGNOSIS In dogs that have chronic tear overflow, the hair around the eyes that has been saturated with tears develops mahogany staining.

To find out whether the nasolacrimal duct is blocked, a vet instils fluorescent dye on to the surface of the eye. If the system is open, or patent, then the dye will appear almost immediately in the nostril. If no dye is seen, however, the duct is blocked. In this case, the vet will anaesthetize the dog and insert a small tube, or cannula, into the eye end of the nasolacrimal duct, then gently instil more dye. If the duct is patent, this dye will be seen in the nose.

TREATMENT Tear overflow can only be corrected once the underlying cause has been treated. If the problem is due to a bacterial infection, the vet will prescribe antibiotics. There is no surgical treatment for correcting tear ducts that are malformed at birth.

The best way to control facial staining in dogs suffering from chronic tear overflow is to clean away the overflow twice daily (morning and evening) with a saline eye wash. Some books, and some breeders, recommend using chemicals such as hydrogen peroxide or even bleach to clean stained hair. These chemicals are, however, highly dangerous substances – never use them near a dog's eyes.

Brown staining at the corner of the eye, known as "poodle eye", affects some breeds, such as poodles and the Maltese, Pekingese, and Pomeranian. Breeders sometimes treat affected dogs with long-term oral antibiotics if they are being shown professionally. This measure reduces mahogany staining, but constant use is not recommended. A safer alternative is to apply a water-based barrier ointment, such as petroleum jelly, to the skin below the eyes to prevent tears from coming into contact with hair. Some handlers apply white chalk powder before showing their dogs, but it can irritate the eyes.

DRY EYE

If the lacrimal glands fail to produce enough tears, the eyes become dry and dull-looking. This problem is called dry eye or keratoconjunctivitis sicca.

The lack of tears initially causes conjunctivitis. The risk of infection increases enormously, as does the risk of corneal damage such as ulceration. A little later in the course of the disease, a sticky discharge of mucus replaces the tears, and becomes thick and tenacious. In many cases, a secondary bacterial infection that produces pus develops. The eyes turn dry and opaque. If the cornea becomes inflamed and ulcerated, keratitis (*see pp.215–16*) results.

Many conditions can trigger dry eye. Immune-mediated disease, in which a dog's immune system "attacks" its own lacrimal glands, is the most common cause of the problem in West Highland White Terriers as well as in several other breeds. Other disorders that reduce the production of tears include viral infections such as distemper; bacterial infections, such as those

BREEDS AT RISK

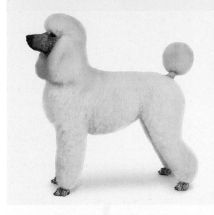

Breeds that have an inherited predisposition to blocked tear ducts include:

- Brachycephalic (flat-faced) breeds
- Bichon Frise
- Maltese
- Lhasa Apso
- Poodles (above)
- Pomeranian
- Toy breeds

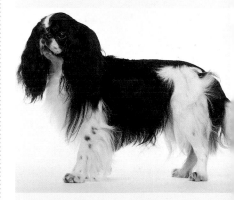

The breed most prone to dry eye is the West Highland White Terrier. Other affected breeds include:

- Bulldog
- King Charles Spaniel (above)
- Cavalier King Charles Spaniel
- Cocker Spaniel
- Lhasa Apso

TEAR STAINING

When the eye produces too many tears, or if the lacrimal drainage system is blocked or too narrow, the tears spill over the lower eyelids, particularly around the corner of the eye. Over time, the tears create an unsightly, mahogany-brown stain on the facial hair.

caused by *Staphylococcus*; and underactivity of the adrenal glands. Dry eye may also follow a physical injury to the lacrimal glands, or may develop when the nerves to the glands are damaged by middle ear infection. In addition, dogs that are being treated with a course of sulfa drugs, such as sulphonamides or trimethoprim-sulfa, can be predisposed to dry eye.

DIAGNOSIS Simple conjunctivitis is a common canine eye problem; for this reason, early dry eye, in which the only visible sign is inflammation, may not be accurately diagnosed unless the vet measures tear production. An accurate diagnosis is made by gauging tear production with a Schirmer test. A special strip of sterile filter paper is placed in the corner of the eye for a minute. The tears will wet the strip a small distance. A normal tear test wets the strip up to 20 mm (¾ in), while in dry eye the moisture travels up the strip only to 10 mm (½ in) or less.

TREATMENT The treatment for dry eye varies according to the severity of the

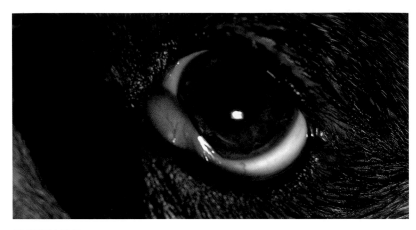

CHERRY EYE
A dog's third eyelid is not normally visible. If the gland behind the third eyelid swells for any reason, the gland and the eyelid protrude, producing so-called "cherry eye".

condition. In the mildest cases, applying artificial tears four or more times a day for several weeks is the only measure needed. This treatment keeps the cornea and the conjunctiva sufficiently moist and lubricated to prevent further, more complicated conditions from developing. More commonly, affected dogs need artificial tears together with antibiotic eye drops to eliminate secondary eye infection. In dogs with dry eye caused by immune-mediated disease, immunosuppressant drugs have successfully eliminated the need for surgical intervention. Corticosteroids and cyclosporin ointment are used; cyclosporin appears to reverse the destruction of the lacrimal glands.

CONDITIONS OF THE THIRD EYELID

The third eyelid, also called the haw or the nictitating membrane, does for a dog's eyes what our index fingers do, less effectively, for ours. The third eyelid moves up from within the lower lid and mechanically sweeps the eye, removing small foreign bodies and minor irritants. If you watch your dog as it falls asleep, you can see the third eyelid move over the eye even before the eyelids are completely closed. The

lower lacrimal gland, which forms part of the the third eyelid, produces roughly half of the eye's tears.

THIRD EYELID PROTRUSION

The third eyelid (nictitating membrane) consists of mobile cartilage covered by conjunctiva. Behind the cartilage, on the eyeball side, is the lower of the lacrimal glands, which is properly called the "nicitating membrane gland". For reasons that are poorly understood, this gland sometimes swells to five or more times its normal thickness. As it does so, it lifts the nictitating membrane away from the surface of the eye. Once this problem occurs, the continued swelling of the nictitating membrane gland causes the third eyelid to flip over. The gland appears as a round, glistening, pink mass in the corner of the eye; for this reason, the condition is called "cherry eye". Once exposed, the gland can irritate the cornea, causing conjunctivitis until the cherry eye is treated. Protrusion of the gland can affect one or both eyes.

TREATMENT Using local anaesthetic drops, vets can often rotate the gland back into its normal position in the third eyelid. The problem is likely to recur, however, unless a minor surgical procedure is carried out to fix the

---

Q   **ONE OF MY DOG'S THIRD EYELIDS IS DARKER THAN THE OTHER. WHAT DOES THIS MEAN?**

A   It does not mean anything. In some individuals there is pigmentation on the edge of one third eyelid but not the other; this feature may make the two eyes appear different, but it is of no medical consequence.

Q   **CAN I USE HUMAN EYE-CARE PRODUCTS ON MY DOG'S EYES?**

A   Generally speaking, you can. There is little difference between human and canine tears, so artificial tears intended for our eyes are excellent for a dog. Similarly, soothing eye washes for humans are the right pH for a dog's eyes.

position of the gland. Neither the third eyelid nor its associated lacrimal gland should be removed unless there are overwhelming reasons to do so.

EVERSION, OR SCROLLING, OF THE THIRD EYELID

In this condition, the edge of the third eyelid curls outwards in a scroll, causing mild conjunctival irritation. Eversion of the third eyelid may occur in one or both eyes. Some breeds are particularly prone to it (*see right*).

TREATMENT The scrolled-over cartilage is surgically removed.

CORNEAL CONDITIONS

The smooth, transparent cornea allows light rays to pass through to the lens and reach the retina. It also acts as a barrier that protects the delicate internal structures of the eye. Any change or damage to the surface of the cornea will diminish a dog's eyesight. Some problems of the cornea are insidious – for example, when light-occluding pigmentation occurs. They cause no pain and a dog does not complain. Other corneal damage and conditions, such as keratitis, do cause pain and, consequently, can be diagnosed earlier.

CORNEAL DAMAGE

Dogs are prone to scratches (abrasions) of the cornea. These injuries cause local swelling that makes the corneal surface appear hazy, cloudy, or opaque. Abrasions are likely to develop into ulcers. Corneal damage may result from disease as well as abrasions, and may lead to ulcerative keratitis (*see below*).

Corneal damage is usually painful. The dog squints or keeps the affected eye slightly closed. The eye becomes inflamed and initially produces excess tears. Secondary infection is common and generates a purulent discharge.

DIAGNOSIS The full extent of corneal injury becomes visible if fluorescent dye is applied to the cornea. All of the damaged areas take up the dye. Even

the slightest abrasion needs immediate veterinary attention.

TREATMENT An antibiotic may be given prophylactically to prevent infection. Topical atropine may be used to dilate the pupil and relieve pain.

ULCERATIVE KERATITIS

Keratitis is inflammation of the cornea. The condition may either be superficial or penetrate deep into the bottom layer of the cornea. In addition, it may involve superficial or deep ulceration. Ulcerative keratitis is more serious than non-ulcerative keratitis (*see below*), because it can lead to collapse of the eye. Ulcers can cause extreme pain. They may be accompanied by squinting and excessive production of tears. In addition, the dog may become over-sensitive to light.

Ulcers may be due to physical injury but are also associated with the following disorders: dry eye; underactive adrenal glands; sugar diabetes (*see p.336*); underactive thyroid glands; slow-healing ulcers; and inherited corneal dystrophy (*see p.216*).

DIAGNOSIS Fluorescent dye dropped into the eye will reveal small ulcers. Larger ulcers can be seen as spots or depressions on the cornea.

TREATMENT Surgery is often necessary for ulcers. Soft contact lenses, specially designed for a dog's eyes, may also be used as protection. A bubble-like bulge within an ulcer shows that it is about to burst, causing the liquid in the anterior chamber to discharge; urgent surgery will be needed to save the eye.

NON-ULCERATIVE KERATITIS

Other forms of keratitis do not involve ulcers. In interstitial keratitis ("blue eye"), the cornea becomes cloudy and a bluish film appears. This condition may be due to infectious canine hepatitis (*see p.148*). In non-ulcerative pigmentary keratitis, melanin (dark pigment) is deposited in the cornea.

In some dogs with dry eye, blood vessels grow over the cornea, creating

BREEDS AT RISK

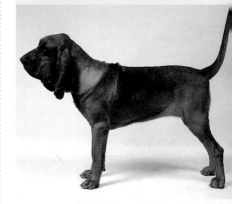

Protrusion of the third eyelid, or cherry eye, occurs most frequently in these breeds:

- Beagle
- Bloodhound (above)
- Boston Terrier
- Boxer
- Bulldog
- Cocker Spaniel
- Lhasa Apso
- Shar Pei

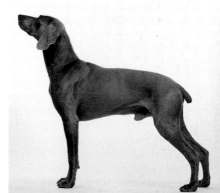

Eversion or scrolling of the third eyelid occurs most frequently in these breeds:

- Great Dane
- Irish Wolfhound
- Neapolitan Mastiff
- Newfoundland
- Weimaraner (above)

a condition called vascular keratitis. Other dogs inherit a predisposition to a condition called chronic superficial keratitis, which is often known as pannus (*see below*).

DIAGNOSIS AND TREATMENT Most dogs spontaneously recover from interstitial keratitis without treatment. Progressive pigmentary keratitis, however, can lead to loss of vision and blindness, although there is some evidence that topical cyclosporin will slow down the process by which pigment is deposited. In dogs with vascular keratitis, the condition usually improves spontaneously once the irritating cause is controlled.

PIGMENTED KERATITIS

The Pekingese often develops a general form of pigmented keratitis, which begins at the nasal side of the eyeball and spreads across to the other side. This keratitis is caused by a chronic irritation from the nasal fold.

TREATMENT Trimming the hair on the nasal skin fold usually reduces corneal irritation. The best way to treat this condition is to remove the fold of nasal skin surgically.

CHRONIC SUPERFICIAL KERATITIS (PANNUS)

Pannus is a form of vascular keratitis mediated by the dog's immune system. A brown patch of pigment, which is reddened by blood vessels, develops on the cornea and, if it is left untreated, will spread over the entire surface.

Once thought to be confined to German Shepherd Dogs, this condition has since been recognized in various other breeds, including the Australian Shepherd, Border Collie, Tervueren (Belgian Shepherd), Greyhound, and the Siberian Husky.

TREATMENT Topical corticosteroids, applied over a long period, shrink the corneal blood vessels and stop them from spreading. In instances where long-term corticosteroid treatment cannot be administered, surgical intervention is often possible.

CORNEAL DYSTROPHY AND DEGENERATION

In corneal dystrophy, off-white, crystalline, opaque areas develop in the same places in the corneas of both eyes. There is no pain, discomfort, or inflammation. Most dystrophies are superficial and cause no problems. Some, however, are deep; they cause diffuse swelling of the cornea that interferes with vision and may cause blindness. Certain breeds are prone to corneal dystrophy (*see opposite*).

Corneal degeneration can look exactly like corneal dystrophy, but it occurs only in one eye and is the result of a physical or metabolic injury. There may be some associated pain.

TREATMENT No effective treatment for corneal dystrophy exists. Surgical removal may improve eyesight, but only temporarily. Corneal degeneration may deteriorate further to form an ulcer. The associated spread of blood vessels may be treated with topical corticosteroids and antibiotics. Serious opacity caused by degeneration can be surgically removed, but subsequent scarring can interfere with vision.

LENS CONDITIONS

The transparent lens focuses light rays on to the retina at the back of the eye. In young dogs, the lens functions very well because it is flexible and crystal-clear. As a dog grows older, however, the lens becomes hardened and hazy, or sclerotic. Injury or disease may cause the lens to slip from its moorings – a process called luxation. Disease, or an inherited defect, can cause a lens to become opaque and form a cataract.

CATARACT

When the proteins in a lens become cloudy, the lens loses part or all of its transparency. The affected area, called a cataract, may become mildly foggy or completely opaque. This problem may affect only part of the lens or may fill it completely. A complete cataract results in a white, crystalline lens with a slightly yellow cast. The development of a cataract is irreversible.

Most cataracts develop as a result of inheritance; however, trauma and metabolic disease, specifically sugar

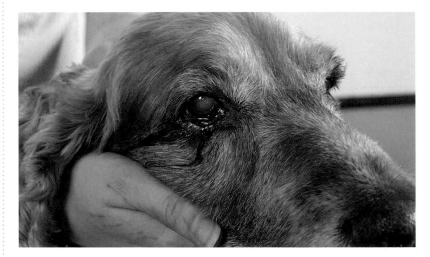

CATARACT
When a dog loses the normal transparency in a lens, an opaque spot or spots appear on the eye. The opacity is often white, but sometimes there is a faintly yellow cast. A cataract has no distinctive shape or size and may fill the whole lens. In some cases, the cataract scatters light rays within the eye and causes squinting.

diabetes (*see p.336*), may also cause them to form. Hereditary juvenile cataracts occur in over 80 breeds, including the Boston Terrier, Golden Retriever, Labrador Retriever, Cocker Spaniel, Miniature Schnauzer, West Highland White Terrier, Siberian Husky, and Old English Sheepdog. Diabetic cataracts can develop within weeks; they may even be the first indication to an owner that a dog has developed sugar diabetes.

DIAGNOSIS An owner or vet may suspect that a dog has a cataract if the lenses appear opaque or if the animal seems to have failing vision. Cataracts are often confused, however, with the clouding of the eye that can be seen in corneal disease (*see above*). A vet will confirm the presence of a cataract by ophthalmoscopic examination.

TREATMENT Surgery will be considered if the dog is blind or on the verge of blindness. There are many methods for removing cataracts, but surgery is only undertaken when it is likely to restore or significantly improve vision. To establish whether it will be beneficial, the retina should always be examined by electroretinography as early as possible. While it is normal for humans to have an artificial lens inserted to replace a damaged lens, the procedure is far more complicated in dogs and so is not frequently undertaken.

PREVENTION All individuals intended for breeding should have their eyes examined for incipient cataracts. Juvenile hereditary cataracts may not develop until six years of age in some breeds, so it is even more important that the parents, grandparents, and great-grandparents of breeding animals are known to be free from cataracts.

NUCLEAR SCLEROSIS

This is the most common eye problem in dogs. It is not a disorder as such, but is a result of normal aging. Over time, in dogs aged eight years and older, the centre of each lens becomes more sclerotic – in other words, harder and more dense. This hardness begins to reflect light rather than refract it on to the retina. The result is an increasing bluish-grey appearance in the lenses.

It is safe to assume that dogs lose their near vision to roughly the same extent as humans, who naturally develop sclerosis at 45 to 50 years of age and often need reading glasses. The older a dog becomes, the less likely it is to see objects that are right in front of its eyes. Distant vision, however, is unaffected.

DIAGNOSIS AND TREATMENT It is easy to mistake nuclear sclerosis for a developing cataract; however, cataracts prevent your vet from clearly seeing the retina with an ophthalmoscope, but nuclear sclerosis does not.

LUXATION OF THE LENS

When the lens luxates, it falls forwards into the anterior chamber of the eye or backwards into the posterior chamber. A partial change (subluxation) or a complete shift (luxation) of the lens can be caused by trauma (from dog fights to road traffic accidents), inflammation in the anterior chamber, glaucoma, aging, or inheritance.

Luxation may be painful and cause glaucoma (*see p.218*). The sclera (the white rim around the cornea) becomes inflamed, and the cornea may turn hazy or opaque. Subluxations are more difficult to diagnose. They may cause no signs other than mild inflammation and increased tear production.

Breeds with a known hereditary predisposition to luxation of the lens include the Sealyham Terrier, Parson Russell Terrier, Tibetan Terrier, Border Collie, and both Wire-haired and Smooth Fox Terriers.

DIAGNOSIS AND TREATMENT Your vet will diagnose partial or full luxation by examining your dog's eyes. A fully luxated lens will be removed as soon as possible to save the remaining vision. Subluxation of the lens is usually treated with medications to reduce associated inflammation.

BREEDS AT RISK

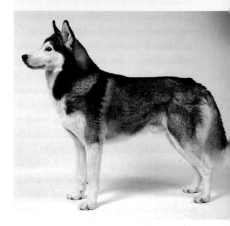

Superficial corneal dystrophy occurs in many breeds including:

- Beagle
- Cavalier King Charles Spaniel
- Collies
- German Shepherd Dog
- Siberian Husky (above)

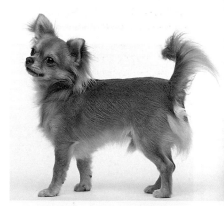

Deep corneal dystrophy may occur in these breeds:

- Boston Terrier
- Chihuahua (above)
- Dachshund

EARS AND HEARING
anatomy and care

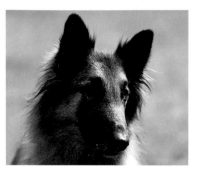

German Shepherd Dog with erect ears

There was a time when dogs' ears came in only one size and shape, just like those of their wolf ancestors. This natural ear has a flap, or pinna, that is erect and highly mobile, well-insulated with hair on the outside, and very smooth on the inside. When we began to breed dogs to suit both our practical purposes and our visual preferences, we created the amazing variety of ear shapes and sizes that dogs have today. But in changing the design of the dog's ear, we have increased the risks and the incidence of ear problems.

The most obvious changes made by breeding are those to the shape or size of the ear, such as the lopped ears of spaniels or the excessively long ears of the Basset Hound. Other, less noticeable changes have been problematic, however, especially the unwitting breeding of dogs such as Schnauzers and Poodles to grow hair all the way down their ear canals to the ear drums.

Ear problems are among the most common reasons why dog owners visit vets, but many problems can be prevented or treated at home. As a general rule, dogs with erect ears that have no hair inside are less prone to ear infections and other problems than those with hairy ear canals or with droopy ears.

CARING FOR A DOG'S EARS
The anatomy of the ear protects the actual organ of hearing from injury. At the same time, however, the length of the ear canal and simple gravity together encourage the accumulation of wax, debris, and foreign material, such as grass seeds, which cannot easily be shaken out of the ears.

Keep your dog's ears in as natural a condition as possible. For most dogs this means doing nothing other than occasionally removing visible wax on the inside of the ear flap.

Always check your dog's ears after it has been playing in tall grass. Look for grass seeds or other plant material, such as the awns of barley, that might travel down the ear canals and get caught in the hair. This is a particular problem with spaniels. Keeping the hair clipped directly below the ear

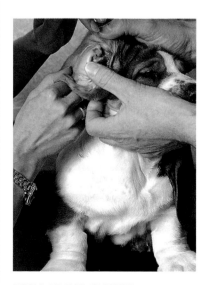

REGULAR EAR CHECKS
Regular checks to detect parasites or a build-up of wax are important for all dogs, but especially for those with lopped ears.

opening will reduce the risk of grass seeds catching in it and working their way into the ear canal.

If your dog has hair in its ear canals, routinely pluck small amounts with your fingers and afterwards instil a proprietary ear cleaner. Train your dog from puppyhood to accept this as a weekly routine. If your dog has been in a fight, check the ears for injuries. Blood can trickle down the canal, predisposing it to external ear canal infection (*see p.226*).

CLEANING A DOG'S EARS
If your dog's ears are clean, leave them alone. Routine cleaning is unnecessary. To remove wax, moisten a cloth with mineral oil and, using your finger, wipe all accessible parts of the ear. Only use a cotton bud (dipped in mineral oil) with extreme caution. If you push it too far it turns into a plunger, pushing debris deeper into the ear canal.

If wax has accumulated in the visible part of the ear canal, instil a few drops of mineral oil or baby oil, leaving it in the ears for a few hours to soften the wax. Alternatively, use a proprietary wax remover made with a dilute salicylic acid solution. After the solution has had a chance to work, gently flush the ear canal with a

ANATOMY OF THE EAR

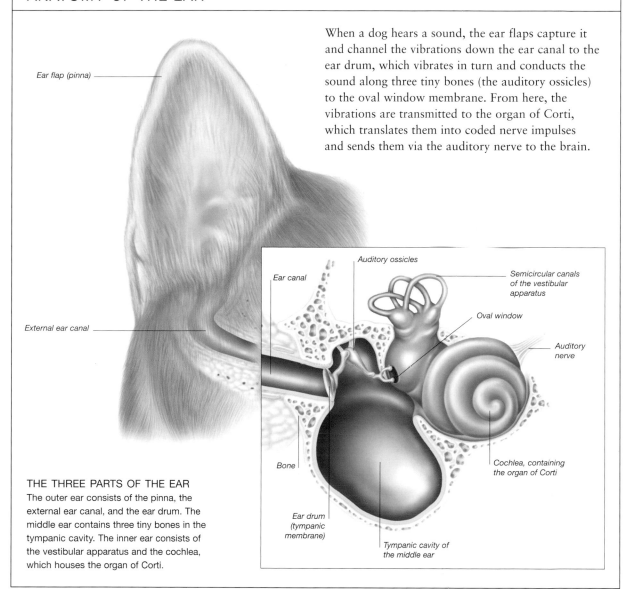

When a dog hears a sound, the ear flaps capture it and channel the vibrations down the ear canal to the ear drum, which vibrates in turn and conducts the sound along three tiny bones (the auditory ossicles) to the oval window membrane. From here, the vibrations are transmitted to the organ of Corti, which translates them into coded nerve impulses and sends them via the auditory nerve to the brain.

Ear flap (pinna)

External ear canal

Auditory ossicles

Ear canal

Semicircular canals of the vestibular apparatus

Oval window

Auditory nerve

Cochlea, containing the organ of Corti

Bone

Ear drum (tympanic membrane)

Tympanic cavity of the middle ear

THE THREE PARTS OF THE EAR

The outer ear consists of the pinna, the external ear canal, and the ear drum. The middle ear contains three tiny bones in the tympanic cavity. The inner ear consists of the vestibular apparatus and the cochlea, which houses the organ of Corti.

solution made of equal portions of lukewarm white vinegar and distilled water. Make sure you use only the gentlest pressure. When you have finished, press cotton wool inside the ear to dry up the solution.

Never use alcohol-based solvents in your dog's ears because they may cause intense irritation.

KEEPING THE EARS DRY

Warm, moist conditions encourage the organisms that cause ear infections, so do not let water remain in your dog's ears and enter the ear canals. Insert a tight ball of cotton wool in each ear before you bathe your dog, and always dry your dog's ears thoroughly after it has been swimming.

CARING FOR DROOPY EARS

Reduce the weight of thick hair by routinely clipping or shaving the hair from the inside surfaces of the flaps. This allows better air circulation in breeds such as spaniels. Such dogs may benefit from having their ears taped back for a few hours each week, especially in hot and humid climates.

DIAGNOSIS AND TREATMENT

If you think your dog has a problem in one or both of its ears, try to identify it from one of the early signs or the diagnostic information in the following pages. You will also find advice about what you can do to help relieve certain problems. But if you are in any doubt, consult your vet at once.

Your vet will try to determine which part of the ear – the outer, middle, or inner ear – is affected. He or she may then look in your dog's ears with an otoscope (*see below*). This device is used to shine a light into the ear and down the ear canal and to magnify anything that might be hidden there.

What is done next depends upon what the vet finds, on the dog's medical history, and on the circumstances in which you have brought your dog to the vet. A swab may be inserted into the ear and the retrieved material examined under the microscope for mites or their eggs, bacteria, yeast, white blood cells, and other unusual cells. The vet may take a biopsy of tissue or an X-ray to see if the middle ear is infected and filled with debris.

CLASSIFYING PROBLEMS

Vets classify ear problems in two ways. Primary conditions (*see pp.226–28*) are due to an injury to, or a disease in, the ear itself. Problems of the ear flap are a sub-division of these (*see pp.228–29*). Secondary conditions of the ear (*see pp.229–30*) are caused by a problem originating elsewhere in the body; allergies are the most common cause of these ear disorders.

EARLY SIGNS OF EAR PROBLEMS

You can help prevent ear problems or at least spot them early enough so your vet can diagnose and treat your dog quickly and prevent the problem from getting worse. Ear problems that persist for a long time without treatment can result in severe irritation, impaired balance, or deafness.

The following are some early signs of ear problems:
• Head and ear shaking, or scratching one or both ears, can indicate mites, infection, a foreign body, or allergies.
• An unpleasant odour emanating from one or both ears can indicate mites or an infection.
• A yellow, brown, or mahogany-coloured ear discharge can indicate mites (especially if the discharge is dark) or an infection.
• Inflammation of the ear flap or of the opening of the ear canal can indicate mites, infection, a foreign body, or allergy.
• A yelp or other indication of pain if a dog is touched around the ears can indicate an infection or a foreign body.
• If the head is tilted to one side, there could be a middle ear condition.
• Apparent loss of hearing can indicate excessive wax build-up, an injury, or brain damage.
• Swelling on an ear flap is usually a haematoma.
• Stumbling or circling to one side can indicate infection in the inner ear or even brain damage.

TREATING EAR CONDITIONS

If a foreign body such as a grass seed is seen by your vet when the ear is examined, it will be removed with long alligator forceps. If the ear is too painful, a short-term anaesthetic is given while the ear is examined and flushed to the ear drum with a special catheter.

Most infections are treated with antibiotics. Ear mites are eliminated with proprietary ear mite medications. Non-prescription ear drops containing pyrethrins, natural insecticides made from chrysanthemums, are effective against ear mites if they are used for a long enough period.

Wax can be softened using mineral oil or proprietary wax-softening ear drops. In addition, a mild acidifying solution may be used once or twice a week to reduce glandular secretion and lower the humidity in the ear canal, especially in lop-eared dogs. These

VET'S ADVICE

Look inside your dog's ears every time you groom them. Your vet will inspect your dog's ears with an otoscope (pictured) as part of a regular check-up, especially if the breed has "unnatural" shaped ears or is one with hair growing inside the flap and ear canal. Never ignore any early signs of ear problems (see above). The sooner a vet looks at the ear the better the outcome of any treatment is likely to be. Small problems that are neglected can lead to worse conditions and more damage to the ear.

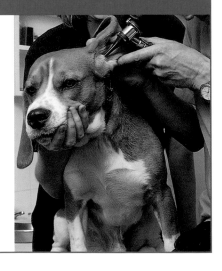

solutions may sting if your dog has broken skin or an inflammation of the ear canal.

In some circumstances, the only solution to a chronic ear problem is surgical alteration of the ear canal to allow better aeration. If the ear drum has been ruptured and a chronic middle ear infection exists, it may be beneficial to remove the entire ear canal and drain the middle ear – an operation called a bulla osteotomy.

HOW TO GIVE EAR DROPS

Although one person can carry out this treatment alone (*see below*), treating any ear condition is often easier as a team effort, especially when dealing with larger dogs. While one person holds and reassures the dog, the other instils the drops and massages them throughout the ear. After softening the wax with a cleansing solution, follow up with prescribed drops.

As with any medicines, never call your dog to you when giving ear drops, because coming to you should always be associated with enjoyment and is a vital part of training. Instead, go to your dog, command it to sit, instil the appropriate medication, massage it thoroughly around the ear canal, then give your dog a food treat and plenty of praise.

ADVERSE REACTIONS

If your dog's ear condition appears to improve as a result of medication but then get worse again, it may have a contact allergy to the medication. One drug that may cause a contact allergy response is neomycin sulphate, which is an effective ear antibiotic but is known to provoke itching and inflammation. Propylene glycol, the inert base component of many ear medications, may also cause contact allergy itchiness in susceptible dogs.

Q WHY CAN DOGS HEAR SOUNDS THAT ARE INAUDIBLE TO US?

A This is part of the wolf in dogs. Small prey such as mice and rats make high-pitched sounds, and these animals are part of a wolf's summer diet. A bonus is that vampire bats in Central and South America seldom feed on dog blood – dogs hear them coming.

Q DO DOGS ENJOY LISTENING TO MUSIC?

A Ivan Pavlov found that dogs can distinguish between two notes that differ by only one eighth of a tone. Whether they enjoy or dislike music is another matter. I know one Dachshund who attacks her owner's ankles each time he practises his Shostakovich!

HOW TO APPLY DROPS TO YOUR DOG'S EARS

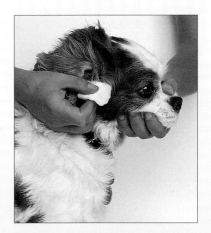

1 With your fingers under the lower jaw and your thumb between the eyes and the nose, hold your dog's head firmly but without squeezing. Dampen some cotton wool with warm water or a wax-removal solution, then lift up the ear flap and wipe away any wax you can see. Do not attempt to remove wax from the ear canal.

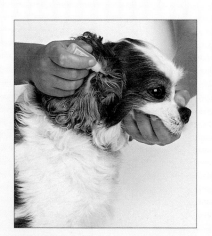

2 Keep holding the head still with one hand and lay back the flap of the ear with your other hand. It is best to do this with the bottle of ear drops ready. Hold the nozzle of the bottle over the opening of the ear canal and point it towards the tip of the nose. Squeeze the prescribed number of ear drops into the ear canal.

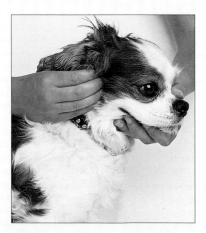

3 Keep holding the head steady and prevent your dog from shaking its head. Remove the bottle and let the ear flap drop down again. Gently but firmly massage the cartilage at the bottom of the ear for no more than 30 seconds; this will spread the drops throughout the canal. Finish off by giving your dog a food treat and plenty of praise.

PRIMARY CONDITIONS

The majority of ear conditions are primary – that is, they are the result of an injury to, or a disease in, one or more parts of the ear. For conditions affecting the ear flap, or pinna, *see pp.208–9.*

EAR MITES

Ear mites (*Otodectes cyanotis*) are tiny parasitic insects that feed on skin debris. They are very common in pups and cause about 10 per cent of cases of ear inflammation in young dogs. Most of the mites remain within the ears but a few spend short periods outside them. These are the source of frequent reinfestations. Ear mites are highly contagious to other dogs and cats, but are not transmitted to humans.

DIAGNOSIS If your pup is scratching its ears and shaking its head, and has a mahogany to black waxy discharge, assume it has ear mites. Mites are white, the size of a pin head, and move vigorously when you shine a light upon them. If you look at an ear swab against a dark background you will see them wriggle.

TREATMENT Treat the ears with an over-the-counter, pyrethrin-based ear drop solution or a prescribed medication for at least three weeks. Most medications kill the adult mites but not their eggs, so you have to continue treatment until all the eggs have hatched and the mites are destroyed. Flea insecticides will kill ear mites that travel outside the ears.

Ear mite problems are often complicated with secondary infections from opportunist bacteria and yeast. As a result, your vet may prescribe an antibiotic to combat the bacteria or an antifungal to stop the yeast. If itchiness is intense, he or she may include an anti-inflammatory.

Ear mites spread very easily, so you need to treat all your dogs and cats; if you have any rabbits or ferrets, you will need to treat them as well.

OTITIS EXTERNA

Infections of the outer ear may be bacterial, fungal, or caused by yeast. Dogs do not catch ear infections from other dogs. External ear canal infections are caused by opportunist microorganisms already in your dog's ears. Given the opportunity, they will multiply in excess and displace the beneficial bacteria.

Malassezia is possibly the most common cause of otitis externa. This yeast is a prime opportunist, taking advantage of mite infestations, allergy, or other causes of ear canal inflammation. *Malassezia* often occurs concurrently with a bacterial ear infection. The ear may be smelly, inflamed, hot, or painful. Affected dogs shake their heads and scratch either behind or in their ears.

Pseudomonas is an opportunist bacterium that causes ear infection when there is chronic otitis.

DIAGNOSIS The dog shakes its head and scratches or rubs the ear, which is painful. It may tilt the head down on the affected side. There is usually a waxy discharge with a bad smell. Your vet will carry out a culture and sensitivity test or examine the ear discharge under the microscope to investigate the underlying cause.

TREATMENT A lotion that combines an antibiotic, an antifungal, and an anti-inflammatory is usually dispensed. Oral ketoconazole may be used for *Malassezia* infection. A drying solution may be recommended for weekly or twice-weekly use to prevent the infection from recurring.

OTITIS MEDIA AND INTERNA

Untreated external ear infection may lead to middle or inner ear infection (otitis media and otitis interna, respectively). These conditions are far more difficult to overcome than a simple external infection.

Vets have observed that some dogs with middle and inner ear infections have intact ear drums and no sign of external problems. These conditions develop because the infection has tracked up from the back of the throat into the middle ears via the Eustachian tubes. These are the tubes that "clear" or "pop" with changing air pressure when we fly on aircraft.

DIAGNOSIS Signs are similar to otitis externa except that pain becomes more intense and hearing can be impaired, especially if both ears are infected.

TREATMENT Effective treatment involves your vet puncturing the ear drum to flush out the hidden infection.

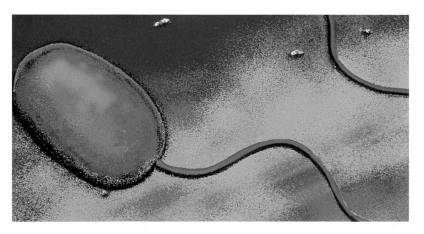

HIGHLY MAGNIFIED PSEUDOMONAS BACTERIUM
Pseudomonas bacteria have a hair-like tail, or flagellum, and are able to take the opportunity to multiply when warm, moist conditions occur in the ear canal.

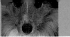

A chronic external ear infection usually leads to a chronic middle ear infection. In both of these conditions, surgery to open the side of the ear canal and permit easier access to the ear drum region beneficially alters the microenvironment. The effect of this is to reduce the risk of infection and, at the same time, improve access to the deeper parts of the ear.

LOSS OF BALANCE–VESTIBULAR SYNDROME

Balance and orientation are controlled by the vestibular apparatus and its connections to the brain. Middle or inner ear infections and conditions may lead to damage and loss of balance. Older dogs may commonly suffer from a sudden loss of balance, often accompanied by a head tilt, nystagmus (ticking movement of the eyes), bad coordination, circling, loss of appetite, and vomiting. The cause of canine vestibular syndrome is not yet known. This condition is sometimes erroneously mistaken for a stroke.

DIAGNOSIS AND TREATMENT Almost invariably, the signs of vestibular syndrome diminish rapidly within one week, and have disappeared within a month, although a residual head tilt is not uncommon. Only symptomatic treatment is necessary, to control nausea and prevent accidental injuries.

GRASS SEEDS AND FOREIGN BODIES

All kinds of grass seeds and other foreign bodies can get stuck in your dog's ears. For example, bristly awns of barley, often called foxtails, can work their way down the ear canal. Your dog will usually shake its head vigorously to try to dislodge them.

DIAGNOSIS Your vet will use an otoscope to identify and locate the grass seed or foreign body.

TREATMENT To prevent the sharp tip of the awn from penetrating the delicate ear drum, instil about ten drops of mineral oil in the affected ear; this

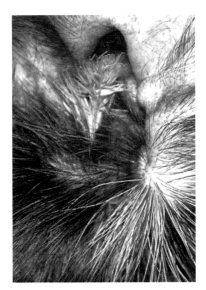

GRASS SEED
Some grass seeds are equipped with tiny hooks to attach themselves to the hair and coats of passing animals. When lodged in an ear they cause intense irritation.

gives temporary relief while you arrange to visit the vet. Your vet will remove the foxtail with alligator forceps passed through an otoscope.

EAR DISCHARGES

Ear discharges are not so much a condition in themselves as a symptom of any one of several problems. For example, ear mites usually produce a dry, gritty "coffee granule" substance in the ears; this is a mixture of wax and mite excrement.

Malassezia wax is usually dark brown and soft. A moist, light yellow, fruity-smelling paste indicates a bacterial infection. Itchiness and redness without discharge is often a sign of allergic otitis (*see p.230*).

EAR TICKS

The ear tick (*Otobius megnini*) is a rare tick that attaches itself to the wall of the ear canal, where it sucks blood.

TREATMENT The ear tick is removed by your vet using alligator forceps passed through an otoscope.

Q CAN I USE COTTON BUDS TO CLEAN MY DOG'S EARS?

A Yes, but take great care when using a cotton bud. Use it only to clean out wax and debris from visible areas. Never insert a cotton bud down the ear canal. The tip acts like a plunger, compacting debris onto the ear drum, and this makes any ear condition more serious and more difficult to treat.

Q CAN I PREVENT GRASS SEEDS FROM GETTING INTO MY DOG'S EARS?

A This is a seasonal problem, which occurs when grass matures and the seeds become brittle and dry. There is little you can do other than avoiding areas of dense vegetation and clipping the hair near the opening of the ear canal (and between the toes – another area where grass seeds penetrate). It is more important to check your dog's ears and toes immediately after the dog has been outdoors; any grass seeds will usually be visible and will still be easy to remove.

Q SHOULD I LET MY DOG SCRATCH ITS EARS?

A Yes, in moderation. Scratching or rubbing the skin is part of routine grooming. Watch carefully; you will see that if your dog has dew claws, these are used to clean the nooks and crannies under the ear flap, then sniffed, licked, or rapturously sucked. A little routine maintenance of this kind is fine. If you think your dog is paying more attention than usual to its ears, however, look at and sniff around them. If anything appears unusual, arrange to take the dog to your vet.

RUPTURED EAR DRUM

Ear drums that have been torn by trauma or damaged due to infection have a remarkable capacity to heal themselves, providing the underlying cause is removed. If using standard ear medicines on a dog with a ruptured ear drum, however, take great care because these can cause further damage. Certain drugs used to treat ear infections, such as the aminoglycoside group of antibiotics (including gentamicin and neomycin sulphate), can cause deafness by damaging the nerve tissue.

DIAGNOSIS AND TREATMENT Your vet will determine the severity of the rupture and, if necessary, will treat the underlying infection or infestation. Minor ruptures will spontaneously heal. In more permanent ruptures, hearing may be moderately impaired but the risk of middle or inner ear infection will increase markedly.

TUMOURS

Squamous cell carcinoma is a common kind of skin cancer that can occur on the edge of the ear flap (and the bridge of the nose), triggered by constant exposure to intense sunlight. Less common is a ceruminoma, a tumour of the wax-producing cells lining the ear canal. Ceruminomas are benign and small, with the potential to become malignant if left untreated.

DIAGNOSIS Squamous cell carcinoma initially resembles a crusty fly bite. Ceruminomas, pinkish-white growths, are usually diagnosed after they become infected or bleed in the ear.

TREATMENT The affected part of the ear is surgically removed.

EAR FLAP (PINNA) PROBLEMS

Dogs such as spaniels, with floppy or excessively hairy ears, are more susceptible to ear flap problems than dogs such as the German Shepherd Dog, with erect and hairless ears.

HAEMATOMAS

When blood accumulates between the skin and the cartilage of the ear flap, a blood-filled blister called a haematoma develops. This is a fluctuating swelling under the skin of the ear flap that is hot and soft to the touch.

Haematomas usually occur as a consequence of vigorous head shaking, especially in older dogs. They may also be caused by a blood clotting disorder, warfarin poisoning (*see pp.420–23)*, or trauma. There is some evidence that both Labrador Retrievers and Golden Retrievers have a genetic predisposition to haematomas.

DIAGNOSIS Visual examination of the affected ear flap is usually all that is necessary for diagnosis.

TREATMENT Routine treatment by your vet will include draining the fluid from the haematoma. This is often followed by applying temporary stitches to prevent the ear flap from refilling with blood or serum.

Injecting cortisone directly into the empty cavity is therapeutic for some dogs. In other cases, however, a decent-sized drainage hole has to be made on the inner surface of the ear flap to allow continuous drainage. Haematomas have a tendency to recur.

BITES AND OTHER PHYSICAL INJURIES

Ears are frequently bitten during dog fights. The edges and tips of the ear flap, in particular, bleed profusely.

TREATMENT Clean wounds thoroughly. Avoid covering a bite wound because it will always be heavily infected and covering only encourages infection. Other wounds, however, may be covered (*see p.395)*. If you think that the cartilage of the ear is damaged, consult your vet.

EXTERNAL PARASITES

A variety of skin mites, including *Demodex canis* and *Cheyletiella yasguri*, can affect the skin on the ear flap. Another mite, *Sarcoptes scabei*, is responsible for causing scabies. None of these mites should be confused with ear mites (*see p.226)*.

Scabies mites, in particular, have an affinity for ear tips, causing hair loss and a crusty and intensely itchy reaction. Refer to External Parasites for more detail (*see pp 158–65)*.

DIAGNOSIS Visual examination is usually all that is necessary.

TREATMENT The dog's entire body must be treated to be certain of eliminating these parasites.

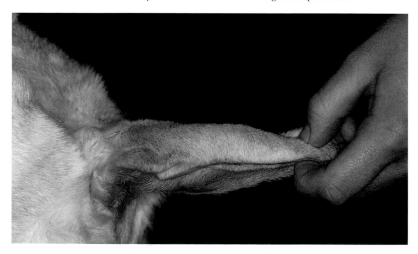

HAEMATOMA
Vigorous shaking of the head can cause a blood blister (haematoma) between the skin and the cartilage of the ear flap. When you touch it, this haematoma feels hot and soft.

FROSTBITE

Prolonged exposure to winter conditions, when the wind chill factor is severe, puts the tips of the ears, especially those with little hair cover, at risk of frostbite.

DIAGNOSIS The skin of the ear flap is pale or sometimes blue. If a clear line develops between the normal healthy skin and dead, black skin, contact your vet immediately.

TREATMENT If your dog has been exposed to prolonged cold, pad the ears with cotton wool dampened with a little lukewarm water. Do not rub the ears because this will only make them itchier.

ALLERGIES

Some ear antibiotics may cause your dog to experience an allergic reaction in which the ear flap becomes hot and slightly swollen. An allergic reaction to an insect bite, or to food or medicines given by injection or by mouth, may also cause the ear flap to become thickened and inflamed.

VET'S ADVICE

Ears are exasperating. Once changes have occurred in the ear canals (such as the stimulation of excess activity by wax-forming cells) it may take months before normal activity returns. Do not expect an ear problem to be cleared up completely after one visit to your vet. It is common for a follow-up examination to be necessary, usually to discover what was hidden the first time because of the wax, discharge, and other debris. By the time of your second visit, pain, swelling, and debris should be minimal. Your vet may now change the treatment and ask to see your dog yet again to ensure that the condition has disappeared.

TREATMENT An antihistamine or corticosteroid injection will reduce discomfort and inflammation. In some cases, the allergic reaction can progress to anaphylactic shock (*see p.388*), and an adrenaline injection must be given.

FLY BITE

Some flies irritate and bite the tips of the ears, causing black, crusty scabs to develop. Dogs with erect ears, such as German Shepherd Dogs and collies, are particularly susceptible, as are dogs living in areas where these flies are found, such as Australia.

TREATMENT To be on the safe side, keep your dog indoors when flies are a nuisance. Alternatively, protect your dog from bites with a relatively safe insecticide such as a pyrethrin.

SUNBURN

Dogs with white coats seem to be more prone than most to sunburn. To prevent sunburn of the ear flaps, apply a sun block of SPF 30 or higher before letting your dog out in direct sunshine for prolonged periods. (*See also p.197.*)

SECONDARY CONDITIONS

Sometimes, a disease or illness that affects another part of the body will show up as a symptom in the ear. These secondary conditions include food allergies, inhalation allergies, and hormonal problems.

If your vet thinks an ear problem is secondary, he or she may take a blood sample to check the function of the thyroid gland. The vet may suggest allergy testing if an inhalation allergy is suspected, or diet restriction if food allergy is a possibility.

Your dog's medical history and perhaps even its breed may influence the occurrence of secondary problems. For example, Cocker Spaniels are more prone to ear problems caused by food allergies than are other breeds. Such problems can only be resolved when

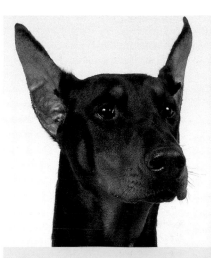

Q IS IT EVER NECESSARY TO CUT A DOG'S EARS OR TAIL?

A Ear cropping is a procedure that was carried out originally on breeds of German origin, such as Boxers, Dobermans, Great Danes, and Schnauzers, and on fighting dogs such as Bull Terriers. It was done to protect the ears from injury and to make dogs look more fierce.

There is no medical or ethical justification for this procedure; it is still carried out only because some breeders hate the idea of change. Vets with a genuine interest in the welfare of dogs will not carry out this unnecessary and uncomfortable amputation. In many countries – for example, all of Western Europe (including Germany) and Australia – ear cropping is illegal.

Tail amputation (docking) is also unnecessary for all except some working gun dogs. In some countries the practice is illegal; in others, it may only be carried out by a vet, or breeders may dock their own pups. If you would like a new dog to have its natural ears and tail, ask your vet's staff to recommend breeders in your area, or look on the internet. There are breeders of almost every breed who do not interfere with either ears or tails.

ALLERGIC OTITIS

This condition is usually associated with itchiness and inflammation but no discharge. If a dog damages its ear while scratching, a secondary bacterial infection may result. Excess wax production in the ears may be a form of seborrhoea – an allergic response to a perceived challenge from something that has been eaten or inhaled.

DIAGNOSIS The dog may be sensitive to, or intolerant of, a particular food, so your vet may initially suggest an elimination diet for at least six weeks to identify the potential source. Alternatively, the dog's skin or lungs may be hypersensitive, so intradermal skin testing for inhaled and contact allergens such as dust mites, human dander, flea saliva, and pollens may also be considered.

TREATMENT Corticosteroid drops are often used to reduce itchiness. Only when the cause of the allergic reaction is eliminated does this form of waxy otitis resolve. This can be a frustrating and lifelong condition.

HORMONAL PROBLEMS

Hair loss on the ear flaps is a hereditary condition in some breeds, such as Dachshunds and Yorkshire Terriers. In other breeds it may be a sign of an underactive thyroid gland, indicating that insufficient amounts of thyroid hormone are being released into the bloodstream. This condition, which is called hypothyroidism, may also cause an excess production of tenacious ear wax.

Some breeds – particularly the Yorkshire Terrier and the Smooth Dachshund but also the Boxer, Boston Terrier, Chihuahua, Italian Greyhound, Manchester Terrier, and Whippet – develop a progressive and permanent hair loss to their ear flaps. Some Toy and Miniature Poodles experience periodic hair loss from the ears.

DIAGNOSIS AND TREATMENT Diagnosis is by clinical signs, such as a blood test to check thyroid function. Hair loss due to hypothyroidism may respond to a course of thyroid hormone. Given time, the hair often regrows at the next growing season. Inherited hair loss cannot be rectified, although selective breeding can reduce its incidence in future generations.

HEARING PROBLEMS

A dog's hearing is remarkable. While some dogs' ears are better tuned than others, dogs can hear a sound four times further away than humans, and can detect and locate the source of a sound in six hundredths of a second.

They can also distinguish sounds that are particular to their owner from the multitude of sounds all around them – often from the depths of sleep.

Deafness is particularly disturbing for a dog and its owner because it eliminates an important form of communication between people and dogs. With effective training, however, deaf dogs can easily learn to understand and respond to sign language.

Dogs can be born deaf. They can also lose their hearing as a result of old age, infections of the middle and inner ears, an injury to the head, a tumour, or through the use of some drugs and antibiotics. Loss of hearing can be temporarily caused by excessive wax in the ears or hair blocking the ear canal.

CONGENITAL DEAFNESS

Deafness existing from birth is caused early in foetal development, when the sound receptor cells in the ear fail to form properly. Pups may have hearing at birth but lose it within a few weeks. Breeders are often unaware of the problem until training sessions begin.

A link seems to exist between congenital deafness and the genes for the colour of a dog's coat, which means that some breeds are more prone to deafness than others.

HANDLING DEAFNESS

Always keep a deaf dog on its leash. With patience and food rewards with strong odours, use simple but flamboyant hand signals to train your dog to come, sit, stay, and lie down. A deaf dog's other senses often become more acute. Use floor vibrations or a flashing light to get its attention. The most natural way for a deaf dog to cope with its disability is by having a hearing companion. Your deaf dog understands what is happening by watching the body language of its buddy.

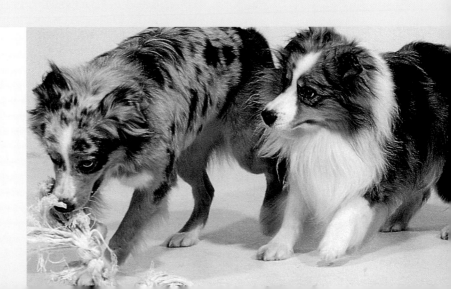

THE BAER TEST

The BAER (brain-stem auditory evoked response) test is designed to assess the hearing in both ears. It records the electrical activity in the cochlea and the auditory pathways in the brain. The test is painless and easy to perform on a relaxed dog, and may only require anaesthesia if the dog becomes very agitated. It lasts for 10–15 minutes. Tiny electrodes, placed under the skin of the scalp, are linked to a computer that sends signals to the dog via foam insert earphones. The interpretation of the test should be conducted by a vet who has training in this technique.

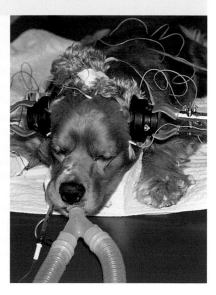

A BAER test on an anaesthetized dog

ACQUIRED DEAFNESS

Dogs that lose their hearing usually do so gradually. Their ability to hear low-frequency sounds is thought to remain longest, although some dogs who lose their hearing in old age may still be able to hear high-pitched sounds. As deafness sets in, dogs become less active, appear reluctant to awaken from sleep, and increasingly seem to ignore commands.

Acquired deafness may be due to tissue damage, caused either by a severe infection to the middle or inner ears or as a consequence of drug toxicity. Antibiotics such as neomycin sulphate and gentamicin, which are used to treat ear infections, can damage the nerves conducting auditory signals from the organ of Corti and the vestibular apparatus to the brain.

Less commonly, a tumour of the inner ear, or an injury sustained to the head, may cause deafness by damaging the cochlea and the organ of Corti within, or harming the auditory nerve.

Deafness resulting from old age is common (see p.375). It is usually a gradual process that starts around ten years of age.

DIAGNOSIS When your dog fails to respond to your commands, do not assume that its behaviour is due to petulance or an unwillingness to obey. Deafness is often gradual and develops insidiously in older dogs.

When only one ear is damaged or defective, you may not notice for some time because dogs manage to compensate so well as other senses take over. Try using a dog whistle to attract the animal's attention, or find some other way to handle the deafness.

If you suspect that your dog might be going deaf, test it by clapping your hands while standing behind it and watching the reaction. With normal hearing, your dog should turn directly towards the sound. If it has impaired hearing, it will hear something but will be unsure of the direction of the sound. If the dog is completely deaf it will simply not respond.

A vet will be able to carry out a technical procedure called a BAER test (see above) to find out if your dog is clinically deaf.

TREATMENT Although hearing aids have been developed for dogs, few dogs are willing to tolerate them.

BREEDS AT RISK

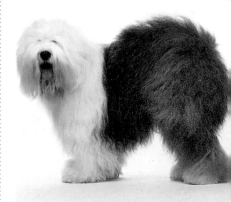

Over 30 breeds of dog are at risk from congenital deafness in one or both ears, with the highest incidence in Dalmatians. Predominantly white dogs, and dogs with merle coats, are particularly susceptible. Genetic evidence suggests that this form of deafness is associated with the colour of the coat and is linked with either the merle or the piebald gene.

Breeds with the merle gene include the Collie, Shetland Sheepdog, dappled Dachshund, American Foxhound, Old English Sheepdog, and Norwegian Dunker.

Breeds with the piebald gene include the Dalmatian, Beagle, Bulldog, Samoyed, Bull Terrier, English Setter, Greyhound, Sealyham Terrier, and Pyrenean Mountain Dog.

Breeds most likely to be affected by deafness

- Australian Shepherd Dog
- Border Collie
- Boxer
- Bull Terrier
- Collie
- Dalmatian
- English Setter
- Old English Sheepdog (above)
- Shetland Sheepdog

RESPIRATORY SYSTEM
how your dog breathes

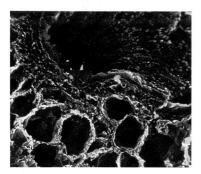

Air sacs in lung tissue

Every living cell in your dog's body needs a constant supply of oxygen to survive. Cells must also dispose of the metabolic waste product carbon dioxide. The job of the respiratory system, together with the circulatory system, is to deliver oxygen from the air inhaled into the lungs to all the body cells, and to remove carbon dioxide and return it to the lungs to be exhaled. This exchange of oxygen and carbon dioxide is very effective because the lungs have a vast surface area, containing millions of tiny air sacs, and a rich supply of blood.

Air that is inhaled passes through the respiratory tract, a series of branching, semi-flexible tubes, until it reaches the alveoli, where gas exchange occurs. The respiratory tract is divided into two parts. The upper respiratory tract consists of the nasal passages, throat, larynx (voice box), and trachea (windpipe). The lower tract consists of the bronchi (the two airways that branch from the trachea) and the lungs, which are soft, spongy organs surrounded by a double-layered membrane called the pleura.

Q WHY DO DOGS PANT AFTER EXERCISE?

A Breathing is controlled by the respiratory centre in a part of the brain known as the medulla. From there, messages travel down nerves to the diaphragm and rib muscles to make them contract and relax, enabling breathing. Nerve cells in the respiratory centre, and in the arteries, are sensitive to levels of carbon dioxide in the blood. A rise in carbon dioxide levels, which occurs when a dog is physically active, increases the breathing rate to return the level back to normal, causing panting.

UPPER RESPIRATORY TRACT

The nose has two functions. It is a dog's most sophisticated sensory organ, able to detect the faintest of odours. The part of the nose that smells (the olfactory portion) contains sensory cells. Cavities in the bones around the nose, called sinuses, help to improve the sense of smell. The nose also filters, warms, and moistens inhaled air before it passes into the throat.

The throat, or pharynx, is divided into upper and lower sectors: the upper nasopharynx (above the soft palate) and the lower oropharynx. The larynx contains the vocal cords, which vibrate with the passage of air to make sounds.

The trachea further moistens and warms air as it passes into the lungs. Horseshoe-shaped rings of cartilage encircle and support the structure, and bands of muscle allow the trachea to stretch during breathing.

LOWER RESPIRATORY TRACT

The trachea divides in two just before it reaches the lungs. Each resulting tube is called a bronchus. The bronchi further divide within each lung into smaller and smaller bronchioles, which terminate in tiny, bubble-like sacs called alveoli.

The lungs contain millions of alveoli, which are surrounded by a network of blood capillaries. The alveolar walls are only one cell thick; they enable oxygen and carbon dioxide to pass between the sacs and the bloodstream.

HOW BREATHING OCCURS

The ribs and muscles of the chest, along with the diaphragm (the dome-shaped sheet of muscle that separates the chest from the abdomen), act like bellows, rhythmically contracting to suck air into the lungs and relaxing to push air out. The rate at which these muscles contract and relax is controlled by a special respiratory centre in the brain.

DEFENCES

The respiratory tract has direct access to the outside world; for this reason, defensive mechanisms have evolved to protect it from damage by inhaled foreign particles. The respiratory tract is lined with microscopic, hair-like cilia that sweep mucus and debris from the airways. This "mucociliary escalator" can be damaged by infection, irritants, and inflammation. Coughing, gagging, and sneezing are natural reflexes that expel irritants from the airways. The bands of muscle in the trachea contract when the airway is irritated so that foreign particles are prevented from entering the delicate lungs.

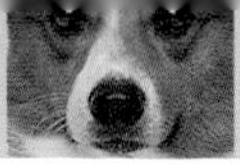

RESPIRATORY SYSTEM

The upper part of the respiratory system includes the nasal passages, the pharynx (throat), the larynx (voice box), and the main airway, called the trachea or windpipe. The trachea is a long tube supported by horseshoe-shaped rings of cartilage. This tube divides into the two bronchi, one bronchus entering each lung. The lungs are soft, spongy, elastic organs, each encased in a membrane called the pleura. Within the lungs, each bronchus divides many times into smaller bronchioles, which end in tiny air sacs called alveoli.

OXYGENATING THE BLOOD

In the alveoli, the air in the lungs meets the blood capillaries and exchange of oxygen and carbon dioxide occurs. Each alveolus is surrounded by many capillaries and by a very thin membrane so gas exchange can take place effectively.

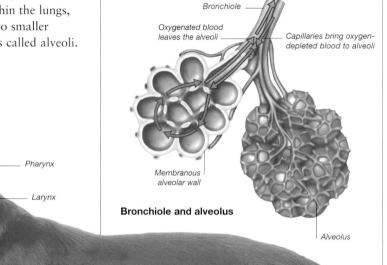

Bronchiole

Oxygenated blood leaves the alveoli

Capillaries bring oxygen-depleted blood to alveoli

Membranous alveolar wall

Bronchiole and alveolus

Alveolus

Nose

Pharynx

Larynx

Rings of cartilage

Trachea

Trachea divides into two bronchi

Lung

Heart

Diaphragm muscle

CONTROLLING BREATHING

When the diaphragm contracts and moves downwards, it expands the chest cavity and draws air into the lungs. When the muscle relaxes, it squeezes air out of the lungs.

DIAGNOSING RESPIRATORY DISORDERS

Problems may arise anywhere along the respiratory tract. Conditions affecting the upper part of the respiratory tract include foreign bodies in the nostrils (*see p.237*) or the throat (*see p.241*) and infections such as kennel cough (*see p.240*). Lower respiratory tract disorders include bronchitis, pneumonia, and accumulation of fluid in the chest cavity (*see p.242*).

Virtually all respiratory disorders cause changes in an affected dog's breathing pattern. Unusual breathing is often the first sign of a respiratory problem and therefore may be an important diagnostic clue.

MONITORING BREATHING

Your dog takes breaths between 10 and 30 times a minute. The normal breathing rate is dependent on size, being slower in large individuals and faster in smaller ones. You need to become accustomed to your dog's usual breathing pattern, including the normal sounds that the dog makes as

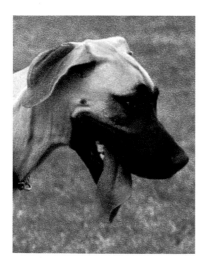

HEALTHY PANTING
Dogs lose more of their body heat through their mouths than we do. It is normal for them to pant after exertion or in hot weather.

it breathes in and out. This knowledge will make it easier for you to detect any changes from the normal pattern. (*See also pp.402–05.*)

RAPID BREATHING

Like humans, dogs breathe faster after exercise. They may also pant in hot weather and when excited or nervous. Rapid breathing also occurs, however, in dangerous conditions such as shock, poisoning, or heatstroke. Contact your veterinary surgeon immediately if your dog's breathing rate has suddenly increased for no obvious reason.

SHALLOW BREATHING

This sign means that something is interfering with the normal expansion and contraction of the chest. A dog with shallow breathing compensates by breathing more rapidly. Pain (for example, from bruising or damage to the ribs) can cause this problem. If your dog has developed shallow breathing, and particularly if it has suffered an injury, contact your vet immediately.

VET'S ADVICE

Do not mistake normal panting for laboured breathing. Panting, which is shallow, rapid, open-mouthed breathing, is not a medical problem; it is what hot, nervous, excited, or exhausted dogs do. Vigorous exercise will induce panting. Do contact your vet, however, if your dog starts panting for no apparent reason. Pain sometimes causes a dog to pant, as can drugs such as corticosteroids. One indicator of whether panting is healthy is the colour of the tongue: a pink tongue indicates plenty of oxygen in the blood.

LABOURED BREATHING

Difficulty breathing is always a cause for concern. Possible causes include heart failure (*see p.250*), lung disease or a build-up of fluid in the chest (*see p.242*), trauma such as a torn diaphragm (*see p.244*), and tumours. Contact your vet immediately.

NOISY BREATHING, WHEEZING, AND COUGHING

Any change in a dog's breathing sounds is significant. Possible causes include obstructions in the upper respiratory tract and paralysis of the vocal folds. Contact your veterinary surgeon if your dog develops noisy breathing.

Wheezing is not as common in dogs as it is in people. When it does occur, it usually indicates a problem affecting the lungs, or inflammation of the bronchi (*see p.242*) caused by allergy, irritation, or infection. Wheezing dogs should receive veterinary attention within 24 hours.

Coughing indicates irritation in the respiratory tract. During coughing, the trachea contracts by about one-sixth of its normal size, forcing air out at high speed to dislodge any foreign matter from the airways. A dog that is coughing persistently should be taken to see a vet within 24 hours.

DIAGNOSTIC METHODS

There are various techniques that your vet can use to find out what is causing your dog's breathing problems.

PHYSICAL EXAMINATION

Depending on the clinical signs, the vet may check inside the dog's mouth or nostrils for any foreign objects, feel the chest and ribcage, and listen to the lungs using a stethoscope. The vet may also take the dog's temperature; a raised temperature may indicate a respiratory tract infection.

IMAGING TECHNIQUES

X-rays are often used to detect foreign bodies in the airways, and also to look for structural abnormalities of the respiratory tract, fluid build-up in the lungs, or tumours in the lung tissue.

BACTERIAL CULTURE

The vet may take a swab of nasal discharge or of fluids from the throat to make a culture, which will reveal the organisms responsible for infection.

STOOL ANALYSIS

A stool sample will be analysed if a parasitic infestation is suspected to be the cause of lung damage. Worm eggs can be seen in the stools.

BRONCHOSCOPY

A bronchoscope is an instrument used to look inside the trachea and the bronchi and to collect tissue samples for examination under the microscope.

TRACHEAL WASH

Also called lavage, this procedure is a method of obtaining cells and other material from the inside of the dog's trachea for analysis. A tracheal wash is generally performed in conjunction with bronchoscopy.

The dog is first anaesthetized and a needle is inserted through the throat. Saline fluid is then flushed through the needle into the trachea. This small amount of fluid is withdrawn into a syringe, and the cells that it now contains are examined by a specialist called a cytologist. Other portions of the fluid sample are retained for bacterial culture (*see above*).

The material collected from the dog's trachea may be examined under a microscope or may be cultured for microorganisms, depending on the nature of the symptoms.

ALLERGY TESTS

Although allergies in dogs, even those that are due to inhaled substances, are more likely to show up as a skin complaint, they can also manifest themselves in the form of respiratory symptoms (*see p.124*).

Procedures such as intradermal skin tests or ELISA tests (*see p.181*) may be carried out if a dog's breathing problems are thought to be due to an allergy to a particular substance.

DISTINGUISHING CHOKING AND GAGGING

Although these two conditions may look similar, they have different causes. A dog that is choking has something stuck in its windpipe that is interfering with breathing and needs to be removed urgently. Choking is potentially life-threatening. A dog that is gagging has something stuck or irritating in its mouth or in the top of its throat and is in more discomfort than immediate danger.

CHOKING	GAGGING
• Choking sounds	• Pawing at the mouth
• Severe distress	• Mild distress
• Difficulty breathing	• No breathing difficulties
• Loss of consciousness	• Rubbing the face on the ground
• Bulging eyes	• Unpleasant breath
• Blue tongue	• Spasms of the throat

Seek urgent veterinary treatment and take first-aid measures (*see box, right*).

Look for object stuck in the mouth and remove it (*see box, right*).

Q WHAT IS THE BEST WAY TO REMOVE AN OBJECT SAFELY FROM A DOG'S MOUTH?

A If your dog has something stuck in its mouth and is gagging, restrain it, without using a muzzle. Then open the mouth, with one hand grasping the upper jaw and pressing the upper lips over the teeth and the other hand holding open the lower jaw. Look at the roof of the mouth, the back of the throat, and around the teeth to locate the object. Use a spoon handle, or similar implement, to remove it gently. Try to do this as quickly and firmly as possible to reduce the risk of being bitten.

Q WHAT SHOULD I DO IF MY DOG IS CHOKING?

A First, distinguish choking from gagging (*see box, left*). Choking is an emergency, needing your immediate treatment. If your dog is conscious, put your arms around the dog's belly, make a fist, and squeeze firmly upwards and forwards just behind the ribcage. For a small dog, place your hands on either side of the animal's belly and then squeeze the body firmly upwards and forwards.

If the dog has lost consciousness, place it on its side. Put the heels of both your hands just behind the dog's back ribs. Press sharply to expel the blockage. Use your finger to remove debris from the mouth. Give artificial respiration and cardiopulmonary resuscitation if necessary (*see p.389*).

Never give cough medicine to a dog that is gagging or choking, because it may prevent expulsion of the foreign object and make the problem worse.

Q MY DOG ALWAYS SEEMS TO HAVE A DRIPPY NOSE. SHOULD I BE WORRIED?

A Some dogs have naturally drippy noses. Drip without sneezing, particularly if the fluid is clear and watery, usually occurs when the individual is nervous or excited but may also occur even when a dog is asleep. This drip is a normal condition, not a problem. An abnormal nasal discharge (which may be cloudy or profuse), accompanied by sneezing, can be caused by minor conditions such as hay fever or by more serious problems such as nasal tumours. (Remember, sneezing itself is not an illness, but a reflex action to rid the nasal passages of irritants.) Persistent or severe sneezing along with a drippy nose may indicate a disorder, and should be investigated by a veterinary surgeon.

Q WHAT IS THE BEST WAY TO STOP A NOSEBLEED?

A Keep your dog quiet and confined. Apply a cold compress (in an emergency, you could use a bag of frozen peas) for about five minutes to the top of the nose, between the eyes and nostrils. Cover the bleeding nostril with absorbent material. Do as little as possible, and try to calm and soothe your dog if it is distressed.

If the bleeding does not stop within a few minutes, and especially if the cause of the nosebleed is unknown, contact your veterinary surgeon as soon as possible. Do not muzzle your dog or tilt its head back to prevent blood from dripping out of the nostrils. In addition, do not attempt to pack the bleeding nostril with anything such as cotton wool or gauze because this action is very likely to stimulate sneezing.

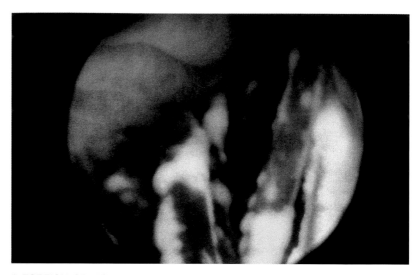

A FOREIGN OBJECT BLOCKING A NOSTRIL
Blockage of a nostril by a foreign object can interfere with breathing. It may also cause local pain and inflammation and a nasal discharge or bleeding. Vegetation inhaled by sniffing is a common external cause of nasal blockage.

NASAL CONDITIONS

The nose leather (exterior of the nose), a specialized part of the skin, can be affected by a variety of conditions (*see pp.196–97*). The nose is also the port of entry to the respiratory system. Problems with the nostrils can interfere with the dog's breathing.

ALLERGIC RHINITIS
Overwhelmingly, the most common cause of abnormal nasal discharge is allergy (*see p.124*). Nasal irritation due to an allergy is called allergic rhinitis. This condition may occur in response to a variety of substances, but grass seeds and pollens are a common cause of allergy; the resulting condition is known as hay fever.

Allergic rhinitis produces a clear nasal discharge, often accompanied by sneezing and runny, itchy eyes.
DIAGNOSIS AND TREATMENT Avoiding whatever causes the allergic nasal discharge is the treatment of choice, but it is often extremely difficult to determine the cause or, once the problem has been identified, to avoid

it. Allergy tests such as ELISA (*see p.181*) may be performed. Allergic rhinitis is usually treated with antihistamine drugs.

INFECTION OF THE NASAL CAVITY AND SINUSES
A bacterial, viral, or fungal infection of the nasal cavity eventually produces a nasal discharge of mucus or pus. If the infection spreads from the nasal cavity into the facial sinuses, a condition called sinusitis ensues. Infection involving the sinuses causes a nasal discharge into the back of the throat: so-called "post-nasal drip". Affected dogs may gag or retch. There may be an accompanying foul odour.
DIAGNOSIS AND TREATMENT A culture and sensitivity test of the discharge is performed to identify the type of microorganisms involved.

Bacterial nasal discharge is treated with a broad-spectrum antibiotic, usually for at least two weeks, while fungal infections are treated with oral antifungal medication for several months. Chronic infection, especially if it involves the sinuses, is often difficult to treat. In some severe cases, the nasal cavity or the affected sinus is opened surgically so that the area can be thoroughly cleansed.

FOREIGN OBJECTS

Discharge from one nostril only usually shows there is something stuck in that nostril. Blades of grass and grass seeds are the most common foreign bodies found in the nostrils, but anything small enough to be sucked in through sniffing may cause a problem.

A foreign object in a nostril usually causes a sudden paroxysm of sneezing and pawing at the nose. The affected nostril may also bleed.

DIAGNOSIS X-rays and scans are sometimes necessary to determine the cause of a discharge. An endoscope may be used to look for a foreign object.

TREATMENT If you can see something protruding from your dog's nostril, such as a blade of grass, carefully remove it with tweezers. If you cannot remove the object yourself, contact your vet immediately. The vet may need to sedate or anaesthetize the dog before attempting to extract the foreign object. Antibiotics may be prescribed to prevent infection.

POLYPS AND TUMOURS

These growths can develop inside the nostrils. A polyp is an enlargement of a nasal mucus-producing gland and is not cancerous. Most nasal tumours, on the other hand, are cancerous, and tend to be fast-growing.

Both polyps and tumours cause a discharge or bleeding from the nostril, accompanied by noisy breathing. A tumour may also result in a bulge on the affected side of the nose and obstruction to the airflow.

DIAGNOSIS X-rays and endoscopy may be used to look for an abnormal growth. A sample of tissue is usually taken from a tumour and examined to determine whether it is cancerous.

TREATMENT Polyps are surgically removed, although these growths have a tendency to recur, requiring further treatment. All tumours, whether they are cancerous or not, are surgically removed. If a tumour is found to be cancerous, radiotherapy may also be given (*see p.133*).

CLEFT PALATE AND ORAL-NASAL FISTULA

A pup that sneezes or has a nasal discharge after eating may have a cleft palate, a defect in which the two sides of the palate have not fused by birth, leaving an open passageway between the mouth and the nasal cavity.

Older dogs with severe tooth decay (*see p.263*) may also develop an oral-nasal fistula (a channel joining the mouth and nasal cavity) when one of the upper canine teeth or premolars is lost through infection, injury, or surgery.

TREATMENT For both cleft palate and oral-nasal fistula, the abnormal channel is surgically reduced.

NOSEBLEED

Nosebleeds are often accompanied by sneezing in a "chicken or egg" fashion. Which comes first? Intense sneezing may cause a nosebleed, while a bleeding nose certainly stimulates sneezing.

The possible causes of nosebleeds include a foreign object in a nostril; paroxysmal or violent sneezing from hay fever; bacterial, fungal, or viral infection causing inflammation of the nasal membranes; nasal polyps or tumours, especially in older dogs; blood clotting disorders such as von Willebrand's disease (*see p.258*); and rodent bait (warfarin) poisoning.

DIAGNOSIS AND TREATMENT If bleeding is persistent or occurs without any obvious cause, contact your vet. The vet will examine the dog to check for foreign objects in the nostril, or may take a swab of the discharge if an infection is suspected.

Most nosebleeds clear up after a few minutes when a cold compress is applied (*see opposite*), or when the cause of the nosebleed is treated.

BREEDS AT RISK

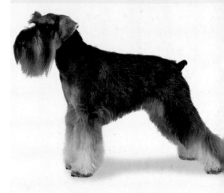

Breeds most prone to inherited cleft palate include:

- Beagle
- Boston Terrier
- Bulldog
- Cocker Spaniel
- Miniature Schnauzer (above)
- Pekingese

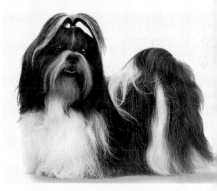

Small nostrils are a particular problem in brachycephalic (flat-faced) and moderately flat-faced breeds such as:

- Boston Terrier
- Bulldog
- Cavalier King Charles Spaniel
- Chow Chow
- Pekingese
- Pug
- Shih Tzu (above)

SMALL NOSTRILS

Some pups, most commonly those belonging to flat-faced breeds, are born with narrow nostrils (a condition called stenotic nares). This problem makes breathing difficult. Other pups have moderately wide nostrils but the nasal cartilage is soft and floppy, and, as a result, the nostrils collapse as the affected pup breathes in.

The degree of severity varies from mild, producing few signs, to severe, causing affected pups to breathe noisily or breathe through their mouths and possibly to have a nasal discharge. Severely affected pups fail to thrive and are poorly developed.

TREATMENT When necessary, small nostrils are enlarged by removing a wedge of nasal skin and cartilage. When possible, a decision to operate is postponed until a dog is physically mature. Some flat-faced pups outgrow their anatomical defects.

THROAT CONDITIONS

Pharyngitis (inflammation of the pharynx), usually caused by infection, affects a dog's ability, although not necessarily its desire, to eat. In addition, foreign objects such as bones or toys can become lodged in the pharynx, causing retching and gagging.

Conditions involving the larynx and the trachea generally cause a change of voice quality, coughing, or gagging. Anything that blocks the larynx or the trachea causes choking.

LARYNGEAL INFLAMMATION

The inside of the larynx is lined with a mucous membrane; however, unlike that of the trachea, the membrane does not contain cilia (the protective, hair-like structures that remove mucus and debris). Any condition that increases mucus production in this area will cause a dog to "clear its throat" in an attempt to remove debris. This action may lead to laryngitis (inflammation of the laryngeal tissue). Laryngitis may also be caused by excessive barking or infection. It causes a hoarse change of voice or even the loss of barking sounds. **DIAGNOSIS AND TREATMENT** Diagnosis is by the clinical signs and inspection of the throat. Laryngitis is treated by removing the cause of barking and retraining the dog, or treating the cause of coughing.

LARYNGEAL PARALYSIS

This is an unusual condition mainly affecting older dogs, especially Labrador Retrievers. In Bouviers des Flandres, Bull Terriers, Dalmatians, and Siberian Huskies, the condition is thought to be hereditary. In retrievers and setters, the cause is unknown. Dogs with laryngeal paralysis develop a progressively weak bark, leading to a harsh noise as a dog inhales. Eventually, breathing becomes laboured and difficult, particularly in hot weather. An affected individual has reduced capacity for exercise and may collapse in a faint on exertion. The paralysis may lead to laryngeal oedema (swelling of the larynx). **DIAGNOSIS AND TREATMENT** Paralysis is usually diagnosed with an endoscopic examination. Surgical procedures have been developed for correcting laryngeal paralysis, but all have serious post-surgical drawbacks, including food getting into the respiratory tract.

DEBARKING

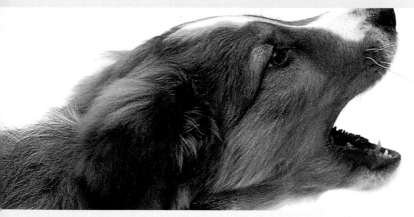

Debarking is a surgical operation that is carried out more frequently in some countries than in others. In this procedure, the fold of tissue on each side of a dog's larynx (voice box), which naturally becomes tightened when the dog barks, is removed. The operation leaves the dog with a quiet, "whispery" bark. Complications after this type of surgery are common, and can be life-threatening; for example, scar tissue that forms in the larynx can block the airway, causing breathing difficulties and pain. Even after debarking, the bark may return after several months. Debarking is inhumane because it deprives a dog of one of its natural means of communicating with people and with other dogs. Dogs are supposed to bark when something is wrong. Excessive barking may be a problem, but it is usually a problem with the environment, not the dog. A dog that barks constantly may be badly socialized or trained, stressed, lonely, fearful, or frustrated. In these cases, it is essential to deal with the cause of the problem, not simply to suppress the symptom by surgically "turning the volume down". There are several effective training techniques that, with some effort and patience, will discourage a dog from barking excessively.

USING CHOKE CHAINS SAFELY

A full choke chain is commonly used as a safety device to prevent a dog from slipping its collar. It should never be used simply to control a dog's behaviour, however, because it may cause compression of the windpipe, especially in small breeds such as the Yorkshire Terrier. If using a choke chain, make sure that you use it correctly, so that it releases instantly after pulling. If put on "backwards", it can lock in a way that constricts the neck. Dogs should, ideally, be controlled by good training, rather than just by a collar.

GOOD PRACTICE

Full choke chains must be used with care. When other means of control are not appropriate, a half-choke collar can be used. This type of collar does not carry as much risk of damage to the larynx as a full choke chain.

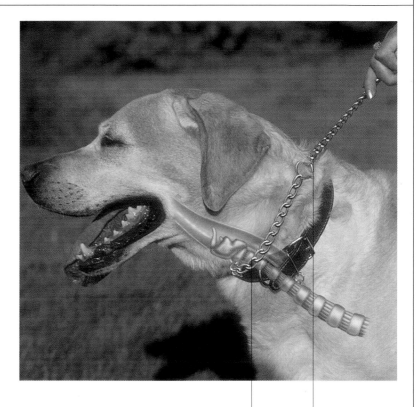

Compression of the larynx | Choke chain

LARYNGEAL OEDEMA

Laryngeal oedema, or swelling of the larynx, is most commonly caused by heatstroke (*see p.408*) or an allergic (anaphylactic) reaction to an insect bite (*see p.427*). It may also be caused by laryngeal paralysis. Laryngeal oedema is a life-threatening condition. The clinical signs include difficult, rapid, laboured breathing, cyanosis (blue gums), and collapse.

DIAGNOSIS AND TREATMENT Laryngeal oedema requires urgent treatment, using corticosteroids to reduce the swelling. Adrenaline may be given in the case of an allergic reaction. Antihistamines may relieve the clinical signs. Surgery to make a temporary opening in the trachea may be needed.

LARYNGEAL TUMOUR

This uncommon condition causes coughing, laboured breathing, a swelling in the larynx that may be felt through the skin, and a change or loss of voice. Malignant squamous cell carcinoma (*see p.136*) is the most common type of laryngeal tumour.

DIAGNOSIS AND TREATMENT Tumours are usually diagnosed by endoscopic examination and tissue sampling. All tumours, cancerous or not, are removed. Surgery leaves a permanent opening in the trachea, called a tracheostomy, which requires special care.

REVERSE SNEEZING

This curious condition, also called laryngospasm, is fairly common in

small breeds, particularly in Yorkshire Terriers. The dog snorts inwards in a sometimes violent paroxysm that may last for up to a minute.

The exact cause of reverse sneezing is unknown. The problem often occurs whenever a dog becomes excited – for example, when the owner returns home. Episodes of reverse sneezing may be frequent but they are never prolonged. After an episode, the dog behaves completely normally.

No treatment is usually needed, although massaging from the larynx forwards may shorten an episode. If your dog has an attack of reverse sneezing and collapses, see your vet to ensure that there is not a foreign object obstructing the larynx.

ELONGATED SOFT PALATE

The soft palate extends backwards from the hard palate (at the roof of the mouth). This area of soft tissue closes off the back of the nasal cavity during swallowing. Some dogs of flat-faced breeds have elongated soft palates that interfere with breathing. Others are prone to the structural defect of small nostrils (*see p.238*). Some have both.

Although this condition is called an "elongated" soft palate, the problem is in fact due to a normal soft palate in a "truncated" face. The soft palate in flat-faced dogs is just as long as that in other dogs of the same size and weight. The compression of the face, however, produces compression of the soft palate, causing it to hang down, sometimes touching or even obstructing the cartilage of the larynx.

This defect leads to gagging or retching, and snoring when the dog is relaxed or sleeping. The intensity and frequency of snoring increases with age. The condition worsens over time, as the soft palate tissue loses its elasticity. More severely affected dogs may snort, gag, or even faint, especially on exertion. In addition, an elongated soft palate predisposes to inflammation of the throat and tonsils.

TREATMENT An elongated soft palate that is causing breathing difficulties is shortened surgically. If possible, the operation is postponed until the dog is physically mature, because some flat-faced pups outgrow their anatomical defects. In breeds such as the Bulldog, Pekingese, and Pug, an operation in which the nasal openings are enlarged to improve the breathing may be performed at the same time.

COUGH

Coughing is a defence mechanism that naturally removes unwanted material from the air passages. The mechanism is also triggered by damage or irritation to the lining of the airways. Coughing may be brought on by various causes, including pressure from collars, allergy, pollution, poisons, infections, worms (*see pp.168–71*), heart conditions, lung diseases, injuries, respiratory tract tumours, or a collapsing trachea.

DIAGNOSIS AND TREATMENT A dog with a severe or persistent cough should be seen by a vet. The type of cough often suggests the diagnosis; for example, a deep, dry, hacking cough suggests infection of the throat or trachea; a spasm of prolonged coughing when the dog is lying down may indicate heart disease; a "goose-honk" cough is likely to be caused by a collapsing trachea. Diagnosis may also require X-rays, analysis of a stool sample for worm eggs, and bronchoscopy and/or tracheal wash, especially if mucus or blood is expelled with the cough.

Treatment is given for the cause of the cough. Short-term medications for severe cough include expectorants and cough suppressants.

KENNEL COUGH

Kennel cough or canine cough are popular names given to a variety of infections that cause damage to the larynx, trachea, and bronchi. These

DAMAGE TO CILIA IN THE WINDPIPE

Kennel cough damages the cilia – the tiny, hair-like structures that line the trachea (windpipe) and normally sweep mucus and debris out of the respiratory tract. In a dog with kennel cough, the cilia appear stunted or "clubbed", and they are no longer able to carry out their function properly. As a result, foreign particles and excess mucus irritate the trachea, causing coughing and inflammation of the tracheal lining.

FUNCTION OF THE CILIA
The cilia are extensions of the cells that line the trachea. They move in a coordinated and forceful wave-like motion (called the mucociliary escalator) to remove excess mucus and inhaled matter from the trachea.

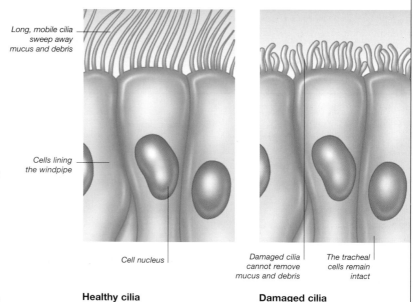

Long, mobile cilia sweep away mucus and debris

Cells lining the windpipe

Cell nucleus

Healthy cilia

Damaged cilia cannot remove mucus and debris

The tracheal cells remain intact

Damaged cilia

diseases include infection with the bacterium *Bordetella bronchiseptica* and infection with a variety of viruses, including parainfluenza and adenovirus types CAV-1 and CAV-2 (*see p.148*). Other infections that damage the trachea and bronchi include distemper (*see p.147*) and mycoplasma (*see p.143*).

An affected dog is bright and alert but has a harsh, dry, non-productive cough. Pinching the dog's windpipe triggers a cough.

Puppies, small dogs prone to tracheal collapse, individuals suffering from chronic bronchitis, and those with reduced immunity are susceptible to secondary bacterial infection in the lungs (*see p.242*). This is a serious complication. Affected dogs have a fever, are lethargic, and may be uninterested in food. If pneumonia develops, the cough becomes more moist-sounding. There may also be wheezing and rapid breathing.

DIAGNOSIS AND TREATMENT For details of diagnosis and treatment, refer to Infectious diseases (*see pp.142–57*).

COLLAPSING TRACHEA

Tracheal collapse is the result of an anatomical defect in toy breeds, particularly the Yorkshire Terrier but also the Chihuahua, Pomeranian, and Toy Poodle, which becomes evident with increasing age. The normally rigid structure of the trachea becomes weakened and prone to collapse on internal or external pressure.

An affected dog coughs like a honking goose. Coughing is triggered by excitement or physical activity. It is more likely to occur in overweight individuals or in those suffering from respiratory conditions such as chronic bronchitis (*see p.242*).

DIAGNOSIS Your vet will first eliminate other possible causes of the coughing, such as heart disease. A collapsing trachea is confirmed by X-rays.

TREATMENT Treatments vary depending on the severity of the condition. Weight loss is important if excess weight has contributed to the problem. Training to reduce excited behaviour, or mild sedation, may be recommended to prevent the condition from worsening. Drugs such as bronchodilators, cough suppressants, and corticosteroids may be given to suppress coughing and reduce secretions. Antibiotics may also be given to prevent infection. In addition, eliminating any pollutants, such as cigarette smoke, from the dog's environment may be helpful. In some cases, surgery to insert a tubular support for the collapsed trachea is performed, but this is only practical for the section of the trachea situated in the neck, not for the section in the chest cavity.

OBSTRUCTIONS IN THE TRACHEA

Anything that obstructs the trachea causes choking. Small objects that are ingested and become stuck in the back of the throat are a common cause of choking. Another cause is an allergic reaction to an insect bite or sting in the mouth that causes the tongue to swell.

Q DO DOGS GET COLDS LIKE HUMANS?

A Dogs cannot catch human common cold viruses. They do, however, suffer from canine infections of the upper respiratory system, which cause sneezing and coughing. These infections include the group commonly called "kennel cough" as well as the more serious distemper virus. If your dog has a runny nose and is coughing persistently, contact your vet.

Q WHEN IS A COUGH A CAUSE FOR CONCERN?

A Coughing is a natural reflex response to clear the airways of excess mucus and debris. It is a cause for concern only if it is severe or persistent, or if it sounds unusual (for example, a honking cough may suggest tracheal collapse).

VET'S ADVICE

Dogs, especially pups, chew things as a natural means of investigation, to relieve boredom, to exercise the teeth and gums, or simply for the fun of it. Never leave small chewable articles in places where dogs can find them. Pups, in particular, may swallow small objects and are at risk of choking on them.

Never use small balls in retrieving games with your dog. A golf ball, for example, may easily lodge in the back of the throat, obstructing the trachea. Even larger balls, such as tennis balls, may be potentially dangerous for some dogs.

Dogs naturally need to chew. Ensure that they have chew-toys that are durable or digestible.

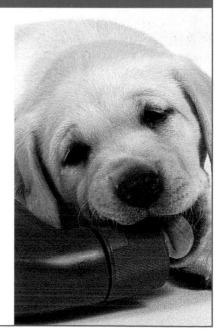

Q DO DOGS SUFFER FROM ASTHMA?

A Asthma is an allergic reaction in the lungs that causes narrowing of the smaller airways, which makes it difficult to breathe out. While it is common in humans and fairly common in cats, asthma is very rare in dogs. There are, however, other conditions that dogs can develop that cause wheezing and lung congestion.

Q WHAT IS THE OUTLOOK FOR A DOG WITH PNEUMONIA?

A Bacterial and parasitic forms of pneumonia respond well to immediate treatment with antibiotic and antiparasitic drugs. Viral (distemper) pneumonia is more serious, due to damage in other areas of the body, and has a poorer outlook. Systemic fungal pneumonia must be treated very aggressively, but even with treatment the outlook is only fair. Aspiration pneumonia usually responds to antibiotics and symptomatic care. In all instances of pneumonia, full recovery takes many weeks or months.

Q IS A COLLAPSED LUNG PAINFUL?

A Yes, it is. While a build-up of air in the chest cavity may occur spontaneously in some dogs, it is more likely to be due to trauma such as a road traffic accident, gunshot injury, or even falling from a window. Regardless of the cause, part of your vet's initial routine treatment for a collapsed lung is pain control. A narcotic such as morphine or pethidine may be used.

FLUID IN THE LUNGS

A build-up of fluid within the lungs is called pulmonary oedema. This condition is usually caused by failure of the left side of the heart (see p.250). Other possible causes include trauma to the head, near-drowning, inhalation of smoke or chemical fumes, and some forms of poisoning. An affected dog has a moist cough.

DIAGNOSIS AND TREATMENT Pulmonary oedema is usually diagnosed from the clinical signs and an examination. Imaging techniques may be performed to confirm the diagnosis in some cases. Treatment with diuretics and other medications eliminates the fluid in the lungs and associated coughing.

COLLAPSED LUNG

Any chest trauma that results in a penetrating injury to the chest wall, from a dog bite to a bullet, will allow air to enter the chest cavity. Air may also enter the cavity from the lungs if there is lung damage from trauma or disease. In either instance, the lung collapses. The dog will gasp for breath. The condition is life-threatening.

DIAGNOSIS AND TREATMENT A collapsed lung is suspected when there is known chest trauma. X-rays will confirm the diagnosis. Treatment usually involves surgical repair of the trauma, during which the surgeon reinflates the lungs to fill the chest cavity. In other cases with no obvious penetrating injury, the vet reinflates the lungs by removing air from the surrounding pleural cavity.

RUPTURED DIAPHRAGM

The diaphragm is the dome-shaped sheet of muscle that separates the chest and abdominal cavities. The muscle may easily be torn, especially in road traffic accidents and in falls.

Although there may be no visible external injuries, the rupture causes a loss of negative pressure in the chest cavity and immediate lung collapse, which may be life-threatening. Affected dogs suffer from severely laboured breathing. In some instances, a lobe of liver slips through the tear, sealing the

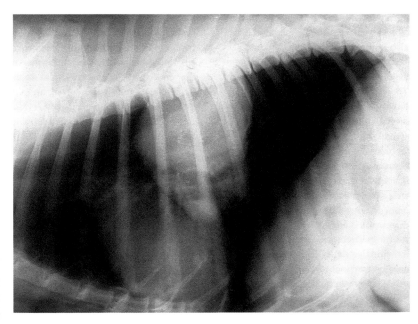

LUNG TUMOUR
This X-ray shows the chest and abdomen of a Golden Retriever that has lung cancer. The rounded white mass is a tumour in one of the lungs.

wound; when this happens, breathing difficulties may be less dramatic.

TREATMENT A ruptured diaphragm is surgically repaired through an incision in the abdominal wall.

LUNG TUMOURS

Almost all tumours of the lungs are cancerous. Primary lung tumours (those that originate in the lung tissue) are uncommon in dogs, perhaps because they do not smoke. On the other hand, secondary, or metastatic, lung cancers (those that have spread to the lungs from cancers originating in other parts of the body, such as the breast, bone, thyroid gland, or skin), are not unusual (*see pp.130–41*). Both primary and secondary lung cancers mainly affect older individuals.

A lung tumour tends to produce vague signs – usually only a non-productive cough that develops from soft to harsh. There may be reduced tolerance of exercise. In advanced cases, fluid may accumulate in the chest cavity (*see p.243*), leading to increasingly laboured breathing.

DIAGNOSIS AND TREATMENT Chest X-rays are used to diagnose a lung tumour, and a tissue sample from the growth may be taken endoscopically to confirm the diagnosis. Almost all lung tumours are cancerous and occur in older individuals; for these reasons, surgery is rarely an option. For similar reasons, aggressive chemotherapy is not often a viable option. Palliative therapy to ensure comfort is usually the most that can be done. The outlook for a dog with lung cancer is poor.

ALLERGIC LUNG DISEASE

An allergic lung disease may be due to a reaction to an inhaled substance such as grass seeds (*see p.124*). In addition, the heartworm *Dirofilaria immitis* (*see p.254*) may cause a lung condition called allergic pneumonitis, in which the lung tissue becomes inflamed and fluid accumulates in the alveoli (the tiny air sacs within the lungs).

PARASITES

A variety of worms that live in the respiratory tract, or that migrate to the airways from other areas of the body, can cause damage to the lungs. These parasites include roundworms, whipworms, hookworms (right), and lungworms (*see p.171*). Dogs with heavy infestations of these worms may develop a dry cough, lose weight, and show reluctance to exercise and shortness of breath. Another lung parasite is the lung fluke *Paragonimus kellicotti*, which is found on the east coast of North America and usually contracted by eating crayfish or aquatic snails. The flukes produce cysts in the lung tissue. All of these types of parasite can be diagnosed from stool samples or from tracheal washes. Wormers such as fenbendazole are given to eliminate the parasites. Treatment is usually effective within a few days.

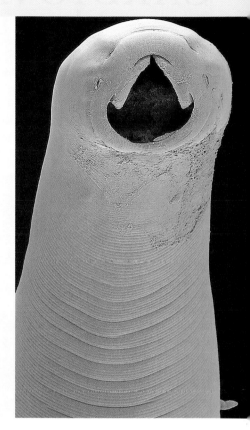

Dogs with allergic lung disease have a cough, breathe rapidly, and may develop a fever and lose weight. In severe cases, excitement may lead to laboured breathing and even collapse.

DIAGNOSIS A tracheal wash will reveal large numbers of eosinophils, a class of white blood cells that increase in number during an allergic reaction. Large numbers of eosinophils will also be seen in a blood sample. These blood cells also multiply in the presence of parasites, so a stool sample may be examined to check for worms.

TREATMENT Affected dogs are given corticosteroid drugs, the dose being gradually reduced over three to four weeks. Relapses are not uncommon, requiring a further course of treatment. If worms are present, additional treatment with wormers is necessary.

VET'S ADVICE

Parasite-triggered respiratory conditions are most common in young pups. The pup inherits worms from its mother. If there is a heavy load and the worms are not treated with effective anthelmintic drugs, they migrate through lung tissue and may cause conditions ranging from mild bronchitis to severe or life-threatening pneumonia. This problem is completely avoidable. Worm pups with an effective drug that destroys all stages in the worm's life cycle, including the migratory larval stage that moves through the lungs.

INVESTIGATION AND TREATMENT

The signs of canine cardiovascular or blood disorders are usually quite vague. The most common sign is increasing lethargy and an associated inability to perform normal activities, such as jumping, as well as before. Coughing or fainting are more obvious signs of a problem. Heart disease is often first diagnosed as an incidental finding when an affected dog has an annual health check-up.

DIAGNOSTIC AIDS

Your vet will use some of the following to help make an accurate diagnosis of your dog's heart condition.

STETHOSCOPE

The simplest and still most valuable diagnostic tool, the stethoscope is a flexible rubber tube with a sound-detecting device at one end and a pair of earpieces at the other. With a good stethoscope, your vet listens to the rate and rhythm of heart beats and hears the distinctive sounds made as the heart valves open and close during the pumping cycle. Electronic stethoscopes magnify or clarify heart sounds.

BLOOD PRESSURE MEASUREMENT

The measurement of blood pressure is under-used as a diagnostic tool in veterinary medicine. Once a dog's normal resting blood pressure has been established, the subsequent finding of a raised or lowered blood pressure can be a vital diagnostic aid.

In comparison to people, dogs do not have as many suitably round body parts where a blood pressure cuff can be wrapped. The tail is usually the best location. Blood pressure is measured in millimetres of mercury (mmHg). It is recorded at systole, when the ventricles of the heart are contracting and the pressure is at its highest, and diastole,

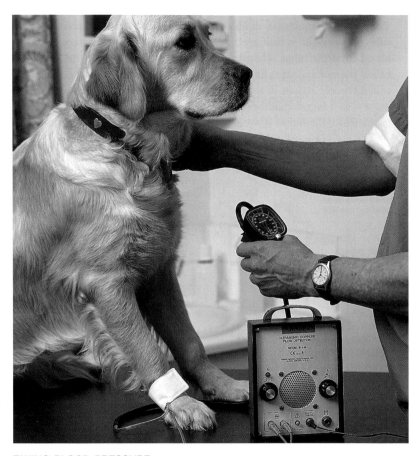

TAKING BLOOD PRESSURE
This Golden Retriever is having its blood pressure taken with the cuff wrapped around its foreleg. This positioning is a viable alternative to wrapping the cuff around the tail.

BLOOD PRESSURE

In contrast to humans, normal blood pressure in a dog depends on breed. Differences between breeds can be dramatic. Sight hounds have normally high resting blood pressure, while giant breeds average much less.

BREED GROUP	TYPICAL RESTING BLOOD PRESSURE
Sight hounds	147 mmHg (systole) over 76 mmHg (diastole)
Toy breeds	134 mmHg (systole) over 75 mmHg (diastole)
Giant breeds	121 mmHg (systole) over 67 mmHg (diastole)

when the ventricles are relaxing and refilling and pressure is lowest. The result is expressed as "X" mmHg (systole) over "Y" mmHg (diastole).

ELECTROCARDIOGRAPHY

Electrocardiography (ECG) has dramatically improved the rapid and accurate diagnosis of heart disease. ECG effectively measures electrical changes in the heart. Interpreting an ECG reading gives your vet a good three-dimensional understanding of pacemaker, valve, and muscle changes.

IMAGING TECHNIQUES

X-rays are excellent for showing heart enlargements, while echocardiography (ultrasound imaging of the heart) can visualize the inside of the heart. Using an echocardiogram, your vet can watch the heart valves work and can see the thickness of the muscular wall.

BLOOD TESTS

Blood tests tell your vet whether a dog is anaemic (a cause of an audible heart murmur) or whether the kidneys may be failing due to inadequate output from the heart. A bacterial culture of blood can reveal any microbes responsible for heart valve infection. In areas where heartworm disease is endemic, blood tests for microfilariae (one form of the heartworm parasite) may be performed before preventative treatment begins.

TREATMENT

The treatment of canine heart diseases is based mainly on medication. A wide variety of drugs originally developed to treat human heart conditions can also be used in dogs. These medications include drugs to lower blood pressure and drugs to aid the heart's pumping action. The drugs are classified into various groups, such as beta blockers, calcium channel blockers, ACE inhibitors, and diuretics. The ACE inhibitors are a particularly useful group that reduce blood pressure and ease the workload of the heart by widening blood vessels.

There are no surgical treatments for the most common forms of canine heart disease. Some rare conditions, however, can be treated in large dogs through the surgical implantation of an artificial pacemaker.

Q WHAT IS THE DIFFERENCE BETWEEN HEART DISEASE AND HEART FAILURE?

A A heart disease is any abnormal condition affecting the heart. A dog may have a heart disease but show no sign of illness and never need medical treatment. Sometimes, the disease leads on to "heart failure", a condition in which the heart cannot keep up with its workload of pumping blood to the lungs and around the rest of the body. Heart failure always has noticeable effects, such as reduced tolerance of exercise, coughing, or even collapse.

Q DO DOGS EVER HAVE HEART ATTACKS?

A Coronary artery disease leading to a "heart attack", though common in humans, is rare in dogs. It may occur in individuals with conditions that cause very high blood cholesterol levels, such as advanced hypothyroidism.

HOW ACE INHIBITOR DRUGS WORK

In the body, an enzyme called ACE (angiotensin-converting enzyme) binds to a protein in the blood called angiotensin I, and converts it into angiotensin II, a substance that constricts blood vessels. ACE inhibitors block the action of the enzyme, thus reducing the production of angiotensin II and lowering blood pressure.

BLOCKING ACTION

To produce angiotensin II, an ACE molecule first binds to angiotensin I. The ACE inhibitor prevents this process by locking itself on to the ACE molecule.

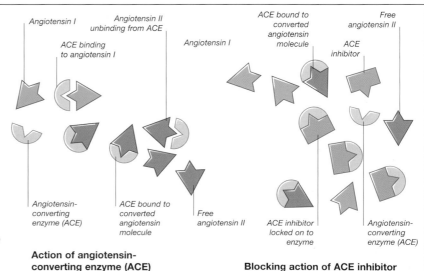

Angiotensin I

ACE binding to angiotensin I

Angiotensin II unbinding from ACE

Angiotensin I

ACE bound to converted angiotensin molecule

Free angiotensin II

ACE inhibitor

Angiotensin-converting enzyme (ACE)

ACE bound to converted angiotensin molecule

Free angiotensin II

ACE inhibitor locked on to enzyme

Angiotensin-converting enzyme (ACE)

Action of angiotensin-converting enzyme (ACE)

Blocking action of ACE inhibitor

DISORDERS ASSOCIATED WITH THE HEART VALVES

Problems associated with the heart valves constitute the most common form of heart disease in dogs.

CHRONIC VALVE DISEASE

For unknown reasons, the leaflets of the valves between the atria (upper heart chambers) and ventricles (lower chambers) can become thickened and distorted until their edges no longer meet when the valve shuts. This defect allows some blood to be forced back into one or both of the atria when the ventricles contract to expel blood from the heart. The seepage increases as the valve defect worsens. Sometimes, some of the muscular cords (chordae tendinae) holding the valve leaflets in place rupture. If this happens, that part of the valve becomes useless.

DIAGNOSIS During the initial stages of valvular heart disease, there may be no obvious signs that anything is wrong. The condition is usually discovered during a routine examination, when a vet hears a heart murmur. When valve disease is present, the mitral valve, which lies between the atrium and the ventricle on the left side of the heart, is usually affected. The equivalent valve on the right side of the heart, the tricuspid valve, is affected in only about one third of cases.

TREATMENT Chronic valve disease is an important cause of heart failure, a condition in which the heart cannot keep up with its workload. Treatment of heart failure is described below. There is no evidence that treatment of valvular heart disease before the earliest signs of heart failure prolongs a dog's life expectancy.

CONGESTIVE HEART FAILURE

A heart affected by a disease that reduces its pumping efficiency (most often chronic valve disease) can usually "compensate" for months or years. It

---

EFFECT OF VALVULAR HEART DISEASE

In chronic heart valve disease, the flaps, or leaflets, that make up a valve become distorted and thickened so that they no longer form a tight seal when the valve closes. This reduces the heart's efficiency as a pump. The basis of the problem is illustrated schematically on the right.

NORMAL AND FAULTY VALVE

Blood that has just passed through a normal valve cannot return, because back pressure causes the valve flaps to come together, forming a seal. In a faulty valve, some blood seeps back.

Blood exerts back pressure

Blood exerts back pressure

Flaps forced together, closing valve

Some blood leaks back through valve

Normal valve   **Faulty valve**

---

usually does so by increasing in size. Eventually, the underlying disease leads to congestive heart failure, in which blood becomes backed up in the veins. This build-up, in turn, forces fluid out of the circulation into the body tissues, in the lungs and elsewhere.

Congestive heart failure can occur gradually or suddenly. The early signs include reduced exercise tolerance (becoming out of breath very quickly during exercise) and lethargy. Because congestive heart failure occurs in older dogs, these signs are often mistaken as natural age-related changes. Soon, a dry, non-productive cough develops, initially after exercise and at night.

As heart failure persists, more changes are noticed. Some dogs lose their appetite, may lose weight, and may breathe more rapidly. In some cases, fluid that has been forced out of the veins may cause ascites (swelling of the abdomen) and swelling of the limbs. Eventually, fluid back-up in the lungs may cause a frothy cough or production of a bubbly pink fluid.

In the late stages of heart failure, a dog braces itself on its elbows and

extends its head to breathe. The dog's gums and tongue become blue. The pulse becomes rapid and may become irregular. Fainting easily occurs with the slightest exertion.

DIAGNOSIS A vet diagnoses congestive heart failure when the typical signs are present and are consistent with known heart disease. If there is no known heart disease, chest and abdominal X-rays, ECG, and echocardiography are performed. If the heart failure primarily affects the right side of the heart, a blood test may be carried out for heartworm infestation.

TREATMENT Dogs with heart disease but no signs of heart failure should be treated normally and given a full exercise routine. When the first signs of heart failure develop, a dog benefits from treatment with a combination of ACE (angiotensin-converting enzyme) inhibitors and diuretics such as frusemide. The ACE inhibitors reduce the workload on the heart by causing blood vessels to widen. The diuretic is a "water pill"; it makes your dog urinate more, which clears fluid congestion from the lungs and veins.

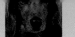

Other medications that act on the heart and circulation, such as digitalis, calcium channel blockers, beta blockers, and anti-arrhythmic drugs, may also be used in some cases. Nitroglycerine (a drug that widens blood vessels) may be recommended in some advanced cases.

Dietary treatment for heart failure remains controversial. Excess salt in the diet should be avoided, but the benefit of low-salt diets is, as yet, not proven. Essential fatty acid (EFA) supplements may be of value for some dogs with congestive heart failure; so, too, may the antioxidants selenium and vitamin E. Routine, daily light exercise is beneficial as long as it does not cause the dog to cough, tire easily, or breathe rapidly.

BACTERIAL ENDOCARDITIS

This condition is an infection of the heart valves and the lining of the heart muscle. Bacteria enter the bloodstream from wounds or infections elsewhere in the body and invade the heart valves, where they produce cauliflower-like masses called vegetations. Some of the vegetations break off and spread via the bloodstream to infect other parts of the body. Gum disease is one possible source of bacteria. In addition, dogs being treated with immunosuppressant drugs, including corticosteroids, are at increased risk of bacterial infection.

The fact that infection can and does affect other parts of the body means that dogs often have non-specific signs suggestive of a number of diseases. These signs include lethargy, loss of appetite, fever, shaking, lameness, and personality changes.

DIAGNOSIS An affected dog usually has a heart murmur, often changing in intensity from day to day. Chest X-rays, ECG, and echocardiography are used to confirm a diagnosis. A blood culture identifies the bacteria and the antibiotic drugs that are likely to be effective against them.

TREATMENT An appropriate antibiotic, selected according to bacterial culture,

BREEDS AT RISK

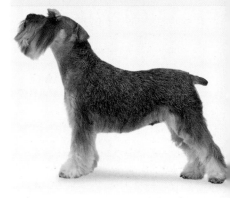

The risk of valvular heart disease is related to the type of dog. While the condition is known to affect around 50 per cent of Cavalier King Charles Spaniels, it is relatively uncommon in medium, large, and giant breeds. A vet may take into account the breed of the dog (as well as other factors, such as the animal's age) in making a diagnosis of valvular heart disease. The causes of the difference in

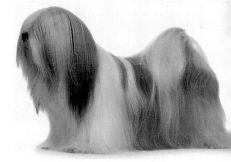

susceptibility between one breed and another are genetically based, though not, as yet, fully understood.

Breeds with a high incidence of valvular heart disease include:

- Miniature Schnauzer (top)
- Cavalier King Charles Spaniel
- Chihuahua
- Lhasa Apso (above)
- Miniature and Toy Poodles
- Yorkshire Terrier

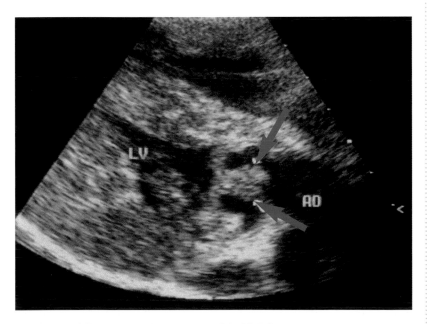

ECHOCARDIOGRAM IN BACTERIAL ENDOCARDITIS

An echocardiogram gives a "real-time" view of what is happening in the heart. The vet can watch the valves perform and measure blood flows. This "frozen" echocardiogram image shows disease changes on a heart valve (arrowed) in a dog with bacterial endocarditis.

is given intravenously for the first week (through a tube called an indwelling cannula). Oral antibiotic therapy will continue for the long term. Affected dogs are monitored closely. Repeat X-rays and echocardiography will show the vegetations shrinking in size. Even so, the outlook is not good; congestive heart failure may occur at any time.

HEART MUSCLE DISEASES

Diseases of the heart muscle are less common than disorders of the valves. Dilated cardiomyopathy is, however, the second most common form of canine heart disease. Hypertrophic cardiomyopathy, although a common condition in cats and people, is rare in dogs; so, too, is myocarditis.

DILATED CARDIOMYOPATHY

This condition, also called DCM, affects relatively young dogs, usually

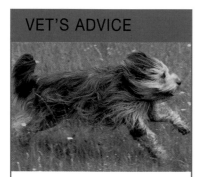

VET'S ADVICE

The risk of heart disease is inherited, particularly in certain breeds. It can be reduced by breeding from dogs whose families are free of disease. In this way, for example, Swedish breeders have postponed the onset of heart disease in Cavalier King Charles Spaniels by several years. Some heart muscle diseases may be linked to overactivity of the immune system; reducing challenges to the immune system may reduce the risk of disease.

under seven years old, and sometimes as young as two years of age. In Cocker Spaniels it may be associated with hypothyroidism (see p.331), a condition in which the dog's immune system attacks its own thyroid gland, resulting in diminished thyroid hormone production. DCM may also be associated with the immune system in the Doberman. The breeds most commonly affected include the Boxer, Doberman, Irish Wolfhound (all high-risk), and also the Afghan Hound, Great Dane, Old English Sheepdog, and Saint Bernard. The condition is now also being diagnosed in smaller breeds, including Cocker Spaniels and Dalmatians. Curiously, DCM affects more males than females.

Affected dogs are lethargic, tire easily from routine exercise, and often go off their food and lose weight. They may have a cough, especially at night. Congestive heart failure develops; as a result, fluid accumulates in the lungs and/or the belly, causing the abdomen to swell. Both Boxers and Dobermans may die suddenly without showing any previous signs of ill health.

DIAGNOSIS An ECG will show changes in the heart's rhythmic contraction, while a chest X-ray will reveal that the heart has become enlarged and dilated (expanded). Echocardiography will confirm that the heart wall is thin and the heart chambers are enlarged.

TREATMENT The dog is given treatment for congestive heart failure (see p.250). Diuretic drugs such as spironolactone or frusemide (furosemide) diminish the build-up of fluid in the lungs and abdomen, while ACE inhibitors and a new drug, pimobendan (Vetmedin), improve the heart function and circulation. There is nutritional logic in supplementing the diet with taurine and L-carnitine, although the benefit of these nutrients has never been properly studied. The long-term outlook for an affected dog is rather poor, although the use of pimobendan has increased survival time threefold in Dobermans.

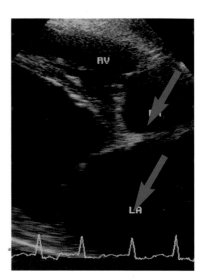

ECHOCARDIOGRAM DIAGNOSIS
Echocardiography allows the thickness of the heart wall to be measured; it is required for a diagnosis of dilated cardiomyopathy. This echocardiogram shows a thinned heart wall and enlarged chambers (arrowed). A simultaneous electrocardiograph (ECG) trace has been superimposed.

HYPERTROPHIC CARDIOMYOPATHY

In this condition, the heart wall becomes thickened. It usually affects the ventricles (the lower chambers of the heart). As the muscle thickens, it reduces the space inside the heart for blood. The most common sign is reduced exercise tolerance. While the heart rate, rhythm, and sounds may be normal when a dog is resting, the rate suddenly increases with exercise.

DIAGNOSIS AND TREATMENT
Hypertrophic cardiomyopathy is diagnosed by echocardiography. Treatment with the calcium channel blocker drug diltiazem appears to prolong life expectancy. Strenuous exercise should be avoided.

MYOCARDITIS

This rare inflammation of the heart muscle has many possible causes. When canine parvovirus infection first occurred, the virus caused a fatal form of myocarditis in pups, but this cause is now extremely rare. Other causes of myocarditis include distemper virus; Lyme disease; other viral, bacterial, and microbial infections; and trauma.

DIAGNOSIS AND TREATMENT Clinical signs of myocarditis include lethargy, fainting, and heart rhythm disturbances. The treatment for this condition is similar to that for congestive heart failure (*see pp.250–51*).

CONGENITAL HEART DEFECTS

These heart defects are structural abnormalities that are present at birth. They often, but not always, have a genetic origin. All forms are rare.

DIAGNOSIS A congenital defect will initially be diagnosed by a vet listening to a pup's heart with a stethoscope. Diagnosing the exact form of the birth defect requires more sophisticated investigation. Once the initial diagnosis is made, the severity of the defect is determined through further testing. An ECG and X-rays are beneficial, but the most accurate diagnosis is made using a special form of echocardiography called Doppler ultrasound. This type of imaging demonstrates the defect and can measure the velocity of blood flow in selected areas of the heart.

TREATMENT The treatment depends on the severity of the defect, which is determined according to the results of Doppler ultrasound. In the United States and Canada, the Orthopedic Foundation for Animals gathers data on congenital cardiac defects; breeding stock found to be free of congenital defects are issued with certificates.

PATENT DUCTUS ARTERIOSIS (PDA)

In this most common of congenital defects, the connection between the aorta and pulmonary artery, necessary before birth to bypass the developing pup's non-functioning lungs, fails to close down at birth as it should. As a result, some of the blood pumped by the left side of the heart and intended for the body flows instead through the open duct to the lungs. This abnormal blood flow puts a strain on the heart.

DIAGNOSIS AND TREATMENT Dogs with PDA benefit from relatively uncomplicated open chest surgery in which the open duct is tied shut.

VALVULAR AND SEPTAL DEFECTS

Structural abnormalities of the heart valves include narrowing (stenosis) and malformation (dysplasia). A septal defect, or "hole in the heart", is an abnormal opening in the septum, the wall between the chambers of the heart.

Some pups are born with mild valvular or septal defects, of which the only evidence is a heart murmur. These dogs grow up to lead normal lives. In others, the defect is more significant. Though fit and robust as pups, they may not grow as expected, be prone to fainting, or have reduced exercise tolerance. Heart failure occurs suddenly. In the most severely affected dogs, signs of heart disease develop early. These animals do not usually survive for more than one year.

DIAGNOSIS AND TREATMENT Pulmonary stenosis (narrowing of the pulmonary valve, on the right side of the heart) can be successfully treated with surgery, but other valve defects have a poor outlook. Surgery is usually not practical. Septal defects are difficult to repair and require coronary bypass facilities needed for open heart surgery.

TETRALOGY OF FALLOT

This is a rare heart condition, which consists of four congenital defects: pulmonary stenosis; a septal defect; thickening of the wall of the right ventricle; and an abnormally placed aorta. Affected dogs have a bluish discoloration of the skin at rest and very quickly become out of breath during exercise. Surgery is the only way of effecting a cure.

BREEDS AT RISK

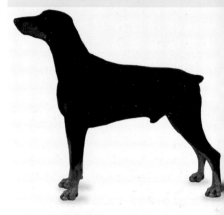

Breeds known to be susceptible to congenital heart defects include:

- Basset Hound
- Beagle
- Bichon Frise
- Boxer
- Boykin Spaniel
- Bull Terrier
- Chihuahua
- Chow Chow
- Cocker Spaniel
- Collies
- Doberman (above)
- English Bulldog
- English Springer Spaniel
- German Shepherd Dog
- German Short-haired Pointer
- Golden Retriever
- Great Dane
- Keeshond
- Labrador Retriever
- Maltese
- Newfoundland
- Pomeranian
- Poodles
- Rottweiler
- Samoyed
- Schnauzers
- Shetland Sheepdog
- Weimaraner
- Welsh Corgis
- West Highland White, Yorkshire, and other terriers

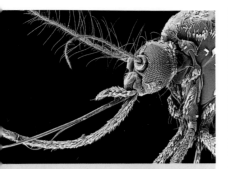

Q HOW DO I KNOW IF MY DOG IS AT RISK OF HEARTWORMS?

A Heartworm disease is associated with certain areas. In Europe, dogs are at risk in the Mediterranean region, especially in the Po River valley of northern Italy. The disease occurs throughout Australia, including the colder areas, and in many other regions of the world, including parts of North America. Any dog that lives in an affected area and is not treated preventatively is at risk.

Q CAN HEARTWORMS BE SURGICALLY REMOVED?

A Surgery is considered only when drug therapy is not possible and the risk of liver failure is high. Surgery to remove heartworms is a dramatic procedure. Accessing the heart via the jugular vein, the surgeon uses a special instrument to remove the worms.

Q WHAT IS MEANT BY THE TERM OCCULT INFECTION?

A An "occult" heartworm infection is a situation in which no microfilariae (microscopic forms of the heartworm) are present in the blood, but there are adult worms in the heart. A dog will then have a negative test for microfilariae but a positive test for adult worms. There are various possible causes, such as the presence of only male worms in the heart.

PARASITIC PROBLEMS

There is only one parasite that causes heart problems: the heartworm. This parasite causes a particularly horrible disease. Other parasites, such as hookworms (*see p.169*) and ticks (*see p.163*), can take enough blood from a dog to cause anaemia (*see pp.256–57*).

HEARTWORMS

These worms, of the species *Dirofilaria immitis*, are transmitted to dogs (and sometimes to cats) through mosquito bites as microscopic larvae. They mature into male and female adults, which are the size of earthworms and live in the right side of the heart, particularly the right ventricle and the pulmonary arteries (from which blood is carried to the lungs). In a heavy infestation, the right side of the heart contains a mass of worms, and this obstruction leads to heart failure. In some cases, worms may overflow into the right atrium (the top right chamber of the heart) and even into the large veins that return blood from the liver to the heart. When worms occupy the pulmonary arteries, the obstruction to the blood flow can cause blood clots to develop in the lungs.

The severity of disease depends on the number of worms and the size of the dog. Small dogs suffer more from small worm loads than do large dogs. Affected individuals show signs indicating varying degrees of heart failure, from reduced exercise tolerance through soft coughing to weight loss, visible pulsation of blood flow in the veins of the neck, fainting, and even sudden collapse and death. If the pulmonary arteries are affected, a dog may cough up blood-tinged phlegm. If the veins from the liver are involved, a dog may show signs of liver failure, including jaundice, anaemia, and ascites (a swollen, fluid-filled abdomen).

DIAGNOSIS A blood test called a heartworm antigen test identifies the presence of adult female heartworms.

Occasionally, a false negative test occurs (failure to detect worms when they are present). This result may occur in light infestations or when all the worms are males.

A microfilarial concentration test relies on identifying microfilariae (microscopic forms of the parasite, produced by adult females) under the microscope. Again, a false negative sometimes occurs. About 10 to 25 per cent of infected dogs do not have microfilariae in the bloodstream.

A chest X-ray may show an enlarged right ventricle and pulmonary arteries. ECG sometimes shows a disturbance of the heart rhythm. Echocardiography (examination of the heart structure by ultrasound scanning) reveals the adult worms themselves.

TREATMENT The most effective initial treatment is to stop all exercise. Medical treatment depends on the level of complication associated with the disease. Compounds containing arsenic are given to kill adult worms, although arsenic causes a variety of side effects. The usual drug given is melarsomine (Immiticide) by injection; it has the widest margin of safety and kills over 90 per cent of adult worms. Safer than previous treatments, melarsomine therapy may lead to other problems. Dead worms may cause blood clots to form in the lungs; to break up any clots, your vet may dispense aspirin, which acts to inhibit blood clotting. You should allow the dog only limited exercise for the month following treatment.

Arsenic treatments are dangerous for elderly dogs. If your dog is old, your vet will discuss the pros and cons of their use. You and your vet may decide to treat only with daily low-dose aspirin and restricted exercise. Heart failure caused by heartworms is treated as for other forms of heart failure (*see pp.250–51*).

Four to five weeks after drug therapy, a heartworm antigen test is performed. A negative test usually means that all adult worms have been destroyed. (If the test is positive, your vet will discuss re-treatment.) A microfilaria concentration test follows. If it is negative, no more treatment is needed and routine prevention can begin. If it is positive, the next step is to kill circulating microfilariae. Either milbemycin (Interceptor) or ivermectin (Ivomec) are used "off label" (outside their normally approved use). Ivomec is most effective and has the fewest complications, but is dangerous for some breeds (see below).

PREVENTION Keep your dog indoors at times when mosquitoes are feeding (especially at dusk). If it is not practical to do so, use heartworm preventative medication (see p.256). Keep your dog

on prevention treatment during the mosquito season in any part of the world where heartworm disease is endemic (permanently established). The usual advice is that in areas where mosquitoes are seasonal, medication should be started one month before the mosquito season and continued until one month after the first frost. For the whole of Australia, however, and in any area where mosquitoes are a year-round nuisance, dogs must have preventative medication all year round. In endemic areas, keep newborn pups indoors and begin medication within eight weeks of them first venturing outdoors. When travelling with your dog to an endemic area, begin prevention one month

before travel and continue until one month after returning home. If your dog is more than seven months old and is from, or has visited, an endemic area, ask your vet to carry out an antigen test for heartworm before starting preventative medication.

ADVICE Ivomec is frequently used and very effective, but is not licensed for use in dogs. It is potentially lethal in certain sheepdog breeds, where the drug crosses the barrier that separates the bloodstream from the brain. Ivomec should not be used in the Rough or Smooth Collie, Shetland Sheepdog, Old English Sheepdog, Australian Shepherd, or other herding breeds or crosses including these breeds. The

HEARTWORM LIFE CYCLE

Mosquitoes ingest microfilariae (microscopic forms of the worm) when feeding on an infected dog's blood. The microfilariae develop through three stages in the mosquito, becoming larvae, and move to the insect's mouth. Larvae spread to an uninfected dog when the mosquito feeds again, and burrow under the dog's skin, where they moult through two more larval stages. Now immature worms, the parasites migrate through the bloodstream to their preferred home, the right side of the heart. Over the next six months they mature into adult males and females. These worms produce more microfilariae, so completing the life cycle.

HITCHING A RIDE
The heartworm has a classic parasite's life cycle, spreading from one dog to another by way of mosquitoes, in which its early development takes place.

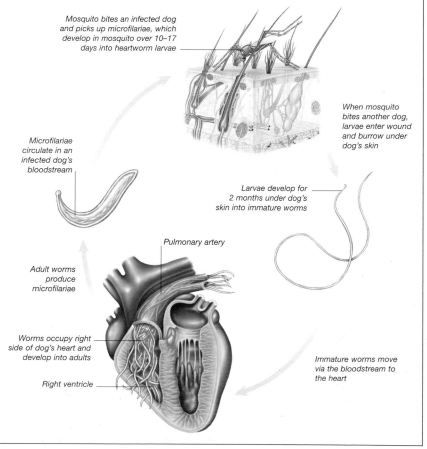

Mosquito bites an infected dog and picks up microfilariae, which develop in mosquito over 10–17 days into heartworm larvae

When mosquito bites another dog, larvae enter wound and burrow under dog's skin

Microfilariae circulate in an infected dog's bloodstream

Larvae develop for 2 months under dog's skin into immature worms

Pulmonary artery

Adult worms produce microfilariae

Worms occupy right side of dog's heart and develop into adults

Right ventricle

Immature worms move via the bloodstream to the heart

HEARTWORM PREVENTATIVE MEDICINES

A variety of medicines are effective for the prevention of heartworm disease. Some have additional effects against other external and internal parasites. The timing of treatment is vital: the heartworm is vulnerable to these drugs at a larval stage, when it is present in the dog's tissues and before it develops into an immature worm and travels to the heart.

NAME	PROPRIETARY (BRAND) NAME	APPLICATION
selamectin	Stronghold Revolution	Monthly "spot-on" treatment applied to the skin between the shoulders. This drug also controls fleas, roundworms, ear mites, the American dog tick, and canine scabies mites.
milbemycin	Interceptor	Monthly oral treatment. It also controls roundworms, hookworms, and whipworms.
milbemycin and lufenuron	Program Plus	As above. It also prevents fleas from hatching.
ivermectin	Heartgard, Ivomec	Monthly oral treatment.
moxidectin	Proheart	Monthly oral treatment. Yearly injections also available in some regions, such as Australia.

branded medicine Heartgard contains the same drug, ivermectin, but at a much lower dose. Heartgard is safe and fully licensed for prevention of heartworm infection.

OTHER MICROFILARIAE

Another worm, *Dipetalonema*, which lives harmlessly under a dog's skin, produces microfilariae that look almost identical to those of *Dirofilaria*, the heartworm. Its only importance is that it can be a cause for mistaken identity in an otherwise heartworm-free individual.

ANAEMIC CONDITIONS

Circulating red blood cells, made in the bone marrow, carry oxygen from the lungs around the body. A deficiency in the numbers of red blood cells is called anaemia. External and internal bleeding are the most obvious causes of anaemia, but there are other possible causes, including premature destruction of healthy red blood cells (haemolysis)

and suppression of red cell production in the bone marrow. Anaemia thins the blood. This development sometimes produces an audible heart murmur (which is distinct from the type of murmur caused by heart disease). Lethargy and weakness are common signs of anaemia; the dog will seem subdued. A seriously affected dog pants more than normal. Its gums become pale and its pulse quickens.

Some specific causes of anaemia include gastrointestinal conditions such as stomach ulcers; metabolic disorders such as hypothyroidism (*see p.331*); treatment with certain drugs, such as paracetamol (*see p.109*); ingestion of warfarin and other poisonous chemicals (*see p.422*); and some cancers, such as leukaemia (*see p.141*).

ANAEMIA DUE TO BLOOD LOSS

The main causes of blood loss leading to anaemia are external injury and internal bleeding. The latter may result from stomach or duodenal ulcers,

including those brought on by drugs (such as aspirin); inflammatory bowel disease (see *pp.285–86*); tumours; or parasites such as heartworms. Fleas and hookworms can cause chronic blood loss in puppies.

DIAGNOSIS External bleeding from injuries causes obvious blood loss and associated anaemia. Internal bleeding may cause a dog to vomit visible blood or pass bloody diarrhoea; an affected dog is also likely to pass stools that are tarry and black due to the presence of dried blood. Black stools (melaena) strongly suggest serious bleeding in the stomach or the duodenum (the first part of the intestines).

TREATMENT The first objective of treatment is to stop further blood loss and, when possible, eliminate the cause. A blood transfusion is usually given for anaemia caused by serious blood loss. Blood replacer fluid is often used because of the lack of readily available and compatible canine blood. The outlook is good once the cause of blood loss has been eliminated.

PREVENTION Internal and external parasite control prevent the occurrence of anaemia as a result of parasitic infestation. Never give drugs licensed for humans to your dog without first speaking to your vet, because some medications may be dangerous.

HAEMOLYTIC ANAEMIA

A haemolytic anaemia is any condition in which healthy red blood cells are destroyed prematurely. There are many causes. Some bacteria produce powerful toxins that destroy red blood cells, and haemolytic anaemia may follow a severe infection with these organisms. Tick-borne blood parasites such as *Babesia* also destroy red blood cells. Inherited genetic defects may lead to haemolytic disease in pups. The most common cause, however, is the body's immune system mistakenly attacking its own red blood cells; this type of anaemia is called immune-mediated haemolytic anaemia (IMHA).

INHERITED FORMS The inherited forms of haemolytic anaemia are rare and restricted to a few breeds. They cause serious or fatal illness in young dogs. There are two main types. Pyruvate kinase deficiency affects some West Highland White Terriers, Basenjis,

and Beagles. Phosphofructokinase deficiency affects some American Cocker Spaniels and English Springer Spaniels. Tests have been developed for detecting whether particular dogs are affected by these conditions or are carriers of the genetic defect. Clubs associated with affected breeds are good sources of up-to-date information on testing for these conditions.

IMHA Frustratingly, the cause of immune-mediated haemolytic anaemia (IMHA) is rarely discovered. All breeds are susceptible but some, including the Cocker Spaniel, Irish Setter, Old English Sheepdog, and poodles, are more predisposed than others. In the 1990s, researchers at the University of Pennsylvania found a statistical link between IMHA and vaccination. On reviewing their records, they found that IMHA occurred more frequently within a month of vaccination than a mathematical model would suggest. When British researchers carried out a similar survey, however, they found no statistical link between the two.

DIAGNOSIS Haemolytic anaemias are more difficult to diagnose than those that are caused by blood loss. Sudden haemolytic anaemia results in a rapid accumulation of the products of red

cell breakdown (such as bilirubin) in the bloodstream. This may cause jaundice, a yellow colouring of the gums and conjunctiva (the covering of the whites of the eyes). The dog's urine may become dark-brown in colour. On examination, the vet will usually find that the spleen is enlarged, sometimes dramatically so. The liver and lymph nodes may also be enlarged, and the vet may hear a heart murmur. A red blood cell count confirms anaemia, while microscopic examination of the blood indicates how the body is responding to the problem. Further blood tests will reveal whether the condition is immune-mediated, which is a vital piece of information for a vet to know when planning treatment.

TREATMENT In IMHA, priority is given to reducing the rate at which the dog's immune system is destroying red blood cells. This treatment is carried out with high doses of corticosteroids and other drugs that suppress the immune system. A blood transfusion before the drugs start working may or may not make the condition worse (the value of a transfusion in these circumstances is controversial). The transfusion may be performed with oxygen-carrying blood replacer fluid rather than donated

RED BLOOD CELL PRODUCTION

Millions of erythrocytes (red blood cells) are made every minute in the bone marrow, a fatty tissue that occupies the interior of bones. All types of blood cells originate from a single kind of cell called a haematocytoblast. Red cells are formed as shown on the right.

PRODUCTION LINE
During the process of red cell formation, the original cell's nucleus is lost and the cell becomes packed with the oxygen-carrying substance haemoglobin.

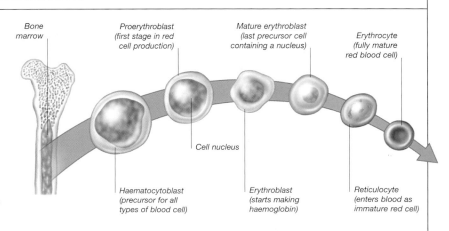

Bone marrow

Proerythroblast (first stage in red cell production)

Mature erythroblast (last precursor cell containing a nucleus)

Erythrocyte (fully mature red blood cell)

Cell nucleus

Haematocytoblast (precursor for all types of blood cell)

Erythroblast (starts making haemoglobin)

Reticulocyte (enters blood as immature red cell)

Stages in red cell production

canine blood. Removing the spleen (splenectomy) is sometimes useful once it has been confirmed that the spleen is a centre of red blood cell destruction.

The outlook for a dog with IMHA is, unfortunately, not promising. Even with rapid diagnosis, treatment, and apparent recovery, relapse (recurrence of the condition) is common, often within the following eight weeks. Up to half of affected dogs have relapses, some of which are fatal.

PREVENTION Until the causes of IMHA are better understood, there is no known prevention of this form of anaemia. In breeds that are known to be predisposed, including the Cocker Spaniel, it is prudent, when your dog has its annual health check-up, to discuss with your vet the efficacy of previous vaccinations, local disease incidence, and known risks of IMHA and other immune-mediated diseases.

BONE MARROW SUPPRESSION ANAEMIA

Red blood cells are manufactured in the bone marrow. Any problem that interferes with their production can cause a bone marrow suppression anaemia. Causes include: chronic illness, especially illness involving the kidneys or liver; iron deficiency, as a result of chronic bleeding from the stomach or intestines or a chronic parasitic infestation; female hormone (oestrogen) given as medication, or from an oestrogen-producing ovarian or testicular tumour; anti-cancer drugs and other drugs that suppress activity in the bone marrow; and cancers that affect the bone marrow.

DIAGNOSIS AND TREATMENT A bone marrow suppression anaemia is diagnosed by examining a sample of bone marrow. The anaemia disappears once the cause is eliminated, provided that it has not resulted in permanent shutdown of red blood cell production. Recovering dogs may be given iron supplements, although this treatment may cause constipation.

BLEEDING AND CLOTTING DISORDERS

Blood clotting depends on a cascade of chemical reactions taking place in the blood after an injury. These reactions, in turn, depend on the presence of substances called coagulation factors in the blood. If any of these coagulation factors is missing or deficient, the clotting process is delayed, and the result is excessive bleeding. Fortunately, bleeding and clotting disorders are uncommon in dogs.

VON WILLEBRAND'S DISEASE

The most common bleeding disorder is von Willebrand's Disease (vWD). This condition has been diagnosed in over 50 breeds. Although rare in all breeds

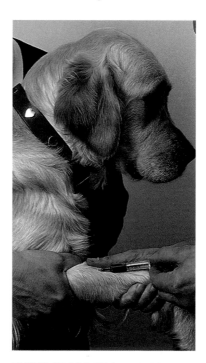

TAKING BLOOD FROM A DOG
Blood samples are routinely taken from a superficial vein on a foreleg. If the blood circulation has collapsed, or when the superficial veins are too small (as in many toy breeds), one of the jugular veins, on either side of the neck, is used.

other than the Doberman, in which it is common but mild, it may cause severe and often fatal bleeding in young Scottish Terriers and Pembroke Welsh Corgis. Bleeding is more severe in young dogs, causing unexpected bruising, nosebleeds, or blood in the urine or faeces. The disease quite frequently occurs in association with hypothyroidism (*see p.331*).

DIAGNOSIS AND TREATMENT Von Willebrand's disease is diagnosed by blood tests. Animals at risk of having the disorder (siblings and offspring of affected dogs) should undergo a blood test for it before having any elective (non-urgent) surgery. DNA testing is available to detect the presence of the defective gene in some breeds. If severe bleeding occurs, blood transfusions or blood replacer fluids are given.

HAEMOPHILIA

This rare inherited condition, which occurs in different forms, affects only male dogs. Canine haemophiliacs have inherited the defective gene from their mothers, who are unaffected "carriers" of the gene. The different forms of haemophilia are caused by deficiencies in the different coagulation factors needed for blood clotting. The most common, Haemophilia A, occurs most frequently in the German Shepherd Dog and the Airedale. Bleeding may occur into the joints or body cavities.

DIAGNOSIS AND TREATMENT Haemophilia is diagnosed by analysis of the coagulation factors in a dog's blood. The condition is treated with supplements of the missing coagulation factor. When bleeding occurs, the dog will be given a blood transfusion; in less threatening situations, blood replacer fluids are used.

COAGULATION DISORDERS

Shock, severe infections, wounds, burns, and even some tumours may lead to a condition called disseminated intravascular coagulation, or DIC, in which microscopic blood clotting occurs throughout the capillaries (smallest blood vessels) of the body. The tiny clots use enormous quantities of coagulation factors; once these are consumed, bleeding follows. DIC is extremely serious and often fatal.

Another type of coagulation disorder is caused by ingestion of warfarin and other anti-coagulant rodent poisons. These substances cause vitamin K deficiency, leading to spontaneous bleeding. Newer anticoagulant rodent poisons are 100 times more toxic than warfarin. (*See p.422.*)

DIAGNOSIS AND TREATMENT DIC is life-threatening. The precipitating cause must be identified and treated. Blood transfusions or heparin may also be needed. Warfarin poisoning responds to injections of vitamin K.

THE THREE STAGES OF BLOOD CLOTTING

When a blood vessel is cut or torn, the damage triggers a series of events that lead to the formation of a clot to seal the injury. In stage 1, immediately following the injury, the damaged blood vessel narrows. Small blood cells called platelets become "activated" on contact with damaged blood vessel walls. Their surfaces become sticky and they start to adhere to the vessel walls near the site of injury. In stage 2, the platelets clump together. The damaged tissue and platelets release chemicals that start a cascade of chemical reactions in the blood. In stage 3, these reactions cause the release of a sticky, thread-like substance called fibrin, which binds the red cells and other blood cells together into a solid clot.

CLOTS AND CLOTTING

The stages in the formation of a blood clot following internal rupture of a blood vessel are shown on the right. The final, crucial stage involves the production of fibrin from a protein called fibrinogen in the blood. Fibrinogen is one of a series of chemicals, called coagulation factors, that must be present within the fluid part of blood for clots to form.

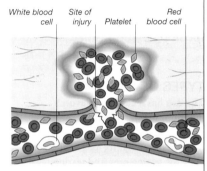

White blood cell · *Site of injury* · *Platelet* · *Red blood cell*

Stage 1

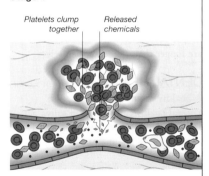

Platelets clump together · *Released chemicals*

Stage 2

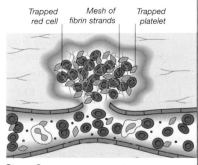

Trapped red cell · *Mesh of fibrin strands* · *Trapped platelet*

Stage 3

Q HOW LONG DO RED BLOOD CELLS LIVE?

A Typically, a red blood cell has a working life of a few months. New cells are made in the bone marrow. (If sudden blood loss occurs, immature red cells, called reticulocytes, are released from the marrow. Your vet will look for these cells in a blood sample. When they are seen, the anaemia is called "regenerative".) When red cells wear out, they are trapped and removed in the spleen. Important parts of the cells, such as iron, are recycled for use in newly manufactured cells.

Q CAN DOGS RECEIVE BLOOD TRANSFUSIONS?

A Yes, they can. The only restriction preventing more widespread use of transfusions is the availability of canine blood itself. Like humans, dogs have different blood types. Compatibility between the blood of the donor and that of the recipient is vital to prevent a dangerous transfusion reaction. Many animal hospitals keep lists of donors – large, healthy dogs with owners willing to have their dogs donate blood. An oxygen-carrying blood replacer fluid, Oxyglobin, is licensed for use in dogs in North America and some parts of Europe but not Australia.

Q WHY AREN'T THERE ANY CANINE BLOOD BANKS?

A Human blood transfusion services are run by health services or by charities such as the Red Cross. The only reason there are no similar canine blood banks is that no canine organization has chosen to create one. Private canine blood banks exist, but their costs indicate that provision of such a service is expensive.

They may occur on the gums, the tongue, and the roof of the mouth, and in the salivary glands.

DIAGNOSIS AND TREATMENT Diagnosis is by veterinary examination. Viral warts do not require any treatment. Tumours of the salivary glands, which are most common in poodles, need to be surgically removed and the dog given radiotherapy afterwards. Other mouth tumours are also treated by surgical removal, possibly combined with chemotherapy or radiotherapy. For any malignant mouth tumour, a dog has the best chance of recovery if the tumour is diagnosed early and treated quite aggressively with wide excision surgery (in which the tumour is removed together with an area of normal tissue). Personally, I had considerable worries about the ethics of, for example, removing half a lower jaw or half a tongue until I saw how comfortable and "normal" dogs became afterwards.

EPULIS

An epulis is a tumour that develops from the periodontal ligament of the tooth, a layer of tiny fibres attaching the root of the tooth to the bone of the jaw. It looks like a firm enlargement of the gum. Several growths may occur at the same time. An epulis rarely becomes malignant. The tumour is most common in breeds such as Bulldogs and Boxers.

DIAGNOSIS Biopsy and X-rays are used to identify an epulis and distinguish it from other types of tumour.

TREATMENT The epulis is surgically removed together with wide margins of tissue that include underlying bone.

SALIVARY GLAND RUPTURE

Four pairs of salivary glands produce saliva, an alkaline and antibacterial liquid that lubricates the mouth and helps with mixing food. The largest of the glands is the parotid gland, located beneath the ears on the sides of the head. Trauma, but also other unknown reasons, may cause one of the salivary

glands to tear and leak saliva into the surrounding tissue; this may cause a soft, fluctuating swelling in the neck.

DIAGNOSIS AND TREATMENT Diagnosis is made by withdrawing saliva from the swelling using a syringe and then examining it. A ruptured salivary gland produces stringy, sometimes blood-stained, material. The damaged gland is surgically removed.

ELONGATED SOFT PALATE

The soft palate separates the oral part from the nasal part of the throat. When it is elongated, the soft palate hangs down, partially obstructing the airway at the back of the mouth.

DIAGNOSIS AND TREATMENT This abnormality is corrected by means of surgery. (*See also p.240.*)

CLEFT PALATE

Some pups are born with a cleft palate. This problem results from a failure of the sides of the palate to fuse down their midline as the pup is developing

in the womb. The more severe the cleft, the more difficulty a pup has in suckling. Trauma to the face or jaw may also cause the palate to split.

TREATMENT Usually, a surgical repair is needed. This is easier on a traumatic injury than on an inherited cleft palate.

CONDITIONS OF THE THROAT

The respiratory and gastrointestinal systems intersect in the throat, which is technically divided into the respiratory part (the nasopharynx) and the gastrointestinal part (the oropharynx). Medical conditions from either system can involve both parts of the throat.

SORE THROAT

Also called pharyngitis, a sore throat is rarely a local condition but is usually associated with other infections in the mouth, sinuses, or respiratory tract. Affected dogs may have a fever, be lethargic, or cough, sneeze, or gag.

DROOLING SALIVA

Drooling excessive amounts of saliva is considered normal for some dogs, especially those with loose, slack lower lips such as Italian Spinones (right) and St. Bernards. Excessive drooling, known as hypersalivation, is a natural response to stimuli such as fear and anxiety. It may also, however, indicate a variety of medical conditions, including disorders of the mouth or oesophagus; motion sickness; heatstroke; liver disease; poisoning or diseases such as rabies; pseudorabies; and distemper. Certain drugs, including anaesthetics and flea-control treatments, may also trigger drooling. In addition, the problem may be a sign that a dog is about to vomit or has a foreign body stuck in its mouth. Lastly, drooling can be a response to localized mouth pain from problems such as periodontal disease, stomatitis, and tooth abscesses.

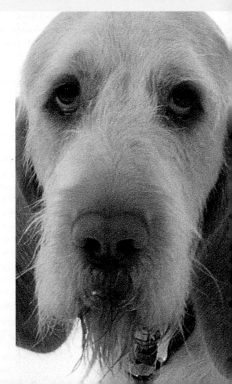

DIAGNOSIS The throat appears red and inflamed, and pus is sometimes seen.

TREATMENT This depends on the cause of the overall infection. Non-steroidal anti-inflammatory drugs (NSAIDs) are used to relieve discomfort. Antibiotics are given to eliminate bacterial infection. In addition, affected dogs need to be fed for a week on soft food that does not irritate the throat.

ADVICE The bacteria that causes "strep throat" in humans can be carried, without clinical signs, by dogs. If your family is being treated for strep throat, ensure that your dog is also treated.

TONSILLITIS

Tonsillitis can occur in any breed but appears to affect small breeds more frequently. The condition is usually part of a generalized infection of the throat or the respiratory system (see p.152). Affected dogs are feverish, depressed, and usually lose their appetite.

DIAGNOSIS The tonsils look angry red and are often enlarged and swollen. The swelling leads to gagging (see box, right) and retching; it can become so great that the tonsils eventually touch each other. Other causes of swelling in the throat include tumours, especially carcinomas and lymphomas. In very rare circumstances, tumours can develop on the tonsils.

TREATMENT Affected individuals are treated with NSAIDs and antibiotics. The surgical removal of chronically infected tonsils (tonsillectomy) is a rare procedure except in Cavalier King Charles Spaniels; if done, associated soft palate and adenoid tissue problems may be corrected at the same time.

FOREIGN BODIES

Bones and other objects, especially sticks, can become lodged at the back of a dog's throat, where they cannot be removed with a spoon handle. A dog with something in its throat gags, paws at its mouth, and may drool or vomit.

DIAGNOSIS AND TREATMENT Contact a vet immediately. A foreign body in

the throat may cause swelling that interferes with breathing. If the object blocks the voice box, the dog will choke and faint (see p.390).

CRANIOMANDIBULAR OSTEOARTHROPATHY

This is a painful developmental joint disease of the upper jaw (mandible) and skull (cranium). Technically, it is not a mouth condition. Some breeds of terrier, particularly Scottish and West Highland White Terriers, develop transient but considerable pain when using their jaws; the pain is most intense from four to ten months of age.

DIAGNOSIS AND TREATMENT The condition is diagnosed according to the signs, age, and breed of the individual. X-rays confirm diagnosis. Treatment involves controlling the pain until the individual outgrows the condition.

SLACK JAW

The lower jaw consists of two separate parts (hemi-mandibles), one on each side. It is joined at the middle of the chin by a firm cartilage. The union of the lower jaw bones sometimes fails, particularly in toy breeds. As a result, the two sections of the jaw remain separate and unstable, causing the jaw to be "slack". The incisor teeth in the region are usually loose.

TREATMENT Any diseased teeth are removed. Secondary infection is treated with antibiotics. In some instances, the joint between the two lower jaw bones is stabilized with screws and wire.

JAW LUXATION AND FRACTURES

Luxation is a condition in which the lower jaw slips out of its joint with the skull. It is a rare problem, most likely to occur in Irish Setters and Basset Hounds. Fractures are more common, and can be due to a variety of traumas.

TREATMENT Jaw luxation usually requires a surgical correction. Surgical repairs to jaw fractures usually involve securing the bones with wire or pins.

CAUSES OF GAGGING

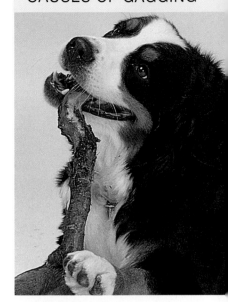

Gagging occurs when the pharynx is irritated and muscles at the back of the throat contract. It can also result from problems in other areas:

Nose, palate, or nasal sinuses

- Cleft palate
- Parasites
- Tumours
- Foreign bodies or obstructions

Respiratory tract

- Tracheal collapse
- Laryngeal paralysis
- Kennel cough or canine cough
- Parasites
- Tumours
- Foreign bodies

Oesophagus or stomach

- Megaoesophagus
- Inflammations
- Tumours
- Foreign bodies

Elsewhere in body

- Fluid build-up around the heart (pericardial effusion)
- Middle ear disorders
- Kidney disease

OESOPHAGUS AND STOMACH
initial breakdown of food

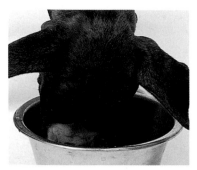

Dogs can swallow with the head down

Once food has been chewed and broken up in the mouth by the teeth, it is swallowed, passing from the back of the mouth over the larynx and into the oesophagus. Waves of muscular contraction then push food and liquids into the stomach, even against the force of gravity. The stomach itself is a holding tank where food is kept and released gradually into the small intestine. Dogs are prone to eat indigestible things accidentally, so vomiting the contents of their stomach is not an uncommon occurrence.

Digestion begins in the first part of the gastrointestinal tract, from the mouth via the oesophagus to the stomach. Essentially, this part of the system is concerned with physically breaking down the food, at first by chewing and then by chemical means in the acidic environment of the stomach.

THE OESOPHAGUS
The oesophagus is a muscular tube through which food and liquids, once swallowed, are transported from the throat to the stomach. Swallowed mouthfuls of material do not simply move passively along the oesophagus,

but are actively pushed and squeezed along by rhythmical contractions of its muscular walls. These movements, which are not under conscious control, are called peristalsis. Aided by the lubricating mucus produced by the walls of the oesophagus, they effectively drive the food towards the stomach independent of the force of gravity. As a result, a dog can stand and eat or drink with its head down.

The dog's oesophagus is a highly elastic organ and allows large chunks of meat to be transported to the stomach. This elasticity, however, also allows sizeable foreign bodies and other objects to be swallowed.

A variety of problems can develop in the oesophagus, many of them painful. The most common problem is regurgitation, which is different from vomiting (*see p.272*).

THE STOMACH
A dog's stomach is relatively large, which is ideal for an animal that feeds and scavenges opportunistically. Dogs are ambitious eaters; when food is available, dogs will eat more than they need – and they have the stomach to store it. Because dogs "taste" life, vomiting is an active feature of many stomach conditions.

A dog's stomach has a considerable capacity to expand when food is plentiful. It can hold between 100 and 250 ml (4–10 fl oz) of contents per kilogram (2.2 lb) of a dog's body weight. This means that my Labrador Retriever's stomach has a capacity of up to 8 litres (14 pints). Any Labrador owner knows that the dog will use this stomach capacity to its limit, which is why some owners say that a Labrador is a life-support system for a stomach.

The stomach is a reservoir for mixed and predigested food, a holding tank where hydrochloric acid and certain enzymes, under the control of gastrointestinal hormones, are secreted. The stomach lining is protected from its own acid by a layer of mucus and by chemicals called prostaglandins. If prostaglandin production is reduced or impaired, stomach inflammation and ulceration occur.

Gastric acids begin the process of breaking down the food for digestion. Muscular waves in the stomach mix and move the food, contributing to its breakdown, before it is passed into the intestines where digestion is completed and the molecular components of food are absorbed (*see p.278*).

Q **WHY DO DOGS SO REGULARLY HAVE PROBLEMS WITH STUCK FOREIGN BODIES?**

A Dogs will eat absolutely anything. That is why so many pharyngeal (throat) problems are caused by penetrating foreign bodies such as shards of bone and pieces of stick. Overwhelmingly, the most common cause of both oesophagus and stomach problems is this basic and natural need to investigate with the mouth. Control what your dog puts in its mouth – it will save visits to the vet.

THE PASSAGE OF FOOD

Each swallowed, mouthful of food enters the oesophagus and is propelled towards the stomach. At the top of the stomach, a tight ring of muscle called the cardiac sphinter opens to allow food in. At the other end of the stomach, another ring of muscle, called the pyloric sphincter, opens at intervals to allow food to pass into the intestines.

STOMACH LINING

Cells in a multitude of glands, embedded deep in the folds of the stomach lining, secrete substances such as mucus, hydrochloric acid, and enzymes into channels called pits.

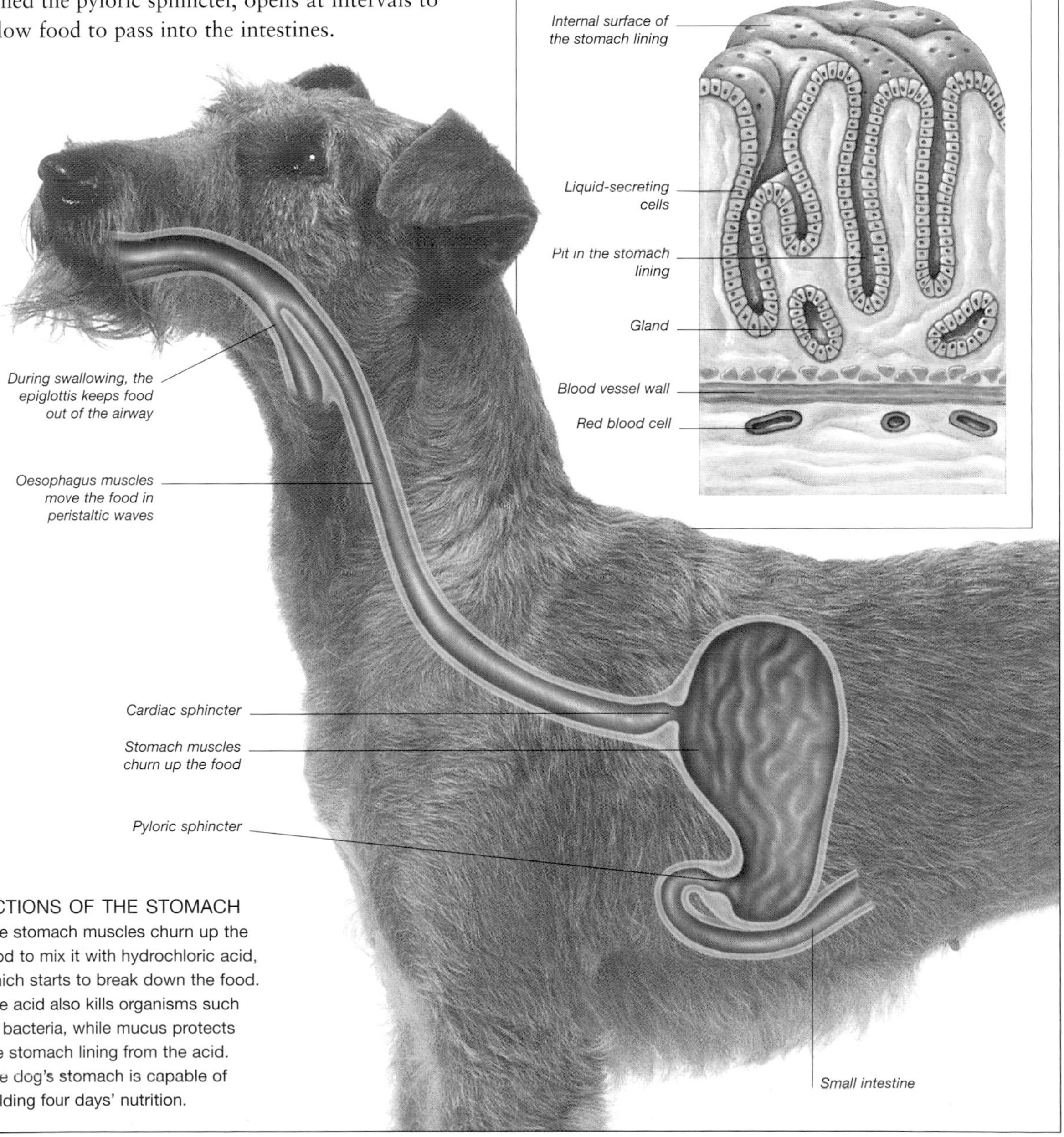

Internal surface of the stomach lining

Liquid-secreting cells

Pit in the stomach lining

Gland

Blood vessel wall

Red blood cell

During swallowing, the epiglottis keeps food out of the airway

Oesophagus muscles move the food in peristaltic waves

Cardiac sphincter

Stomach muscles churn up the food

Pyloric sphincter

Small intestine

ACTIONS OF THE STOMACH

The stomach muscles churn up the food to mix it with hydrochloric acid, which starts to break down the food. The acid also kills organisms such as bacteria, while mucus protects the stomach lining from the acid. The dog's stomach is capable of holding four days' nutrition.

SYMPTOMS AND DIAGNOSIS

The most common clinical signs of oesophageal or stomach problems are regurgitation and vomiting. Other signs include difficulty with swallowing and an unusual increase in appetite. It is important to distinguish regurgitation from vomiting; you also need to know whether vomiting comes on suddenly or slowly, and if it is persistent or intermittent. In most cases, it is wise to contact your vet the same day so that the cause of the vomiting can be diagnosed and treated.

REGURGITATION AND VOMITING

Regurgitation occurs when food in the oesophagus is almost effortlessly – and without retching – expelled through the mouth. This sign can be mistaken for vomiting, when food that has passed through the oesophagus into the stomach is forcefully brought up by muscular contractions.

Vomiting may be triggered by a problem that occurs inside or outside the gastrointestinal system (*see box*,

p.274). The different ways in which a dog vomits can give clues to the cause of the underlying condition.

There are three stages to vomiting. Nausea is the first stage, and its signs include: listlessness, shivering, hiding, yawning, lip-smacking, increased salivating, and increased swallowing. Nausea is often followed by retching, during which muscular contractions occur in the stomach but nothing is produced. During the final stage – vomiting – the contents of the stomach are expelled through the mouth and sometimes through the nose.

ACUTE VOMITING

Dogs "cure" themselves of their scavenging indiscretions by vomiting back foods and foreign bodies that should not be in the stomach. Worms may also be removed in this way. Acute vomiting may also result from motion sickness. With an otherwise healthy dog, all you should need to do is withhold food and water for several hours after a single vomiting episode.

INTERMITTENT AND PERSISTENT VOMITING

Intermittent vomiting may be caused by a food allergy but also by more serious conditions such as metabolic diseases, ulcers, or tumours. See your vet within 48 hours if your dog has been vomiting intermittently over a period of several days.

Repeated and persistent vomiting may be caused by a simple stomach irritation or by a life-threatening obstruction. It warrants an immediate veterinary visit for treatment to inhibit vomiting and to determine its cause.

PROJECTILE VOMITING

This forceful type of vomiting is often caused by an obstruction preventing food from leaving the stomach. It may also, however, be caused by a brain condition, so you need to see your vet the same day.

VOMITING BLOOD OR BILE

Vomiting blood suggests an ulceration in the stomach or small intestine, but also poisoning, a foreign object, a tumour, or a serious infection. See your vet the same day.

If your dog vomits bile, a condition called reflux gastritis, the cause may be a mild allergy. Affected dogs often vomit at the same time each day, but are otherwise healthy. The vomiting is usually controlled with an anti-nausea drug such as metoclopramide.

FOOD RESTRICTIONS FOR VOMITING DOGS

Withhold food for 4–24 hours after vomiting stops, depending on the cause and severity of the vomiting but also the age and fitness of the individual. During this period, give small but frequent amounts of water or ice cubes. Soda water may neutralize the build-up of acid in the stomach of a vomiting dog. Powdered electrolyte

TEDDY BEAR IN A DOG'S STOMACH
This X–ray reveals a teddy bear lodged in the stomach of a dog, behind the diaphragm. It is an illustration of the kinds of objects and foreign bodies that a curious dog will inadvertently swallow as it explores the world around it.

VET'S ADVICE

A single episode of vomiting may be unpleasant for you to clean up and unpleasant for your dog, but in the absence of further vomiting or other clinical signs it is usually of little medical significance. The most common reason for a single vomiting episode is to rid the stomach of something that should not have been there in the first place. Whenever possible, check the contents; this action gives you good clues about what your dog has been doing. It there are any foreign objects in the vomit, such as plastic bottle caps, it tells you that your dog is a scavenger and needs to be watched more carefully in future.

solution mixed in drinking water is always beneficial.

When reintroducing food to your dog after the vomiting has subsided, avoid high-fat, high-protein meals. Feed small but frequent amounts of low-fat, low-protein soft food to avoid stretching the stomach and to help facilitate food leaving the stomach and entering the intestines. A good home-made diet is one part low-fat cottage cheese and two parts boiled rice.

DIFFICULTY SWALLOWING (DYSPHAGIA)

Painful conditions that cause regurgitation (foreign objects, strictures, tumours, inflammations) may also cause difficulty swallowing. As pain increases, eating decreases.

DIAGNOSIS AND TREATMENT While X-rays will help in diagnosing a problem, the solution often involves removing something. Endoscopic examination is the treatment of choice.

INCREASED APPETITE

An increased appetite, or polyphagia, is normal in growing pups, pregnant or lactating females, in cold weather, and when dogs have increased exercise or are fed low-calorie diets.

Polyphagia is also associated with the use of several types of drugs, particularly corticosteroids and anticonvulsants, but also diazepam, antihistamines, and progesterone.

Increased appetite is associated with a variety of medical conditions including brain damage, an overactive thyroid gland (*see p.332*), sugar diabetes (*see p.336*), and a variety of conditions affecting the digestive tract, including megaoesophagus (*see p.274*) and pancreas and bowel disorders (*see pp.278–91* and *pp.292–97*).

DIAGNOSTIC AIDS

The most valuable diagnostic aid for examining the oesophagus, or for looking deeper into the digestive tract, is the endoscope. This is either a fixed or a flexible instrument that can be passed into hollow parts of the body. Using an endoscope, a vet can view internal tissues with a light or a tiny video camera and, with the aid of miniature instruments, can carry out surgical procedures within the tissue. Endoscopy is the best way to collect biopsies or remove foreign bodies lodged in the oesophagus.

A gastroscope is an endoscope that is used to explore the internal surface of the stomach. The gastroscope will allow a vet to see what is happening inside the stomach, and, if necessary, to take biopsy samples and even to carry out minor surgery.

Other diagnostic tools include X-rays and imaging techniques such as ultrasound. X-rays, which may be taken after the dog has ingested a contrast material such as barium, are useful both for locating foreign bodies and for showing oesophageal stricture (narrowing).

Q **CAN FOREIGN BODIES IN THE OESOPHAGUS CAUSE PERMANENT DAMAGE?**

A The longer a foreign body sits in the oesophagus, the greater the risk of permanent damage. Peach or nectarine stones, for example, can lodge in the distal oesophagus, near the entrance to the stomach, virtually embedding in the wall. An affected dog can drink and sometimes still eat without vomiting, but the stone will cause intense local inflammation. Even after the stone is removed, a tight stricture of tissue may develop, causing more chronic regurgitation.

Q **IF A STRICTURE DEVELOPS, CAN IT BE TREATED?**

A Strictures can be "treated" but may be difficult to cure. A special endoscope is passed down to the stricture and then inflated. This is called balloon dilatation – the soft balloon breaks down adhesions. More dramatic surgery may also be needed, or drugs such as sucralfate, cimetidine, ranitidine, omeprazole, and cisapride may be prescribed.

Q **CAN OESOPHAGEAL CONDITIONS BE DIAGNOSED WITHOUT AN ENDOSCOPE?**

A Contrast X-rays can be used to make a diagnosis of most oesophageal or stomach problems. A plain X-ray is taken, looking for foreign objects made of metal, stone or other hard material. Barium is then fed by mouth and another X-ray taken immediately to see if any of this contrast material has remained in the oesophagus. It also shows whether the passage is dilated. There are some instances, however, when an endoscope is vital for either a relatively non-invasive diagnosis or treatment.

OESOPHAGEAL PROBLEMS

The most common cause of sudden regurgitation in dogs is a foreign body lodged in the oesophagus. Drooling may occur because the obstruction prevents saliva from being swallowed.

In cases in which regurgitation is chronic, with a slow onset, the most common cause is an enlargement of the oesophagus (*see below*).

Other causes are lead poisoning, myasthenia gravis or other neuro-muscular abnormalities (*see p.370*); botulism; an underactive thyroid (*see p.331*); underactive adrenal gland (*see p.335*); or an immune-mediated disorder called systemic lupus erythematosus.

ENLARGED OESOPHAGUS

When a section of the oesophagus fails to contract properly or is partially blocked by a foreign body, food cannot progress to the stomach. Instead, it collects at the point where the blockage occurs and forces the oesophagus to expand. Known as megaoesophagus, this is the most common condition that causes dogs to regurgitate food immediately after eating.

Megaoesophagus is an inherited condition in some breeds (*see box, right*). The exact cause is rarely found, however. In older dogs it is an aquired condition; myasthenia gravis is a known cause but in most cases, which usually occur when a dog is over seven years old, the cause remains a mystery.

DIAGNOSIS This inherited condition is frequently diagnosed when pups move from milk to solid food. An X-ray confirms it, while blood biochemistry tests help to determine possible causes.

TREATMENT Ideally, the underlying cause is treated. If this is not possible, dogs are treated with frequent feeds of small, high-calorie meals provided on elevated platforms so that gravity assists the food along the oesophagus. Drugs such as metoclopramide are given to try to stimulate peristalsis in the oesophagus.

FOREIGN BODIES

Bones, string, fish hooks, needles, splintered wood, small toys, and even whole bread knives have been found as foreign bodies in the oesophagus. With dogs virtually anything is possible. A foreign body causes sudden gagging, retching, and possibly drooling. Small articles such as wood splinters cause regurgitation and difficulty swallowing for several days. There may be an accompanying fever and cough. Some dogs stand rigid, unwilling to relax.

A foreign body may cause damage to the wall of the oesophagus, creating a tight stricture. Oesophageal stricture usually causes regurgitation and leads to oesophagitis.

DIAGNOSIS AND TREATMENT Foreign bodies may be seen on plain X-rays. With the dog under general anaesthesia a foreign object can be located, seen, and removed with an endoscope and its grasping instrument.

OESOPHAGITIS

The acid contents of the stomach may back up, or reflux, into the oesophagus and cause inflammation known as oesophagitis. This problem may also result from a hiatus hernia, when the stomach protrudes via the diaphragm.

CAUSES OF VOMITING

The most common cause of vomiting is scavenging, a condition politely called a "dietary indiscretion". If food is vomited undigested, the cause of vomiting is likely to be located in the stomach. If the vomit contains yellow bile the problem may be in the intestines. Blood in the vomit may indicate ulcers or erosion to the lining of the digestive system.

DIETARY CAUSES

- Scavenging (dietary indiscretions)
- Overeating
- Food intolerance
- True allergy

DIETARY CAUSES

- Inflammation (gastritis)
- Parasites
- Ulcers
- Foreign bodies
- Tumours
- Bloat (dilatation volvulus)
- Motility problems

INTESTINAL DISORDERS

- Inflammation (inflammatory bowel disease, colitis)
- Parasites
- Foreign bodies
- Tumours
- Infections (parvovirus, distemper)
- Bacterial overgrowth (SIBO)
- Telescoping of intestines (intussusception)
- Constipation

OTHER ABDOMINAL DISORDERS

- Inflamed pancreas (pancreatitis)
- Inflamed peritoneum (peritonitis)
- Abdominal tumours

OTHER DISORDERS

- Kidney failure
- Liver diseases
- Diabetes
- Underactive adrenal gland (hypoadrenocorticism)
- Overactive thyroid gland (hyperthyroidism)
- Blood poisoning (septicaemia, endotoxaemia)
- Electrolyte and acid-base upset
- Anxiety, fears, phobias

FORMS OF POISONING

- Lead
- Antifreeze (ethylene glycol)
- Strychnine
- Heart medications (digitalis)
- NSAIDs
- Chemotherapy drugs
- Some antibiotics

DIAGNOSIS AND TREATMENT Endoscopic examination reveals the inflammation from the reflux. Sucralfate is a common medication for oesophagitis. Surgery may resolve the hernia.

OESOPHAGEAL TUMOURS

Oesophageal tumours, although rare, are usually malignant. Growths caused by the oesophageal worm *Spirocerca lupi*, found only in the southern areas of the United States, are also rare; in time, however, these benign lumps can become malignant fibrosarcomas or carcinomas (*see p.140*).

TREATMENT Tumours are surgically removed, and the worms are treated with anthelmintic drugs.

STOMACH PROBLEMS

Many of the stomach problems that affect dogs cause vomiting as a main clinical sign. The most efficient way to diagnose problems is through the use of X-rays, ultrasound, or gastroscopy. When a gastroscope is not available, exploratory surgery is a valuable but more invasive alternative.

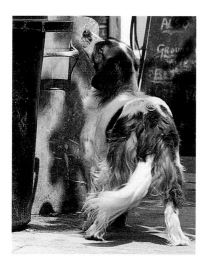

SCAVENGING DOGS
Dogs are persistently curious about the world and are prone to rummaging around in dustbins, which may cause dietary indiscretions and lead to acute gastritis.

ACUTE GASTRITIS

Gastritis is usually caused by dietary indiscretions but also by infections, parasites, and poisons. Affected dogs vomit and go off their food.

DIAGNOSIS AND TREATMENT Diagnosis is usually based on the clinical history and a physical examination. Treatment involves removing any known or obvious cause of the gastritis and also correcting any complications, such as electrolyte imbalances. Feeding the affected dog is restricted.

CHRONIC GASTRITIS

Dogs with chronic gastritis vomit sporadically over a period of time. The problem may be caused by persistently eating grass or by foreign bodies, chemical irritations, or food allergies.

DIAGNOSIS Blood sampling may reveal an increased level of eosinophils, a type of white blood cell that is involved in the immune response to parasites but is also implicated in allergy. If a biopsy obtained by gastroscopy reveals the presence of eosinophils in the wall of the stomach, a diagnosis of eosinophilic gastritis is made.

TREATMENT Treatment may include anti-emetics such as metoclopramide to control further vomiting, and fluid therapy. Corticosteroids are used in cases of eosinophilic gastritis. Anti-ulcer drugs, such as cimetidine and ranitidine, and protectors of the mucous lining of the stomach, such as sucralfate and misoprostol, work in dogs as they do in people.

ULCERS

The most common cause of stomach ulcers is drugs: corticosteroids and nonsteroidal anti-inflammatory drugs (NSAIDs). Shock, stress, severe illness, and allergy may also cause ulcers.

Dogs suffering from ulcers vomit intermittently, appear unhappy, and lose weight. Fresh or old blood may appear in the vomit. The stools may be black (melaenic) due to blood passed from the stomach or duodenum.

BREEDS AT RISK

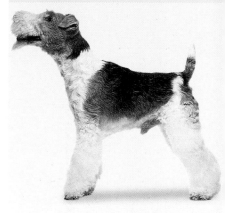

Megaoesophagus is a rare condition. It is a known inherited trait in certain lines of Miniature Schnauzers and Fox Terriers (above). The most common cause of megaoesophagus, however, is acquired damage as a consequence of a foreign body in the oesophagus.

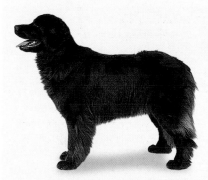

Megaoesophagus also occurs with increased incidence in the following breeds:

- German Shepherd Dog
- Great Dane
- Irish Setter
- Labrador Retriever
- Newfoundland (above)
- Shar Pei

Q DO DOGS SUFFER, AS WE DO, FROM ULCERS CAUSED BY HELICOBACTER BACTERIA?

A The bacterium *Helicobacter pylori*, which has been implicated in human stomach ulcers, does not occur in dogs, although *Helicobacter heilmannii* does. This bacterium is found during some gastroscopic examinations but it is not thought to be associated with any canine gastric problems.

Q CAN DOGS SUFFER FROM STOMACH ULCERS CAUSED BY WORRY?

A Unpleasant (and what today would be unethical) and unacceptable experiments carried out over 60 years ago on a variety of animals showed that chronic stress induces stomach ulcers in many different mammals. A little stress is good for dogs, as it is for us, but chronic stress can lead to stomach ulcers. Fortunately, drugs such as omeprazole, developed to treat our stress-related stomach ulcers, are equally effective in dogs. The fact that no drug company at this time has applied for a veterinary product licence for any of these safe and effective "H2 antagonist" drugs is a good indication of how infrequently the condition occurs in canines.

Q WHY DO NSAIDS INCREASE THE RISK OF STOMACH ULCERATION?

A Each species has its own idiosyncratic reaction to medications. Dogs' stomachs are more sensitive to NSAIDs than are human stomachs. This is why NSAIDs such as carprofen, meloxicam, and ketoprofen have been developed specifically for veterinary use. These drugs are potentially less irritating than drugs such as ibuprofen, licensed for human use.

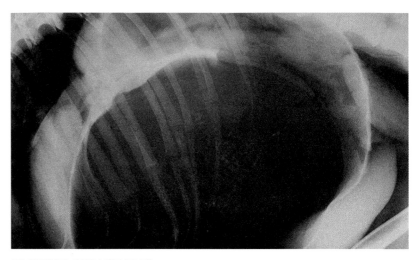

DILATATION AND VOLVULUS
This X-ray shows the (black) air-filled stomach dilated under the ribcage, pushing the liver, to the left, against the diaphragm. The (white) spleen at the bottom right is swollen. These changes lead to rapidly developing, life-threatening clinical shock.

An unusual cause of stomach ulcers comes from the presence of mast cell tumours on the skin. These tumours release large quantities of histamine, which, in turn, triggers hydrochloric acid secretion in the stomach. Any dog with several mast cell tumours should be assumed to be at risk from stomach and duodenal ulcers.

DIAGNOSIS The most accurate way to diagnose the presence of ulcers in the stomach is through the use of gastroscopy. Contrast X-rays and ultrasound may also help.

TREATMENT The cause of the ulcer needs to be eliminated. Severe anaemia due to blood loss is treated with a blood replacer and a combination of drugs is administered to protect the mucous lining of the stomach and to enhance tissue repair. Medication continues until gastroscopy shows that all ulcers have healed.

ADVICE Dogs are more sensitive than humans to the ulcer-inducing capacity of non-steroidal anti-inflammatory drugs (NSAIDs). Only give NSAIDs that have been licensed for veterinary use; these drugs are safer for dogs than many NSAIDs licensed for people.

OBSTRUCTIONS

Various obstructions are caused by foreign bodies, tumours, and scarring, or by contractions around the pyloric canal (where food moves from the stomach into the duodenum). Affected dogs vomit, lose weight, and often appear uncomfortable.

DIAGNOSIS AND TREATMENT Contrast X-rays show little or no emptying of stomach contents into the duodenum. Ultrasound may show an enlarged, fluid-filled stomach. Gastroscopy reveals the exact cause of obstruction. A surgical correction is usually needed.

MOTILITY DISORDERS

The stomach may empty its contents into the intestines too quickly or too slowly. Delayed emptying is a common cause of vomiting and loss of appetite.

DIAGNOSIS AND TREATMENT When the exact cause of delayed emptying is unknown, dogs are treated according to their clinical signs. Metoclopramide inhibits vomiting, while cisapride stimulates emptying of the stomach. Easily digested food (one part low-fat cottage cheese to two parts boiled rice) is fed frequently in small quantities.

POLYPS AND TUMOURS

Stomach polyps are fairly common but are usually benign. Malignant tumours, such as adenocarcinomas and lymphosarcomas, are rare but do occur. Affected dogs show signs of foreign bodies, ulceration, or obstruction.

DIAGNOSIS AND TREATMENT Viewing the stomach with a gastroscope yields the most accurate diagnosis. Surgical removal of the part of the stomach containing the tumour is effective for benign tumours. The outlook for malignant tumours is very poor.

BLOAT (DILATATION VOLVULUS)

Bloat (dilatation) followed by stomach rotation (volvulus) is a life-threatening condition. Partial or complete rotation prevents food from entering or leaving the stomach. The abdomen swells. The affected dog may drool, retch, wander restlessly, become listless, or show signs of pain. Symptoms of shock quickly develop (see p.388).

Bloat is an acute condition with a high fatality rate even for dogs that receive immediate medical attention. Early diagnosis and swift surgical intervention, combined with aggressive medical therapy increases the chances of survival. This condition, however, is as serious as it gets.

DIAGNOSIS X-rays confirm diagnosis. The dog may be just uncomfortable or may be in advanced, life-threatening shock. Reducing pressure inside the stomach is vital. If a tube cannot be passed down the oesophagus into the stomach, your vet will insert a large-diameter needle through the abdominal wall directly into the stomach.

TREATMENT Emergency therapy with fluids, corticosteroids, antibiotics, drugs to control related heart arrhythmias, and drugs to limit the release of large quantities of tissue-damaging free radicals starts immediately.

At the same time, surgery is used to rotate the stomach back and to secure it down into its normal position. The spleen, because it acts as a pendulum and is often damaged by a gastric rotation, is usually (although probably needlessly) removed.

PREVENTION If you have a dog that is known to be at risk of bloat (see box, right), you can take steps to prevent the problem. Limit water consumption for an hour before or after each meal. Do not allow the dog to drain the bowl of its contents: water should be consumed in moderate quantities. Do not allow rolling or other exercise after meals. Dividing food into small meals has not been shown to reduce the risk of further bloating.

BREEDS AT RISK

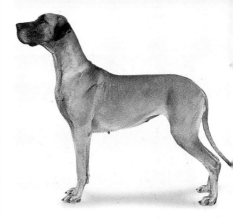

The risk of bloat runs in families. Middle-sized, large, or giant breeds with deep, narrow chests are most at risk from this condition.

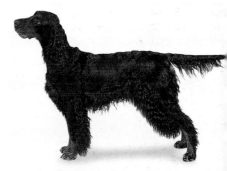

Breeds at risk of bloat include:

- Doberman
- Gordon Setter (above)
- Great Dane (top)
- Irish Setter
- Irish Wolfhound
- Standard Poodle
- Weimaraner

VET'S ADVICE

The drug metoclopramide is an excellent anti-emetic but in some individuals, particularly Yorkshire Terriers, it may cause temporary behaviour changes, including restlessness, hyperactivity, and frenetic behaviour. While disturbing to watch, the effects wear off within a few hours. If your dog has an adverse reaction to metoclopramide, keep it away from stimulations such as light and sound. Phone your vet and report what is happening.

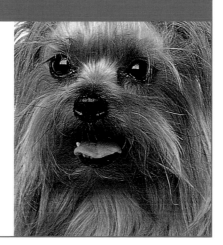

DAMAGED MUCOSAL VILLI

The villi lining the mucosa (inner surface) of the small intestine can be damaged by infections such as parvovirus. They become stunted and are less able to absorb nutrients, and this problem leads to malabsorption (*see below*).

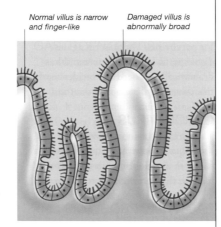

Normal villus is narrow and finger-like

Damaged villus is abnormally broad

STUNTED VILLUS
Compared with normal villi, damaged villi are shorter and broader. As a result, the overall surface area for absorption of nutrients is reduced.

Q **WHAT IS THE DIFFERENCE BETWEEN COLITIS AND INFLAMMATORY BOWEL DISEASE?**

A Colitis is an inflammation of the colon (the largest part of the large intestine) and is the cause of over half of all cases of chronic diarrhoea. Inflammatory bowel disease (IBD) is any of a group of diseases, each characterized by an increase in a specific type of inflammatory cell in the large or small intestine, and is a possible cause of colitis. IBD can only be diagnosed by a vet examining a biopsy specimen and finding these characteristic inflammatory cells.

Q **CAN STRESS CAUSE DIARRHOEA IN DOGS?**

A Many vets believe that dogs can suffer from stress-induced acute diarrhoea, sometimes called "nervous colitis", "spastic colitis", or "irritable bowel syndrome". This may be a motility disorder (one that affects muscle action in the intestine) triggered by anxiety.

called a protein-losing enteropathy, or PLE. It is a life-threatening condition. There is a net loss of body protein, leading to vomiting and diarrhoea but also to fluid build-up under the skin (oedema) or in the abdomen (ascites). PLE may be caused by intestinal infection, inflammation, a tumour, parasites, or bleeding. Treatment depends on eliminating the underlying cause of the disease.

MALABSORPTION SYNDROME

In malabsorption, the intestines either cannot digest food or cannot absorb the nutrients from it. The syndrome is not a disease but is the consequence of a small intestine or digestive enzyme (pancreatic) disorder. Malabsorption is most often caused by damage to the villi of the small intestine; this damage may result from food sensitivity or from parasitic, bacterial, or viral infection, especially parvovirus (*see p.145*). It may also be due to inflammatory bowel disease (*see right*) or exocrine pancreas insufficiency (*see p.294*). Dogs suffering from malabsorption look malnourished, although they eat voraciously. Their stools are large,

greasy, and smelly. Because fat is not digested but instead passes through the entire digestive tract, the hair around the dog's anus may be oily.

DIAGNOSIS AND TREATMENT
Malabsorption syndrome is generally diagnosed by a vet after examining the affected dog and blood testing for the vitamins B12 (cobalamin) and folic acid. A biopsy of the lining of the small intestine is often needed to determine an exact cause. Treatments are appropriate for the specific cause of malabsorption, but usually involve dietary management.

FOOD ALLERGIES

Signs of food allergies sometimes involve the digestive tract, sometimes appear on the skin, and sometimes affect both areas. Gastrointestinal signs include vomiting (of stomach contents or blood), diarrhoea, abdominal pain (colic), and changes in appetite. More general signs include lethargy and weight loss. Skin signs include itchiness, self-inflicted skin damage, scaly or inflamed skin, pimples leading to secondary infection, and inflammation within the ear canal (otitis externa).

DIAGNOSIS AND TREATMENT To identify a food allergy, the vet may arrange for your dog to be fed a diet consisting of foods that the dog has never eaten before, for at least three weeks. If the dog's stools return to normal but diarrhoea returns when the old diet is fed, this confirms the diagnosis. To prevent a recurrence, the dog will need a hypoallergenic diet (*see below*).

INFLAMMATORY BOWEL DISEASE (IBD)

Inflammatory bowel disease (IBD) is a group of diseases causing inflammation of the intestinal lining and resulting in malabsorption. Each disease is defined by a specific type of inflammatory cell found in the lining of the intestines and involved in that disorder (*see p.286*). Affected dogs have chronic diarrhoea, pass stools more frequently, experience

CAUSES OF BLACK, TARRY STOOLS (MELAENA)

Black, tarry, sticky stools indicate that bleeding is occurring in the gastrointestinal tract. Some main causes are listed below. Melaena is not a disease but rather a sign of disease. Effective treatment involves finding and eliminating the cause of bleeding.

CATEGORY	SPECIFIC CAUSES
Swallowed blood	Injury or disease in the nose, mouth, or oesophagus
Bleeding in the stomach or intestines	Stomach or intestinal inflammation, ulcers, tumours, or presence of hookworms or whipworms
Internal bleeding caused by ingestion of drugs or poisons	Nonsteroidal anti-inflammatory drugs (NSAIDs), corticosteroid drugs, warfarin
Internal bleeding caused by foreign body	Swallowed foreign objects such as toys, peach stones, pebbles, or small bones

pain when they pass stools, lose weight, look malnourished, and are often anaemic.

DIAGNOSIS AND TREATMENT Diagnosis is by endoscopic examination of the intestine and examination of a biopsy specimen. The types of cells involved suggest that IBD is an immune-mediated disease and that food allergy should always be considered part of the problem. An affected dog should be fed a "hypoallergenic" diet, which does not contain proteins, carbohydrates, or fats that the intestinal immune system may class as "foreign". Several dog food manufacturers produce these

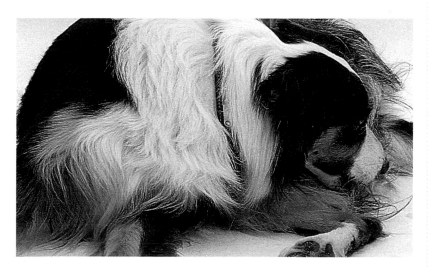

LICKING THE REAR END
This behaviour may be due to worms, particularly tapeworms, but more commonly results from anal sac discomfort. Licking empties the sacs, resulting in relief for the dog but a very unpleasant smell for anyone nearby. Open perianal tumours and injuries also induce licking.

BREEDS AT RISK

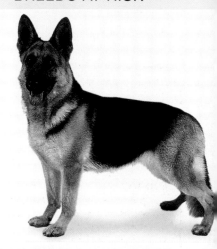

The world's most popular breed, the German Shepherd Dog (above) also has probably the highest incidence of bowel disorders. A variety of malabsorption problems affect the breed, especially small intestinal bacterial overgrowth (SIBO), inflammatory bowel disease, and exocrine pancreatic insufficiency.

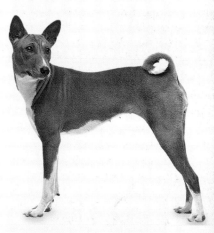

Breeds prone to protein-losing enteropathy include:

- Basenji (above)
- Shar Pei
- Soft-coated Wheaten Terrier
- Yorkshire Terrier
- Norwegian Lundehund

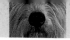

Q **CAN DRINKING MILK CAUSE DIARRHOEA IN DOGS?**

A Any change in diet may potentially cause diarrhoea. Milk, in particular, may cause diarrhoea in adult dogs because, unlike pups, they no longer produce sufficient amounts of the enzyme lactase, which breaks down milk. If your dog likes milk but suffers from diarrhoea when drinking it, try giving lactose-free milk, which is available in supermarkets for lactose-sensitive people.

Q **WHAT DO THE LETTERS "SIBO" MEAN?**

A SIBO stands for "small intestine bowel overgrowth". It is a specific condition in which, for a variety of reasons, a pure culture of bacteria increases and displaces other beneficial bacteria in the intestine. There is a dramatic increase in the number of bacteria in the small intestine, and this interferes with normal absorption of nutrients. The result is chronic intermittent diarrhoea and weight loss or failure to gain weight. SIBO is most often seen in German Shepherd Dogs, but can affect other breeds as well. It may develop in association with exocrine pancreatic insufficiency, and may also be seen with inflammatory bowel disease, although vets are not always able to determine which came first.

Q **WHAT IS MEANT BY GLUTEN-SENSITIVE DIARRHOEA?**

A This condition is a sensitivity to a wheat protein called gluten. It occurs in some lines of Irish Setters, but is otherwise rare. Gluten-sensitive diarrhoea is treated with metronidazole and by feeding the dog a gluten-free diet.

diets. Rice is a preferred carbohydrate because it is highly digestible. Potato, corn, and tapioca are all gluten-free.

Immunosuppressant drugs such as corticosteroids are routinely used to treat IBD. Anti-inflammatory drugs such as sulphasalazine are used when inflammation is restricted to one part of the colon. Increasing the amount of fibre in the diet improves stool consistency and colon motility (muscle action), and supports the growth of intestinal bacteria that aid digestion.

CONSTIPATION

A constipated dog passes only small amounts of faeces, tries to defaecate but is unsuccessful, or does not even try. A vet will diagnose the condition by physical examination. He or she is able to feel a full colon through the abdominal wall or by a digital rectal examination. Treatment depends on the cause. Specific known causes are eliminated. Blockages are broken down using laxatives and enemas.

AGE-RELATED CONSTIPATION

Many old or middle-aged dogs are prone to constipation. A common predisposing cause is that the dog does not drink enough water.

TREATMENT To treat age-related constipation, soak dry food in an equal volume of water and leave it for 20 minutes for the water to be fully absorbed. This increases the dog's fluid consumption. Use an osmotic laxative such as lactulose or a stimulant laxative such as senna, as instructed by your vet, or add a little cow's milk to the diet, because this may act as a natural laxative. Let your dog out frequently, to give it more chances to defaecate. Your vet may administer an enema: do not try to give your dog an enema yourself. Common phosphate (Fleet) enemas may be toxic for a small dog's kidneys.

PREVENTION Prevent your dog from eating undigestible material such as grass. Provide routine exercise, a digestible diet, and plenty of water.

TYPES OF INFLAMMATORY BOWEL DISEASE

Inflammatory bowel disease (IBD) is perhaps the most common cause of chronic vomiting and diarrhoea in dogs. There are several different types, each of which characterized by an increase in a specific type of inflammatory cell found in the intestines. The various types and their treatment are listed below. Dog breeds that are prone to developing inflammatory bowel disease include the Basenji, Shar Pei, and German Shepherd Dog (lymphocytic-plasmocytic colitis) and the Boxer (histiocytic ulcerative colitis).

TYPE	TREATMENT
Lymphocytic-plasmocytic colitis	Hypoallergenic diet, antibiotics, corticosteroids
Eosinophilic colitis	Parasite control, corticosteroids
Granulomatous enteritis	Corticosteroids, metronidazole
Neutrophilic colitis	Antibiotics, corticosteroids
Histiocytic ulcerative colitis	Hypoallergenic diet, antibiotics, corticosteroids

Consider feeding a commercially prepared diet for older dogs that contains added fibre, or feed a high-fibre diet available through your vet. Alternatively, add bulk laxatives, such as unprocessed wheat bran or a dietary fibre supplement, to your dog's food (one to five teaspoons daily).

Liquid paraffin (mineral oil) is an effective preventative but can be dangerous. Never give it directly by mouth: because it is tasteless, there is a risk that it may get into the windpipe. Instead, mix it in once or twice a week with your dog's food, using one tablespoon for every 30 kg (65 lb) of the dog's weight. Do not use mineral oil more frequently than this because it can interfere with the intestinal absorption of fat-soluble vitamins.

OTHER INTESTINAL CONDITIONS

Certain other conditions may partially or completely block the intestines or may stimulate excess gas production.

INTESTINAL OBSTRUCTION

Dogs foolishly swallow things, some of which are not digestible and form blockages. These include toys, bones, pebbles, fruit stones, pieces of corn cob, fabric, food wrappers, and just about anything else they come across. Small items usually pass through uneventfully, although accompanied by soft stools or diarrhoea. Foreign objects that have left the stomach but lodged in the first part of the intestine usually cause vomiting; if the pancreas is disturbed, there will also be pain. Other items stop at the junction between the small and large intestines.

Foreign bodies with string attached are particularly damaging. The object can anchor in one location and the extended string acts as a saw in the intestines, eventually breaking through the intestinal wall and producing life-threatening peritonitis (inflammation of the membrane lining the abdomen).

CAUSES OF CONSTIPATION

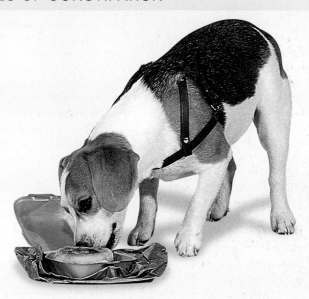

Some of the most common causes of constipation in dogs are listed below. One of the most common causes is the dog simply not taking in enough fluids. If a dog is just mildly dehydrated, water is drawn into the bloodstream from the colon, and this process dries and hardens the faeces.

DIET

- Eating grass or plant material, hair, rubbish, and other indigestible materials
- Not drinking enough fluids

DRUG-INDUCED

- Antihistamines (e.g. chlorpheniramine)
- Antacids (e.g. aluminium hydroxide)
- Diuretics (e.g. frusemide)
- Anticancer drugs (e.g. vincristine)
- Kaolin-pectin

PAIN

- Injury to the hips, pelvis, or spine
- Wounds or infections around the anus
- Impacted or infected anal sacs

DEHYDRATION

- Problems associated with any fluid or electrolyte imbalance

NEUROLOGICAL

- Spinal cord diseases
- Megacolon
- Pelvic nerve damage

ENVIRONMENT

- Changes in routines, such as a home change or hospitalization
- Unusual inactivity
- Lack of an acceptable toileting site

OBSTRUCTION

- Perineal hernia (a type of hernia affecting the anus and rectum)
- Strictures
- Foreign bodies
- Enlarged prostate gland in males
- Tumours
- Pelvic fractures

OTHER

- Hypothyroidism

The small intestine can telescope into the large intestine, causing a total blockage called an intussusception. This situation, occurs particularly in pups, is extremely damaging to the telescoped tissue, and clinical shock will develop.

Tumours are another, uncommon cause of obstruction. Initially, they can lead to decreased motility of the intestines (a condition called ileus).

DIAGNOSIS Intestinal obstructions, including intussusceptions, can often be felt through the abdominal wall, especially in pups and young dogs. Plain or contrast X-rays are useful in fat dogs or for partial obstructions. Partial obstructions can be difficult to diagnose even with contrast X-rays.

TREATMENT Surgery is usually needed to remove a foreign body. If there is a tumour, the lungs and liver are X-rayed to see whether any secondary tumours are present before surgery is performed.

MEGACOLON

A permanent distension of the colon, called megacolon, is very uncommon in dogs. When it does occur, it is most often as a result of chronic constipation. Treatments include the use of stool softeners and dietary fibre.

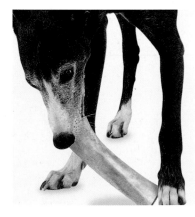

BONES AND CONSTIPATION
Pieces of bone can cause intestinal blockages. In addition, too high a level of bone in the diet can cause the stools to become solid and lead to constipation.

BURPING AND FLATULENCE

The passage of gas from the stomach (burping) or from the anus (flatulence) are quite common when a dog has been eating highly fermentable foods, such as soya (tofu), or undigestible carbohydrate, as in raw vegetables. Flatulence can also occur with all forms of malabsorption.

Several types of gas are produced in the intestinal tract, but the big stinker is hydrogen sulphide. Nuts, and vegetables such as broccoli, cabbage, cauliflower, mustard, radishes, and turnips, can all increase hydrogen sulphide production in the intestines. This chemical is also about as toxic as cyanide, and there is some evidence that it may be a factor in ulcerative colitis – a serious intestinal disease of humans and dogs.

DIAGNOSIS AND TREATMENT Underlying conditions that cause malabsorption are treated. For fast eaters, feed several small meals of easily digestible, low-fibre food daily. Adding some activated charcoal, or the over-the-counter product simethicone, to your dog's food may significantly reduce the odour of the gas produced.

RECTAL AND ANAL CONDITIONS

The rectum and anus form the final part of the gastrointestinal tract. They are prone to a number of specific and quite common conditions.

PERINEAL HERNIA

A perineal hernia is a peritoneum-lined sac that protrudes through weakened muscles on either side of the anus. This type of hernia usually occurs in older male dogs. The presence of the sac allows the rectum to balloon out into the hernia. This leads to visible bulging beside the anus and to constipation.

DIAGNOSIS A vet usually diagnoses the condition by means of a digital rectal examination. A barium enema confirms the diagnosis.

TREATMENT Surgical correction, combined with neutering (spaying or castration), is the most effective treatment. After surgery, stool softeners and a low-residue diet help normal bowel evacuation.

RECTAL AND ANAL OBSTRUCTIONS

The most common cause of rectal obstruction in male dogs is an enlarged prostate. Other causes of obstruction include constipation or interference from a perineal hernia (*see above*). Stool accumulates in the hernia, diverting it to the left or right.

DIAGNOSIS A digital rectal examination (physical examination using a finger) will usually enable a vet to make this diagnosis. Endoscopic examination of the rectum (proctoscopy) or X-ray imaging may also be necessary.

TREATMENT The objective of treatment is to remove the obstruction. Dogs with enlarged prostates are given drugs to shrink the prostate or, preferably, are neutered (castrated). Perineal hernias are surgically repaired; because the development of the hernia is related to sex hormones, neutering is usually carried out at the same time.

RECTAL POLYPS AND TUMOURS

After the mouth, the colon is the most usual site in the digestive tract for tumours to develop. The most common types of digestive tract tumour are adenocarcinomas and lymphomas. Fortunately, both are uncommon. Rectal polyps (adenomas) are also uncommon, but they account for half of all growths in the rectum or the colon. Tumours occur predominantly in older individuals.

DIAGNOSIS AND TREATMENT A vet will diagnose the presence of rectal polyps or a tumour by physical examination, endoscopy, and biopsy. Benign polyps are surgically removed. Tumours are also usually surgically removed; in addition, lymphomas may be treated

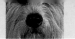

ADDING CHARCOAL TO FOOD

If your dog is flatulent and produces some noxious smells, you might think about adding charcoal to its diet. This will absorb some of the bad-smelling gases produced in its intestines (such as hydrogen sulphide). Activated charcoal is sold over the counter at most pet stores. If you wish to give your dog charcoal, take the following steps:

• Ask your vet's opinion first.

• Do not give it for more than two or three days at a time, because as well as absorbing noxious gases, it may also absorb nutrients, robbing your dog of essential vitamins and minerals.

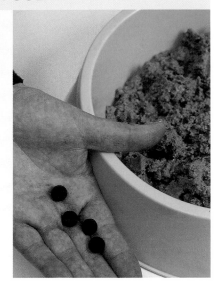

with anticancer drugs. Local surgical excision of lymphomas results in an average survival time of between six and 12 months.

RECTAL PROLAPSE

Forceful straining may cause the rectum to protrude from the anus. This problem is most common in pups under four months of age and in small dogs with associated severe diarrhoea. Other causes of rectal prolapse include straining due to constipation, intestinal blockage, bladder obstruction, and giving birth. If only the lining of the rectum (mucosa) prolapses, a swollen, doughnut-shaped, red ring of tissue protrudes from the anus. Some owners mistake this tissue for haemorrhoids. In a complete rectal prolapse, a small, sausage-shaped piece of red tissue extends from the anus.

DIAGNOSIS AND TREATMENT A mucosal prolapse is less severe than a complete rectal prolapse. The underlying cause is removed. A local anaesthetic and a lubricant are applied to the mucosa. The dog is fed a low-residue diet.

Complete prolapse requires urgent attention. Keep it moist with water-soluble jelly. Your vet will insert a temporary purse-string suture to hold the rectum back in its normal position. Further surgery may be necessary.

PERIANAL SKIN DISEASE

Repeated bouts of diarrhoea, especially in pups, can lead to inflammation around the anus. Other causes of inflammation are dragging the bottom

VET'S ADVICE

Some dogs, Yorkshire Terriers in particular, suffer from pieces of passed stool sticking to the long hair around the anus. This causes painful contact irritation and inflammation to the anal region. The dog acts as if it is constipated – scooting, failing to find a comfortable position, and sometimes whining. To deal with this problem, carefully clip the matted hair and faeces from the region. Apply a topical antibiotic/anti-inflammatory cream or ointment.

Q MY DOG IS FAECALLY INCONTINENT. WHAT ARE THE POSSIBLE CAUSES?

A Loss of control over bowel movements has a very wide range of possible causes. These include aging, inflammation, tumours or injuries to the large intestine, constipation or diarrhoea, perianal fistulas, and anal damage from surgical intervention. A range of nerve conditions may also cause loss of bowel control, including spinal cord damage, loss of anal sphincter control, and infections or tumours leading to nerve damage. See your vet to have the cause of your dog's problem investigated.

Q WHAT IS MEANT BY THE TERM "ILEUS"?

A The intestines do not like being irritated, either by conditions that cause inflammation or by being harshly handled during surgery. A common response is for the intestines to "go quiet", to stop peristaltic movement. They act as if there is an obstruction, but there is none. This condition is called ileus. Diseases such as parvovirus and pancreatitis (inflammation of the pancreas) can cause ileus. Very rarely, just touching the intestines during routine surgery may cause this condition.

Q MY DOG SEEMS TO HAVE FLUID COLLECTING IN ITS ABDOMEN. WHAT COULD BE THE CAUSE?

A This problem, called ascites, has a number of possible causes. They include heart failure; liver disease; severe malabsorption; severe intestinal or pancreatic disease; bowel perforation; a ruptured lymphatic duct; ruptured bladder; and internal bleeding. See your vet immediately.

(scooting) on rough surfaces and irritation from tapeworm segments. Skin allergies may also manifest itself in this region.

DIAGNOSIS AND TREATMENT Eliminating the cause of irritation usually results in an improvement in this condition. Topical antibiotic/anti-inflammatory lotions may need to be used.

PERIANAL TUMOURS AND PERIANAL ADENOMA

These growths are very common benign tumours seen in older male dogs. Cocker Spaniels and Beagles have a higher incidence than some other breeds. Rarely, a dog develops a malignant form called a perianal adenocarcinoma. These growths are usually first seen on a routine annual veterinary examination. If a tumour has already ruptured, the dog will lick the bleeding open wound. Other dogs will take a greater than normal interest in the affected dog's bottom. Perianal adenomas can occur anywhere in the tissue surrounding the anus.

DIAGNOSIS AND TREATMENT The tumours are diagnosed on visual inspection. They usually need male hormone (testosterone)to grow; for some reason, neutering (castration) at the same time that the tumours are removed is by far the most effective treatment. Drugs such as delmadinone may be used to shrink the tumours temporarily. Medical management is useful when surgery is not possible. Microscopic examination of a sample of the removed tumour will confirm that it is either an adenoma or the more dangerous adenocarcinoma. If adenocarcinoma is revealed, surgery is followed by radiation therapy.

ANAL SAC CONDITIONS

The anal sacs are part of a dog's territory-marking apparatus. Each time a dog passes a stool, it anoints the faeces with a few drops of a substance produced within the sacs. Other dogs

ANAL SACS

The anal sacs are situated on either side of the anus. They contain a cocktail of smelly fatty acids, each of which has a specific role in communication between dogs. After a dog defaecates, muscles around the anus squeeze drops of the fluid on to the stool. The smell of this substance is what primarily interests dogs when they sniff other dogs' droppings.

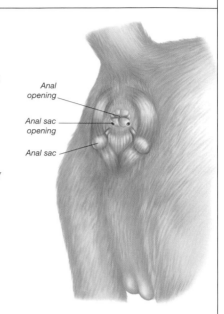

Anal opening

Anal sac opening

Anal sac

LOCATION OF SACS

If you raise your dog's tail to the "flagpole" position, the anal sacs are located under the skin at the "four and eight o'clock" positions.

come along and sniff this material. It is like reading the daily paper.

Estimates about the incidence of anal sac problems vary; while veterinary schools report an incidence of 12 per cent in the general dog population, vets in general practice see a higher incidence. The most common sign is increased licking or scooting. Some affected dogs simply jump up from a resting position as if they have been startled or felt a sudden pain.

BLOCKED ANAL SACS

Anal glands are most likely to become blocked if the stools are soft, because the contents will not be squeezed out.

DIAGNOSIS AND TREATMENT

Uncomplicated blocked anal sacs are diagnosed by squeezing the sacs to feel if they are full. They can be emptied by external or internal pressure. Some dogs need to have their anal sacs emptied frequently – as often as every month. Your vet can do this, or you can do this at home if you are willing and your dog is not overweight.

First, put on disposable latex or plastic gloves. Raise your dog's tail to the flagpole position, which causes the anus, and the anal sacs, to protrude (see box, above). Next, place your fingers on either side of the anus, at the "four and eight o'clock" positions. You will feel two lumps like single grapes if the anal sacs are full. Gently but firmly squeeze each sac with your thumb and forefinger, milking upwards and outwards. Your fingers will be at "three and nine o'clock" when they complete their squeezing action. The anal secretions will be discharged on to your glove and may drip on to the floor. Wipe the secretions from the anus with cotton wool, then clean the area with damp tissue. Only empty the anal sacs if they need emptying. Always give your dog a food treat immediately afterwards for allowing you to do something so intimidating.

If your dog's anatomy prevents external emptying, visit your vet, who will empty them by pressing from inside and outside the anus. You should always contact your vet if the anal sacs are blocked or if the substance secreted is overwhelmingly smelly, yellow, green, or blood-tinged.

INFECTED ANAL SACS

Anal sac infection (anal sacculitis) causes a painful swelling on the affected side, to the left or right of the anus. Usually only one side is affected.

DIAGNOSIS Gently squeezing the anal sac produces repellent, purulent (pus-filled) material that is yellow, green, or blood-tinged. A bacterial culture and an antibiotic sensitivity test are usually undertaken.

TREATMENT Infection is treated by flushing the sac with an appropriate antiseptic or antibiotic while the dog is deeply sedated or anaesthetized.

ANAL SAC ABSCESS

If the anal sac canal (leading from the sac to the mucosal lining just inside the anus) is blocked, the sac may swell and burst through the skin on either side of the anus, producing a draining abscess. The painful swelling is initially red; it becomes purple just before rupturing. Rupture of the abscess reduces pain.

DIAGNOSIS AND TREATMENT If an abscess has not already ruptured it is treated by being lanced (cut open), often under general anaesthesia. The abscess and sac are flushed with a solution containing an antiseptic or antibiotic. Oral antibiotics and pain control medication are also given. In rare circumstances, surgical removal of the anal sacs is necessary.

PERIANAL FISTULA/ANAL FURUNCULOSIS

In this condition, ulcerating, bleeding, painful tracts of infection, from which a smelly fluid drains, develop in the tissue surrounding the anus. Perianal fistula/anal furunculosis may not in itself be very painful, but dogs with this condition often have inflammatory bowel disease as well, which does cause pain.

DIAGNOSIS AND TREATMENT Simply lifting an affected dog's tail can be very painful. Pain control and sedation are useful to help with a diagnosis, which is usually made when a vet visually inspects the region.

Surgical correction is sometimes necessary, and long-term treatment with corticosteroid drugs or the immunosuppressant drug cyclosporin is effective. Recurrences are common but can be contained with further medical management.

PERITONITIS

Peritonitis is not a disorder but a serious condition in which the lining of the abdominal cavity becomes inflamed. It occurs when any irritating or infectious substance, such as urine, bile, blood, digestive enzymes, bacteria, or the contents of the intestines, leaks into the abdominal cavity. The leakage may be caused by penetrating wounds; rupture of organs such as the bladder; perforations from foreign bodies or ulcers in the stomach or intestines; bleeding from tumours or injuries; bloat; acute inflammation of the pancreas (pancreatitis); or suture breakdown after surgery. Peritonitis is extremely painful. Dogs are listless and often reluctant to move. Some groan. Others vomit. Most affected dogs collapse from shock.

DIAGNOSIS AND TREATMENT A vet will usually diagnose the condition simply by examining the dog. When the peritonitis is localized, X-rays may be useful in locating the site.

Affected dogs are treated for shock and dehydration with intravenous fluids, antibiotics, and corticosteroids. An exploratory operation is performed to find and repair the source of the peritonitis. All unwanted material is removed, and the abdominal cavity is flushed with a solution containing an antibiotic. Part of the incision may be left open to drain further infected material and then closed at a later date.

BREEDS AT RISK

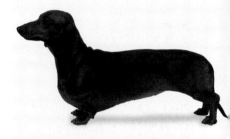

Breeds prone to anal sac problems include:

- Dachshunds (above)
- Retrievers
- Spaniels

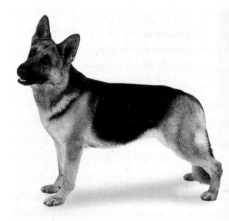

Perianal fistula and anal furunculosis are rare except in the following breeds:

- German Shepherd Dog (above)
- Irish Setter

PANCREAS AND LIVER
vital support for digestion

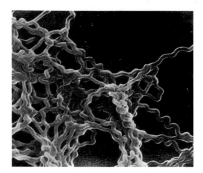

Leptospiral organisms

Food is mechanically digested in the stomach, then it passes into the duodenum (the first part of the small intestine), where chemical digestion takes place. This process depends on a supply of enzymes, which break down food into substances that the body cells can use. Most of these enzymes are manufactured in the pancreas. The liver is also vital for digestion; it produces bile, which helps to break down fat so that it can be absorbed by the body. In addition to helping with digestion, the liver removes toxins from the bloodstream.

The liver has several vital functions. It stores nutrients, detoxifies the blood, and helps to regulate circulation and body temperature. In particular, it makes bile, a liquid that is necessary for fat digestion in the intestines. Bile is stored in the gall bladder and enters the duodenum via the bile duct.

Medical conditions develop if the liver cannot carry out a particular task. Some disorders develop because the liver cannot store a certain nutrient effectively, as in copper storage disease. In others, the liver loses its ability to break down harmful products from microbes or man-made substances such as drugs. Digestion problems occur when bile does not circulate properly.

The liver may also suffer physical damage. Circulatory diseases may cause it to swell and leak fluid into the abdominal cavity. The liver has an excellent ability to repair itself after acute inflammation; however, chronic inflammation leads to cirrhosis, a condition in which repeated repairs lead to a build-up of scar tissue.

The pancreas secretes powerful enzymes that break down protein, fat, and carbohydrate. A lack of these enzymes leads to poor digestion and malabsorption conditions. The enzymes should seep through the pancreatic duct directly into the small intestine; if they escape into any other areas, they cause intense, painful inflammation.

In addition to its digestive function, the pancreas secretes various hormones, including insulin, into the bloodstream. This function is covered in disorders of the hormonal system (*see pp.336–38*).

DISEASES OF THE PANCREAS AND LIVER

Not all pancreas and liver conditions occur on their own; your dog may have two or more of them concurrently. All of these diseases require veterinary treatment for the complete control or elimination of problems.

BLOOD VESSELS FROM LIVER TO HEART

Nutrient-rich blood from the intestines travels via the portal vein to the liver, where it is cleansed of toxins. The blood then leaves the liver via the hepatic vein, and travels to the heart via the vena cava. If blood is not cleansed, toxins can circulate throughout the body.

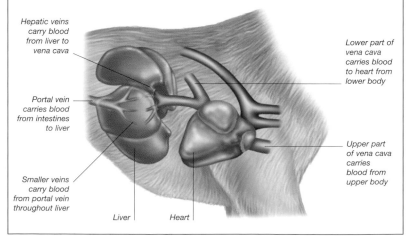

Hepatic veins carry blood from liver to vena cava

Portal vein carries blood from intestines to liver

Smaller veins carry blood from portal vein throughout liver

Lower part of vena cava carries blood to heart from lower body

Upper part of vena cava carries blood from upper body

Liver   Heart

LIVER AND PANCREAS

The liver is the body's largest internal organ. It consists of several lobes that surround the upper part of the stomach, separating the stomach from the diaphragm. When the liver increases in size, as happens with many disease conditions, a vet performing a physical examination can feel that the edges of these lobes are more rounded. If the diaphragm is ruptured by serious trauma, it is possible for a lobe of the liver to slip into the tear. Bile is manufactured in the liver, stored in the gall bladder, and secreted from the liver or gall bladder into the intestines via the common bile duct. The pancreas lies in contact with the duodenum, the first part of the small intestine. Its digestive enzymes enter the duodenum via the pancreatic duct.

LOCATION AND FUNCTION

The liver and pancreas surround the stomach. Both of these organs add digestive enzymes to food that has left the stomach for the intestines.

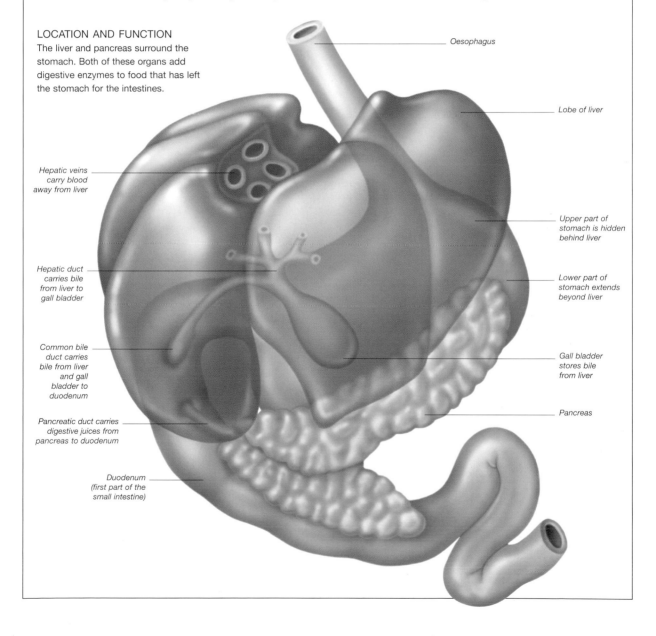

Oesophagus

Lobe of liver

Hepatic veins carry blood away from liver

Upper part of stomach is hidden behind liver

Hepatic duct carries bile from liver to gall bladder

Lower part of stomach extends beyond liver

Common bile duct carries bile from liver and gall bladder to duodenum

Gall bladder stores bile from liver

Pancreatic duct carries digestive juices from pancreas to duodenum

Pancreas

Duodenum (first part of the small intestine)

DISEASES OF THE PANCREAS

A variety of problems may affect the pancreas. It may become inflamed (pancreatitis), or unable to produce enzymes. Cancer may also develop.

PANCREATITIS

The exact causes of pancreatitis remain a mystery; however, there is a direct relationship between the severity of attacks and a high-fat, low-protein diet. There is also evidence that certain drugs, including corticosteroids, diuretics, and some ulcer-healing drugs (such as cimetidine), are associated with it. In addition, damage to the pancreatic duct may cause enzyme seepage and painful inflammation in surrounding tissues. While the true incidence of pancreatic disease is not known, on routine post mortems about one per cent of dogs have signs of pancreatitis.

Acute pancreatitis is a very painful condition typically affecting overweight, middle-aged females. It causes extreme pain. The dog tucks up its belly, vomits, and develops signs of shock (see p.388). In less severe instances, the dog drops its front half into a position like a "play-bow", but is reluctant to drop its hind quarters. Milder pancreatitis

Q WHY ARE FEMALES MORE PRONE TO PANCREATITIS?

A Obesity, which affects females more than males, is thought to be the major risk factor for the disorder. Another factor is sugar diabetes (see p.336), which is more likely in overweight females.

Q IS DIET IMPORTANT IN TREATING PANCREATITIS?

A A more important measure is withholding food, which should usually be done for three days. Dogs that are fed sooner are more likely to have relapses.

causes lethargy, vomiting, diarrhoea, and a fever. Acute pancreatitis occurs most commonly in Miniature Poodles, Miniature Schnauzers, Cocker Spaniels, and West Highland White Terriers.

Chronic pancreatitis is more difficult to diagnose, and most of the clinical signs involve the intestines.

DIAGNOSIS X-rays and ultrasound may show anatomical changes to the duodenum. Blood analysis shows higher levels of white blood cells and increased activity of liver and pancreas enzymes – a result of inflammation.

TREATMENT The aims of treatment are to control pain, overcome the effects of shock, and reduce pancreatic activity. The latter is achieved by withholding food for a short period of time; the dog may be fed intravenously as a safe alternative. Unlike in people, antibiotics are rarely used in dogs with pancreatitis. Corticosteroids are used only if there is clinical shock. Once vomiting has been controlled, a low-fat maintenance diet is given, usually in small, frequent meals.

EXOCRINE PANCREATIC INSUFFICIENCY (EPI)

For still unknown reasons, the exocrine (outer) part of the pancreas may lose its ability to make digestive enzymes. This problem, called exocrine pancreas insufficiency, may be an autoimmune condition, in which the immune system attacks its own tissue. Autoimmune conditions are the most common cause of canine diabetes; the immune system destroys the ability of the pancreas to produce insulin (see p.336). EPI is a particular problem in families of German Shepherd Dogs, in which it is an inherited condition. Scar tissue from previous bouts of pancreatitis may also trigger EPI.

Affected dogs eat voraciously but lose weight. They pass large quantities of grey diarrhoea like cow manure.

DIAGNOSIS The appearance of the stool and microscopic examination for undigested fat are often diagnostic. Also, blood tests show low levels of

digestive enzymes.

TREATMENT Affected dogs are given commercially produced dried pancreatic extracts. If this measure is not effective, your vet may suggest feeding fresh cow pancreas from an abbatoir, although public health regulations make this a difficult solution. Dogs should also be fed supplements of fat-soluble vitamins, especially vitamin E. Antibiotics (metronidazole, oxytetracycline) and corticosteroids are used in some cases.

PANCREAS TUMOURS

These tumours are adenocarcinomas (see p.140), which are uncommon but usually highly malignant. The signs of cancer are non-specific: weight loss, vomiting, and lethargy. At present there is no treatment. Even with surgery the outlook is poor.

DISEASES OF THE LIVER

Few conditions affecting the liver produce consistent clinical signs. This is because the liver has a superb ability to regenerate new cells, so if small or moderate numbers of liver cells are destroyed due to injury or disease, no signs appear. In fact, over 80 per cent of liver function may be lost before a dog shows signs of liver failure.

Generally speaking, regardless of the cause of liver disease, there are two important facts that vets will consider. The first is whether the condition is acute or chronic. The second is whether it is a primary liver condition, in which a harmful agent such as an infection or toxin has a direct effect on the liver, or a "secondary" condition, resulting from a problem elsewhere in the body. An example of the latter is when a dog's heart fails to pump efficiently and, as a result, the liver swells as blood collects in it to be transported to the heart.

ACUTE LIVER FAILURE

Severe liver necrosis (tissue death), an uncommon condition, causes acute liver failure (rapid loss of liver function).

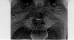

The signs include depression, vomiting, diarrhoea, and nervous conditions such as twitching or seizures. Acute liver failure can be due to infectious diseases such as canine infectious hepatitis or, in the UK, canine acidophil cell hepatitis virus. The condition can also be caused by various types of drug, including anticonvulsants, antibiotics, and analgesics. In addition, it may result from shock, trauma, heatstroke, acute circulation failure, or septicaemia.

DIAGNOSIS Acute liver failure may be mistaken for acute gastroenteritis (*see p.282*), but blood tests usually reveal elevated liver enzyme activity, low blood sugar, excess cholesterol, and bile. X-ray images may show that the liver is enlarged.

TREATMENT An affected dog will be hospitalized and given intravenous fluids, together with other medications, to control the clinical signs.

CHRONIC LIVER DISEASE

This condition causes a build-up of inflammatory cells and fibrous tissue within the liver. Almost invariably, it causes liver enlargement; if it is not treated or controlled, it finally leads to cirrhosis (formation of scar tissue in the liver) and liver failure. Chronic liver disease is difficult to diagnose in its early stages because it seldom causes signs. All the causes of acute liver failure may also cause chronic liver disease; in addition, the infectious disease leptospirosis (*see p.151*) is a common cause in certain localities.

Early signs of liver disease include loss of weight, loss of appetite, and increased drinking and urinating. In later stages, once nearly all of the liver function has been lost, the following signs occur. Body tissues develop a yellow staining (jaundice). The urine is dark and the colour of tea, due to the presence of bile, and the faeces are greyish-white and loaded with fat. Internal bleeding leads to blood in the urine or the stools and bruising on the skin. The dog has a swollen abdomen

due to fluid accumulation (ascites) and swollen legs (dependent oedema). The animal also shows behavioural changes such as disorientation, loss of coordination, twitching, or seizures, due to ammonia-induced brain inflammation (hepatic encephalopathy).

DIAGNOSIS A variety of blood tests are used for diagnosis, including tests for enzymes, bilirubin, and bile acids. Images of the liver may be produced using X-rays (including contrast X-rays), ultrasound, CT, and MRI. A needle biopsy or a fine-needle aspiration, in which liver cells are withdrawn using a needle and syringe, provides the most accurate diagnosis.

TREATMENT There are numerous causes of liver disease, many of which arise outside the liver; effective treatment therefore depends on treating the primary condition or removing the cause of disease. The treatment varies with the severity of the disease. Physical activity is kept moderate, and a specially formulated diet, containing small amounts of high-quality protein, is fed. Dextrose saline may be given intravenously, and diuretics used to remove fluid from the abdomen.

INFECTIOUS CAUSES OF HEPATITIS

Infectious canine hepatitis (CAV-1) and various forms of *Leptospira* bacteria cause hepatitis, as does the rare canine acidophil cell hepatitis virus. CAV-1 may cause sudden death. In other cases, it causes a high fever, abdominal pain, vomiting, diarrhoea, depression, and liver enlargement. The signs of leptospiral hepatitis depend on which form of the bacterium has caused the infection. Some forms cause severe hepatitis, jaundice, and kidney damage, while others cause more chronic, mild liver disease. CAV-1 and leptospiral hepatitis are prevented by routine inoculation. Canine hepatitis vaccine may provide immunity for several years, while leptospirosis vaccine offers protection for 6 to 12 months.

COPPER STORAGE

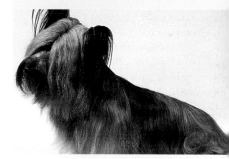

The liver is responsible for storing copper and excreting it in the bile. If it is not excreted properly, a dog develops copper-storage disease or copper hepatopathy.

Bedlington Terriers can inherit a predisposition to a copper-storage disease. Carriers are diagnosed by genetic testing; a liver registry of carriers and non-carriers exists at Purdue University, Indiana, USA. Affected dogs are fed copper-restricted and zinc-supplemented diets. Skye Terriers (above) are prone to a similar disease. West Highland White Terriers have a moderately high incidence of mild copper-storage disease, but seldom have problems. Middle-aged Dobermans may also be affected.

Q WHY DOES LIVER DISEASE CAUSE BEHAVIOUR CHANGES?

A There are several suggested explanations. One is that liver disease leads to accumulation in the brain of natural depressant substances. Whatever the theory, liver disease leads to the barrier between the bloodstream and the brain becoming inefficient. Hepatic encephalopathy (brain inflammation associated with liver problems) may cause signs such as anxiety, loss of vision, pacing, or circling.

Q DOES ALCOHOL CAUSE LIVER CIRRHOSIS IN DOGS?

A Yes, it does. Dogs that routinely drink the beer slops behind a bar often have elevated liver enzyme levels similar to those seen in humans who drink alcohol in excess. Alcohol, however, is not the only cause of cirrhosis. In urban environments, many dogs over ten years of age that are blood-tested as part of their yearly health check-ups have liver enzyme levels higher than those thought to be "normal". Unknown environmental factors account for these instances of mild to sometimes severe cirrhosis.

Q CAN THE LIVER BE SAFELY OPERATED ON?

A Yes, it can, although surgery is only an option when at least one large lobe is not affected by disease. Common reasons for liver surgery are local abscesses or tumours in single liver lobes.

Q DO DOGS EVER GET GALL STONES?

A Yes, but gall stones are much less common in dogs than in humans. Treatment is rarely needed.

BREED-ASSOCIATED CHRONIC LIVER DISEASES

Dobermans, especially middle-aged females, are at risk of chronic hepatitis and cirrhosis, that is thought to be immune-mediated (see p.124). Treatment often involves use of corticosteroids. Cocker Spaniels and American Cocker Spaniels, especially young males, have an increased risk of chronic hepatitis. Disease is more serious in these breeds, often with a grave prognosis.

Bedlington Terriers and Skye Terriers may inherit a predisposition to copper-storage disease (see p.295). West Highland White Terriers have an increased risk of chronic hepatitis and later cirrhosis, which may be linked to copper storage problems.

DRUG-INDUCED CHRONIC HEPATITIS

Liver poisoning is a fairly common problem. Drugs known to be potential poisons include inhaled anaesthetics such as halothane, the antibiotic trimethoprim-sulfa, the heartworm treatment diethylcarbamazine, and the painkiller paracetamol. In addition, anticonvulsants such as phenobarbital, antifungal drugs such as itraconazole, the antiparasitic drug combination oxibendazole and diethylcarbamazine, and the NSAID (painkiller and anti-inflammatory drug) carprofen (Rimadyl) have been associated with an increased risk of hepatic disease in some dogs.

Liver poisoning may also be caused by toxins in food (endotoxins); toxic chemicals such as phenols; heavy metals; chlorinated compounds and aflatoxin from mouldy seed; or drugs that are usually therapeutic but may be toxic in excess or in particular dogs.

DIAGNOSIS AND TREATMENT Liver toxins cause signs of acute or chronic liver failure. Blood tests for liver enzyme activity are not diagnostic for differentiating poisoning from other causes of liver damage.

Antibiotics such as enrofloxacin may be used when opportunist infection

occurs. Corticosteroid drugs are sometimes helpful, as is a substance called ursodeoxycholic acid, which promotes bile circulation.

LIVER SHUNT

This condition is an abnormal opening between the portal vein (which carries blood from the intestines to the liver) and the posterior vena cava (carrying blood back to the heart). As a result of the shunt, some of the blood from the intestines fails to filter through the liver and be purified of toxins such as ammonia. This blood then circulates to the brain, where the toxins cause inflammation (hepatic encephalopathy).

In some breeds there is a genetic predisposition to liver shunt. Unborn pups have a natural link between the portal vein and the vena cava, because the digestive system is not yet in use; this link should close at birth, but in some newborn pups it fails to do so. Affected breeds include the Miniature Schnauzer; Yorkshire, Maltese, and Cairn Terriers; Old English Sheepdog; and Irish Wolfhound. Dogs can also acquire shunts from trauma to the liver.

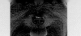

MISDIRECTED BLOOD VESSELS IN LIVER SHUNT

Blood from the intestines is normally transported to the liver, where it is cleansed of impurities and toxins. Either because of a congenital anatomical defect or as a result of liver damage, blood can bypass the liver, moving directly from the intestines to the heart without being cleansed. This condition is called liver shunt (or liver bypass, portosystemic shunt, or hepatic encephalopathy). It can lead to toxin-induced inflammation of the brain.

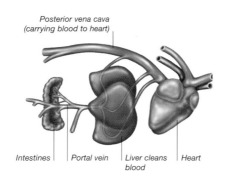

Posterior vena cava
(carrying blood to heart)

Intestines | Portal vein | Liver cleans blood | Heart

NORMAL SYSTEM

Normally, blood from the gastrointestinal tract is brought into the liver via the portal vein. The blood is cleansed of toxins in the liver, then the clean blood is passed on to the heart via the posterior vena cava.

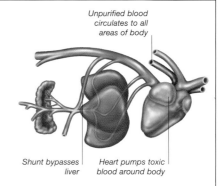

Unpurified blood circulates to all areas of body

Shunt bypasses liver | Heart pumps toxic blood around body

LIVER SHUNT

In newborn pups the link from the portal vein to the vena cava fails to close as it should, or in older animals an abnormal link opens, allowing blood containing toxins to pass directly to the heart.

Affected dogs show signs associated with brain inflammation, including staggering, twitching, lethargy, and seizures. Some individuals may be thirsty and may vomit.

DIAGNOSIS AND TREATMENT Diagnosis is based on blood samples, bile acid measurement, X-rays, and ultrasound. The liver shunt is tied off surgically. Antibiotics such as neomycin and metronidazole are used to control the bacteria that produce ammonia.

Specially formulated veterinary diets are available for dogs that have liver conditions. These diets contain the necessary extra nutrients as well as restricted levels of high-quality, very digestible protein.

Vincent Biourge, a French veterinary nutritionist, also recommends this home-made diet:
1.5 cups low-fat cottage cheese
3 cups cooked rice (cooked from raw, not pre-cooked rice)
25 g (1 oz) cooked beef liver
1 teaspoon calcium carbonate
1 tablespoon corn oil
250 mg vitamin C
1 capsule B complex plus iron.

HEPATIC TUMOURS

A wide variety of tumours develop in the liver. They may be either primary, originating in the liver, or secondary, as metastases (migrating cancer cells) from regions such as the mammary tissue or spleen. Signs of liver tumours are non-specific, and include weight loss, vomiting, and lethargy.

DIAGNOSIS AND TREATMENT Physical examination, X-rays, ultrasound, and CT and MRI imaging are all used diagnostically. A biopsy is necessary to make an accurate diagnosis and to assist with decision-making for any possible treatment.

HEPATIC AMYLOIDOSIS

This is a rare condition, seen only in the Shar Pei. In hepatic amyloidosis, fatty deposits accumulate in a variety of organs, including the liver and kidneys. It occurs as a consequence of chronic infection, inflammation, or an immune-mediated disorder.

DIAGNOSIS AND TREATMENT Clinical signs include fever (Shar Pei Fever) and swollen hocks. Scientists are still searching for an effective treatment.

GALL BLADDER AND BILE DUCT DISEASE

The gall bladder stores bile, a digestive liquid consisting of acids, cholesterol, and certain other substances absorbed from the intestines and processed in the liver. Normally, bile is excreted from the gall bladder (or directly from the liver) back into the intestines via tiny ducts. Any part of this system may suffer obstruction, inflammation, or rupture.

Bile duct obstruction is most often due to pancreatic disease (see p.294); it may also be caused by tumours or stones in the gall bladder. Bacteria from the intestines may cause bile duct inflammation (cholecystitis). Severe cholecystitis, or traumatic injury, may cause a bile duct to rupture.

DIAGNOSIS AND TREATMENT The system is examined by X-ray, blood analysis, and ultrasound. The underlying disease is treated. Gall stones are only removed if there is associated disease. Antibiotics are used for most gall bladder diseases. A ruptured bile duct will leak bile, causing rapid, severe tissue damage, and need immediate surgical repair.

URINARY TRACT
clearing fluid and cleaning blood

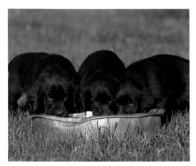

Puppies drinking from a bowl

The main function of the urinary tract is to filter the blood, excreting waste products of metabolism and excess water as urine. It also regulates the level of fluid and of certain salts in the dog's body and maintains the acid-base balance. The urinary tract consists of a pair of kidneys, located either side of the spine just under the last rib; the bladder; the ureters, which connect each kidney to the bladder; and the urethra, through which urine leaves the body. The prostate gland in male dogs is sometimes also considered part of the urinary tract.

All the activities that a dog performs, from eating and breathing to running and jumping, are made possible by chemical reactions in its body cells. Wastes produced as a result of these reactions collect in the bloodstream. For a dog to stay healthy, its urinary tract must filter out these wastes from the blood and excrete them.

THE KIDNEYS
This cleansing process starts in the kidneys. These organs are supplied with blood by the renal artery, and clean blood leaves the kidneys via the renal vein. Each kidney contains about 400,000 individual cleansing units called nephrons. (Each human kidney has about 1 million nephrons, while a cat's kidney has roughly 190,000.) Each nephron is made up of a globe of capillaries (tiny blood vessels), called a glomerulus, and a long, thin tube called the renal tubule. Pores in the glomerulus allow only some substances in the blood to pass through; for example, red blood cells are too large to pass through the pores. Smaller molecules and fluids can pass from the glomerulus into the renal tubule, where useful substances such as glucose are reabsorbed into the bloodstream. The fluid remaining in the renal tubule, called urine, is a mixture of wastes, such as urea (produced by protein metabolism), and other substances not required by the body, such as excess water and salts.

This constant filtration of the blood helps to regulate fluid levels. If a dog drinks more water than is needed for its body's requirements, the excess is excreted in urine; if the dog needs to conserve water, the kidneys make the urine more concentrated by reabsorbing more water from the renal tubules. The amount of water reabsorbed or excreted by the kidneys is controlled by a hormone called anti-diuretic hormone (ADH), which is produced by the pituitary gland, at the base of the brain, in response to the concentration of the blood. As well as regulating water balance, if the blood becomes too acidic or alkaline the kidneys change the urine's acidity level to restore the correct balance.

The kidneys also secrete hormones, such as erythropoietin, which stimulates the production of red blood cells.

PASSING URINE
Urine from the nephrons collects in the hollow centre of each kidney, the renal pelvis, before travelling down the ureters to the bladder, where it is temporarily stored. A ring of muscle applies pressure to the urethra at the exit from the bladder to stop leakage.

When the bladder stretches to a certain size (or is inflamed by disease), nerves in the wall send signals to the spinal cord and brain. Signals are then sent back to the bladder, making it contract and expel urine. The timing of urination is under the conscious control of the brain. When a well-trained dog feels the urge to pass urine, it asks to go out, the muscles around the urethra relax, and the dog urinates.

Q HOW MUCH URINE DOES A DOG PRODUCE EACH DAY?

A A healthy dog excretes about 0.25–1.0 litres (½–2 pints) of urine each day, although this varies between individuals.

Q WHAT IS THE BEST WAY TO HOUSE-TRAIN A PUPPY?

A Teaching a dog when and where to pass urine is the basis of successful house-training. The key is for the puppy to become aware of its urge to urinate, so this can be brought under conscious control (see p.32).

THE URINARY TRACT

Urine passes from the kidneys, where it is made, through the ureters to the bladder. When the bladder is full and its walls become stretched, the dog feels the need to pass urine, which it does through the urethra. This passage opens at the tip of the penis in males, and between the folds of the vulva in females. In male dogs, the prostate gland encircles the urethra just below the bladder.

BLOOD FILTRATION IN THE KIDNEYS

The kidneys cleanse the blood. Blood entering the kidneys is filtered through clusters of capillaries called glomeruli. In each glomerulus, impurities and excess water are removed from the blood to be excreted as urine.

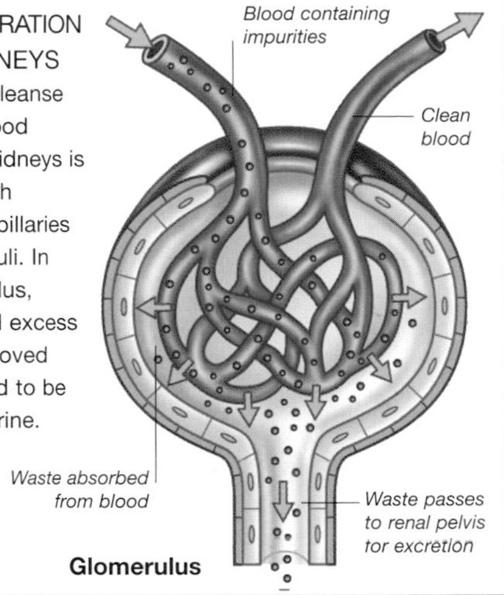

Blood containing impurities

Clean blood

Waste absorbed from blood

Waste passes to renal pelvis for excretion

Glomerulus

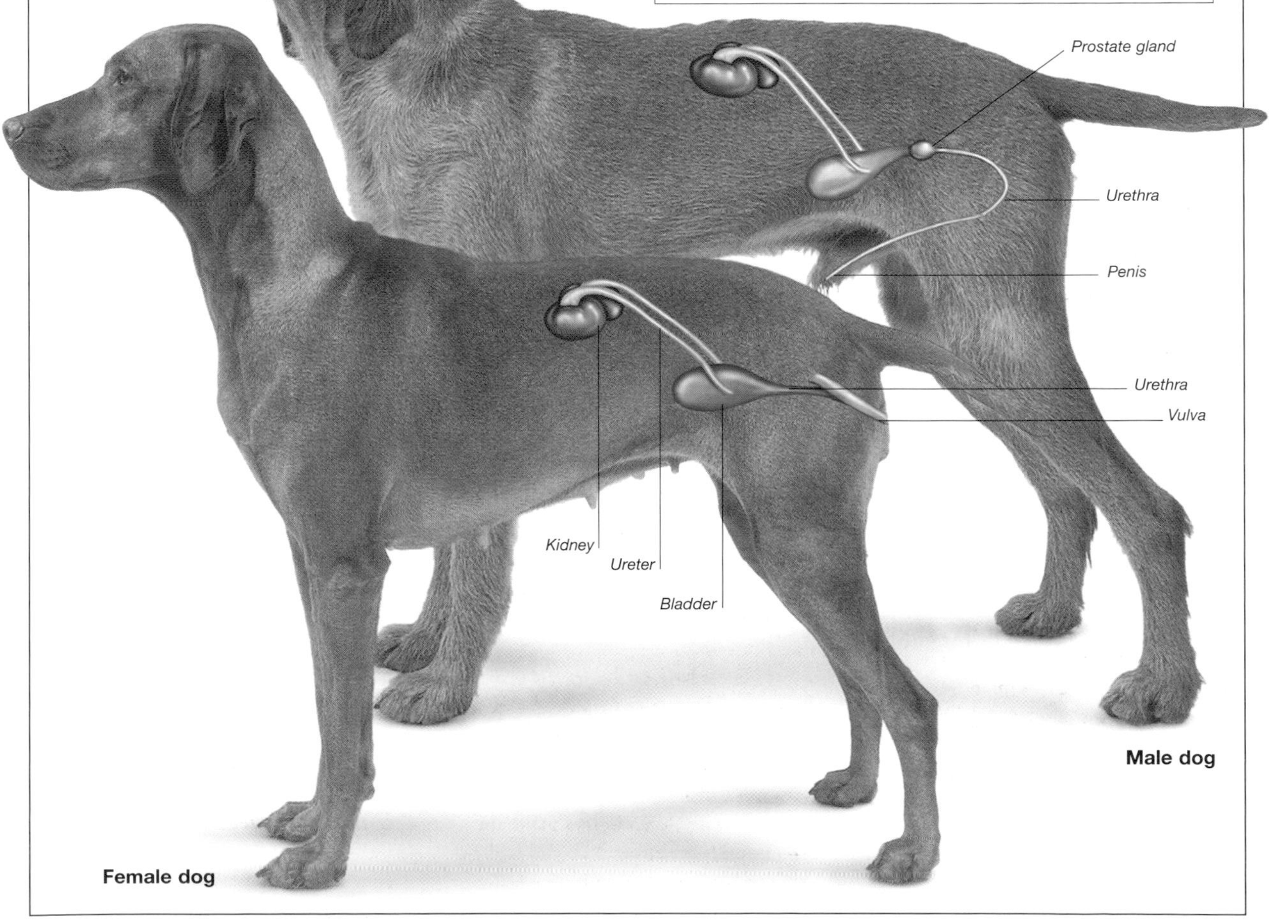

Prostate gland

Urethra

Penis

Urethra

Vulva

Kidney

Ureter

Bladder

Male dog

Female dog

CLINICAL SIGNS

Disease in the urinary tract can affect the efficiency of kidney filtration, the quantity and quality of the urine, the frequency of the need to urinate, or control over when urinating occurs. Mineral crystals or stones can develop anywhere in the tract. Lower urinary tract disease, involving the bladder and urethra, is relatively common and can usually be controlled by altering the dog's diet and the acidity of the urine. Kidney failure may be brought on by injury, disease, or immune system disorders, but it also occurs simply as a result of advancing years.

Most urinary tract disorders cause changes in the normal pattern of drinking and urinating. Such changes are typically the first sign that there is a problem. The opposite is not necessarily the case, however: not all changes in drinking or urinating are caused by urinary tract disease.

INDICATIONS OF URINARY TRACT PROBLEMS

Changes in a dog's habits of urination may indicate a problem in the urinary tract, but may also occur for a variety of reasons unrelated to urinary function.

INCREASED OR MORE FREQUENT URINATION

The passing of large amounts of urine – more than 50 ml (2 fl oz) per kilogram (2.2 lb) of body weight daily – is called polyuria. This condition is often a sign of kidney disease.

Causes of increased urination arising within the urinary tract include kidney infection, kidney insufficiency or failure (*see p.307*), or a lack of kidney response to anti-diuretic hormone (ADH). Causes originating outside the urinary tract include diabetes mellitus (*see p.336*); ADH deficiency due to a pituitary gland disorder; liver disease; uterine infection in females; overactive or underactive adrenal glands (*see p.335*); an underactive thyroid gland (*see p.331*); excess calcium in the blood; insufficient potassium in the blood; congenital disorders; trauma; certain drugs; or a change in diet.

Frequency refers to how often a dog urinates, not how much. While increased urination usually increases frequency, there are many conditions in which frequency is increased but quantity is not. Bladder, urethral, or lower genital tract inflammation; bladder sediment or stones; and prostate conditions may trigger only slightly increased urine volume but an obvious increase in urinary frequency.

INCREASED THIRST

A marked increase in thirst is termed polydipsia. In veterinary practice, this word is used of an animal consuming more than 100 ml (4 fl oz) of water per kilogram (2.2 lb) of body weight daily.

Very few of the causes of polydipsia actually arise in the urinary tract; the problem is almost always triggered by conditions outside the tract. Examples include fever and pain, which can upset the ADH and water balance; altered behaviour (causing so-called psychogenic polydipsia); or physical brain conditions (encephalopathies). In many cases, polydipsia inevitably leads to an increase in urination.

PAIN OR DIFFICULTY PASSING URINE

Pain or difficulty urinating, called dysuria, may cause various signs of distress. An affected dog may strain; dribble urine; squat or lift a leg but pass nothing; lick the penis or vulva more frequently; cry out; resent being touched; pass small quantities of urine frequently; or pass blood, sediment, or

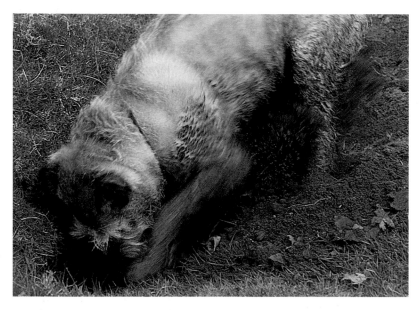

DOG DOWN A RAT HOLE
Some dogs love chasing rats, mice, and other small animals. They could be at risk of poisoning from warfarin, a substance often put down by farmers and landowners to kill rats and other vermin. Warfarin poisoning can produce blood in the urine along with other potentially serious clinical signs.

mucus. Dysuria is usually associated with lower urinary tract disease, including bladder sediment or stones, trauma, inflammation of the bladder or urethra, urinary tract tumours, and prostate conditions in males.

INCONTINENCE

Incontinence means an inability to control the discharge of urine. A dog that is incontinent may constantly leak urine or may release urine only in certain circumstances, such as when lying down or when excited. There are different forms of incontinence, which have different causes (*see p.307*). Incontinence may or may not be associated with increased urination.

BLOOD IN THE URINE

Blood in the urine, a condition called haematuria, is always significant. It has many possible sources. Bleeding accompanied by pain usually indicates a disorder of the lower urinary tract. Blood without pain suggests kidney disease. Haematuria may also result from bladder or kidney stones, severe urinary tract inflammatory disease (*see p.304*), poisoning by warfarin (rat poison), autoimmune haemolytic anaemia or thrombocytopenia (*see p.127*), oestrus in the female or sexual overexcitement in the male, tumours, or trauma to the genital tract.

CONSULTING YOUR VET

Consult your vet if you notice a marked or persistent change in your dog's urinary habits, and certainly if you see blood in your dog's urine. Take a fresh sample of urine that your dog has passed that day to the vet. Collect it from the dog's midstream flow (a few seconds after it starts urinating) if possible, in a clean container such as a jar. Be ready to answer questions about the frequency of urination, any incontinence, the typical amount of water drunk in a day, and whether your dog eats wet or dry food.

URINE COLOUR

The intensity of urine colour is directly related to its concentration. A morning flow is often darker than flow from later in the day because of overnight concentration. Only clear yellow to amber is normal. Drugs, diet, and eating certain plants can cause urine colour to change. Below are some typical causes of colour changes.

APPEARANCE	CAUSED BY
Orange	High concentration Liver disorders
Pink, red, or red-brown	Blood or broken-down red blood cells Warfarin poisoning Consumption of foods such as beetroot or blackberries
Brown or black	Broken-down red blood cells Bile due to liver disorders
Milky white	Pus due to trauma or inflammation Mineral crystals Fats due to a metabolic disorder Sperm
Clear or colourless	Low concentration

Q **IS IT HARMFUL IF MY DOG DOES NOT URINATE FOR A WHOLE NIGHT?**

A If your dog is young and healthy, no it is not. Most individuals have no difficulty or discomfort controlling their bladders for up to 12 hours. Later in life, however, this is too long an interval. It is in your dog's interest that it has access to its toileting site no less often than every 6–8 hours.

Q **HOW DO I KNOW IF MY DOG IS STARTING TO FEEL PAIN WHILE URINATING?**

A If a dog has mild pain, such as a burning sensation, it will continue to maintain its urinating position after it has finished passing urine. This is the first sign of a potential lower urinary tract disorder. If you see your dog doing this, make an appointment to see your vet and take a recent urine sample from your dog with you. Severe pain will cause obvious signs of distress, such as whimpering.

Q **IS THERE A RELATIONSHIP BETWEEN FEEDING DRY DOG FOOD AND URINARY DISORDERS?**

A Basically, there is not. Some urinary conditions, however, such as urine sediment or stones, are made worse by concentrated urine; feeding wet food (usually about 80 per cent moisture) is likely to dilute the urine more than feeding dry food (about 15 per cent moisture). Each individual dog's needs vary. If your dog has a urinary tract disorder, discuss diet changes, including the merits of wet versus dry food, with your vet.

DIAGNOSING URINARY DISORDERS

More than for any other body system, the diagnosis of most urinary tract diseases can be made from careful examination of a fresh urine sample and from accurate information that you can provide about your dog's drinking and urinating habits.

DIAGNOSTIC TESTS

Your vet will use one or more of the following tests to determine the cause of your dog's urinary problem.

ANALYSIS OF URINE SAMPLES

A routine urinalysis will probably be the first test carried out if a urinary tract disorder is suspected from the clinical signs. In this procedure, the vet can quickly test a sample of urine in the surgery to detect a range of substances (see box, below). The test is carried out using a dipstick with a series of patches along its length that test for different chemicals. When the stick is placed in the urine, chemicals in these patches react with substances in the urine to produce a colour change. The colours of the patches are then compared to a chart to confirm whether or not specific substances are present. The depth of the colour change gives a rough indication of the amount of the substance present in the sample.

A sample of urine can also be spun in a machine called a centrifuge to separate out sediment. The sediment is then examined under a microscope for crystals (from the kidneys or bladder); casts (plugs of debris flushed down from the kidneys); cells from the urinary tract lining; sperm (from intact male dogs); blood cells; and microorganisms.

If your vet needs to make a culture to identify a suspected microorganism, he or she will need an uncontaminated urine sample. Bacteria naturally inhabit the urethra, so the only way to obtain this type of sample is by a procedure called cystocentesis. The vet cleans the dog's abdominal skin, then passes a fine needle directly into the bladder to collect the urine sample.

ANALYSIS OF BLOOD SAMPLES

A variety of blood tests may be used to diagnose urinary tract conditions. They include blood counts, to assess the numbers of each type of cell in the sample (a large number of white blood cells indicates infection); measurement of metabolic waste products such as urea and creatinine, which gives the vet an idea of how well the kidneys are functioning; and measurement of mineral levels, because these levels may be altered in kidney disease. Other blood tests are used to help diagnose the cause of increased urination.

IMAGING TECHNIQUES

Plain X-rays can be taken to reveal physical abnormalities such as bladder or kidney stones or malformation of the urinary tract. In contrast X-rays, a material that is opaque to X-rays is injected intravenously to outline the inside of the kidneys and the ureters, or air is introduced via a urinary catheter to outline the wall and contents of the bladder and urethra. An intravenous pyelogram (IVP) is an X-ray procedure in which contrast dye is injected into a vein; the dye is excreted by the kidneys and outlines the renal pelvis and ureters.

Ultrasound imaging is useful for three-dimensional examination of the kidneys, bladder, and prostate gland. CT scans may also be used for this purpose, and provide detailed images of these organs.

URINALYSIS

Urine consists of waste products that are filtered from the blood by the kidneys, in a mixture of water, salts, and other chemicals. Abnormal levels of chemicals in the urine, or the presence of substances not normally found in urine, may indicate a problem with the filtering ability of the kidneys. Urinalysis can also help diagnose certain hormonal disorders, infection, and diseases affecting other organs.

ABNORMAL READINGS	INDICATION
Very high or low concentration	Kidney problems
High acidity or alkalinity	Kidney problems
Nitrites	By-products of bacteria; bacterial infection
Protein	Damaged urinary tract lining
Red and white blood cells	Bleeding in the urinary tract or infection
Ketones	Chronic fever or advanced kidney disease
Bile	Liver problems
Sugar	Diabetes mellitus

ENDOSCOPY

An endoscope is the best diagnostic aid for examining the lining of the urethra and bladder. The viewing instrument is inserted into the urethral opening, and surgical instruments may be passed down the endoscope to collect samples of tissue or perform minor surgery. The use of endoscopy is generally restricted to larger female dogs, because it is easier to perform the investigation in these dogs and causes them only minimal discomfort.

INTERNAL DIGITAL EXAMINATION

"Low-tech" but highly diagnostic, a digital rectal examination involves the vet inserting his gloved finger into the dog's anus to feel the size and shape of the prostate gland and urethra. A digital vaginal examination may be done to assess the condition of the urethral opening in females.

WATER DEPRIVATION OR SYNTHETIC ADH

In healthy dogs, the concentration of urine increases when water is withheld, because the pituitary hormone ADH prompts the kidneys to conserve water. The water deprivation test detects whether the pituitary gland is releasing ADH and the kidneys are responding to it. A good alternative to water deprivation is to monitor the dog's response to treatment with synthetic ADH given by eye drops or injection.

RENAL BIOPSY

A biopsy is undertaken only when other diagnostic tests have failed to determine the cause of a kidney disorder and when it is thought that the results are likely to improve the management of a kidney condition. The dog is anaesthetized and a needle is inserted through the skin to remove a sample of kidney tissue, which is then examined under a microscope.

URODYNAMIC MEASUREMENTS

A variety of urine flow studies can be used to investigate problems with urine control, such as severe incontinence. They are available at referral centres such as veterinary school teaching hospitals. In these studies, probes are inserted into the bladder and rectum or vagina to monitor pressure changes while the bladder is being filled through a catheter and emptied. X-rays may also be taken during the procedures.

VET'S ADVICE

While urinalysis sticks provide a clear grading of what is present in urine, the meaning of these results is not always straightforward, and it is important to consult your vet rather than attempt diagnosis yourself. For example, protein may come and go at different times and for different reasons; a sustained raised level is a cause for concern. If using the sticks to monitor a condition over some time, it is important to take the samples at the same time each day, preferably first thing in the morning.

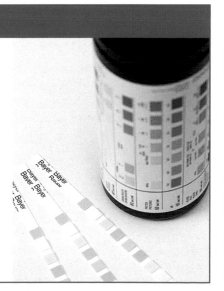

Q HOW DO I COLLECT A URINE SAMPLE FROM MY DOG?

A Males are easy. Just clean a glass jar under hot water, then put on a washing-up glove and catch a sample in the jar as he lifts his leg. For a female, slip a clean saucer under her as she urinates, then transfer the urine to a jar. This is difficult with very small dogs; in this case, ask your vet for a syringe so that you can immediately draw up a sample from a relatively clean surface. (To do a urine stick test and measure specific gravity, your vet needs no more than a teaspoonful of urine.)

Take a sample a few moments after the dog has started urinating to avoid contamination by bacteria from the urethra.

Q IS INCREASED THIRST USUALLY DUE TO A PROBLEM IN THE URINARY TRACT?

A Kidney disease is a common cause of increased thirst, but there are other equally common causes, including sugar diabetes, liver disease, and an overactive adrenal gland. One of the most common causes of temporary increased thirst is therapeutic drugs; both corticosteroids and diuretics trigger increased drinking. A more unusual possibility is a psychological problem. For inexplicable reasons, some physically healthy dogs go through short episodes of dramatically increased drinking. The problem is almost always self-correcting.

BLADDER AND URETHRAL INFLAMMATION

Bacterial infection, mineral deposits, injuries, tumours, and even stress can cause cystitis (inflammation of the lining of the bladder) or urethritis (inflammation of the urethra). These inflammatory conditions often occur together and are then called lower urinary tract disease (LUTD).

Bladder and associated urethral conditions can affect dogs of all ages. Infection of the lower urinary tract is more common in females than in males because they have a shorter urethra, which means a shorter distance for bacteria to travel from the outside of the body to the bladder.

Both cystitis and urethritis cause pain. An affected dog will urinate and lick the vulva or penis more frequently than normal. The urine may appear cloudy and often has a sour smell. Mineral crystals in the bladder or urethra can develop as a result of bacterial infection (see below).

Infection is the most common cause of cystitis or urethritis. In addition, prolonged corticosteroid drug therapy increases the risk of cystitis. Persistent emotional stress may be another cause; it has been shown in humans and cats that stress somehow causes a malfunction in the normal chemical process by which neurotransmitters (nerve cell signal chemicals) are broken down in the body. In males, cystitis is often associated with prostate gland infection (see p.306).

DIAGNOSIS Urinalysis usually reveals high levels of white blood cells, nitrites, and alkalinity of the urine rather than the normal acidity (because of bacterial fermentation).

TREATMENT Antibiotics are given, usually for a minimum of two weeks. Subsequent urinalysis should be normal before antibiotic treatment ends. If another episode of cystitis occurs shortly afterwards, bladder sediment or stones may be present.

STONE BLOCKAGE IN THE MALE URINARY TRACT

The structure of the urinary tract in male dogs places them at greater risk of urethral blockage than females. Stones that form in the bladder may pass down the urethra and become lodged behind the bone in the penis, completely blocking the outflow of urine. This condition causes pain and considerable straining with inability to pass urine.

URETHRAL OBSTRUCTION
Mineral stones most often develop in the bladder. They may form for a variety of reasons, including infection or breed predisposition. When large stones travel from the bladder down the urethra, they may become stuck behind the os penis (penile bone), preventing the flow of urine out of the body.

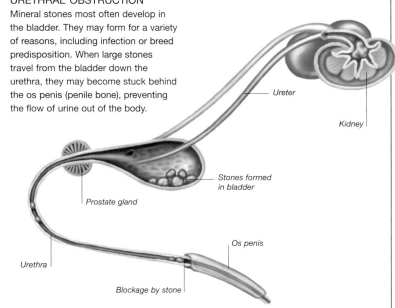

Ureter

Kidney

Stones formed in bladder

Prostate gland

Os penis

Urethra

Blockage by stone

BLADDER SEDIMENT, STONES, AND URINARY TRACT BLOCKAGES

Dogs of any age or breed can develop mineral sediment, called crystals, or mineral stones, called uroliths, in any part of the urinary tract. Stones most commonly develop in the bladder and pass down into the urethra; kidney stones are rare in dogs.

The composition of urinary tract stones varies. The most common type of stone, struvite, usually results from lower urinary tract infection. Other stones develop for different reasons; many of the rarer types are due to inherited metabolic disorders.

While some dogs with bladder stones have no signs, others have lower urinary tract pain, which may cause them to adopt a crouching posture. A stone passing down the urethra can lodge behind the the os penis (the bone in the penis), completely blocking the urethra (see box, above). This blockage causes considerable straining, failure to pass urine, and dramatically increasing pain leading to shock as the bladder increases in size.

A diagnosis is made by examining urine sediment. Large stones may actually be felt when a vet palpates the abdomen, while others are revealed by plain or contrast X-ray or ultrasound. The treatment varies according to the type of stone, but always involves eliminating the underlying cause, such as bladder infection, and reducing the quantity of sediment or preventing its recurrence though diet management. Large stones or those causing urethral blockages are surgically removed.

STRUVITE STONES

These urinary tract stones are made of a substance called magnesium ammonium phosphate, which is most frequently called struvite. They are the most common type of canine bladder or urethra stone.

Their development is usually triggered by staphylococcal or proteus bacterial infection of the lower urinary tract. The bacteria create alkaline urine, the ideal environment for struvite stones to form.

TREATMENT Persistent and efficient antibiotic treatment is vital if infection is the cause. Special veterinary diets are available that promote acidic urine and reduce the amounts of calcium, phosphorus, and magnesium in the diet. Given time, small struvite stones will dissolve in dogs on this diet, although the diet is designed for short-term use only. Large stones are surgically removed.

Dogs that suffer from recurring urinary tract infection are very likely to develop more struvite stones. In some cases, preventative antibiotic therapy is necessary.

CALCIUM OXALATE STONES

These are the second most common type of bladder or urethra stone in dogs. They may develop as a result of chronic mild dehydration. Large stones may become lodged in the urethra, or behind the os penis in males, causing severe pain and complete blockage of the urine flow.

TREATMENT Dogs with these stones should be encouraged to drink more water. The simplest way to do this with dogs that eat dry food is to switch them over to wet food diets.

The stones cannot be dissolved, but only controlled by dietary means. To control calcium oxalate stones, feed a diet with reduced protein, calcium, and sodium that promotes acidic urine. Avoid excess vitamin D or ascorbic acid, which encourages the formation of calcium oxalate stones. Avoid giving the dog treats containing chocolate because it contains oxalates. Fortify the diet with vitamin B6, vitamin K, vitamin A, and the amino acid lysine. Urinary acidifying diets, the preferred treatment for struvite stones, actually promote growth of calcium oxalate stones and should be avoided.

Large stones, or those causing a blockage in the urinary tract, are surgically removed.

CYSTINE STONES

These rare stones occur most frequently in male Dachshunds. They have also been found in Bulldogs. Cystine stones are the result of a metabolic disorder leading to a condition called cystinuria.

TREATMENT A specially formulated, very low-protein diet, supplemented with a little sodium bicarbonate to boost the urine pH just above neutral, is the usual treatment.

URATE STONES

These stones develop almost uniquely in the Dalmatian. They rarely occur in other breeds, although the Bulldog seems to have a slight predisposition. Urate stones result from inherited alterations in urate metabolism.

TREATMENT The aims of treatment are to maintain a neutral urine pH and to restrict dietary sodium and purine (a

BREED PREDISPOSITION TO BLADDER STONES

Struvite crystals and stones most often develop in the bladder subsequent to urinary tract infection. The anatomy of the female urinary tract increases the risk of infection, and therefore the risk of struvite stones. Other, less common types of bladder stones form as a result of dehydration, dietary factors, or metabolic disorders. These types of stone tend to be more common in males. Below is a table comparing incidence of the various types of stone according to breed and sex.

BREED	MOSTLY MALE	MOSTLY FEMALE
Basset Hound	Cystine	
Bichon Frise	Calcium oxalate	Struvite
Bulldog (English)	Urate, cystine	
Cocker Spaniel	Calcium phosphate	Struvite
Dalmatian	Urate	
Dachshund	Cystine	
German Shepherd Dog	Silica	
Golden Retriever	Silica	
Labrador Retriever	Silica	
Lhasa Apso	Calcium oxalate	
Miniature Poodle	Calcium oxalate	
Miniature Schnauzer	Calcium oxalate	Struvite
	Calcium phosphate	
Shih Tzu	Calcium oxalate	
Yorkshire Terrier	Calcium oxalate	
	Calcium phosphate	

ACUTE KIDNEY FAILURE

Sudden interruption of efficient renal filtration causes acute kidney failure. Local infection may directly damage the kidneys; however, most cases of kidney failure result from problems outside the kidneys, such as shock or a systemic disease, that have a devastating secondary effect on kidney filtration.

The general signs of acute kidney failure are quite obvious but do not specifically indicate the source of illness. Signs include loss of appetite, vomiting, diarrhoea, lethargy, and weakness. Because there are so many underlying causes of acute kidney failure, these signs are mixed with those of the triggering condition. There is seldom any weight loss or change in the hair or coat. Dogs are, however, dehydrated. Temperature is often below normal (hypothermia). There may be ulcers in the mouth and a typically sweet (uraemic) smell to the dog's breath. The whites of the eyes may be bloodshot. Dogs with acute kidney failure breathe faster and have faster heart rates than normal.

DIAGNOSIS Urinalysis and urine sediment examination are performed. A high urine concentration strongly suggests that the kidney problem is secondary to another disorder arising elsewhere in the body. White blood cells, casts, and other matter in the urine indicate damage in the kidneys themselves or elsewhere in the urinary tract. Blood tests may reveal infection and metabolic disease, and may be used to assess kidney function. X-rays and ultrasound scanning may help the vet to determine the nature of changes in the kidneys.

TREATMENT The initial objectives of treatment are to sustain life and to eliminate the cause of kidney failure. Intravenous fluid therapy is essential. The aim of this therapy is to replace fluid losses, maintain good fluid balance, and promote urine formation. If the dog starts to urinate, it is responding to this treatment.

Diuretic drugs such as frusemide are effective when used early in acute kidney failure. Mouth ulcers caused by uraemia are treated with chlorhexidine mouthwash several times daily. Nausea is controlled with metoclopramide. Most affected dogs are unwilling or unable to eat, so nourishment is added to the intravenous drip. Alternatively, food may be given by stomach tube if there is no vomiting.

Where facilities exist, acute kidney failure is treated with dialysis. In peritoneal dialysis, a special fluid is introduced into the peritoneal cavity (inside the abdomen), which draws waste material out through the peritoneal lining. After a certain period of time, waste fluid is removed and fresh fluid is added. In this way, the peritoneal lining temporarily takes on the function of the kidneys. Repeat sessions are needed. In haemodialysis, the blood is filtered through a

CAUSES OF ACUTE KIDNEY FAILURE

Vets usually classify the causes of kidney failure as: prerenal, resulting from conditions arising outside the kidneys, such as shock, that then affect blood flow or pressure in the kidneys; renal, affecting the kidneys themselves, such as infections of the kidneys; or postrenal, resulting from partial or complete urinary tract obstructions causing a back-up of urine and consequent kidney damage.

CATEGORY	EXAMPLES OF CAUSES
Infections	Lower urinary tract infection that moves up the tract into the kidneys, causing pyelonephritis (a serious infection in the filtering nephrons) Leptospirosis (bacterial disease) Septicaemia (blood poisoning)
Shock	Burns Trauma Haemorrhage Heatstroke Urinary tract obstruction
Heart conditions	Low blood pressure Blood clots
General diseases	Liver failure Peritonitis (inflammation of the abdominal lining) Pancreatitis (inflammation of the pancreas)
Other	Tumours
Chemicals and drugs	Ethylene glycol antifreeze Amphotericin B (an antibiotic that is toxic to the kidneys) In some dogs with low blood pressure, certain non-steroidal anti-inflammatory drugs

machine. Haemodialysis is available in only a few veterinary hospitals.

Dietary management to reduce the demands on the kidneys is vital. A variety of low-phosphorus renal support diets are available through veterinary practices (*see p.310*).

The prognosis depends on the cause of the kidney failure and on the aggressiveness and efficiency of treatment. Unfortunately, most dogs (60 per cent in a recent study) do not recover. Of those that do, many go on to develop chronic kidney failure.

CHRONIC KIDNEY FAILURE

While chronic kidney failure develops insidiously, it invariably ends with the signs of uraemia (*see p.308*). As it develops, a dog drinks more and loses first body fat, then muscle mass. The coat sheds, loses its sheen, and looks unkempt. The dog generally slows down and has fatigue, increasing listlessness, and a loss of interest in its surroundings. Mild retching begins, followed by vomiting froth or meals. Body tremors or loss of fine balance become noticeable. Eventually, seizures may occur. This point is called end-stage kidney failure.

DIAGNOSIS The vet may be able to feel small, shrunken kidneys, hear a slight heart murmur with a stethoscope, and detect the uraemic smell to the breath. The gums may look drier than normal. Blood chemistry tests show elevated blood urea, nitrogen, and creatinine, as well as raised blood phosphorus levels. Anaemia is often detected, and the dog may have raised blood pressure.

TREATMENT Diet is central to treatment (*see below*). Plenty of fresh water is also important. Fluids are sometimes given intravenously or, in certain cases, subcutaneously (under the skin). High blood pressure is managed with ACE inhibitors such as enalapril, or with calcium-channel blockers such as amlodipine besylate.

DIET AND KIDNEY FAILURE

Diet management is the primary treatment for chronic kidney failure. The aims of this treatment are to minimize clinical signs of kidney failure, help maintain the dog's well-being, and, if possible, prolong its life.

A diet for dogs with kidney failure should have the following features,

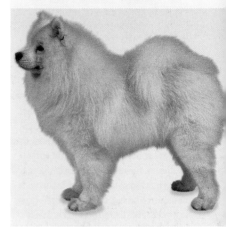

BREEDS AT RISK

Some breeds of dog inherit a genetic predisposition to developing juvenile kidney failure.

Disease develops early, shortening life dramatically, in these breeds:

- Cocker Spaniel
- Samoyed (above)
- Shar Pei

The development of disease is not so acute in other breeds, although the following breeds share the same tendency:

- Alaskan Malamute
- Basenji
- Beagle
- Bernese Mountain Dog
- Bull Terrier
- Cairn Terrier
- Chow Chow
- Doberman
- English Foxhound
- German Shepherd Dog
- Golden Retriever
- Lhasa Apso
- Miniature Schnauzer
- Norwegian Elkhound
- Rottweiler
- Shih Tzu
- Soft-coated Wheaten Terrier
- Standard Poodle
- Welsh Corgis

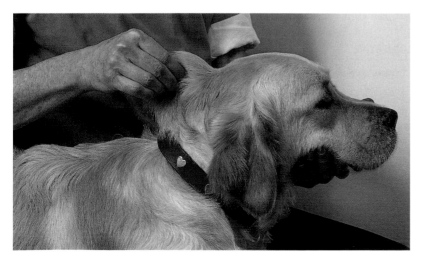

VISUAL CHECK FOR DEHYDRATION
In a healthy dog, the loose skin on the back of the neck is elastic and quickly springs back into shape after it has been pinched. In a dog that is dehydrated, the skin loses its elasticity, and the pressure marks made when a person pinches the skin remain for a minute or so afterwards.

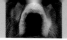

REPRODUCTIVE SYSTEM
male and female problems

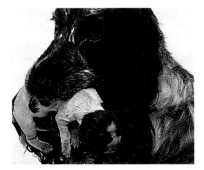

A mother retrieves her pup

While females ovulate and become interested in sex approximately every six months, male dogs are lifelong sexual opportunists. This is a practical arrangement with sociable canines, allowing mothers to concentrate on pregnancy, birth, and initial care of the young pups. Neutering (desexing), often an emotional issue because it seems unnatural to some people, is the most effective way to prevent the common medical problems that affect the reproductive system. In females, it can prolong life expectancy.

Reproduction is the very essence of life. Strip away all other concerns and it is the core reason for existence. By domesticating the dog, we took control over its destiny – but in a wonderfully perverse way, our control of the dog's reproductive system has meant the dog has spread around the world in a way it could never have done on its own. It is a reproduction success story.

FEMALE EGGS
A female pup is born with the potential for producing about 700,000 eggs in her ovaries. By the time she reaches puberty, she has about half this figure. This number falls to about 30,000 when she is five years old; at the age of ten, she has no more than a few hundred left. This means that the best time for a female to breed is

between two and six years of age, after which her fertility begins to decline. As long as she remains healthy she will continue to produce eggs. Unlike female humans, female dogs do not have to go through menopause.

A female releases a number of eggs at the ovulation stage of her sexual cycle, or oestrus. Small breeds release between two and ten eggs and have

Q **IS IT GOOD FOR A BITCH TO HAVE A LITTER BEFORE SHE IS SPAYED?**

A This is a natural question from a species with a life-long need to nurture. Dogs do not think in the abstract as people do. What is psychologically fulfilling for us is not necessarily the same for a dog. Of course, when the mothering hormones are activated a mother gets satisfaction out of suckling and caring for her young, but this is short-lived in dogs compared to us. Maternal behaviour quickly evolves into competitive behaviour. Consider breeding from your dog only if you feel she is physically and mentally sound and you have assured homes for the pups.

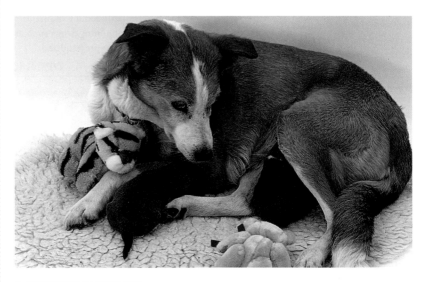

A POSSESSIVE MOTHER
After the birth of her pups, a new mother settles down, relaxes, and allows her litter to suckle. During this early stage of neonatal care, she can become very possessive and defensive – even to the point of gathering around her the playthings she had when she was pregnant.

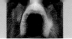

MALE AND FEMALE REPRODUCTIVE SYSTEMS

The male's penis has a bone, the os penis, that strengthens the erectile tissue. Around the middle of the penis is the bulbourethral gland, which enlarges four or five times during an erection. It locks the penis inside the female's vagina during mating and ensures that the ejaculate reaches the eggs. In the female, eggs from the ovaries are released into the fallopian tubes, where fertilization by the sperm takes place. The fertilized eggs then implant themselves in the two "horns" of the Y-shaped uterus. At birth, the pups and their placentas pass out through the vulva via the now-opened cervix and the vagina.

THE TIE

Sexual union between a male and a female is called a "tie". The male's penis swells inside the vagina, while the vaginal muscles constrict around the penis. The dogs may be tied for over half an hour.

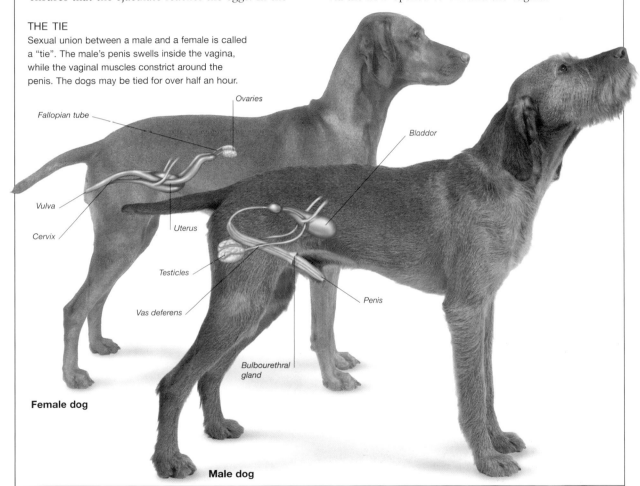

Ovaries

Fallopian tube

Bladder

Vulva

Cervix

Uterus

Testicles

Vas deferens

Penis

Bulbourethral gland

Female dog

Male dog

small litters. Larger breeds release between five and 20 eggs and tend to have bigger litters.

MALE SPERM

As with the males of other mammals, the two testes produce both sperm and testosterone, the male sex hormone.

Under the influence of luteinizing hormone (LH), which is released by the pituitary gland beneath the brain, testosterone and sperm are produced fairly constantly by the testes all year round. This means that males are ready to mate at any time. There is some evidence that male dogs experience a little hormonal "spring fever" as the daylight hours increase.

Prior to ejaculation, the sperm mix with fluid from the prostate gland; this sugar-dense liquid helps the sperm to pass through the female reproductive tract. Once there, sperm can survive and remain viable for up to six days.

SPAYING

This is called an ovariohysterectomy and involves removing the ovaries, oviducts, and uterus of a female. It is more effective than closing off the oviducts or removing the uterus alone because it not only sterilizes a dog but also shuts down the ovarian cycles and prevents the sexual behaviour normally associated with oestrus. It also reduces the medical risks associated with continued hormone production.

An additional advantage of early spaying is the virtual elimination of the risk of mammary cancer. By the time a female has had four oestrous cycles, she is 300 times more likely to develop mammary cancer than if she were spayed before her first cycle.

One disadvantage of spaying is that, in rare circumstances, a female may become incontinent. This problem is most likely in genetically predisposed dogs, especially certain Dobermans and Bearded Collies.

Some immature females have retracted "infantile" vulvas. Many vets feel that spaying should be postponed until after the first oestrous cycle, when natural vulvar swelling overcomes this condition. Other immature females suffer from juvenile vaginitis, but the hormonal changes and discharge of oestrous usually clear it up. Females can be spayed a few months later.

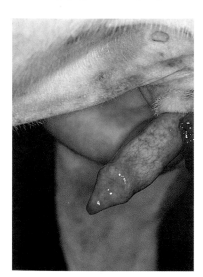

PARAPHIMOSIS
During mating or excitement, an acute difficulty may arise when the male's engorged penis fails to retract in its sheath.

MISMATINGS/CHEMICALLY POSTPONING BREEDING

Sex hormones such as oestrogen can be used to terminate pregnancies, usually several days after a mismating. These drugs are effective when used properly, but frequent use can lead to variety of disorders of the reproductive system. Sex hormones are also used to delay or postpone oestrus. Overuse increases the risk of womb infection later in life.

CASTRATION

Also called orchidectomy, castration is an operation that removes the testes. It stops sperm production and reduces the production of testosterone. The levels of testosterone fall within eight hours, but sperm already in the system may remain active and viable for another 36 hours.

Castration causes the loss of many male characteristics, such as marking with urine and aggression with other males. It also stops young dogs from trying to mount people's legs. Castrating dogs does not prevent rare prostate cancer, but it does avoid any risk of the more common prostatic hyperplasia and testicular tumours.

VASECTOMY

An alternative to castration, this is a relatively simple operation involving the removal of short sections of the vas deferens, which carries sperm from the testicles into the urethra.

Vasectomy is an excellent method of birth control while at the same time perpetuating the male characteristics of the dog. a vasectomy unlike castration, does not stop or reduce urine-marking, "roaming", and inter-male aggression.

MALE MEDICAL CONDITIONS

Unlike in females, few conditions affecting the male are life-threatening. This is why neutering (desexing) does not increase the life expectancy of males as it does for females.

When they do occur, the male's problems will affect the penis, testicles, or prostate gland. The most common problems cause discharge from the foreskin, or prepuce, and changes in the size of the testicles. Conditions of the prostate gland are frequent in older male dogs.

TIGHT SHEATH OPENING (PHIMOSIS)

Some male pups are born with a tight opening in the sheath surrounding the penis. In adults, scar tissue from an injury or infection may cause the sheath opening to tighten. Affected dogs may show signs of pain when urinating and are distressed when sexually excited.

TREATMENT Surgical relief may be necessary for this condition.

PENIS STUCK OUT OF THE SHEATH (PARAPHIMOSIS)

Long hair on the tip of the prepuce can cause the skin to roll inwards when a dog has an erection. During an erection the bulbourethral gland on the penis can swell so much that it is too wide to retract into the sheath. Affected dogs lick their penis and look uncomfortable. Paraphimosis is often a problem of young, oversexed Yorkshire Terriers and is seen occasionally in dogs after castration.

TREATMENT Lubricate the penis with a water-soluble jelly or liquid paraffin. If these items are unavailable, a little vegetable cooking oil will do. Retract the prepuce back, or ease the penis forwards, to release trapped hair that has caused the prepuce to roll over on itself. Slide the penis back into its sheath. If this is not possible, keep the penis moistened with one of the lubricants and get veterinary help immediately. In certain circumstances, surgery may be needed to reduce the "strangling" of the penis. If an erection is prolonged, a lubricant can reduce the difficulty of retraction.

SHEATH AND PENIS INFECTION (BALANOPOSTHITIS)

A male dog normally produces a cream-yellow lubricant (smegma) in the sheath of his penis. In young dogs, this fluid can be quite productive, dripping out from the prepuce when the dog is resting. This preputial drip can be aesthetically unpleasant, but it is not a medical problem.

An inflamed penis and prepuce is a sign of balanoposthitis infection. The preputial drip is excessive and foul-smelling, and the dog increasingly licks the tip of his penis. There are many potential causes of balanoposthitis, including: a bacterial or a herpesvirus infection; a foreign body, such as a grass seed; a physical injury; or a failure to secrete sufficient lubricant.

DIAGNOSIS AND TREATMENT Bacterial infection can be cultured and antibiotic sensitivity determined. Viral infection is much more difficult to diagnose. Failure to respond to the antibiotic treatment increases the risk of herpesvirus infection. Viral infection can be transmitted to females during mating, leading to sterility.

Excess smegma and foreign bodies, such as plant seeds, are flushed from the sheath with warm saline or dilute chlorhexidine antiseptic. Preputial flushing also reduces the quantity of normal preputial discharge.

TUMOURS OF THE PENIS AND PREPUCE

Tumours of the penis and prepuce do occur but are uncommon. They include mast cell tumours, papillomas, fibromas, and transmissible venereal tumours, which are spread by sexual contact in younger dogs. The presence of a tumour usually triggers increased licking of the penis. There may be signs of blood in the dog's urine.

UNDESCENDED TESTICLES

In the foetus, testicles develop inside the abdominal cavity, near the kidneys. They migrate down through the inguinal rings (openings within the groin) into the scrotum (*see box, left*). Migration always occurs by birth or a few days after. If neither testicle migrates, and they remain in the abdominal cavity, the dog is called a cryptorchid. If only one testicle migrates through an inguinal ring, the dog is a monorchid.

It is not unusual for testicles to migrate through the inguinal rings but then remain for a while between the skin in the groin and the inguinal muscles, before continuing their descent into the scrotum. Undescended or partly descended testicles is an inherited condition in many breeds. There is a high incidence of cancer in undescended testicles.

DIAGNOSIS Normally, both testicles should be visible in the scrotum. The tracks under the skin leading from the scrotum up to the inguinal rings in the groin, are carefully felt for partly descended testicles.

TREATMENT Abdominal testicles should be surgically removed. Testicles that have partly descended and have passed through the inguinal ring should be monitored for changes in texture or size and removed if necessary. This condition is inherited, so dogs with partly descended or completely undescended testicles should not be used for breeding. This is the strongest argument for castration.

TESTICLE DESCENT

The testicles develop in the abdominal cavity of the foetus and descend into the scrotum. This usually occurs before the male pup is born or a few days afterwards.

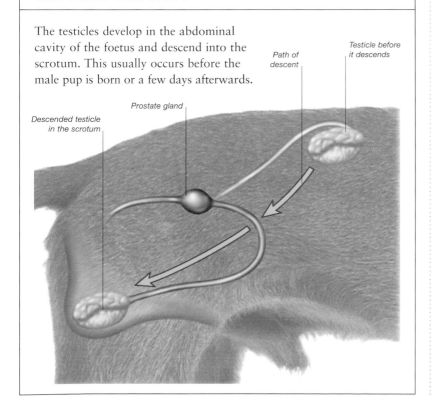

Testicle before it descends

Path of descent

Prostate gland

Descended testicle in the scrotum

TESTICLE ENLARGEMENT

Tumours are the most common cause of painless testicle enlargement. They occur in the testicles of older dogs, usually over seven years old. Infection or injury from dog bites, frostbite, or contact with corrosive chemicals may cause painful enlargement.

A moist scrotal skin infection that causes weeping skin damage and heals into a hard, carapace-like scab can give the impression of testicle enlargement.

DIAGNOSIS Tumours seldom cause any symptoms, although female hormone-producing tumours cause changes such as hair loss, increased pigmentation in the skin of the groin, and enlargement of the mammary glands.

Unless they are enormous, tumours are frequently diagnosed during an annual routine physical examination. If a dog has a pain-producing testicular injury or an infection (orchitis), he will stand and walk with his legs spread. Testicular tumours are surgically removed and identified by a pathologist. Metastasis is very rare.

TREATMENT Penetrating injuries are treated with painkillers and antibiotics. Cold packs are sometimes used. Skin infection is cleaned with skin antiseptic such as chlorhexidine, and dogs are given painkillers and antibiotics. Elizabethan collars are often necessary to prevent the dog from licking the protective scab off damaged skin.

REDUCTION IN TESTICLE SIZE (HYPOPLASIA)

Some testicular tumours secrete female hormones that cause the testicle on the opposite side to shrink and become small (hypoplasia). After a penetrating wound or infection (orchitis), the testicles may also shrink and become non-functional. Sperm that enter the bloodstream can trigger the immune system to attack the testicles, so testicular shrinkage after a penetrating injury is an immune-mediated disease. Rarely, the testicles of young dogs fail to mature into sperm-producing

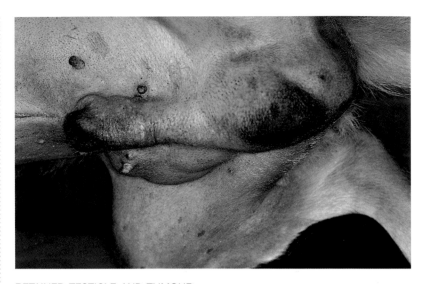

RETAINED TESTICLE AND TUMOUR
Before birth the two testicles descend through the inguinal canal in the groin and into the scrotum. Occasionally, a testicle fails to complete its passage, remaining in the abdomen or, as here, in the groin. There is a high risk of tumour development in such cases.

organs. At the other end of a dog's life, ageing can lead to a reduction in the size of the testicles.

DIAGNOSIS Tumours may be the main cause, so report any shrinkage to your vet. In breeding dogs, semen analysis used to monitor fertility may also detect the presence of tumours.

PROSTATE CONDITIONS

The prostate gland, which is wrapped around the urethra at the point where it emerges from the bladder, produces a nourishing liquid for transporting sperm in the ejaculate.

Diagnosis of prostate conditions relies on detecting signs associated with partial or complete obstructions caused by the enlarged gland. (Most prostate conditions cause enlargement of the gland. Aggressive antibiotic treatment is often necessary.)

PROSTATIC INFECTIONS

The prostate gland commonly becomes inflamed when there is an infection of the bladder or the urethra. Prostatic infections cause swelling. There may be signs of constipation but also more frequent urinating, with pus or blood in the urine.

DIAGNOSIS AND TREATMENT Prostatic infections are identified by bacterial culture and treated with antibiotics.

BENIGN HYPERPLASIA

The prostate gland naturally increases in size (hyperplasia) with time. When it reaches a maximum size, usually between six and ten years of age, it swells and pushes on the floor of the rectum. This benign hyperplasia causes a bottleneck for stools to pass through. Initial symptoms include ribbon-like stools or a difficulty in passing stools.

In rare instances, hyperplasia can produce small to enormous cysts of the prostate gland. In even rarer instances, a prostate tumour may develop.

DIAGNOSIS Hyperplasia is diagnosed by examining the rectum. Cysts are confirmed by X-ray or ultrasound.

TREATMENT Severe hyperplasia is arrested and reduced by castration. Injections of delmadinone often temporarily shrink the hyperplasia. Prostatic cysts that are causing problems are surgically corrected.

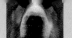

FEMALE MEDICAL CONDITIONS

Many, if not most, of the medical conditions affecting the reproductive tract of the female are painful and/or life-threatening. This alone is sufficient reason to spay females not intended for breeding early in life. Reproductive tract infections are not uncommon in maiden females. Surprisingly few medical problems are associated either with conception or pregnancy.

VAGINAL INFECTION (VAGINITIS)

Vaginitis can be caused by a bacterial mycoplasmal, or viral infection, or by an anatomical abnormality that permits urine to pool in the vagina. An affected dogs licks her vulva more than normal. The interior of the vagina is often inflamed. Male dogs are sexually attracted to females with vaginitis.

DIAGNOSIS AND TREATMENT Analysis of the urine will eliminate urinary tract disorders. A culture and sensitivity test, together with an analysis of the cells of the vagina, confirm diagnosis. Accumulated discharge is flushed out by a very dilute antiseptic lavage such as chlorhexidine. Bacterial infection is treated with an appropriate antibiotic. Severe anatomical abnormalities are surgically corrected. There is no specific treatment for vaginitis that is caused by herpesvirus.

JUVENILE VAGINITIS

Some pups develop a sticky, greenish-yellow vaginal discharge before they are two months of age. This juvenile vaginitis causes no obvious discomfort, although the hair on the tip of the vulva can dry into a hard, crusty wick.

TREATMENT The region is cleansed with very dilute, tepid salt water or a mild, non-irritating and very dilute antiseptic solution. The condition almost always clears spontaneously when a pup has her first oestrus. For this reason, if you are not planning to breed from your dog, spaying should be postponed until three months after the first oestrus cycle.

UTERINE INFECTION (PYOMETRA)

A uterine infection, or pyometra, is a potentially life-threatening event. It may occur at any time in the days, weeks, or months after an oestrous cycle and requires immediate veterinary attention.

The earliest sign of an impending uterine infection is a discharge of mucus (mucometra) after the oestrus stage of her cycle. To all intents and purposes, the female is clinically fine, yet inside her womb, mucus-producing cells have multiplied and created a condition called cystic endometrial hyperplasia. This may not cause a clinical problem, but mucus is an ideal breeding ground for bacteria. Either in that oestrus or in the next, bacteria do multiply, turning the mucus into pus.

If the cervix remains open, pus escapes from the uterus and dribbles through the vagina and out of the vulva. This is "open pyometra", which can be diagnosed relatively easily.

If the cervix has clamped shut, then pus builds up inside the uterus. This is a "closed pyometra", in which the clinical signs develop faster. They include: increased thirst; decreased appetite; more frequent urination; and the need to rest more than normal.

Females with pyometra often have a normal body temperature and, if the cervix is open, a pale green, creamy to bloody discharge from the vagina.

Later, in the course of infection, the presence of considerable amounts of pus accompanies signs of shock. These include: vomiting; rapid breathing; racing pulse; fever; and collapse.

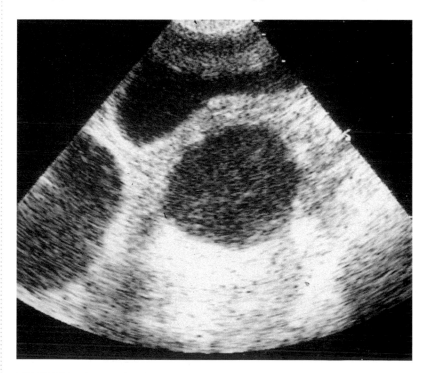

ENLARGED UTERUS DUE TO PYOMETRA

In a closed pyometra, when the cervix is tight and no uterine contents can pass through, pus builds up in the uterus and the uterus expands. This ultrasound image reveals that the uterus is expanded and filled with fluid. The fluid is almost certainly pus.

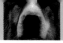

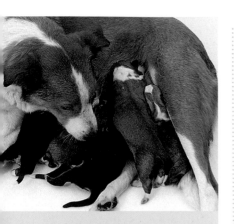

Q HOW COMMON IS PYOMETRA?

A It is one of the most common life-threatening conditions of intact females. While it is most likely to occur in females over six years of age, a pyometra may develop at any age, even after the very first oestrus cycle. The disease is almost invariably associated with metoestrus, the phase of the cycle that is dominated by progesterone. Progesterone drugs may also predispose to pyometra. What happens is not fully understood, but it seems that the lining of the uterus "over-responds" to progesterone, creating an environment in which bacteria can multiply. Left untreated, a closed pyometra is fatal.

Q HOW CAN I PREVENT MY DOG FROM DEVELOPING A PYOMETRA?

A Simple: make sure she is neutered. If she is not, watch out for the signs: vaginal discharge four to eight weeks after oestrus when the pyometra is open, and lethargy, increased thirst, and decreased appetite in females with a tight cervix where there is no visible discharge. A "pyo" can develop earlier, either immediately after ovulating or as late as three months after ovulating.

DIAGNOSIS A vet will diagnose open pyometra from the symptoms. In the early stages, with little or no discharge, a blood sample can reveal the presence of a bacterial infection in the body.

Diagnosis of closed pyometra is confirmed by X-ray or ultrasound, both of which will show an enlarged uterus. The womb can swell to an enormous size, even larger than it does for a full litter of pups. Ultrasound will safely be able to distinguish between pyometra and pregnancy.

TREATMENT If either an open or closed pyometra is diagnosed by the vet, an immediate ovariohysterectomy, or spaying, (*see p.316*) needs to be performed. Intravenous fluids and antibiotics are routinely given.

If the cervix is open so that the pus can drain freely, it is possible to use drugs to induce the womb to contract and squeeze out the pus. To this effect, a prostaglandin called PGF 2 alpha is given on consecutive days by injection. This drug is not, however, licensed for use in dogs. Common side-effects of this treatment include vomiting and apparent foot discomfort. Antibiotics, chosen by culture and sensitivity testing, are given for several weeks.

The likelihood of future womb infections is high. A female should be bred at the next season if recurrence is to be avoided.

PYOMETRA IN YOUNG FEMALES

Cystic endometrial hyperplasia takes years to develop, yet dogs under six years of age can develop pyometra. Many have previously been given oestrogen drugs – for example, for mismating – so there could be a relationship between oestrogen therapy and pyometra in the younger animal.

ENDOMETRITIS

The lining of the womb is called the endometrium. Sometimes, the womb can become "mildly" infected by bacteria that do not produce pus. This may occur after a more serious womb infection. Affected bitches may show no signs of endometritis, but when they are used for subsequent breeding they fail to conceive.

DIAGNOSIS Ultrasound reveals a thicker than normal endometrium, and a biopsy will confirm the diagnosis.

TREATMENT There is no effective medical treatment to enhance the fertility of affected females. Bitches with endometritis are usually spayed to prevent pyometra, which is almost inevitable, from developing.

VAGINAL HYPERPLASIA AND VAGINAL PROLAPSE

During the early stages of oestrus, when the reproductive tract is under the influence of oestrogen, the lining of the vagina thickens and causes the vulva to swell visibly.

This vaginal hyperplasia usually causes swelling in the perineal region but sometimes the vaginal lining becomes so thickened that it bulges out of the vulva. The protruding pink mass stimulates the female increasingly to lick the vulva. At the same time, urination may appear painful.

In the most severe instances, the hyperplasia is so extensive that there is a vaginal prolapse – the vagina emerges out of the vulva as a doughnut-shaped ring of pink tissue. This prolapse can also occur if females that are "tied" during mating are separated before the bulbourethral gland of the male has reduced in size.

Hyperplasia and prolapse are most common during oestrus but may also occur at birth. Very rarely, straining to clear an obstruction in the rectum can cause a prolapse of the vagina.

DIAGNOSIS Veterinary examination is all that is required for diagnosis.

TREATMENT In most instances, the only treatment necessary is to keep the vaginal tissue moistened with a lubricating jelly or liquid paraffin. An antibiotic ointment may also be used to prevent bacterial infection.

VAGINAL POLYP

A vaginal "polyp" is a growth from the lining of the vagina. Technicallly speaking, there is no such thing as a polyp – it is really a "polypoid" vaginal tumour, which may be either benign or malignant. Vaginal polyps are usually classified as a fibroma, fibromyoma, or sarcoma. They are uncommon but are more frequent than other shapes of vaginal tumours.

DIAGNOSIS A polyp is usually only apparent once it has reached a size where it causes the vulva to appear swollen or is visible as a pink mass bulging from the vulva.

TREATMENT Vaginal polyps have to be surgically removed.

TUMOURS OF THE REPRODUCTIVE TRACT

Tumours of the ovaries, uterus, cervix, and vagina are infrequently diagnosed, primarily because neutering of females removes most of the tissue in which these tumours grow. In intact females, a vet also rarely diagnoses the tumours until they have reached an advanced state of development.

TREATMENT The treatment of choice is a complete ovariohysterectomy (*see p.316*), including the cervix.

Secondary spread of these tumours is rarely observed.

PREVENTION Spaying before the female enters her first oestrus will eliminate the risk of mammary tumour. Spaying after multiple seasons, does not reduce the risk.

MAMMARY GLAND DISEASES

A female typically has two rows of five mammary glands. Each row extends from the chest to the groin. The mammary glands in the groin are the most likely to be affected by infection and the most severe form of mammary tumour. Those glands on the chest are the least likely to develop serious medical problems.

MAMMARY ENLARGEMENT

The mammary glands naturally enlarge with milk during late pregnancy, but they also enlarge during a false pregnancy (*see p.314*).

TREATMENT For healthy females in false pregnancy, the best treatment is simply to withhold water for five to ten hours, and food for a day. These steps are often enough to stop the further production of milk.

VET'S ADVICE

The earlier a lump is found, the better the prognosis. If your female has not been spayed, or if she was spayed after having oestrous cycles for several years, get into the habit of carefully examining her mammary tissue. Mammary tumours develop most commonly in the regions closest to the teats. They are similar to "duct carcinomas" in women. Feel under the teats for what start as small, hard, gritty lumps. Lumps in the skin are unlikely to be true mammary tumours.

MAMMARY TUMOURS

These tumours are the most common form of cancer to affect females. Most are so-called "mixed mammary tumours" with the potential to become malignant. While many mammary tumours appear as hard, mobile, pebble-like masses under the skin near the teats, the most aggressive form causes rapid, painful swelling in the breasts in the groin. Visually, it is not possible to differentiate this form

SPAYING FOR HEALTH AND CONVENIENCE

Spaying involves removing not only the uterus but also the ovaries. All diseases of the uterus are triggered by activity in the ovaries. Neutering before the first season also dramatically reduces the risk of mammary tumours. Apart from the impact on the health of a female, the advantage of an ovariohysterectomy is that the individual ceases to experience oestrous cycles and to attract males. Generally speaking, most owners do not want the inconvenience of twice-yearly temperament changes and the nuisance consequences of canine ovulation on the male dog population, even if pregnancy is no longer a consideration.

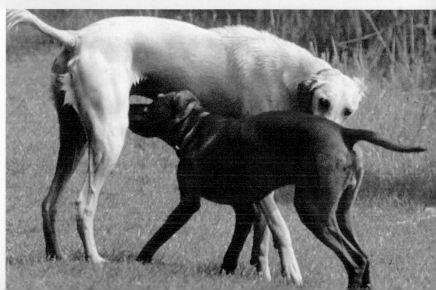

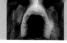

of tumour from mastitis. It is often complicated by a secondary bacterial infection, and so antibiotic treatment will produce an initial reduction in the swelling and the pain.

DIAGNOSIS AND TREATMENT Removal and the histopathological testing of tissue is the only guaranteed way of diagnosing a mammary tumour correctly. Discrete masses of tumour tissue should be removed by a partial or regional mastectomy. Aggressive, inflamed tumours in the mammary glands in the groin area can be particularly unpleasant.

PREVENTION The risk of mammary tumours is negligible in females spayed before their first oestrus. Spaying after the first oestrus still reduces risk by over 99 per cent! Subsequent seasons increase the risk. Spaying after about six oestrous cycles does not reduce the risk but because mammary tumours "feed" on female hormones, reduces the speed of development.

MEDICAL PROBLEMS DURING PREGNANCY

When a pregnant female fails to take one or more pups to full term, the pups die and are either resorbed by the mother's body or else aborted and expelled from the womb.

Take the following special precautions when caring for your pregnant dog.
• Make sure she does not receive any vaccinations during the first four weeks of pregnancy.
• Do not give her any drugs unless they are absolutely necessary.
• Keep her away from any places where she might ingest insecticides.
• Do not administer any herbs unless they are proven safe to use with dogs during pregnancy.
• If she develops worms, treat her only with anthelminthic medicines that are known to be safe and effective for use during pregnancy.
• Do not subject her to any excessive energy demands, such as long walks.
• Do not project human values on to her. Your dog does not need a pregnancy to feel fulfilled.

RESORPTION

Foetal resorption can occur during the first six weeks of pregnancy. One or more pups may die, their remains are broken down, and as much as possible is removed by the white blood cells of the immune system.

If resorption occurs early in the pregnancy, few if any clinical signs will manifest themselves. The female seems perfectly normal. Later on, resorption produces so much waste that she

becomes quiet and listless. Residue of the pup remains may become infected, causing a fever, loss of appetite, and a blood-tinged or purulent vaginal discharge. Oral antibiotics given for several weeks are necessary.

ABORTION

After foetuses die, the muscles of the womb may contract and discharge them and their associated products. This is usually called a miscarriage or spontaneous abortion.

A variety of infectious agents can cause abortion. Carriers of the bacterium *Brucella canis* (see p.151) are usually free of signs of illness until abortion occurs, usually at seven to eight weeks of pregnancy. Loss of foetuses is accompanied by a brown-to-green vaginal discharge. *Brucella* can also cause foetal resorption.

Canine herpesvirus infection (see p.146) early in pregnancy causes death and mummification of the foetuses. Later infection causes either abortion or live births followed by death of the pups soon afterwards.

Toxoplasma gondii (see p.173) may cause premature birth or stillbirth, while pups born with *Neospora caninum* (see p.174) will die soon after birth.

MEDICAL PROBLEMS AT BIRTH

Approximately five per cent of all canine births will involve a medical problem. Some breeds experience few or negligible problems, while in other breeds the incidence of problems is extraordinarily high.

Do not hesitate to contact your vet if your dog appears to be experiencing problems with giving birth, or if you think that there is something wrong with the newborn pups – even if you feel unsure and fear it might only be a false alarm. It is a rare vet who does not derive particular pleasure from helping a mother to deliver her pups as comfortably as possible.

VET'S ADVICE

When a pup is born it will acquire protection against various diseases to which its mother has been exposed. This protection is contained in the mother's first milk, or colostrum, and passed on when the pup suckles at its mother's breast. For example, if its mother has been vaccinated against distemper (*see p.147*), maternal antibodies against this disease are passed on to the pup in the colostrum. This is why it is so important for newborn pups to start suckling their mother's milk straight away. The protection is short-lived and lasts from six to 20 weeks. Do not try to boost this natural protection by vaccinating a dog when she is pregnant. Her immune system is already compromised because she is carrying "foreign protein" – her own pups – in her womb. Never vaccinate housemates of pregnant females – vaccine virus can be shed by these dogs and passed on to the mother-to-be.

Medical problems are most likely to occur in the following circumstances:
• females that are pregnant for the first time;
• the delivery of the first pup of a litter, no matter how many times the mother has been pregnant;
• pregnant females who are fat or overweight;
• females who have become pregnant later in life;
• pregnant females that are nervous, anxious, or excitable;
• small mothers with only a single pup or a small litter;
• breeds with large heads, such as the Bulldog;
• when the father is considerably larger than the mother;
• mothers that have previously suffered an injury to the pelvis.

FAILURE TO CONTRACT (UTERINE INERTIA)

Usually, a pregnancy should not last much longer than 67 days after conception without a female showing some signs of impending labour. (Occasionally, some females will not go into labour until 69 or 70 days.)

Lack of contractions, called uterine inertia, can occur with single-pup litters, faulty hormonal activity in the mother, altered muscle tone in the womb, or low levels of calcium circulating in the bloodstream.

Although it is virtually impossible to do from a physiological point of view, some females, particularly small, nervous individuals, can temporarily inhibit the involuntary muscles that cause uterine contractions. This is called "primary" inertia.

Secondary uterine inertia occurs when the uterus has become tired after it has been contracting for some time.

DIAGNOSIS Any female that has reached 67 days of pregnancy and has not yet started her contractions should be examined by avet. An X-ray or ultrasound scan will reveal the position and number of pups.

ASSESSING BIRTHING PROBLEMS

Most dogs manage to give birth with little difficulty. Expect problems, however, if your female was mated with a larger male, because the large pups may not fit easily through her birth canal. Be prepared for difficult births in breeds with large heads or in very small breeds such as Yorkshire Terriers and Chihuahuas. Some dogs become very distressed at birth and virtually stop contracting, wanting to be on a lap rather than in the whelping box or pen.

PROBLEM	ACTION
Mismatched mating	Contact vet after mating for advice
Dog not in labour after 64 days	Contact vet
Stage one of labour (pacing, nesting, and refusing food) lasts over 36 hours	Contact vet
Water has broken but there are no contractions after two hours	Contact vet immediately
No pup after 30 minutes in stage two of labour (contractions)	Contact vet immediately
Blood or green fluid is passed before the first pup is delivered	Contact vet immediately
Contractions stop with pup visible, and do not resume within ten minutes	Contact vet immediately
Pup not expelled after 20 minutes of contractions	Contact vet immediately
Contractions are weak or intermittent	Contact vet immediately
Pups still retained in uterus after two hours since the last delivery	Contact vet immediately
Mother is apathetic, pale, shivering, or twitching	Contact vet immediately
Rectal temperature is below 37.5°C (97.5°F) or over 39.4°C (103°F)	Contact vet immediately
Foul-smelling bloody or black discharge, or greenish-yellow purulent discharge	Contact vet immediately
Green vaginal discharge immediately after birth	Natural; arrange check-up
Green vaginal discharge more than 36 hours after birth	Contact vet immediately
Number of afterbirths is fewer than number of puppies	Contact vet within 24 hours

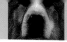

TREATMENT If the cervix is dilated, oxytocin may be given to stimulate contractions. If the cervix is not yet open, an anti-anxiety drug or a tranquilliser may be used.

DIFFICULT LABOUR (DYSTOCIA)

Two of the most common reasons for difficult labour, or dystocia, are to do with the pups. A pup is either too large to pass through the birth canal or is in the wrong position for delivery.

TREATMENT Your vet can rectify some "wrong positions" with fingers and delivery forceps. For others, and for pups that are simply too large, a Caesarean section is the only option.

CAESAREAN SECTION

In a Caesarean, the womb is opened, the pups removed, and the womb sewn shut. It is relatively common and is the treatment of choice for difficult labour where pups cannot or will not pass through the birth canal. A routine Caesarean must take place in a "clean" environment. Any contamination to the area – for example, from the death and decomposition of a pup – makes surgery more difficult and exposes the mother to the danger of infection.

The decision to carry out a Caesarean is influenced by:
• how long the expectant mother has been in labour;
• what X–rays, ultrasound and finger examinations reveal;
• how well the uterus responds to an oxytocin injection;
• the overall medical condition of either the mother or the pups or both;
• whether the anatomy of the mother has any peculiarities.

STILLBIRTH

Fully formed pups die just before birth for a variety of reasons. Entire litters may be affected by infections such as herpesvirus or toxoplasmosis.

PRESENTING POSITIONS OF PUPPIES

A female's litter grows in the two horns of her uterus. At the moment of birth, the position in which the pups present is important to successful delivery. Pups should be delivered head first in a "diving" position. Backwards (back feet and tail first) is also normal, but the elbows may get caught on the pelvic rim. "Wrong positions" include: two foetuses presented simultaneously, one from each horn of the uterus; breech (backwards but with the hind legs flexed forwards); forwards but with the head turned to the side; forwards but with the front feet flexed backwards; and back first.

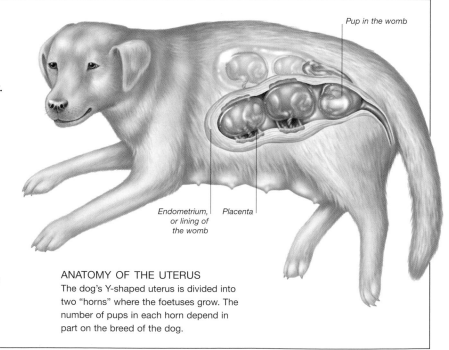

Pup in the womb

Endometrium, or lining of the womb

Placenta

ANATOMY OF THE UTERUS
The dog's Y-shaped uterus is divided into two "horns" where the foetuses grow. The number of pups in each horn depend in part on the breed of the dog.

Single pups in litters may die at birth because of lethal physical defects that prevent survival once the umbilical cord is severed. They may also die because they spend a prolonged length of time in the birth canal after the life-sustaining activity of the umbilical cord has ended and before breathing on its own can begin.

MEDICAL PROBLEMS AFTER BIRTH

The death of a puppy, either just before it is born or during the first week of its life, is sad but it is fairly common. Such deaths account for about one out of seven pups.

Puppy death is inevitable in species, such as the dog, in which the females have multiple births. Most puppy deaths – 65 per cent by one estimate – occur within a week of birth. Typically, between ten and 30 per cent of pups die between birth and weaning.

Mothers, too, can experience one of several "postpartum" conditions, such as bleeding, retaining the placenta, problems with the mammary glands or the uterus, and eclampsia.

BLEEDING

Birth should involve only a small amount of blood loss, and normally there is only mild bleeding. Anything more than this indicates a problem, such as a tear to the vagina. Alert your vet immediately.

RETAINED PLACENTA

After birth has taken place, count the placentas and the pups and make sure that there are the same number of each. Remember, a placenta may take up to 24 hours to be delivered. If there are fewer placentas than pups, assume that a placenta has been retained.

DIAGNOSIS AND TREATMENT If necessary, see your vet, who will give the dog oxytocin to encourage further contractions. A retained placenta almost invariably becomes infected.

ACUTE WOMB INFECTION (METRITIS)

After birth, bacteria can easily migrate from the vulva and into the womb, causing metritis. An affected dog becomes lethargic and feverish, is not interested in her pups, has lost her appetite, and is dehydrated. She shows a purulent discharge, which may be bloody, from her vagina. Womb infection often occurs as a result of an owner's attempts to help their dog give birth in non-sterile conditions.

DIAGNOSIS AND TREATMENT A vet will confirm the diagnosis by culture and sensitivity tests. The infected dog needs immediate treatment with intravenous fluids, antibiotics, and oxytocin to stimulate uterine contractions. In some instances, an emergency hysterectomy may be necessary.

MASTITIS

Mastitis is an infection that may occur during lactation (milk production), when opportunistic bacteria enter the active mammary tissue through skin scratches or punctures.

DIAGNOSIS The local area of the gland is hot, inflamed, reddish-blue, and tender. The female may be lethargic, refusing to eat, and running a fever. Squeezing the teat canal may produce stringy, blood-tinged milk.

TREATMENT Acute mastitis is treated with painkillers and antibiotics, and warm compresses applied for 15 minutes several times daily. Suckling pups should not suckle from infected teats – they are unlikely to do so because of the unpleasant smell and taste. If a female is generally unwell because of mastitis, take the pups away and hand feed them until the antibiotics cure her.

RUPTURED UTERUS

The uterus can tear during birth, causing intense abdominal pain and rapidly developing shock. Alert your vet immediately.

TREATMENT Surgery is urgently needed.

BREEDS AT RISK

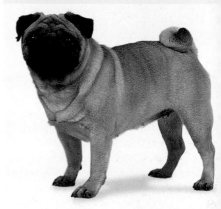

Any small female that is mated to a large dog has an increased risk of a difficult birth requiring a Caesarean. Breed adaptations have made some types of dog more prone to such birth problems, especially those breeds with large heads.

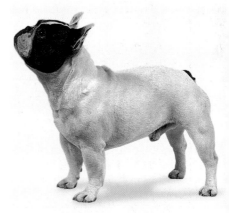

Breeds with an anatomy that increases the likelihood of Caesarean section include:

- Boston Terrier (above)
- Bulldog
- Chihuahua
- Pekingese
- Pug (top)

UTERUS PROLAPSE

While the vagina can sometimes prolapse after birth *(see p. 320)*, so, too, can the entire uterus.

TREATMENT Your vet may try to replace the uterus manually under anaesthesia, but a hysterectomy is usually required.

PLACENTAL SUBINVOLUTION

The wall of the uterus needs to be renewed after the pups are born and their placentas expelled. This renewal of the tissue, called involution, takes approximately 15 weeks.

If the uterine replacement is faulty the condition is called placental subinvolution. This serious condition is more likely to occur in females that are younger than three years of age, after they have given birth to one or even two litters. This subinvolution causes chronic bleeding from the uterus, leading to severe anaemia.

TREATMENT An affected dog needs an emergency hysterectomy.

NO MILK LETDOWN (AGALACTIA)

Before the female gives birth, the hormone prolactin is released from the pituitary gland, stimulating milk production in the breasts. During a natural birth, pressure on the vaginal walls may stimulate the release of the hormone oxytocin. This hormone is thought to be needed for the breasts to release the milk, a state called milk letdown. Certainly, milk letdown appears to activate a brain mechanism that helps with bonding. Mothers may be less likely to reject pups born by Caesarean if they are given oxytocin.

Agalactia is an absence of milk letdown and is caused by a failure to either produce milk or release it. The reasons for it are poorly understood. It may be that nervousness and fear stimulate the fight-or-flight response and release adrenaline, which inhibits the milk letdown action of oxytocin.

DIAGNOSIS Pups not receiving enough milk will cry more than usual. Look at and squeeze each of their mother's teats to see if they are anatomically correct and producing milk.

TREATMENT There is no treatment that will correct the mother's failure to produce milk. Instead, pups should be fed by hand. If milk is present in the mammary gland but is not released, try massaging the teat to stimulate milk flow. If some teats are flowing and others are not, place a good suckler on the poorly-producing teat. This is the best natural stimulus.

An oxytocin injection may prove useful and encourage milk letdown if it is given within a maximum of 48 hours after birth. A vet might try to relax a nervous female with either tranquillizers or mild sedation.

MATERNAL CARE PROBLEMS

There are three possible problems of maternal care: neglect, clumsiness, and exaggerated care. All are potentially lethal to newborn pups.

DIAGNOSIS Maternal neglect is obvious to an owner. The mother may fail to remove the foetal membranes at birth.

Later, when she does not lick, clean, nuzzle, and nurse one or more of her pups, maternal bonding fails to take place. Mothers who take no interest in their pups are, most frequently, first-time mothers and individuals deeply attached to their human family.

Clumsiness may occur at birth or afterwards. A mother can injure her pups as she chews off the placental attachment, or she may roll on them while they are sleeping, a considerable problem with large breeds that produce big litters.

TREATMENT Make sure that the whelping pen offers protection for pups from the weight of a clumsy mother, *(see also p.61)*.

Monitor all new mothers carefully, both at birth and immediately after birth. Give them whatever assistance you think is necessary.

Keep any curious visitors away to reduce distractions and to allow the mother to concentrate on bonding with her pups.

In some cases, your vet will dispense tranquillizers or sedatives.

ADVICE Statistically, one in seven or eight pups is born with a constitutional medical condition. This illness usually

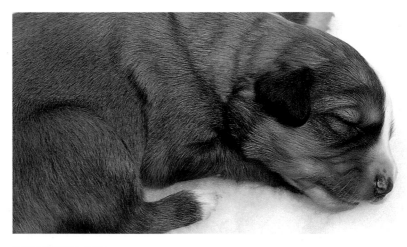

OSTRACIZED PUP
It is not uncommon for a mother to separate out one of her pups and distance it from herself and her litter. She probably senses something wrong with the pup. It is a natural and evolutionarily efficient way for her to devote all her energies to those most likely to survive.

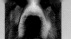

EXAGGERATED CARE

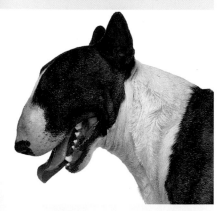

Exaggerated maternal care is a particular concern with Staffordshire Bull Terrier mothers. Maternal licking of the birth membranes can become so exaggerated that it damages the skin around the umbilicus or the puppy's head. In some distressing circumstances, this behaviour can evolve into cannibalism, when a pup's head is consumed. Bull Terrier mothers should be monitored for 24 hours each day for the first several days to ensure that maternal care does not become excessive.

POST-BIRTH PROBLEMS

Most mothers, even novices, are amazingly efficient at giving birth. Without any need for prenatal classes they intuitively know exactly what to do. Mistakes do sometimes happen, however. If any of the problems listed below do occur when your dog has finished giving birth, simply follow the actions and instructions given in the right-hand column. If you are unsure what to do or are worried about either the mother or the pups, call your vet at once. *(See also p.62.)*

PROBLEM	ACTION
Mother has not licked off the placental membranes	Remove membranes.
Pup has not started breathing	Hold the pup upside down to drain fluid. Massage vigorously. If there is no breathing, shake gently and give mouth-to-nose artificial respiration *(see .389)*.
Mother has not chewed off the cord	Tie gauze or thread around the cord 1.5 cm (½ in) from the pup's body. Sever the cord between the tie and the placenta.
Mother is rejecting a pup	Warm the pup in a warm blanket, then place it on a teat. This pup may need feeding by hand *(see p.64)*.

causes a drop in the pup's temperature. A mother naturally disregards any pup with a subnormal body temperature. She may separate it from the rest of the litter. This is her way of supporting the survival of the fittest. From a health perspective it is questionable whether vets and owners should intervene.

ECLAMPSIA (PUERPERAL TETANY)

A mother may develop eclampsia, or puerperal tetany, when the constant production of milk drains too much calcium from her body. This is a potentially life-threatening condition that usually occurs two to four weeks after birth. Giving a female calcium supplements during pregnancy does

not reduce the risk of her developing life-threatening eclampsia.

The low levels of calcium in the mother's blood (hypocalcaemia) are usually the result of an inability to replace the calcium that the mother puts into her milk. Either she is not absorbing calcium properly from her food or the stress of motherhood has reduced her appetite.

The mother becomes restless and pants at first, but soon looks anxious and breathes more heavily. Her panting becomes deep and intense, with her lips pulled well back. Jerky movements develop and muscle spasms resembling those in tetany can be seen. She loses her coordination, then soon develops seizures. Alert your vet immediately.

DIAGNOSIS The symptoms give a clear indication of eclampsia. Rectal temperature is frequently very high. Eclampsia is more likely to occur in poorly nourished individuals, small females, and those with big litters.

TREATMENT Urgent treatment with intravenous calcium gluconate is necessary. High fever is treated as for heatstroke *(see pp.408–09)*.

Pups are temporarily removed from the mother and fed by hand while she recovers. Subsequently, their nursing is restricted to three periods of about 20 minutes each day, with additional hand feeding according to age and needs. The mother is given oral calcium and sometimes corticosteroids. She may be fed by hand until she recovers.

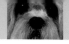

HORMONAL SYSTEM
disorders of the glands

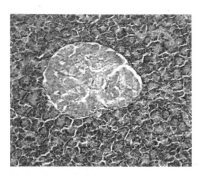

Endocrine cells in pancreas

Your dog's body has a magnificent ability to respond to the opportunities, threats, and challenges of life. While the brain and nervous system initiate instantaneous changes in body function, a small number of important hormones are responsible for the longer-term balance of the body's metabolic activities. These hormones are produced by endocrine glands and released into the bloodstream. Every cell in your dog's body possesses receptor sites that can be switched on or off by one or more endocrine hormones.

Hormones are molecular messengers that influence the chemical activity of cells. During early medical research, scientists concentrated on discovering the molecular messengers produced by the body's glands, which were visible and accessible, and called these products "hormones".

Much later, scientists discovered that other biochemical messengers, such as dopamine and serotonin, helped to conduct nervous impulses in nerves and the brain. These molecules,

called neurotransmitters, are also hormones, but they are present in infinitesimally smaller amounts. Later still, cytokines were discovered to trigger cellular activity; these are also technically referred to as hormones.

In the same way that a thermostat controls temperature, the production of a hormone by an endocrine gland is controlled by a method called biofeedback (*see opposite*).

If, at any stage in the biofeedback process, a hormone is not produced in sufficient amounts or is not turned on or off properly, a variety of medical conditions develop. Some of these are subtle and difficult to diagnose; others are devastating and life-threatening. Treatment of endocrine disorders was one of the great success stories of twentieth-century medicine.

ENDOCRINE GLANDS
Most hormones are produced by the endocrine glands. The activity of these glands is orchestrated by the pituitary (also called the "master gland"). The pituitary, in turn, is linked to and controlled by the hypothalamus, which lies at the base of the brain.

The thyroid and parathyroid glands are situated together in front of the trachea. They produce thyroid and

parathyroid hormones, which help to regulate energy production and calcium metabolism respectively.

The adrenal glands, next to the kidneys, make cortisol and adrenaline. These hormones are central to both an animal's "fight or flight" response and its response to stress.

In females, ovaries make oestrogen and progesterone. In pregnant bitches, the placenta releases hormones that help the foetus develop. In male dogs, the testes produce the male sex hormone testosterone.

The pineal gland, in the centre of the brain, secretes melatonin, which is crucial to maintaining the internal biological clock and the daily rhythms of sleeping and waking.

OTHER HORMONES
As well as glands, certain other body tissues produce hormones, although this is not their primary function. In the pancreas, cells called the islets of Langerhans make insulin, which is vital for the metabolism of glucose. Cells in the stomach lining secrete gastrin, which triggers the release of acid during digestion. The kidneys release vasopressin, to help control blood pressure, and erythropoetin, which aids the generation of red blood cells.

Q **WHAT ARE HORMONES MADE OF?**

A Hormones are simple chemical compounds, usually made from proteins and fats.

Q **WHAT IS THE DIFFERENCE BETWEEN NATURAL AND SYNTHETIC HORMONES?**

A Natural hormones are collected from the glands of animals; for example, forms of insulin are taken from the pancreas of pigs. Synthetic hormones are made in a laboratory. These include L-thyroxine for hypothyroidism.

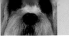

HORMONAL BIOFEEDBACK MECHANISM

The ebb and flow of hormones in the bloodstream is controlled by the biofeedback mechanism. When a hormone is needed, the brain is stimulated and sends a signal to the hypothalamus. This area then signals the pituitary gland to send a stimulating hormone to the relevant gland (the "target gland"). The target gland releases its hormone into the bloodstream. As that hormone circulates, it acts on the relevant tissues. It also passes through the pituitary, giving the gland "feedback" on the level in the bloodstream. When the hormone has performed its function, the pituitary stops secreting the stimulating hormone and, as a result, the target gland also stops production. If the hormone is needed again, the biofeedback cycle is repeated.

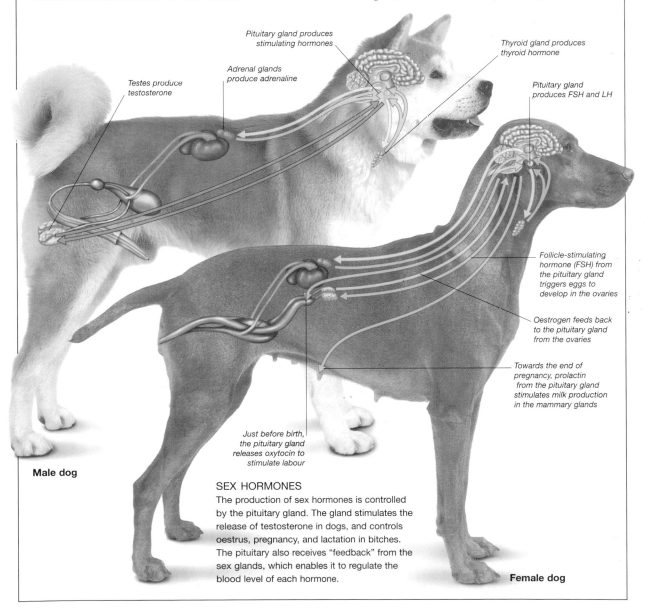

Pituitary gland produces stimulating hormones

Thyroid gland produces thyroid hormone

Adrenal glands produce adrenaline

Testes produce testosterone

Pituitary gland produces FSH and LH

Follicle-stimulating hormone (FSH) from the pituitary gland triggers eggs to develop in the ovaries

Oestrogen feeds back to the pituitary gland from the ovaries

Towards the end of pregnancy, prolactin from the pituitary gland stimulates milk production in the mammary glands

Just before birth, the pituitary gland releases oxytocin to stimulate labour

Male dog

Female dog

SEX HORMONES

The production of sex hormones is controlled by the pituitary gland. The gland stimulates the release of testosterone in dogs, and controls oestrus, pregnancy, and lactation in bitches. The pituitary also receives "feedback" from the sex glands, which enables it to regulate the blood level of each hormone.

Q DO HORMONAL DRUGS FOR HUMANS ALSO WORK IN DOGS?

A Generally speaking, yes, they do. There are, for example, more or less insignificant differences between canine and human sex hormones. Testosterone tablets for humans work equally well for dogs. Many of the therapeutic hormonal drugs used for dogs were, in fact, first licensed for use in humans.

Q WHAT IS A "WATER DEPRIVATION TEST", AND WHY IS IT CARRIED OUT?

A This test is simply an exercise in which water is withheld for a specific period, such as a day. Food is also withheld because of its fluid content. The test is used to detect diabetes insipidus. In healthy dogs, lack of fluids stimulates the pituitary gland to produce ADH, which causes the body to conserve water and makes the urine more concentrated. In diabetes insipidus, however, the water level in the urine does not decrease even when the dog is not taking in any fluids.

Q DOES HYPOTHYROIDISM AFFECT DOGS IN THE SAME WAY AS IT DOES HUMANS?

A Some symptoms do seem to be similar in humans and in dogs. Hypothyroidal people are "weather conscious" – they suffer muscular pain that increases in cold, rainy weather. Affected dogs may have the same problem. There are also similar behavioural changes. In one human study, two-thirds of people with attention-deficit disorder were found to be hypothyroidal, and thyroid supplementation helped to overcome their problem. In dogs, behaviour problems and mood changes have also been traced to thyroid disorders (*see opposite*).

PITUITARY DISORDERS

The pituitary gland produces several hormones that control key functions of the body. Two of these hormones act directly on other parts of the body. Growth hormone (GH) manages the growth of the tissues and organs in puppies, and controls the health of every cell in adult dogs. Anti-diuretic hormone (ADH) acts on the kidneys and regulates urination.

Instructed by the hypothalamus, the pituitary also produces hormones that control the output of the other endocrine glands. These hormones include thyroid-stimulating hormone (TSH), adrenal corticotropic hormone (ACTH), and two sex hormones: follicle-stimulating hormone (FSH) and luteinizing hormone (LH). In females, FSH causes eggs to mature in the ovaries and LH triggers the release of eggs (ovulation). In males, LH triggers the production of testosterone.

Pituitary disorders arise when there is an excess or a lack of particular pituitary hormones. Clinical conditions involving FSH and LH production, however, are very rare.

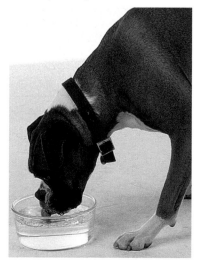

DRINKING TOO MUCH
When a dog drinks water excessively and in large amounts, it is probably suffering from diabetes insipidus.

DIABETES INSIPIDUS

When the pituitary fails to make or release antidiuretic hormone (ADH), or when the kidneys do not respond to it, diabetes insipidus develops.

In young dogs, diabetes insipidus is a functional problem in the pituitary gland. In middle-aged and older dogs, the condition is most likely to be caused by a pituitary tumour.

DIAGNOSIS Affected dogs typically drink almost incessantly, consuming copious amounts of water, and urinate all the time. The specific gravity of their urine (its density relative to the density of water) is 1.001 or less. Disease is confirmed by a monitored water-deprivation test.

TREATMENT This condition is treated with synthetic ADH called DDAVP, given as eye drops twice daily. DDAVP is also available as tablets. The outlook for young dogs is excellent, but it is much less promising for older dogs when a pituitary tumour is the cause.

ACROMEGALY

If the pituitary gland produces an excessive amount of growth hormone (GH), a condition called acromegaly will develop. This condition is extremely rare.

Excessive secretion of GH may occur spontaneously, but it is just as likely to be stimulated by the female hormone progesterone. This hormone may be present in the body either during oestrus, when it is naturally produced, or when it is medically administered. GH triggers proliferation of all tissues, including cartilage and bone. The dog's skin often thickens, especially around the neck. The feet, head, and belly increase in size. The spaces between the teeth increase, and the lower jaw may protrude. Acromegalic dogs are lethargic and pant more than normal.

DIAGNOSIS Visible signs provide a clear diagnosis, especially in middle-aged or older, unneutered (unspayed) females, or in females receiving progesterone

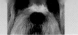

supplements. GH levels in the blood are monitored. There can be associated diabetes mellitus (*see p.322*) with increased blood sugar.

TREATMENT Progesterone-related acromegaly is treated by withdrawing progesterone treatment and spaying.

GROWTH HORMONE (RESPONSIVE DERMATOSIS)

This skin disorder occurs when the pituitary produces too little growth hormone. It affects dogs between the ages of two and five. The condition is extremely rare.

Affected animals are otherwise normal, but develop symmetrical hair loss on the body, neck, ears, and tail. The skin gradually becomes darker. Breeds in which the disease has been recognized include Chow Chows, Keeshonds, Toy and Miniature Poodles, Pomeranians, and Samoyeds.

DIAGNOSIS To confirm the diagnosis, a blood test is carried out to measure the GH level. A substance known to stimulate GH is injected, and further blood samples are then analysed to measure GH levels.

TREATMENT A diagnosis may often be academic, if only because the treatment for the condition (human growth hormone) is extremely expensive and almost impossible to obtain.

THYROID DISORDERS

The two-lobed thyroid gland secretes thyroid hormone, which regulates the body's metabolic activity. Because the hormone's activities and effects are so diverse, symptoms of thyroid disease vary enormously.

HYPOTHYROIDISM

Perhaps the most common hormonal problem in dogs is an underactive thyroid gland, resulting in a deficiency of thyroid hormone. It is reported to affect one out of 250 dogs. In four out of five sufferers, hypothyroidism is an immune-mediated disease, in which the thyroid is attacked and destroyed by the dog's own immune system.

Hypothyroidism is found more often in certain breeds. Cocker Spaniels are overwhelmingly the breed most commonly diagnosed with the condition; Dobermans and Golden Retrievers also have a higher than average incidence. The large number of cases seen in these breeds is partly due to their popularity; however, all three breeds are also known to suffer from various immune disorders. It seems that by selective breeding, using particular lines in each breed, humans may have unwittingly selected for overactive immune systems.

BREEDS AT RISK

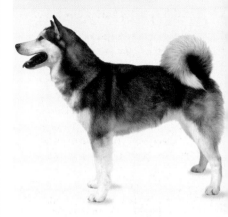

Breeds with a greater than average incidence of hypothyroidism are usually medium to large in size.

The breeds most commonly diagnosed with hypothyroidism are:

- Cocker Spaniel
- Doberman
- Golden Retriever

Other affected breeds include:

- Afghan Hound
- Akita
- Airedale
- Alaskan Malamute (above)
- Beagle
- Borzoi
- Boxer
- Brittany
- Bulldog
- Chow Chow
- Dachshunds
- Great Dane
- Irish Setter
- Irish Wolfhound
- Leonberger
- Miniature Schnauzer
- Newfoundland
- Old English Sheepdog
- Pomeranian
- Poodles
- Shetland Sheepdog

SIGNS OF HYPOTHYROIDISM

The signs of an underactive thyroid gland and the consequent low levels of thyroid hormone can be grouped into very common signs, common ones, and signs that may only appear occasionally.

VERY COMMON	COMMON	OCCASIONAL
Lethargy	Weakness	Oily skin (seborrhoea)
Weight gain	Poor hair quality	Ear inflammation (otitis)
Less tolerance of exercise	Increased skin pigmentation	Skin thickening
Thinning hair	Skin infection (pyoderma) "Tragic" facial expression	Intolerance to cold

There is a range of signs (*see box p.331*), as well as other indicators such as nerve and eye conditions and diarrhoea. There are no obvious signs until about three-quarters of the thyroid has been destroyed, and they may develop very slowly. These facts, as well as other diseases that may also temporarily reduce thyroid activity, probably result in the condition being under-diagnosed.

In addition to physical signs, dogs that have known thyroid disease may show various unusual signs of behaviour. These signs may include unexpected aggression, submissiveness, shyness, fearfulness, passivity, excitability, sensitivity to noise, anxiety, irritability, compulsive activity, chewing, moodiness, lethargy, or apparent depression.

In a survey of 319 dogs with behaviour problems, Professor Nicholas Dodman at Tufts University, Boston, and Dr Jean Dodds found that 208 had thyroid disorders. If your dog has shown signs of a recent mood change, always consider the possibility of a hormone disorder.

DIAGNOSIS Levels of cholesterol and triglycerides (a type of fatty acid) in the blood are raised in about three-quarters of hypothyroidal dogs. A similar number have mild anaemia.

The level of the hormone thyroxine in the blood can be measured. The test results may be difficult to interpret, however, because many illnesses and certain drugs (such as those containing corticosteroids or sulfa) temporarily reduce the blood level of thyroid hormones. Most hypothyroidal dogs have reduced thyroid hormone levels and increased levels of thyroid-stimulating hormone (TSH).

A popular diagnostic test is simply to give extra thyroid hormone and monitor the dog for responses such as better hair quality and activity levels. This is practical but can be misleading – even dogs with normal thyroid glands may grow more hair on this treatment.

TREATMENT Affected dogs respond within days to a synthetic thyroid hormone called L-thyroxine, becoming more alert and willingly taking more exercise. Weight loss is obvious within weeks, but coat changes take much longer – up to 12 weeks. The outlook is excellent. On daily L-thyroxine a dog has a normal life expectancy.

OVERACTIVE THYROID GLAND (HYPERTHYROIDISM)

Overproduction of thyroid hormone is unusual or even rare. Hyperthyroidism is nearly always caused by a hormone-producing tumour. (The majority of thyroid tumours do not produce hormones; however, such tumours are invasive carcinomas (*see p.136*). They often cause other signs, such as coughing and vomiting, because they cause compression of the tissues in the throat and stomach.) Some breeds are particularly likely to develop thyroid tumours (*see box opposite*).

A dog with an overactive thyroid gland has a voracious appetite but loses weight. This is usually, but not always, accompanied by increased drinking and urination. The dog may also become more physically active and show behaviour changes such as increased irritability and aggression.

DIAGNOSIS Affected dogs are usually around ten years old but may be as young as five. If the thyroid gland is enlarged, the vet will be able to feel it in the neck. If hyperthyroidism is suspected, blood samples will be taken; if the condition is present, the results will reveal consistently elevated thyroid hormone levels in the bloodstream.

TREATMENT Surgical removal of the thyroid tumour is the recommended treatment for hyperthyroidism. This measure is very effective for benign tumours but is less helpful for the malignant ones (which occur more commonly). Chemotherapy and radiation therapy both prolong the quantity and quality of life.

ENLARGED THYROID GLAND

The thyroid gland has two lobes and lies beside the trachea. It has one of the richest blood supplies of any tissue in the body. Thyroid enlargement is usually due to tumours. Benign tumours usually cause only a slight enlargement, but malignant tumours turn the gland into a large, solid mass that presses on the trachea, oesophagus, and surrounding tissues.

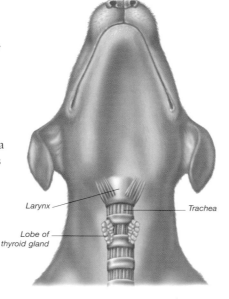

Larynx

Trachea

Lobe of thyroid gland

THE THYROID GLAND
The two lobes of the thyroid gland are situated beside the trachea and just below the thyroid cartilage of the larynx.

PARATHYROID DISORDERS

The parathyroid glands are two tiny areas of tissue, each lying beside a lobe of the thyroid gland. They secrete parathyroid hormone (PTH), which increases the level of calcium in the blood. A hormone called calcitonin, secreted by the thyroid gland, inhibits PTH production if necessary. Medical diseases occur if this balance is upset.

OVERACTIVE PARATHYROID GLANDS

This condition, also called primary hyperparathyroidism, affects older dogs and particularly Keeshonds (*see box right*). It is usually caused by a tumour that makes excess PTH. It can also occur in association with urinary tract disorders that cause the formation of crystals or stones containing calcium. The symptoms are vague; they include increased drinking and urination or urinary incontinence. Many affected animals are listless and lethargic.

DIAGNOSIS This disease is difficult to diagnose quickly. There is increased calcium in the blood, and perhaps urinary tract disease with associated crystals or stones containing calcium. The level of blood phosphorus may be low. The parathyroids are too small to be seen on X–ray or ultrasound.

TREATMENT Affected dogs are treated with diuretics and bicarbonate to manage their excess blood calcium. A parathyroid tumour may be either injected with ethanol to reduce its activity or surgically removed.

UNDERACTIVE PARATHYROID GLANDS

This condition, which is also known as hypocalcemia, leads to a serious lack of calcium in the blood. It causes nerve and muscle problems such as twitching and trembling. Affected

BREEDS AT RISK

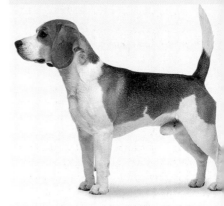

Breeds that may have a higher than typical incidence of thyroid tumours include:

- Beagle (above)
- Boxer
- Golden Retriever
- German Shepherd

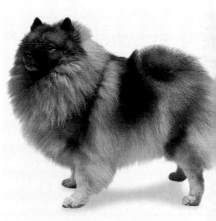

The breed that is most frequently affected by tumours producing an excessive amount of parathyroid hormone is the Keeshond (above). Even within this breed, however, hyperparathyroidism is extremely rare. Although the Keeshond is related to other Spitz breeds, the tendency to develop parathyroid tumours and hyperparathyroidism is not noted in these breeds.

NUTRITIONAL HYPERPARATHYROIDISM

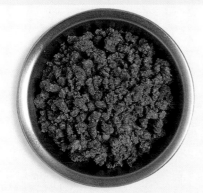

Minced beef

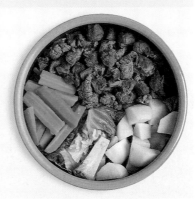

Balanced diet

While it is tempting to think that fresh, home-cooked food will be best for your dog's health, getting the nutrient balance wrong can cause problems. An example of an unbalanced diet is one consisting wholly or mostly of meat, which is high in phosphorus and low in calcium. Dogs need calcium, so the parathyroid gland will attempt to compensate for the lack by raising PTH production and leaching calcium out of the bones. In this condition, called nutritional secondary hyperparathyroidism, the excess PTH activity causes the bones to become thin and the teeth to loosen. Finally, there is no calcium left to leach out and the dog then develops hypocalcemia (see above). Treatment is with vitamin D supplements and, of course, a better balanced diet.

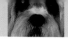
Q WHAT IS THE "FIGHT OR FLIGHT" RESPONSE?

A When an animal is faced by a sudden danger, a series of events takes place inside its body. In particular, the adrenal glands release the hormones adrenaline and noradrenaline.

Adrenaline is sometimes called the emergency hormone because it is released during stress and primes an animal for "fight or flight". It causes networks of minute blood vessels in the body to constrict, but simultaneously stimulates the blood vessels in the muscles and the liver to dilate.

Both adrenaline and noradrenaline stimulate the heart, causing it to pump more blood and raising the blood pressure. The two hormones also affect the digestive system: adrenaline stimulates the breakdown of glycogen to glucose in the liver, raising the level of blood sugar; and both hormones increase the level of fatty acids circulating in the blood. The blood sugar and fatty acids provide extra fuel to enable the dog to fight or run away, or for increased alertness.

Q IS STRESS GOOD OR BAD FOR DOGS?

A A little stress is good and may even be vital for physical and emotional health; however, chronic stress, in which adrenaline is constantly flooding the body, is dangerous because the adrenaline will eventually corrode and disable the immune system. This is why a whole variety of serious conditions, including heart disease, serious infections, and cancer, is more common in chronically stressed animals than in those with normal adrenaline activity.

dogs walk in a stiff or stilted manner. Early signs may be a tense expression on the face or displays of increased nervousness. Face rubbing is common. Underactive parathyroid glands are particularly likely in certain breeds (*see box opposite*).

If they are left untreated, many affected dogs go on to develop the classic convulsions of grand mal epilepsy (*see p.345*), but they do not lose consciousness or urinate excessively.

DIAGNOSIS AND TREATMENT A low level of calcium in the blood is the classic laboratory finding. Affected dogs are given diazepam to control seizures and calcium gluconate intravenously. Long-term treatment consists of vitamin D and calcium supplementation.

ADRENAL GLAND DISORDERS

The two adrenal glands, located beside each kidney, are integral both to life-sustaining metabolic activities and to the body's "fight or flight" response. Adrenal hormones are involved in the following body functions: metabolism of protein, fat and carbohydrate; metabolism of water; regulating blood pressure; and managing sodium and potassium concentrations.

The adrenal glands make adrenaline and noradrenaline, which increase the heart rate and encourage blood flow to the muscles. They also make the male sex hormone androgen. In addition, they produce two types of corticosteroid hormones: glucocorticoids (such as cortisol) and mineralocorticoids. These help to regulate metabolism and reduce inflammation. The latter type, in particular, also regulates sodium and potassium concentration and water balance. An excess of either type or both can supress the immune system.

The "cortisone" that vets give to dogs is a synthetic corticosteroid such as prednisone, prednisolone, or methylprednisolone. The latter has slightly less mineralocorticoid activity. These drugs are hormones, and as such mimic the action of natural hormones. This is what makes them so useful. Corticosteroids are most effective, even life-savers, in two situations: first, when

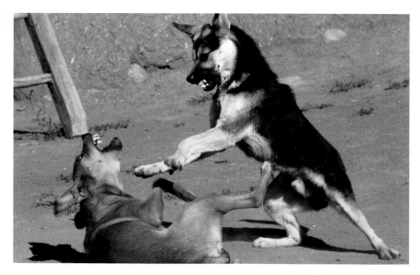

DOG FIGHTING
During a dog fight, the dogs are oblivious to their wounds because their bodies are primed for fighting by adrenaline and their pain is controlled by hormonal painkillers called endorphins. Afterwards, when adrenaline and endorphin levels subside, pain perception returns to normal.

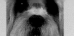
the immune system runs amok and has to be suppressed; and second, when the body is in clinical shock and needs to be revived. My impression is that I have saved more animals' lives with corticosteroids than with antibiotics.

CUSHING'S DISEASE OR SYNDROME

Cushing's disease, also known as hyperadrenocorticism, is overactivity of the cortisol-producing area of the adrenal gland. The most common cause is the pituitary gland producing an excess of adrenocorticotropic hormone (ACTH). Some breeds are genetically predisposed to developing Cushing's disease (*see box, right*).

About half of all dogs affected by pituitary-dependent Cushing's disease have small tumours of the pituitary gland. Cushing's disease may also be caused by a tumour in the adrenal gland itself, or may be due to excessive medical use of corticosteroids (in which case it is referred to as iatrogenic Cushing's disease).

Typically, an affected dog drinks and urinates excessively and is also constantly hungry. It develops a pot-bellied appearance. Hair falls from the body, but not the head or legs; the hair does not regrow if it is shaved. Dogs

pant more, and are weaker and more lethargic, than normal. Skin infection (pyoderma) is common.

DIAGNOSIS Blood tests will reveal changes to white blood cells and increased liver enzyme activity. There may also be excess sugar in the blood. X–rays or ultrasound scans show liver enlargement in most affected dogs. In males, the testicles are often small.

A definitive diagnosis is made by monitoring the cortisol response of the adrenal glands to stimulating and/or suppressing drugs. This test is used to determine whether the source of the disease is either the pituitary gland or the adrenal glands.

TREATMENT Pituitary-dependent Cushing's disease is treated with drugs that suppress pituitary overactivity. Impervious gloves should be worn when handling some of these drugs.

The ideal treatment for Cushing's disease due to an adrenal tumour is surgical removal of the tumour. This is not always possible or practical; if it is not, drugs such as mitotane or, less commonly, ketoconazole are used to suppress the overactivity of the adrenal glands.

Iatrogenic Cushing's disease usually disappears spontaneously once the dose of corticosteroid is gradually reduced.

ADDISON'S DISEASE OR SYNDROME

Addison's disease, which is also called hypoadrenocorticism, is caused by an underactive adrenal gland. This condition is more difficult to diagnose than Cushing's disease (*see above*) because, typically, the illness comes and goes. Addison's disease is usually observed in female dogs between two and seven years old. There is some evidence to suggest it may be an auto-immune disorder.

Breeds predisposed to Addison's disease include the Portuguese Water Spaniel, Leonberger, Nova Scotia Duck Tolling Retriever, and Standard Poodle. I have seen Addison's disease

BREEDS AT RISK

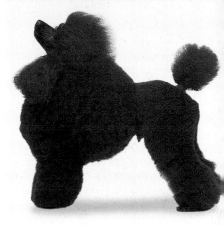

Breeds most frequently affected by underactive parathyroid glands include:

- German Shepherd
- Golden Retriever
- Labrador Retriever
- Miniature Schnauzer
- Poodles (above)
- Terriers

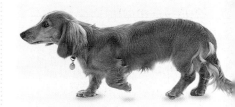

Breeds predisposed to Cushing's disease include:

- Beagle
- Boston Terrier
- Boxer
- Dachshund (above)
- German Shepherd
- Labrador Retriever
- Other terriers
- Poodles – Toy and Miniature

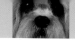
mostly in Leonbergers. The common symptoms of Addison's disease are loss of appetite, lethargy, and depression. Affected dogs lose weight, are prone to vomiting, and become weak.

A related condition, known as an Addisonian Crisis, can be caused by a lack of corticosteroids. This condition can be life-threatening. The symptoms include shivering, shaking, vomiting, dehydration, pounding heartbeat, and collapse. It needs immediate intensive veterinary care with intravenous fluids, usually including glucose, and corticosteroids.

Never abruptly stop long-term corticosteroid treatment of your dog because this is the most common cause of an Addisonian Crisis.

DIAGNOSIS Changes in the levels of electrolytes in the blood serum – low sodium, low chloride, and high potassium – are common. A low response to an adrenocorticotropic hormone (ACTH) stimulation test is the sign used to diagnose the disease.

TREATMENT Dogs are treated with both mineralocorticoid and corticosteroid supplements. Treatment commonly combines prednisolone, which has a low mineralocorticoid activity, and fludrocortisone, which has a high mineralocorticoid activity.

TUMOUR OF THE ADRENAL MEDULLA

The adrenal medulla is the part of the adrenal gland that produces adrenaline and noradrenaline. Rarely, a tumour called a phaeochromocytoma develops in the medulla. The clinical signs that it produces are frustratingly vague, such as weakness, lethargy, loss of appetite, and vomiting.

DIAGNOSIS AND TREATMENT A tumour is usually suspected after other, more common causes of the signs have been ruled out. The diagnosis will be confirmed if a mass is found in the gland and tumour cells are identified following biopsy or surgical removal.

DISORDERS OF THE PANCREAS

Insulin is a hormone produced in the pancreas, in cells called the islets of Langerhans. Its main role is to help the body's cells to absorb glucose. If the pancreas produces an excess of insulin, the level of sugar in the blood will be significantly reduced (*see pp.338–39*); this problem, which is uncommon, leads to collapse and seizures. If the pancreas produces too little insulin, the level of sugar in the blood increases, resulting in diabetes mellitus.

SUGAR DIABETES OR DIABETES MELLITUS

This is the most frequently reported endocrine disorder, affecting about one in 200 dogs. In diabetes mellitus, cells are unable to use glucose, the body's main source of energy, due to impaired action of the hormone insulin.

There are three types of diabetes. Type 1 is caused by a lack of insulin in the blood. In Type 2 there is plentiful insulin in the blood but the cells cannot use it properly. Type 3 results from over-use of corticosteroids to treat another condition.

If sugar remains in the blood but is not absorbed by the cells, affected dogs develop an increased appetite and thirst, increased urination, fatigue, weight loss, recurrent infections, and eye and circulation problems.

Stress plays an important role in diabetes. Some vets think that Type 1, the most common form in dogs, is either an autoimmune disease (in which the immune system attacks and destroys its own insulin-producing cells) or is due to chronically excessive production of corticosteroid hormones by the adrenal glands.

Females, especially fat ones, are twice as likely as males to succumb to diabetes. Some breeds are more likely to suffer from sugar diabetes, including Dachshunds, Miniature Pinschers, Poodles, and small terriers.

DIAGNOSIS Diabetic dogs are often fat or even obese, although after prolonged diabetes they may become thin. They may also develop cataracts (*see p.216*). If diagnosis is delayed any longer, they develop a serious condition called ketoacidosis (*see p.338*). Diagnosis is confirmed by the consistent presence of increased sugar levels in the blood and sugar in the urine. Increased blood sugar alone is not diagnostic because it can be caused by other conditions or even by the most recent meal.

TREATMENT Canine diabetes is almost always treated with insulin injections and a high-fibre diet. Once cataracts

VET'S ADVICE

Once a dog is mature, the number of fat cells in its body is fixed. When it puts on weight, it does not form new fat cells; instead, the existing cells distend. Under stress, cortisol from the adrenal glands acts on fat cells, making them less sensitive to insulin. This process could explain why fat dogs are more likely to develop Type 2 or Type 3 diabetes than lean dogs. You can reduce your dog's risk of sugar diabetes by controlling its weight and diet (*see p.96*), especially if it is female.

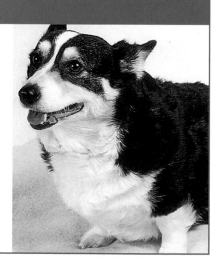

begin to develop, their progress is irreversible even with immediate insulin therapy. Blindness from cataracts is corrected by surgery, which restores vision to over three-quarters of dogs.

DIET MANAGEMENT The aim is to improve the regulation of blood sugar, and specifically to minimize the fluctuation in blood sugar triggered by eating. Blood sugar levels are lower in dogs that are fed high-fibre diets. An added value of complex carbohydrates is that they slow sugar absorption from a meal, reducing the peaks and troughs of blood sugar at and between meals.

Avoid all semi-moist foods because they stimulate the greatest blood sugar increase after eating. Starchy foods require more digestion and this slows the rate of delivery of sugar into the bloodstream. A fibre called CMC (carboxymethylcellulose), for example, helps to slow the emptying of the stomach and, by doing so, to slow the delivery of sugar into the bloodstream.

Some carbohydrates, such as barley, are digested slowly, and as a result they also slow the delivery of sugar into the bloodstream. At the opposite end of the scale, rice is digested quickly, resulting in a blood sugar "peak" and a sudden high demand for insulin.

The best diet for a diabetic dog is one made from a fixed formula with

INSULIN CYCLE

Insulin is vital for digestion. It not only regulates blood sugar levels but also prevents fats from entering or staying in the blood, where they could become dangerous by adhering to artery walls.

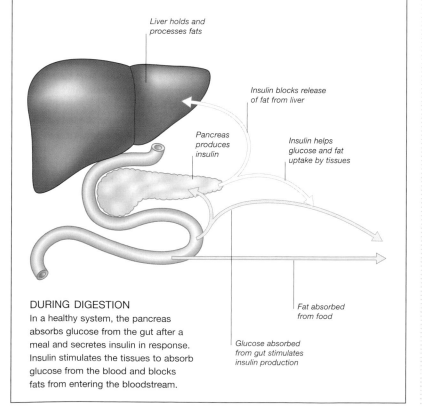

Liver holds and processes fats

Insulin blocks release of fat from liver

Pancreas produces insulin

Insulin helps glucose and fat uptake by tissues

Fat absorbed from food

Glucose absorbed from gut stimulates insulin production

DURING DIGESTION
In a healthy system, the pancreas absorbs glucose from the gut after a meal and secretes insulin in response. Insulin stimulates the tissues to absorb glucose from the blood and blocks fats from entering the bloodstream.

Q **DO ORAL HYPOGLYCAEMIC DRUGS WORK TO CONTROL DIABETES IN DOGS?**

A No, unfortunately they don't. The only effective way to control diabetes is with insulin injections. The amount of insulin your dog needs can be reduced by feeding it with a high-fibre diet.

Q **AREN'T DAILY INSULIN INJECTIONS PAINFUL FOR A DOG?**

A The type of needle used to inject insulin is extremely fine. Injections are usually given into the scruff of the neck, which is one ot the least sensitive parts of a dog's skin. These factors alone ensure that pain is virtually negligible. If you associate the twice-daily insulin injections with food, toys, play, or affection as a reward, the risk of discomfort is further reduced. (A psychological fear of needles is a human, not a canine, foible.)

Q **ARE THERE ANY CLUES THAT A BITCH MAY BECOME DIABETIC?**

A The incidence of sugar diabetes is twice as high in females as in males. Bitches' blood sugar levels are affected by oestrus – which, physiologically speaking, is a dramatic event. During metoestrus, some bitches go through a period of insulin insensitivity, when they drink and urinate more. Blood tests reveal increased blood sugar levels, but urine tests reveal no sugar in the urine. This hyperglycaemia is usually a temporary state needing no treatment. Any female with transient increased blood sugar during its oestrous cycle should be fed a high-fibre diet, have its weight controlled, and be spayed if it is not to be used for breeding.

BRAIN
control centre of the nervous system

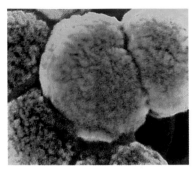

Meningitis bacteria

The brain, together with the spinal cord, is part of the central nervous system. The brain is the source of your dog's consciousness and intelligence, and enables it to experience and communicate emotions. In addition, it controls almost all bodily processes, from sensory perception to regulation of basic functions such as appetite and sleep. To carry out these activities, the brain's billions of cells are able to communicate with every living cell in the body through nerves and through chemicals called neurotransmitters.

Q HOW DO DOGS' BRAINS DIFFER FROM HUMAN BRAINS?

A A dog's brain is structurally very similar to a human brain, although it is about a quarter of the size. Brain activity is, in part, determined by the "hard-wiring" of the genes. Just as our brains are designed to learn language, the dog's brain is set up to learn to interpret scent, and a large part of the brain (in the cerebral cortex) is devoted to this activity in dogs.

Q HOW DOES THE LIMBIC SYSTEM INFLUENCE A DOG'S STATE OF MIND?

A The limbic system influences a dog's emotions through the production of chemicals called neurotransmitters. One of these chemicals is serotonin, which is thought to be associated with mood. In people, a decrease in serotonin leads to depression. Some research in dogs suggests that serotonin is also related to confidence. "Top dogs" have relatively high levels of it, while "underdogs" may produce less of this neurotransmitter.

The brain is composed of specialized structures that have specific functions. The largest part is a two-lobed structure called the cerebrum. In simple terms, the cerebrum is the site of "higher" neural activity such as consciousness, awareness of surroundings, sensory perception (sight, hearing, taste, smell, touch), learning, decision-making, and initiation of voluntary movements. A lower portion of the brain, the cerebellum, is responsible for fine coordination of body movement.

The hypothalamus is a small area of the brain that receives information from the cerebrum and regulates appetite, thirst, body temperature, and sleep cycles. The structure also passes on instructions to the pituitary gland, just beneath the brain; this gland produces hormones that affect growth, reproduction, and stress responses.

The most primitive part of the brain is called the brain stem. This is where the heart rate and breathing rate are controlled. All the nerves that connect to facial muscles and the senses (the 12 cranial nerves) emanate from here. The brain stem narrows at the base to become the spinal cord.

Within the brain are cavities, or ventricles, containing a watery liquid called cerebrospinal fluid, which also fills the core of the spinal cord. This fluid acts as a shock absorber. The brain and spinal cord are also protected by membranes called the meninges.

BRAIN FOOD
Brain cells need plenty of nourishment to function well. Although it makes up only about 2 per cent of a dog's weight, the brain receives around 20 per cent of the blood that the heart pumps out. Its greatest need is oxygen; the brain is overwhelmingly the body's most oxygen-hungry organ. Lack of oxygen, even for as little as 20 seconds, can cause irreversible brain damage. The sugar glucose is also essential; low blood sugar (hypoglycaemia) dramatically interferes with brain function. Other substances, such as the vitamin thiamine, are also required.

THE ROLE OF THE LIMBIC SYSTEM
Mind and body meet in the brain's limbic system. This primitive spider's web of interconnections in the dog's brain orchestrates instincts and emotions. The nervous and hormonal systems are both controlled by the limbic system, through its production of chemical messengers called neurotransmitters.

CROSS SECTION OF THE DOG'S BRAIN

Anatomically, the dog's brain is similar to the brains of most other mammals. The largest part is the cerebrum, which is divided into two halves, or hemispheres. These hemispheres are connected by a bundle of nerve fibres called the corpus callosum. The outer layer of the cerebrum, the cerebral cortex, governs learning and sense perception. In the lower brain, the cerebellum controls muscle coordination, and the brain stem, which joins on to the spinal cord, monitors the heart rate and breathing. The central region of the brain contains the thalamus, through which sensory information passes on its way to the cortex, and the hypothalamus, which regulates bodily processes and influences the hormonal system via the pituitary gland. The brain is protected by layers of tissue called the meninges.

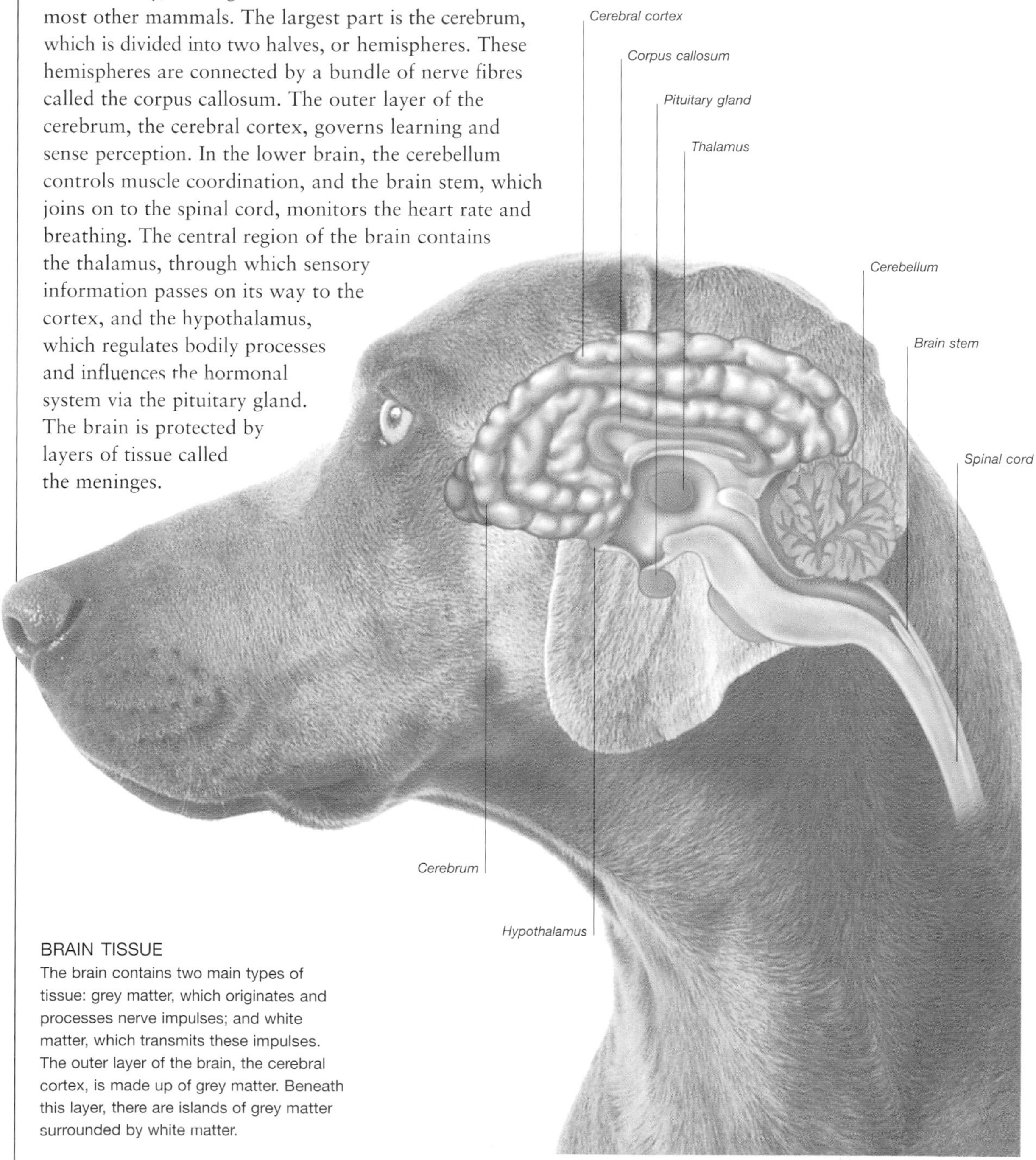

Cerebral cortex

Corpus callosum

Pituitary gland

Thalamus

Cerebellum

Brain stem

Spinal cord

Cerebrum

Hypothalamus

BRAIN TISSUE

The brain contains two main types of tissue: grey matter, which originates and processes nerve impulses; and white matter, which transmits these impulses. The outer layer of the brain, the cerebral cortex, is made up of grey matter. Beneath this layer, there are islands of grey matter surrounded by white matter.

DIAGNOSING BRAIN DISORDERS

Q WHAT IS A VET LOOKING FOR IN A NEUROLOGICAL EXAM?

A Your vet is looking for both physical and behavioural changes suggesting brain damage. If, for example, one eye is dilated but the other is constricted, this raises the possiblity of a brain disorder called Horner's syndrome. In a full neurological examination, a specific sequence of events takes place, leading to a tentative diagnosis of whether or not the brain is affected.

Q HOW WOULD A VET ASSESS A DOG'S MENTAL STATUS?

A The first assessment is based on the dog's response to its name and to simple commands such as "sit". Next, its response to a mild threat, such as a finger flicked in front of an eye, and to a reward such as a food treat or a toy, is observed. The dog is then observed while standing on the floor. A typical relaxed dog will investigate the surroundings, while a nervous dog is likely to move behind his owner for "protection" from the vet. However, a dog with reduced mental status will respond slowly, if at all.

Q WILL MY DOG HAVE TO BE SEDATED OR ANAESTHETIZED TO UNDERGO NEUROLOGICAL TESTS?

A There is no need for the use of anaesthetic during a routine neurological examination, but sedation may be necessary for an effective electroencephalogram. Head scans with either CT or MRI units take time and the patient must remain perfectly still. While humans willingly do so, dogs must be anaesthetized for the procedure.

SOME DEFINITIONS

Your vet may use a variety of words to describe what is happening in your dog's central nervous system, each with a specific meaning.

ATAXIA

This is a lack of muscle coordination, leading to problems with balance or gait. Ataxia may result from a disorder of the cerebellum or of the spinal cord.

PARALYSIS AND PARESIS

Temporary or permanent complete loss of muscle (motor) function results in paralysis. Paresis is an incomplete form of paralysis; for example, with help getting up, a dog with paresis can support itself. Ascending paralysis or paresis starts in the hindquarters and progressively moves forwards to the front limbs and head.

SHIVERING AND TREMBLING

Shivering is high-frequency contraction and relaxation of the muscles, while tremors involve repetitive rhythmic oscillations. Both of these signs are involuntary (automatic) responses.

COMA AND STUPOR

A dog in a coma is unconscious and cannot be aroused. A dog in a stupor is unconscious but can temporarily be aroused before falling back into stupor.

CONCUSSION AND CONTUSION

Both of these conditions usually result from a blow to the head. Concussion kills brain cells. A concussed dog may be unconscious for only a few seconds, but sometimes for much longer. A contusion is bruising of the brain; it may or may not be associated with loss of consciousness. A contused dog is temporarily dazed, confused, and wobbly but quickly recovers.

SEIZURE, CONVULSION, AND FIT

A generalized seizure involves a loss of consciousness accompanied by involuntary activities such as muscle contractions, paddling with the limbs, trembling, and facial twitching. During a seizure, dogs frequently salivate, urinate, and defaecate. The pupils of the eyes are usually dilated. A partial seizure involves only some of these changes and does not necessarily include loss of consciousness. The words "convulsion" and "fit" are used interchangeably with "seizure".

EPILEPSY

In epilepsy, a disturbance in electrical activity in the brain causes a seizure. This term is sometimes also used to refer to a condition in which a dog suffers frequent or recurring seizures.

NYSTAGMUS

This condition is an involuntary and rhythmic movement of the eyeballs, which may appear "jerky". In almost all cases, both eyeballs move together.

DIAGNOSTIC TESTS FOR BRAIN AND NERVE DISORDERS

If your vet suspects from its signs that your dog has a disorder of the nervous system, he or she will ask questions about the dog's current state and any previous illnesses or injuries, and will perform a physical examination. A number of diagnostic procedures are available that help the vet work out what the problem is and where it has arisen in the nervous system.

NEUROLOGICAL EXAM

Your vet may carry out specific tests to observe the dog's head posture; its coordination; ability to walk in a circle clockwise and anticlockwise; stance and gait; menace response when threatened; and facial expression and symmetry. The vet may shine a light into the dog's eyes to check pupil light reflex and symmetry, and will also look for nystagmus. These procedures help to pinpoint the site of possible nervous system damage or disease.

BLOOD ANALYSIS

Routine blood tests can help to identify physical diseases, such as liver failure, that may cause neurological signs.

ELECTROENCEPHALOGRAM (EEG)

An EEG can identify changes in the electrical activity of the brain that may be related to seizures or tumours.

BRAINSTEM AUDITORY EVOKED RESPONSE (BAER)

This test monitors electrical changes in the brain stem. BAER is useful for examining that area of the brain, particularly its ability to process sensory information from the ears.

CEREBROSPINAL FLUID (CSF) ANALYSIS

A needle is inserted into the dog's spinal canal and a sample of cerebrospinal fluid is collected. Specific changes occur in the fluid as a result of infection, inflammation, and tumours. This kind of analysis is, therefore, helpful in diagnosing a range of conditions; for example, changes in fluid pressure may indicate the presence of obstructions.

X-RAYS

Ordinary X-rays reveal any damage to bone and cartilage. In contrast X-rays, a dye is injected to outline the spinal cord (a procedure called myelography).

CT and MRI SCANS

These imaging techniques are the most revealing diagnostic aids, and the best aids for examining the brain itself, but they carry a risk to brain-injured dogs because scans involve anaesthesia.

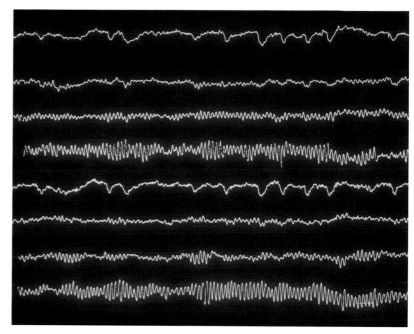

EEG TRACE ON SCREEN

An electroencephalogram (EEG) records the tiny electrical impulses produced by brain activity and shows the results on a screen. By revealing characteristic brain wave patterns, an EEG can help to diagnose epilepsy and brain tumours. This trace shows normal brain waves.

HANDLING A DOG WITH A HEAD INJURY

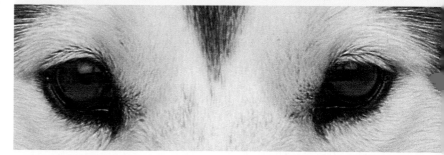

You need to take great care if handling a dog that has suffered a head injury. See First aid (pp.382–401) for guidance on dealing with shock, artificial respiration, and controlling bleeding. You should take the following action.
1 Be as quiet and gentle as possible, and talk soothingly, because any sensory stimulation can trigger pain, fear, or seizures.
2 In temperate or cool weather, cover the dog with a blanket.
3 Assess the dog's level of body control. Pinch the skin between the toes on each leg to check limb movement; lack of pain sensation means spine or nerve damage. Are the eyes moving jerkily, or are the pupils different sizes?
4 Check for and stabilize fractures.
5 Carefully move the dog on to a stretcher, keeping the head higher than the body, and transport the animal immediately to a veterinary surgery.

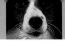
BRAIN DISORDERS

Disorders of the brain can arise as a result of physical injury; through poisoning, either by a substance in the environment or from the effects of a chronic disease elsewhere in the body; through infection, of the brain itself or of its surrounding membranes; or from the growth of tumours in brain tissue. Most brain disorders cause a variety of symptoms and signs, which may include seizures or even coma (loss of consciousness).

BRAIN INJURY

Brain damage may be caused by physical injuries; for example, road traffic accidents may cause concussion or contusion. In such injuries, the brain may be seriously damaged even though the skull is intact; if the head is struck on one side, the brain can be bruised as it is shaken within the skull. If the skull is fractured, fragments of bone may penetrate the brain tissue, causing major bleeding and damage.

Q WHAT SHOULD I DO IF MY DOG HAS A SEIZURE?

A Protect yourself: a dog having a seizure may unintentionally bite. Protect your dog: pull it by the scruff of the neck away from any threats in the environment. Place something soft, such as cushions or a blanket, around and under the dog's head. For short seizures, comfort your dog with soothing words and gentle stroking. For seizures over six minutes in duration, provide comfort yourself but see your vet immediately. After a seizure, provide some water for your dog to drink. Confine your dog and stay with it if it appears disorientated. Touch and a familiar voice are extremely reassuring for many individuals. (It is your turn to be the "companion animal".)

VET'S ADVICE

Collapse is a serious sign of illness and should be treated as an emergency. If your dog collapses, it may be difficult to determine whether the cause is a seizure, a stroke, or heart failure. A dog suffering from a seizure may show rhythmic, jerky movements, and may salivate, urinate, or defaecate. Strokes are not common in dogs. Heart failure usually causes visible blanching of the gums. Whatever the likely cause of collapse, your dog should be seen by a vet as soon as possible.

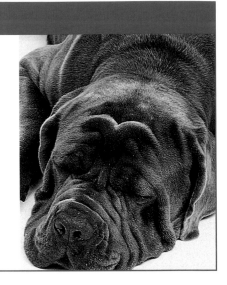

Certain poisons, or toxins, including natural substances such as snake venom and man-made products such as organophosphate insecticides, can damage brain cells if they are ingested or inhaled. (See also pp.414–27.)

Chronic disorders affecting other body organs, such as kidney failure (see p.307), liver failure (see p.294), thyroid gland disease (see p.331), adrenal dysfunction (see p.334), or cancer (see pp.130–41), may lead to brain damage by depriving the brain of substances that it needs to function or by causing toxins to circulate in the bloodstream. Nutritional deficiencies such as lack of the vitamin thiamine can impair brain function and potentially cause permanent damage.

Vascular disease, particularly the "furring up" of cerebral arteries or a stroke (see p.347), can prevent blood from reaching affected parts of the brain. Without an adequate blood supply, those areas of brain tissue will die within seconds.

Brain tumours (see p.346), and other swelling lesions such as polyps and cysts, can compress surrounding brain tissue as they grow. Localized inflammation of brain tissue, such as that caused by meningitis or encephalitis (see p.346), also places pressure on adjacent areas of tissue.

Brain damage can cause changes in a dog's behaviour or physical abilities. The symptoms depend on the region of the brain that has been injured; for example, an injury to the cerebrum may cause changes in mental status or vision, whereas cerebellar injuries often cause ataxia, abnormal head tilt, and nystagmus. The most dramatic behaviour changes involve seizures (see below), stupor, or coma (see below). Paralysis or paresis may result from injury to the brain or to the spinal cord (see pp.350–55).

DIAGNOSIS AND TREATMENT The site and extent of brain damage can be assessed using imaging techniques. The treatment depends on the cause, severity, and location of the damage. For example, antibiotics and/or corticosteroids may be given to reduce inflammation due to infection, and surgery may be helpful to relieve local pressure due to a brain tumour. The prognosis is often unpredictable, especially in the case of head injuries. Painkillers and other drugs can be used to make the dog more comfortable. A dog with overwhelming brain damage is usually put down humanely.

SEIZURES

Epilepsy, the most common cause of a seizure, occurs when there is an abnormal burst of electrical activity in the brain. Seizures may be mild, occur in clusters, or be prolonged (lasting more than five minutes). One possible cause is a physical problem such as a brain injury, the formation of scar tissue in the brain, or a brain tumour (*see p.346*). Other conditions that can provoke seizures are a low level of calcium in the blood, low blood sugar (*see p.338*), hydrocephalus (*see below*), migrating intestinal worm larvae (*see p.168*), post-distemper encephalitis (*see p.146*), poison-induced brain injury, or heat stroke (*see p.408*). In addition, there may be an inherited tendency to seizures in some individuals.

A seizure may be very dramatic, or so subtle that it is easily dismissed as a momentary loss of concentration. Dramatic seizures, often referred to as "grand mal", include three stages.
1. The dog shows behavioural changes, which may include comfort-seeking, restlessness, anxiety, hiding, whimpering, or crying.
2. It collapses and loses consciousness, and the body becomes rigid. These signs are followed by abnormal muscle activity: rhythmic jerking or paddling of the legs, urinating, defaecating, and salivating. This stage lasts for seconds to minutes. In rare instances, it lasts longer and is called status epilepticus.
3. Consciousness returns and the dog is dazed, confused, and temporarily unable to stand. Some dogs appear temporarily blind. This disorientation lasts for minutes to hours.

Milder seizures, called "petit mal" seizures, are of shorter duration. An affected dog may only stumble, losing consciousness for less than a second. In other cases, the only sign of a seizure is unusual behaviour, such as repeated snapping at the air as if to catch a fly or frenzied digging for no apparent reason. This condition is sometimes called psychomotor epilepsy.

The wild frenzy of activity in which some dogs engage after an insect sting may be mistaken for a seizure, but there is no loss of consciousness.

DIAGNOSIS AND TREATMENT The dog's medical history, blood tests, and an EEG are used to diagnose epilepsy. When epilepsy recurs frequently, the drug phenobarbital is the treatment of choice. The level of phenobarbital in the body is regularly monitored by blood tests throughout treatment. Although phenobarbital initially causes sedation, this side effect occurs for only a few weeks. The drug is, however, physiologically addictive, and treatment should never end abruptly.

SLEEP DISORDERS

These disorders are rare in dogs. One such disorder is the canine equivalent of narcolepsy. In humans, narcolepsy causes affected individuals to fall asleep suddenly during waking hours. The canine version was first reported in a family of Dobermans. Dogs with narcolepsy suddenly lose muscle tone for a few seconds while awake, with no other central nervous system signs. They otherwise lead normal lives and do not require any form of treatment.

HYDROCEPHALUS

Hydrocephalus is an accumulation of fluid in the cavities, or ventricles, of the brain. It may lead to seizures and, rarely, vision problems. Seizures caused by hydrocephalus are usually treated with diuretic drugs, which reduce the production of cerebrospinal fluid.

COMA

A coma is usually preceded by signs of confusion, and evolves through a state of stupor (*see p.342*) until the dog has completely lost consciousness. A dog in a coma is insensitive to pain and cannot be roused even temporarily.

The most common primary cause of coma is a condition elsewhere in the body that is "poisoning" the brain, such as kidney failure (*see p.307*),

BREEDS AT RISK

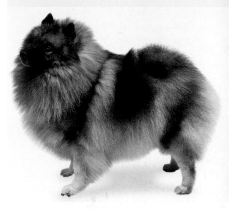

Breeds with a high incidence of or inherited predisposition to epilepsy include:

- Beagle
- Cocker Spaniel
- Dachshund
- German Shepherd Dog
- Golden Retriever
- Irish Setter
- Keeshond (above)
- Labrador Retriever
- Miniature Schnauzer
- Poodles
- Saint Bernard
- Siberian Husky
- Tervueren (Belgian Shepherd)
- Wire-haired Fox Terrier

Toy and flat-faced breeds are prone to hydrocephalus. Such breeds include:

- Boston Terrier
- Chihuahua
- English Bulldog
- Lhasa Apso
- Manchester Terrier
- Papillon
- Pekingese
- Pomeranian
- Toy Poodle
- Toy Spaniel
- Yorkshire Terrier

heart failure (*see p.250*), or liver failure (*see p.294*). Other causes of coma include poisoning by an external agent, such as antifreeze, barbiturate drugs, or carbon monoxide (*see pp.420–23*); brain injury that leads to concussion; fluctuations in blood sugar level, especially in dogs with diabetes mellitus (*see p.336*); infections such as distemper (*see p.147*) or rabies (*see p.144*); or overheating due to heat stroke (*see p.408*) or high fever.

DIAGNOSIS AND TREATMENT Give first aid (*see pp.382–401*). Eliminate any known cause of coma and assess breathing and heart rate. Give artificial respiration and/or heart massage as necessary. If the dog's heart is beating and breathing continues, make sure that the tongue is well pulled out and seek immediate veterinary attention. Your vet will carry out immediate blood tests, set up an intravenous drip, and give appropriate medicines.

MENINGITIS AND ENCEPHALITIS

Meningitis is an inflammatory condition of the meninges, the membranous coverings that protect the brain and the spinal cord. It is usually due to infection. Encephalitis is inflammation of the brain itself. Both disorders are potentially life-threatening.

Bacterial meningitis reaches the meninges via the bloodstream. The infection may enter the body from a bite wound, gum infection, middle ear infection, or other infected site. Aseptic meningitis is a non-bacterial form sometimes seen in dogs under 2 years old that belong to large breeds. Its cause is not known.

Worldwide, distemper (*see p.147*) and rabies (*see p.144*) remain the most common causes of encephalitis. In developed countries, these conditions are prevented by routine veterinary immunization. Other viral causes of encephalitis include pseudorabies and herpes virus. Less commonly, encephalitis is caused by bacteria that

migrate in the bloodstream from head or neck infections, by tick-borne parasites, or by lead poisoning.

A condition called granulomatous meningoencephalitis (GME) is, after post-distemper encephalitis, the second most common form of brain inflammation in dogs. As its name suggests, GME usually affects the meninges and brain tissue. Although the cause remains unknown, it occurs most frequently in young to middle-aged female toy breeds, causing neck pain as well as fever.

Both meningitis and encephalitis may cause depression, behaviour changes, seizures, loss of coordination, and sometimes also a fever.

DIAGNOSIS AND TREATMENT The clinical signs and a physical examination, together with cerebrospinal fluid (CSF)

analysis, help vets to identify the cause of the inflammation.

If the disorder is due to rabies, the dog is humanely euthanized. For other causes of meningitis and encephalitis, treatment is with corticosteroid drugs to reduce inflammation, antibiotics to destroy bacteria, and anticonvulsants to control seizures.

BRAIN TUMOURS

Brain tumours are rare, occurring in about 1 in 6,500 dogs. The most common type is a meningioma, a tumour arising in the meninges (the layer of tissue that covers the brain). Meningiomas tend to be relatively slow-growing, but they can compress surrounding healthy tissue as they grow and divert local blood vessels. Another type of tumour, called a

MENINGITIS AND ENCEPHALITIS

The brain and meninges are in intimate contact with each other; therefore, inflammation to either of them may cause broadly similar clinical signs. The causes of meningitis and encephalitis are, however, often considerably different. The most common cause of encephalitis is canine distemper virus. Meningitis may be caused by infection but it can also be an immune-mediated condition, particularly in adolescent Boxers, Beagles, and Akitas.

MENINGES
The meninges are membranes that act much like clingfilm, surrounding the brain. The blood supply to this area is in intimate contact with the rest of the bloodstream.

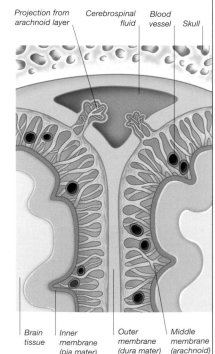

Projection from arachnoid layer · Cerebrospinal fluid · Blood vessel · Skull

Brain tissue · Inner membrane (pia mater) · Outer membrane (dura mater) · Middle membrane (arachnoid)

Detailed view of the meninges

glioma, involves the brain tissue itself. It aggressively invades surrounding healthy tissue and can thus disrupt brain function. Gliomas tend to be more damaging than meningiomas. Tumours may also arise from the tissue of the pituitary gland, at the base of the brain, causing hormonal imbalances and loss of pituitary function (*see p.330*).

The signs depend on the type of tumour and its location in the brain. They may include behaviour changes such as repetitive circling; changes in temperament or mood; seizures; changes to movement and gait; visual disturbances, or even blindness; altered mental abilities; and loss of facial nerve control, causing twitching.

DIAGNOSIS AND TREATMENT A CT or MRI scan of the brain is essential for an accurate diagnosis. Without a scan, it can be difficult to differentiate damage caused by a brain tumour from that due to other conditions such as stroke, metabolic liver or kidney disorders, epilepsy, lead poisoning, or even distemper infection.

Initial treatment of a brain tumour is aimed at controlling the symptoms and improving the quality of life. It often includes the use of anticonvulsant and corticosteroid drugs. The second objective of treatment is, if possible, to prolong good-quality life. Treatments given for this purpose may involve radiotherapy, surgery, or both (*see p.133*). In some cases of meningioma, surgical removal of the tumour provides a cure. Most brain tumours, however, are not operable.

Palliative treatment alone results in a life expectancy of, on average, two months. Radiotherapy often produces dramatic improvements to both the quality and length of life. Average survival rates for the different types of brain tumour are given below.

STROKE

While relatively common in people, strokes are rare in dogs. A stroke may be caused by the rupture of a cerebral blood vessel, with haemorrhage (bleeding) causing local brain damage. More often, a stroke is caused by a blood clot from elsewhere in the body becoming lodged in a brain artery, which prevents the region of the brain served by that artery from receiving the oxygen and nourishment that it needs. This type of interruption in blood supply is called an infarction. Without an adequate supply of blood, brain cells die in a few minutes.

The effects of a stroke appear suddenly. They vary in severity, from confusion and disorientation to seizures and stupor, coma, or paralysis, depending on where in the brain the infarction has occurred. There is usually localized brain swelling. A severe stroke may cause a dog to collapse.

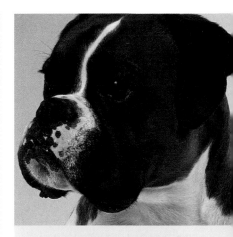

Q ARE ANY BREEDS MORE AT RISK OF BRAIN TUMOURS?

A Brain tumours can develop in any type of dog, and are more common in older individuals of all breeds. Boxers, however, are at greater risk than other breeds.

Q DO DOGS DREAM?

A Dogs dream the same way we do. During deep, or "activated", sleep, dogs may have rapid eye movements (REMs), paddle with their feet, twitch their lips and noses, and sometimes even bark. "Chasing rabbits" during sleep is perfectly normal.

BRAIN TUMOUR SURVIVAL RATES

Statistics from US veterinary teaching hospitals

BRAIN TUMOUR TYPE	MEDIAN SURVIVAL	1 YEAR SURVIVAL	2 YEAR SURVIVAL
All types	11 months	42%	13%
Meningioma	14 months	50%	22%
Glioma	9.5 months	35%	10%

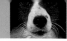

DIAGNOSIS AND TREATMENT A stroke is diagnosed by CT or MRI scanning. Corticosteroid drugs may be used to control brain swelling following stroke, and anticonvulsants may be given to control seizures.

A stroke is a potentially life-threatening condition. The outlook depends on the region of the brain affected and the extent of the brain damage that results. Blood clots are the most likely cause of strokes; for this reason, aspirin may be given on a regular basis to a dog who has suffered a stroke, because it reduces the clotting tendency of the blood and thereby helps to prevent recurrence.

EMOTIONAL DISORDERS

The idea that dogs are capable of having moods and emotional reactions to events, or that each dog has what could be described as its own personality, will meet no opposition from the majority of dog owners. Nor will it seem surprising that dogs show emotional and behavioural problems from time to time, or that they may suffer from a deterioration in their mental function as they grow older. In veterinary science, however, there is some difficulty in classifying and dealing with emotional disorders due to their inevitably subjective nature and the wide range of behaviour that can be regarded as "normal" for a particular individual. We rely on a dog's behaviour to tell us about its emotional state of mind, but the same behaviour can mean many things in different dogs.

SUBJECTIVITY AND DIAGNOSIS

A dog's emotions – its fears and anxieties, its ability to feel sadness or grief – have not been considered an integral part of conventional veterinary medicine until quite recently. As a consequence, many vets feel unsure about using terms that have hitherto been reserved for human psychiatry, such as phobia or depression, to describe behavioural conditions in dogs. Many practitioners feel more certain about diagnoses when they can be backed up by laboratory tests or modern technology. A diagnosis of an emotional disorder is wholly subjective; however, there is an increasing number of veterinary surgeons who have advanced training in behavioural medicine, both in veterinary schools and in general practice.

STRESS – A FINE LINE

Feelings such as anxiety or stress, which we tend to regard as unpleasant emotions, are in fact defensive. They evolved as a means of protection from environmental threats and dangers. In this sense, anxiety is like an emergency chemical first-aid kit. When the cortex of the dog's brain thinks that there is a stress, it communicates through the limbic system (*see p.340*) with the rest of the brain, and triggers a cascade of chemical changes that affect the entire body. During stress, the "fight or flight" hormone adrenaline acts within seconds. The longer-acting hormone cortisol backs up the stress response with increased mobilization of sugar for energy. These chemical changes are vital for the animal's survival, but if they are triggered too easily or last too long, emotional disorders are the consequence. There is no harm in short bouts of stress. If bouts are prolonged, however, or if (like a defective smoke alarm) the stress response is constantly and needlessly triggered, it leads to chronic stress and the sustained release of damaging chemicals in the body that may cause physical illness.

What causes some dogs to react well to even relatively high levels of stress, while some individuals develop behavioural problems after what would seem minor stressors, is an interesting question. The answer is likely to be, at least in part, down to genetic predisposition.

ANXIETY

Dogs often develop rational fears, for example of veterinary clinics, but many also have irrational fears, of men wearing hats, thunder, people limping, or other sights, sounds, or situations that do not in fact present a threat. Such an irrational fear of an object or a situation is called a phobia.

Some dogs become anxious when their owner leaves the room. This distress can lead to panic attacks, in which the muscles become tense and the dog hyperventilates, or compulsive behaviour, in which a dog ritually performs a certain activity such as pacing back and forth or obsessively licking itself. Extreme manifestations of canine anxiety include an inability to relax or to sleep.

Anxiety disorders can be distressing for both the dog and the owner, and it is important to seek veterinary advice if anxiety is persistent or severe.

DEPRESSION

Depression is extremely difficult to diagnose in dogs. It may manifest itself in a decreased or, less frequently, an increased appetite; clinging or "remote" behaviour; irritability; or lethargy. Grieving, a combination of

---

Q **WHAT CAN I DO TO HELP MY DOG STAY MENTALLY ALERT IN OLD AGE?**

A The most important factor here is mental stimulation. Encouraging your dog to use its brain helps to rebuild connections between brain cells and preserve mental abilities. Play with your dog as often as you can. There are various games and exercises that you can set up. Try hiding food items around the home or garden for your dog to search out. You can buy toys that make the dog work at getting a treat contained inside.

depression and sadness, occurs in dogs when an important member of their "family" dies or simply leaves, although this behaviour too is almost impossible to define using standard veterinary medical definitions.

The American neurologist Robert Sapolsky says, "People with chronic depressions are those whose cortex habitually whispers sad things to the rest of the brain." In people and in dogs, the "whispering" takes place through chemicals in the limbic system of the brain (see p.340).

NEW APPROACHES TO TREATMENT

As veterinary surgeons are recognizing the importance of emotional factors to a dog's well-being, there has been a corresponding growth of interest in the development of possible treatments for canine behavioural problems. Increasingly, vets are treating these disorders with a combination of environmental enhancement, special training techniques, and drugs.

Sedatives such as acepromazine are commonly used to tranquillize anxious dogs. These drugs produce a lack of coordination that lasts for about 6 to 12 hours. Anti-anxiety drugs such as diazepam were once commonly prescribed but are now used most frequently for short-term anxiety such as that associated with travel. Newer mood-altering drugs such as clomipramine and amitriptyline, developed to treat anxiety, depression, and obsessive-compulsive disorders in people, are now commonly used in dogs. Only a few of these drugs, however, have been clinically tested and licensed for veterinary use. These drugs affect neurotransmitters such as serotonin. Raising serotonin levels may improve mood or confidence in dogs, as it seems to do in humans with certain psychological conditions. Mood-altering drugs can, however, have profound, and not always anticipated, effects on a dog's behaviour.

Drugs alone do not cure emotional problems. Behaviour therapy is also an important element of treatment. In people, psychotherapy and counselling can affect the state of mind and brain chemistry. In dogs, experiences such as obedience training, desensitizing (for example, exposing a phobic dog gradually to a feared situation until it learns to be calm in that situation), counter-conditioning (in which a dog "unlearns" maladaptive behaviour), and exercise all affect neurotransmitter levels, behaviour, and emotions.

AGE-RELATED BEHAVIOUR PROBLEMS

Most of the signs of senile dementia that we might have also occur in dogs. A typical age-related change in dogs is standing at the wrong place by the door when wanting to go in or out. Some dogs bark "absently". Others seemingly forget why they are where they are. This can be associated with loss of house-training. The term canine cognitive dysfunction (CCD) has been coined to describe the behaviour changes that are typical of old age. The term itself is a mouthful, but it is helpful because its use indicates that this is a medical disorder.

DIAGNOSIS AND TREATMENT Routine, daily mental stimulation is extremely beneficial for older dogs and helps to keep the brain in good working order. The drug selegeline, which was developed for use in humans to delay the development of advanced signs and symptoms of Alzheimer's disease, is licensed for use in dogs with CCD. If your dog is having "senior moments", look carefully at its behaviour. Some aspects of aging are irreversible, but others can be delayed, or even reversed, with regular, frequent mental stimulation and effective use of licensed medication.

VET'S ADVICE

If we feel guilty that we are not giving our dogs enough attention, many of us may interpret changes in our dog's behaviour, such as sulking, not playing heartily, or sleeping more, as "getting even". There is no doubt that dogs have emotions and that sadness is one of them. If your dog seems depressed, give it the benefit of the doubt. Assume that it has a medical condition and see your vet before assuming that it is simply sulking.

NATURAL BEHAVIOUR

Dogs are pack animals. The emotions and behaviour patterns that follow from this characteristic are what make dogs such loyal and affectionate companions. The pack instinct only becomes a problem if it gets out of hand, perhaps manifesting itself as overly clingy behaviour or reluctance to be separated from the owner. In such cases, it may well be that a change in the dog's environment is helpful. Most dogs love attention and being around people. An anxious dog may find familiar human company and petting very reassuring.

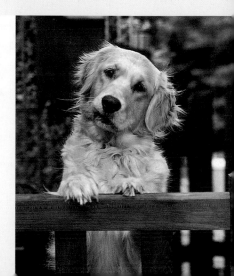

NERVOUS SYSTEM
spinal cord and peripheral nerves

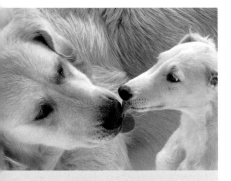

Botulism bacteria cause paralysis

The nervous system is the most complex of the body systems and regulates hundreds of activities simultaneously. It consists of the brain and spinal cord, which together make up the central nervous system, and the peripheral nerves, which branch from the spinal cord and extend throughout the body. The brain is discussed on pp.340–49; in the following section, the spinal cord and the peripheral nerves are considered. These parts of the system pass on sensations to the brain and coordinate action initiated by the brain.

The nervous system is a complex network of cells that enables a dog to receive and process information about its external and internal environment. The system also enables the dog to respond to its environment.

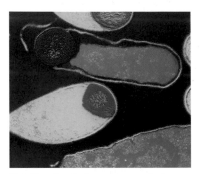

Q **WHY DO DOGS LICK EACH OTHER?**

A Licking does not only send taste messages to the brain. Like the rest of the body, a dog's tongue contains peripheral nerve receptors that are sensitive to heat, touch, and even air movement. The dog doing the licking receives messages in its brain about taste, texture, and warmth. The dog being licked receives sensation messages via its peripheral nerves that it instinctively interprets as soothing.

HOW NERVE CELLS COMMUNICATE

Nerve cells, or neurons, register stimuli from the dog's environment. They also convey information to other cells within the nervous system, as well as to muscle cells and the cells of organs and glands.

Neurons originate, process, transmit, and receive information in the form of electrical impulses. The signals pass from one neuron to another, however, by means of chemicals. For example, sensory nerve receptors convert a sensation, such as a sound, into an electrical signal. This signal passes along the nerve fibre, which projects from the cell. At the end of the fibre, the signal is transmitted by chemical messengers (neurotransmitters) to the next neuron across a tiny gap between the cells (the synapse).

In this way, nerve impulses pass from the receptors in the sense organs, via the peripheral nerves, to the spinal cord, and from there to the brain for processing. Commands for action are sent in the opposite direction – from the brain to the body tissues. These processes take a fraction of a second. As a result, a dog can, for example, hear a loud bang, recognize danger, and activate its muscles to run away.

THE SPINAL CORD

Running like a pipe through the spine, the spinal cord is a cylinder of nerve tissue that links the peripheral nervous system to the brain. It is connected to the brain by the brainstem.

The spinal cord is covered by layers of tissue called meninges. It is further protected by the spinal column. This structure is made up of bones called vertebrae, which are connected by ligaments and muscles. Between most of the vertebrae are intervertebral discs, fibrous pads that cushion the bones and absorb the stresses of movement.

VOLUNTARY AND INVOLUNTARY RESPONSES

Responses to stimuli may be voluntary or involuntary. Voluntary responses, such as barking to get attention, are mainly under conscious control. Involuntary (unconscious) responses fall into two types: autonomic and reflex. The first type is controlled by the autonomic nervous system; this is a sub-section of the nervous system that controls the body's internal environment and regulates vital functions such as the heartbeat. A reflex is an involuntary response, such as withdrawing a paw from a hot surface. Most reflexes are processed within the spinal cord.

THE SPINAL AND PERIPHERAL NERVES

Pairs of spinal nerves branch off the spinal cord and pass through the spinal column between the vertebrae. These nerves divide to form networks supplying all parts of the trunk and the limbs. They carry sensory nerve impulses to the spinal cord and brain; they also carry motor nerve impulses from the brain to the rest of the body. The spinal nerves form several groups along the spinal cord. The cervical nerves, branching from the top, supply the head, neck, and front limbs. The thoracic nerves supply parts of the upper abdomen and muscles in the back and chest. The lumbar nerves supply the lower back and hind legs. The cauda equina, at the end of the spinal cord, controls bladder and bowel function and tail movement.

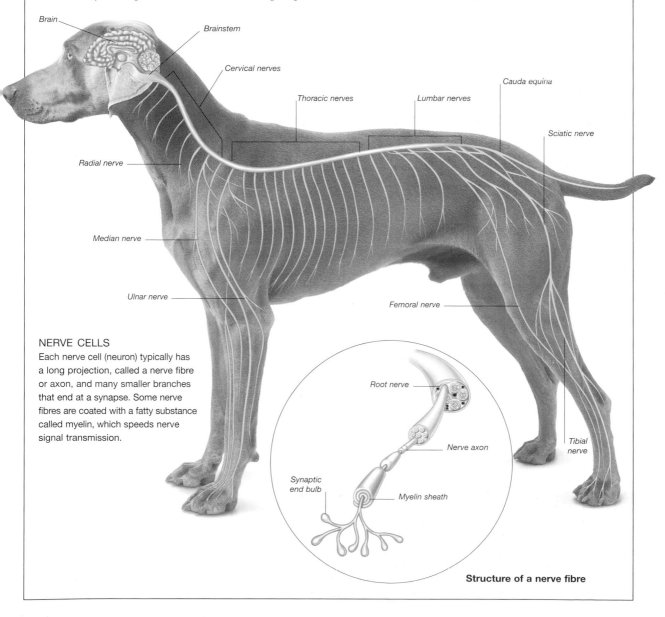

NERVE CELLS

Each nerve cell (neuron) typically has a long projection, called a nerve fibre or axon, and many smaller branches that end at a synapse. Some nerve fibres are coated with a fatty substance called myelin, which speeds nerve signal transmission.

Brain

Brainstem

Cervical nerves

Thoracic nerves

Lumbar nerves

Cauda equina

Sciatic nerve

Radial nerve

Median nerve

Ulnar nerve

Femoral nerve

Root nerve

Nerve axon

Synaptic end bulb

Myelin sheath

Tibial nerve

Structure of a nerve fibre

Any interruption to the constant flow of information from the peripheral nerves to the brain not only prevents the brain from receiving information, but also prevents messages from the brain reaching the muscles and other organs. Injuries and diseases of the spinal cord, or of the peripheral nerves, therefore cause weakness and even paralysis in the affected areas.

The diagnostic procedures and examinations used to evaluate spinal cord and nerve disorders are essentially the same as for conditions affecting the brain (*see pp.342–43*).

SPINAL CORD CONDITIONS

Damage to the spinal cord can cause loss of voluntary muscle movement, changes in spinal reflexes, changes in muscle tone, muscle shrinkage, and loss of touch and pain sensations. Deep inside its protective column of bone, the spinal cord has little or no capacity for repair if it is damaged. The most common causes of damage are physical injuries and slipped or ruptured intervertebral discs (*see below*).

SPINAL INJURY

Injury to the spine can be caused by road traffic accidents, gunshot wounds, or falls. Such injuries often affect other parts of the body as well as the spine. Immediately after a spinal injury, a dog may experience neck and back pain, weakness or paralysis of the legs, loss of feeling in the limbs, and urinary or faecal incontinence. Local tissue inflammation and swelling can cause symptoms to worsen after the injury; they also interfere with the blood supply to the spinal cord and may cause permanent paralysis.

DIAGNOSIS AND TREATMENT A neurological examination and X-rays are required for accurate diagnosis. The drug methylprednisolone is given intravenously to reduce inflammation. Surgical repair of vertebral fractures may stabilize an injured area. Dogs that are severely injured are put down.

ADVICE When transporting a dog with a suspected spinal injury to the vet, first muzzle it if necessary. Take the following steps to minimize the risk of further nerve damage.
• Keep its back as straight as possible.

• Use a hard, flat board, or a thick blanket folded over, as a stretcher (*see p.400*). Gently pull the dog on to the stretcher, then secure it using soft cloth ties or similar material over the hips and shoulders.
• Prevent neck movement if there are neck injuries.

RUPTURED DISC

The intervertebral discs lie just beneath the spinal cord. Injury or wear can cause a disc to degenerate or rupture (*see box below*), compressing the surrounding tissues. In a rupture, the fibrous coating of a disc tears and the inner material escapes. In some larger dogs, the fibrous capsule may remain healthy but the disc suddenly or gradually slips and bulges upwards.

Sudden rupture or displacement of a disc results in pain and often loss of muscle function, which may or may not symmetrically affect both sides of the body. If a displaced disc presses on the spinal cord, there may be complete paralysis beyond the site of damage.

DIAGNOSIS In many cases, a diagnosis is based on a dog's history, breed, and

RUPTURED INTERVERTEBRAL DISC

An intervertebral disc is a pad of cartilage that sits between the vertebrae and acts as a cushion and shock absorber. It consists of an outer capsule of fibrous connective tissue surrounding a gel-like core. When a disc ruptures, the fibrous capsule breaks, allowing the core tissue to spill out of the disc.

BADLY RUPTURED DISC
The fibrous capsule around this disc has ruptured completely, causing the inner disc tissue to escape and press on the spinal cord. This pressure is likely to cause pain and loss of muscle function.

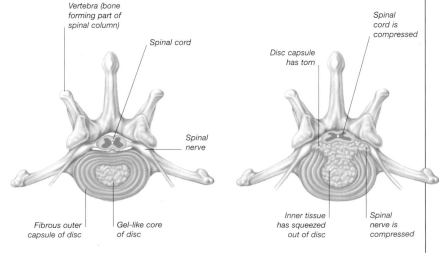

Cross section of normal disc

Cross section of ruptured disc

symptoms. Plain X-rays can show decreased spaces between vertebrae, while contrast X-rays (myelography) reveal the degree of compression on the spinal cord. Analysis of the cerebrospinal fluid can help determine the cause. CT and MRI scans provide detailed images of the displaced disc.

TREATMENT Corticosteroid drugs are beneficial, for most dogs, when given on the same day that injury occurs. After medication, the most important component of treatment is rest, usually for about two weeks, to allow the disc to return to its normal position.

For older, large dogs suffering from chronic bulging discs, continued corticosteroids or analgesics relieve pain but do not lessen the chance of recurrence. While rest is vital, the priority is to prevent the recurrence of disc disease. This may be achieved through surgical interventions.

DEGENERATIVE MYELOPATHY

This progressive condition, also called chronic degenerative radiculomyopathy or CDRM, mainly affects German Shepherds and is fairly common in the breed. It may also occur in other breeds such as Labradors and Retrievers. The disorder tends to appear when the dog is about six years of age.

Affected dogs experience a slow and painless loss of coordination in the hind legs. Early in the course of the disease, many owners assume that weakness in the hind legs is caused by a problem with the hip joint. Over the following years, the weakness evolves into a partial paralysis. The dog seemingly cannot feel where its paws are, but its pain perception remains intact, as does voluntary control over urination and defaecation.

DIAGNOSIS AND TREATMENT This condition is diagnosed by the symptoms and by physical examination. While many treatments have been attempted, none has been shown to slow down or reverse the damage. Weight control is important, as is routine daily exercise

to maintain muscle tone. Anabolic steroids may be given to strengthen the muscles. Protective boots are beneficial if foot-dragging wears the nails down.

WOBBLER SYNDROME

This condition, technically known as cervical spondylomyelopathy, involves progressive loss of coordination in the hind legs. It results from a compression of the spinal cord in the neck caused by vertebral instability. The condition may be complicated by additional changes in the discs, which cause compression and damage to the spinal cord. If untreated, the partial paralysis may spread to the front legs.

Wobbler syndrome occurs most frequently in males, especially in Great Danes under two years old and in Dobermans between three and nine years of age.

DIAGNOSIS A diagnosis is based on the breed affected, the symptoms, and plain and contrast (myelography) X-rays of the spine and spinal cord.

TREATMENT Mild problems are managed with non steroidal anti-inflammatory drugs (NSAIDS) and sometimes also neck braces. In severe cases, early surgery to relieve spinal compression is beneficial, although associated with many complications.

BONE SPURS

In some older dogs, spurs of bone called osteophytes grow on the vertebrae. Although the growths may look quite dramatic when seen on an X-ray, the osteophytes themselves do not cause pain unless (rarely) they project up towards the sensitive spinal cord. Over time, the spurs grow towards each other, eventually joining and fusing the vertebrae together.

DIAGNOSIS AND TREATMENT In itself, a fusion of vertebrae does not cause pain or need treatment. Sometimes, however, it restricts movement of the vertebral column and causes pain and stiffness. This condition, spondylosis deformans, is treated with painkilling drugs.

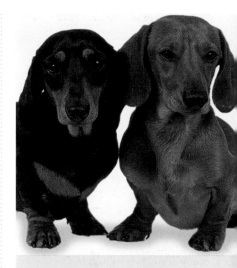

Q IS ACUPUNCTURE USEFUL FOR TREATING PAIN CAUSED BY DISC DISEASE?

A Acupuncture is beneficial for many dogs when pain is moderate or chronic. It is of no value for dogs with serious spinal cord compression. Remember, the objective of any treatment is to reduce mental as well as physical stress and create the best environment for the body's natural power of repair to take effect. Dogs that are distressed by needles, strangers, car trips, and so on will not benefit from acupuncture if they find the procedure itself stressful. The likelihood of distress depends on the personality of the individual.

Q IS DISC DISEASE DUE TO WEAR AND TEAR, AND ARE SOME BREEDS MORE PRONE TO IT?

A The intervertebral discs are most likely to rupture in breeds that have long backs and short legs, such as the Dachshund (above). This is because the dogs' anatomy causes the spine to flex and puts stress on the discs. Disc disease is much less common in dogs that have a more upright, wolf-like build.

PERIPHERAL NERVE CONDITIONS

Peripheral nerve disorders are rare in dogs. Most instances are due to physical injury from road traffic accidents, falls, and gunshot wounds.

Damage to a peripheral nerve causes both a loss of sensation in a particular area and loss of function in the muscles that are served by that nerve. If the nerve to the tail is damaged, for example, there will be temporary or permanent loss of the ability to sense pain in the tail area, to wag the tail, or to lift it when defaecating. In the legs, one peripheral nerve supplies the muscles that flex while another supplies the muscles that extend. Car accidents can damage one or both of these nerves, producing either full paralysis of all the leg muscles or a partial paralysis affecting only a specific group of muscles.

HEREDITARY NERVE DISORDERS

There are a number of rare hereditary diseases in which the nerves degenerate. As with most genetic conditions, there are no specific treatments for these diseases, but in some cases an affected dog may live comfortably for many years.

BREED	AGE OF ONSET	SYMPTOMS AND SIGNS
Cairn Terrier	4 months	Hind limb weakness leading to exaggerated leg movements and head tremors
English Pointer	4–5 months	Progressive paralysis of all legs
German Shepherd	12 months	Hind limb weakness leading to exaggerated leg movements and faecal incontinence
German Shepherd	9 years	Progressive ataxia (loss of muscle coordination) and hind leg weakness (see Degenerative myelopathy, p.353)
Alaskan Malamute	7–18 months	Exercise intolerance and clumsy or exaggerated leg movements
Rottweiler	12 months	Gradual-onset paralysis of all limbs
Boxer	2–3 months	Clumsy or exaggerated leg movements
Dalmatian	2–6 months	Fainting, breathing problems, laryngeal paralysis
Bouvier des Flandres	4–8 months	Breathing problems, laryngeal paralysis
English Springer Spaniel	12–18 months	Behaviour changes and ataxia

DIAGNOSIS AND TREATMENT Pain-response tests can reveal how much sensation has been lost from the area. If a leg is injured, for example, the dog may have pain sensation on one side of the leg but not on the other. Extensor muscle paralysis will cause a leg to be permanently flexed, although the leg still bears weight when straightened. Amputation of an affected limb may be necessary; however, a surgical procedure to transpose muscle attachments and produce a stiff but straight leg is sometimes an alternative.

PARALYSIS

Paralysis is the loss of controlled movement, which may be caused by an inabiliy of the motor nerves to communicate with one or more muscles. Complete paralysis, affecting all of the muscles, rarely occurs in dogs. Partial paralysis affecting the hind quarters is more common. Both types are most commonly caused by spinal cord injury (see p.352). Paralysis can be either temporary or permanent.

TRAUMATIC PARALYSIS

Spinal cord trauma, from a road traffic accident or other injury, is the most common cause of paralysis. A slipped intervertebral disc pressing on the spinal cord can also cause partial or complete paralysis.

DIAGNOSIS AND TREATMENT Treatment is with intravenous methylprednisolone. Surgery may also be beneficial.

TICK PARALYSIS

Certain tick species found in North America and Australia carry a poison in their saliva that affects the motor nerves. Initial signs include hind limb weakness about a week after a tick has attached itself. Full paralysis ensues in one to three days.

DIAGNOSIS AND TREATMENT A dog usually begins to improve within a day of the ticks being removed. Australian tick paralysis, however, can be more

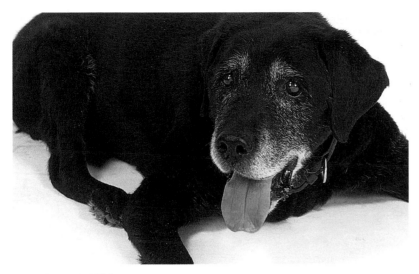

OLD AGE TREMORS

It is not uncommon for older dogs to develop tremors in their hind legs, or sometimes in all four legs, with no other signs of neurological disease or injury. These tremors usually do not cause a dog any problems with movement or gait.

severe. Dogs may continue to deteriorate for another couple of days after the ticks are removed, and may be given hyperimmune antiserum.

COON HOUND PARALYSIS

The cause of this North American disease is unknown. It occurs most often in hunting dogs one to two weeks after contact with a raccoon. Weakness begins in the hind limbs and progresses forward. Even the most severely affected dogs continue to be able to wag their tails. Spontaneous recovery usually occurs within weeks or months.

MYASTHENIA GRAVIS

This condition occurs in three forms. In about 25 per cent of affected dogs, full paralysis and breathing difficulties occur within three days. In another 40 per cent, full paralysis develops more slowly; most of these dogs develop a flaccid oesophagus and therefore cannot swallow. The remaining 35 per cent of dogs with myasthenia gravis do not develop full paralysis; the paralysis affects only specific areas, such as the face, pharynx, larynx, or oesophagus.

DIAGNOSIS AND TREATMENT The most common diagnostic test involves an injection of edrophonium chloride, a drug that prevents the breakdown of neurotransmitters at receptor sites; the drug temporarily increases muscle strength. A more accurate diagnostic serum antibody test is available, but this is less widely used. Affected dogs are injected with the drug neostigmine; the use of other drugs is controversial. Myasthenia gravis persists for months or years, but spontaneous remission sometimes occurs.

BOTULISM

This condition is rare in dogs. It results from a neurotoxin that is produced by *Clostridium botulinum* bacteria, found in tainted canned food and carcasses. Paralysis, ascending from the hind limbs, occurs within hours to days of eating tainted food.

DIAGNOSIS AND TREATMENT Mildly affected dogs often recover without treatment. In other cases, antitoxin halts the progression of the paralysis, but it does not reverse any nerve damage that has occurred before treatment.

Q WHAT CAUSES FACIAL PARALYSIS, AND IS THERE ANY CURE FOR IT?

A In most instances, the cause of facial nerve paralysis is not known, although some affected dogs have associated thyroid gland impairment. The paralysis usually affects only one side of the face, and is first suspected when a dog dribbles excess saliva, eats messily, or loses facial symmetry. Often, a dog cannot close its eyelid on the affected side. While there is no treatment for facial paralysis, the condition seemingly improves as the affected shrunken muscles become fibrous and retract. Drooling usually disappears within a month.

Q WHY DO ONLY SOME DOGS DEVELOP PARALYSIS AS A RESULT OF TICK BITES?

A Certain species of tick (*Dermacentor*, *Amblyomma*, and *Ixodes*) species, found in North America and Australia, carry in their saliva a heat-sensitive neurotoxin that causes paralysis. (Interestingly, cats appear to be resistant to tick neurotoxin.)

The degree of paralysis that a bitten dog suffers will vary with the environmental temperature and the amount of neurotoxin in the tick's saliva. The toxin from the Australian *Ixodes* tick is more potent than that carried by North American ticks. Because the neurotoxin is temperature-sensitive, dogs recover faster when they are kept in air-conditioned premises.

BONES, JOINTS, AND MUSCLES
strength, movement, and flexibility

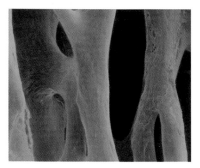
Microscopic view of bone tissue

The bony framework of the skeleton gives the dog's body shape and supports its soft tissues. The skeleton is as strong as steel, yet as light as aluminium. Joints are formed where two or more bones meet and are held together by ligaments. Muscles and their associated tendons make up the bulk of a dog's body and account for half its weight. In a healthy dog, the skeleton is supple, the joints move freely, and the muscles are elastic and powerful. Controlled by the central nervous system (*see pp.340–49*), movement is smooth and coordinated.

The skeleton, the joints between bones, and the muscles are known collectively as the musculoskeletal system.

FUNCTIONS OF BONE
Bone consists of a resilient protein framework strengthened by mineral deposits. While bone may appear to be lifeless and unchanging, it is actually living tissue, supplied with nerves and blood vessels, that is constantly being broken down and rebuilt. Bone is also a storage site for calcium, phosphorus, magnesium, and other minerals the body needs, and the core contains the bone marrow, which makes blood cells (*see pp.258*).

JOINTS CONNECT BONES
Joints are covered with lubricated cartilage that allows them to move smoothly. The range of movement of a joint is determined by its shape and structure. For example, the stifle joint is a hinge joint that simply bends and straightens the leg, while the hip joint is a ball-and-socket joint which allows movement in more directions.

TYPES OF MUSCLE
All mammals have three kinds of muscle. Cardiac muscle is specific to the heart, making up most of its tissue. Smooth muscle controls the movements of the internal organs, and is not under conscious control. Skeletal (striated) muscles are those attached to the skeleton, and are used for active movement.

TENDONS AND LIGAMENTS
Some skeletal muscles attach directly to bones. Others taper into elastic tendons, which in turn attach to the skeleton. Ligaments attach two bones; for example, the cruciate ligaments in the stifle joint hold the long bones of the leg together. Tendon and ligament fibres pass through the surface of the bone and are embedded in the bone itself.

HOW MOVEMENT OCCURS
Movement of the body depends on the interaction of bones, muscles, and joints in response to signals from the brain and nerves. A muscle typically connects two bones and crosses the joint between them. When a muscle contracts, it pulls on the bones to which it is attached and produces movement. Muscles can only pull, not push. Many muscles are arranged in pairs, one on each side of a joint, so that they produce equal and opposing movements.

Q ARE ALL DOGS' BONES EQUALLY STRONG?

A No, they are not. The bones of large dogs in their first year of life are not as strong as those of smaller dogs the same age. Even within breeds, the bones of bigger male pups are not as strong as those of smaller females. In large breeds, the bones have a thinner cortex, larger medullary cavity, and less dense spongy bone (*see p.359*); this may be the reason why such breeds have more skeletal deformities than smaller breeds.

Q CAN I PROTECT MY BIG PUPPY FROM BONE DEFORMITIES?

A The best way to reduce risks is to minimize stresses on joints. While your pup is growing, avoid games that involve jumping, such as ball-catching. Feed your pup carefully so that its skeleton grows slowly. Do not feed a calorie-rich or mineral-rich diet. Such over-nutrition will cause the bones to grow faster but have low density, and the skeleton will be less able to withstand stresses from increasing muscle mass and body weight.

THE SKELETON

The skeleton supports the dog's weight and facilitates movement, providing a superstructure for muscle and tendon attachments. The bones are held together by tough ligaments, and articulated by a variety of types of joints, some of which allow free movement and some of which are fixed and provide stability. The bone ends at movable joints have smooth surfaces of cartilage, and the joints contain lubricating fluid, to reduce friction. The cartilage also acts as a shock absorber for the force exerted with every step.

BONE SHAPES

Bones come in many shapes and sizes, ranging from flat plates that anchor large muscle masses, such as the shoulderblades, to hollow, thick-walled tubes that support weight or act as a lever, such as those in the limbs.

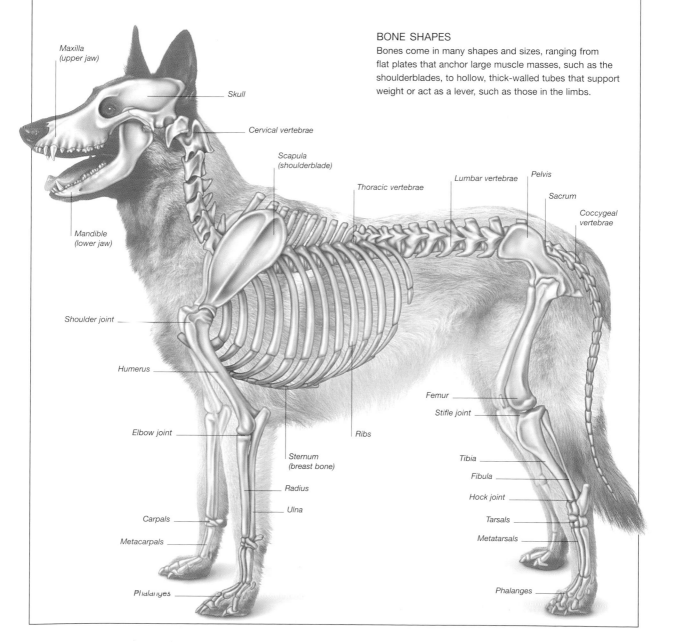

Maxilla (upper jaw)

Skull

Cervical vertebrae

Scapula (shoulderblade)

Thoracic vertebrae

Lumbar vertebrae

Pelvis

Sacrum

Coccygeal vertebrae

Mandible (lower jaw)

Shoulder joint

Humerus

Femur

Stifle joint

Elbow joint

Ribs

Sternum (breast bone)

Tibia

Fibula

Radius

Hock joint

Ulna

Carpals

Tarsals

Metacarpals

Metatarsals

Phalanges

Phalanges

THE MUSCLES

Muscles consist of tissue that can contract powerfully to move the body, maintain its posture, and work the internal organs, including the heart and blood vessels. These functions are performed by three different types of muscle: skeletal muscle, cardiac muscle, and smooth muscle. Skeletal muscle makes up the majority of the muscle bulk. A dog has over 500 skeletal muscles, some of which are shown on the right. Usually, each end of a skeletal muscle is attached to a bone by a tendon (a flexible cord of fibrous tissue). These muscles can be controlled consciously to produce movement. They are sometimes called voluntary muscles, and are also known as striated ("striped") muscles due to their striated appearance under a microscope.

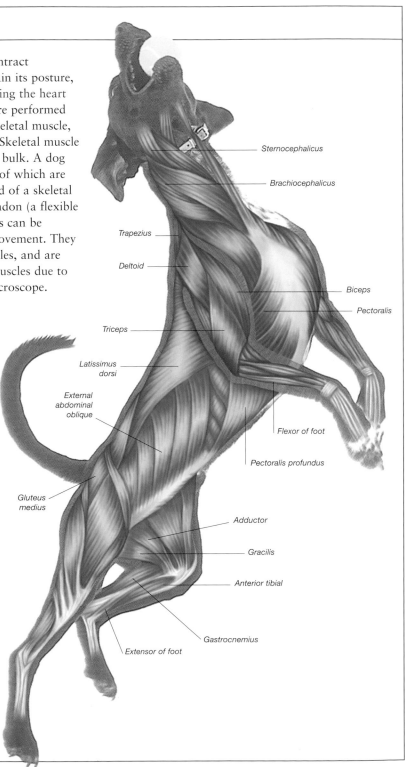

Sternocephalicus

Brachiocephalicus

Trapezius

Deltoid

Biceps

Pectoralis

Triceps

Latissimus dorsi

External abdominal oblique

Flexor of foot

Pectoralis profundus

Gluteus medius

Adductor

Gracilis

Anterior tibial

Gastrocnemius

Extensor of foot

HOW MUSCLES WORK TOGETHER

Most muscles work in what are called "antagonistic pairs", each muscle being paired with a muscle that has the opposite effect. One muscle works to flex or bend a limb, while its opposite in the pair extends or straightens it. In more complex joints, such as the ball-and-socket joint in the shoulder, several pairs of muscles work in different directions to provide flexibility.

SYMPTOMS AND DIAGNOSIS

The most common sign of muscle, joint, or bone disorders is lameness, or limping, although it may also be caused by injury to the foot or the pad of the paw, for example, by thorns or splinters, or by nerve injuries.

LAMENESS/LIMPING

Walking on four legs has great advantages over walking on two. If one leg hurts, there are three more that can carry weight. Dogs naturally carry most of their weight on their forelegs.

If your dog is taking shorter steps than usual, is placing less weight on one leg, or is bobbing its head as it walks, it is lame. Finding the cause of lameness can be more challenging than you might think. Even determining which leg a dog is limping on can sometimes be difficult.

There are many possible causes of lameness, each of which produces specific clinical signs. If your dog is limping, your vet may want to see it walk and will then examine the paws, limbs, and back, looking for injuries or swelling, and flexing and extending all the joints. He or she may ask the following questions:
• Has lameness developed gradually or occurred suddenly?
• Are you aware that your dog has sustained any injuries?
• Is a foot held up or not fully bearing weight?
• Is your dog licking at any area, especially the paw?

DIAGNOSTIC PROCEDURES

If your dog is lame, or has any other signs of bone, joint, or muscle disorders, your vet can employ various techniques to investigate the cause.

EXAMINATION

The vet will examine the affected part for injuries and areas of swelling or tenderness. Lacerations of the foot pad or bite wounds tend to be red, warm, and tender, and may bleed.

IMAGING TECHNIQUES

Plain X-rays are used to detect broken bones and joint dislocations. Contrast X-rays outline joints and the spinal cord. Nuclear scintigraphy (bone scanning) using radioactive isotopes is used at some veterinary schools to picture bone and its surrounding tissue. CT and MRI scans are useful for outlining the extent of bone tumours.

ARTHROSCOPY

In arthroscopy, a fine fibre-optic viewing tube is inserted into a joint, for example the knee joint, so that the vet can examine the tissues directly.

BLOOD TESTS

Blood tests may be performed to help the vet decide whether it is the muscles or the nerves that are damaged.

STRUCTURE OF BONE AND MUSCLE TISSUE

Bones have two layers. The cortex (outer layer) is made up of dense, heavy, compact tissue covered by a membrane called the periosteum. The medulla (inner layer) consists of spongy bone that has many struts (trabeculae); these are arranged to provide maximum support without adding excessive weight.

Muscles that make large, fast movements have long, parallel fibres. Muscles within the torso have shorter fibres that are strong but cannot contract as fast or to the same extent.

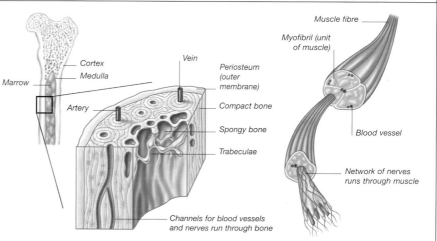

SECTION THROUGH A LONG BONE
A long bone, such as the femur, has a marrow-filled central cavity surrounded by spongy bone and then compact bone.

SKELETAL MUSCLE FIBRE
This type of muscle is formed of long, strong, parallel fibres that can contract quickly and powerfully for short periods.

ANALYSIS OF JOINT FLUID

Synovial fluid is withdrawn from a joint using a needle and syringe. Analysis of the fluid helps vets to differentiate between infection, inflammation, and immune causes of disease.

BIOPSY

Examination of a biopsy specimen under the microscope helps determine the exact cause of an abnormality.

ELECTROMYOGRAM

An electromyogram is a diagnostic aid used to record electrical activity in resting or working muscles.

INJURIES OF THE JOINTS, LIGAMENTS, AND TENDONS

Dogs are curious, inquisitive, and inclined to act before thinking. The environment in which most dogs live, with open roads and open windows, is more risky than the environment in which they evolved. One consequence is that physical injuries, from cuts, bruises, sprains and strains to joint dislocations, and from ligament and tendon tears to broken bones, are fairly common.

Injuries to joints, ligaments, and tendons are usually, but not always,

caused by trauma. A strong force is necessary to dislocate a joint or tear a tendon. Such injuries usually result from road traffic accidents and falls from a height. A sprain (overstretching of a ligament) may be caused by trauma; it may also be due to exuberant running or jumping. Strains (damage to muscle fibres and tendons) have similar causes. Torn ligaments are common in dogs, particularly in the stifle and knee joints. Unlike other joint and tendon injuries, a ligament may tear while a dog is engaged in normal activity, such as walking up stairs or gently trotting.

DIAGNOSING LAMENESS

CAUSE	CLINICAL SIGNS
Cut paw pads	The dog may lick the pad.
Grass seed or other foreign body penetration between the toes	The dog usually licks the area. An abscess can form at the entry site. Lameness progressively worsens until the abscess bursts.
Bite wounds and secondary infections	Licking of wounds. Lameness worsens as swelling and infection increase.
Sprains and strains	Lameness is sudden, sometimes accompanied by swelling or bruising. May last days to weeks.
Degenerative joint diseases	Occurs in older dogs. Worse on waking. Lameness improves with exercise.
Inherited joint diseases	Often occurs in younger dogs. Seldom associated swelling. Worsens over time.
Ligament tears	Lameness is sudden. Pain is usually minimal. Lameness becomes chronic. Minimal weight-bearing capacity.
Fractures and dislocations	Lameness is sudden. Pain is severe. Accompanied by swelling and inability to bear weight.
Bone tumours	Single leg limp in older dogs. Pain worsens with time and does not respond to rest.
Spinal cord damage	Sudden in small dogs, sometimes gradual onset in larger breeds. Moderate to severe pain. Often a symmetrical lameness.
Degenerative nerve diseases	Mostly seen in German Shepherds. Gradual onset in middle-aged dogs. No pain or swelling, but hind paws buckle over.

VET'S ADVICE

Sudden lameness is often the result of damage to bones, muscles, or joints, but there are also other possible causes. Perhaps the most common is a painful broken claw. Equally likely is a grass seed stuck in the skin between the toes. Cut paw pads, and injuries from dog fights, cause pain as well as lameness. If your dog is limping, look for the simplest causes before assuming that there is a major injury.

DISLOCATION

A bone that separates from its adjoining bone at a joint has been dislocated. A complete dislocation, in which the bones come apart, is called a luxation. This causes sudden pain and loss of use of the affected limb. The elbow or knee may be bent, with the leg pointing either towards or away from the body. The affected leg may appear longer or shorter than the other legs. In a subluxation, the bones come only partially out of the joint, and the joint deformity is minimal. Luxation or subluxation can occur in the shoulder, elbow, hip, and stifle joints, and in the small joints that make up the hocks and wrists.

Dislocations often involve ligament tears (*see below*) and damage to the joint cartilage (*see below*).

DIAGNOSIS Luxations – for example, the ball of the femur coming out of the hip socket – are readily diagnosed by examination and X-ray. Subluxations tend to be more difficult to diagnose, even on an X-ray.

TREATMENT Some dislocated bones can be manually replaced under general anaesthesia if a dog is taken for veterinary treatment shortly after an injury. Left too long, retraction of the muscles around the joint and the formation of a blood clot make manual repair very difficult. Surgical repair is then necessary.

After either form of treatment, the affected joint is usually immobilized in a sling or a splint for at least a week. Thereafter, gentle activities such as swimming may help the dog to recover joint strength and flexibility.

DAMAGE TO THE JOINT CARTILAGE

The cartilage cushion in a joint is called the meniscus. Isolated meniscus injuries are rare in dogs. Injuries to the meniscus are usually associated with a dislocation of the knee joint (*see above*) and a torn cruciate ligament (*see below*). In these cases, the

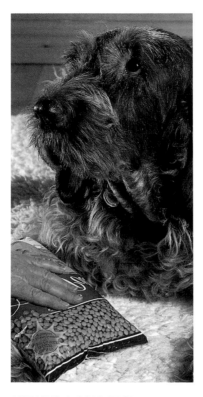

APPLYING A COLD PACK
The application of a cold pack (frozen peas or crushed ice wrapped in a towel) for 20 minutes three or four times a day can help relieve the pain of a muscle or joint injury.

meniscus is repaired during surgery for joint or ligament repair.

If a knee ligament injury is left untreated, secondary damage to the meniscus may occur in the weeks and months that follow. The end result may be degenerative joint disease (*see p.363–65*) and permanent lameness.

SPRAINS AND STRAINS

A strain is damage to muscle fibres and tendons. Strains cause lameness, pain, and local swelling of the muscles. They are often accompanied by slight bleeding, and bruising may be seen beneath the fur. Muscle strain may be accompanied by a mild overstretching of a ligament, called a sprain. Severe overstretching causes ligament inflammation or tendinitis. Muscle or

tendon tears are uncommon other than in working dogs, racing greyhounds in particular, and occur as a result of exaggerated use.

DIAGNOSIS A physical examination locates the source of lameness. X-rays may be taken to eliminate fractures, dislocations, and most but not all instances of degenerative joint disease, confirming that the damage is to the soft tissue.

TREATMENT Overwhelmingly, the most important part of treatment is rest. This cannot be overstated. Physical activity soon after a muscle strain can turn a minor inconvenience into a chronic and major injury.

Immediately after injury, confine your dog to a small space. Apply ice packs (a bag of frozen peas, or crushed ice, wrapped in a tea towel is fine) for 20 minutes three to four times daily. The wrapped bag can sometimes be taped to an injured region using gauze. Cold packs reduce swelling.

After the first 24 hours following injury, switch to warm (not hot) packs three times a day for another two days. This prevents too much muscle contraction. Painkillers are not usually given unless pain is severe. Pain is useful; it is there to tell your dog to rest the joint. When pain control is necessary, meloxicam or carprofen are effective choices.

LIGAMENT INJURIES

By far the most common ligament injury is to the anterior cruciate (knee) ligament. Torn knee ligaments can occur because of injury, but cruciate ligament damage is most likely to occur spontaneously in middle-aged, overweight dogs. Breeds prone to torn cruciates include Boxers (who may develop the condition even while quite young) and Golden Retrievers. Sudden onset of hind leg lameness may be caused by cruciate ligament damage. The meniscus, or cartilage cushion, in the knee is commonly damaged when the ligaments are torn.

Whatever the predisposing causes, ligament injuries, particularly those that do not heal well, are associated with an increased risk of degenerative joint disease (DJD). On X-ray, many dogs with complete anterior cruciate rupture also have evidence of DJD. This sign suggests that a partial rupture may have occurred previously, triggering the DJD. Some experts believe that the angle of the top of a dog's tibia is crucial in determining the risk of cruciate rupture – one author writes that if this angle is greater than 28 degrees, stretching or rupture of the cruciate ligament is predictable.

DIAGNOSIS On physical examination, the vet can usually feel a slackness in the joint. A short anaesthetic may be necessary to relax the leg muscles and feel this slackness. X-rays may be

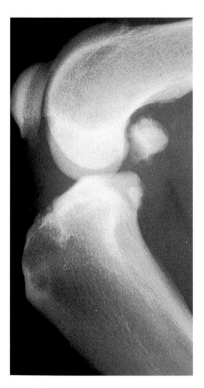

RUPTURED CRUCIATE LIGAMENT
This X-ray shows a ruptured anterior cruciate ligament in the knee joint. Cruciate ligament damage may be caused by injury but often occurs spontaneously in overweight dogs.

performed so that the vet can exclude damage to bones.

TREATMENT In overweight dogs, weight control is of paramount importance to treatment. In small breeds, surgery may be required. Although weight reduction may seem to repair the joint, over the following three months fibrous tissue develops and the joint no longer has the elasticity provided by a ligament.

For larger dogs, and for ligament damage that is due to traumatic injury, surgical repair is definitely required. In this procedure, surgeons may "harvest" some tissue from the hind leg or use synthetic tissue to create a new ligament. A more radical and patented technique called tibial plateau levelling osteotomy is used by some veterinary surgeons. This surgery reconfigures the joint so that it is no longer dependent on the anterior cruciate ligament for stability.

Surgical repair restores good function to the knee joint, usually within two months, but it does not prevent future arthritis, especially when the joint cartilage has been damaged. During the two years following a cruciate tear, the dog may suffer from periods of joint discomfort, but this usually responds to painkillers.

TENDON INJURIES

If overstretched or overworked, a tendon can become inflamed. This condition is called tendinitis. The sheath around the tendon may also become inflamed; this is called tenosynovitis. Both conditions cause local swelling, redness, and lameness. Strained tendons often result from sudden wrenching or twisting movements. The tendons of the forepaws (front and back) are strained most often.

If a tendon is torn, an injury most common in sporting dogs and racing greyhounds, there is severe lameness, pain, and loss of use of the limb. The heel (Achilles) tendon is most prone to tearing injuries and may be severed in dog fights and car accidents. Rupture

of the Achilles tendon causes a dropped hock.

DIAGNOSIS Diagnosis is by physical examination and manipulation of the affected area. X-rays are usually taken to exclude a fracture or dislocation.

TREATMENT The affected part should be rested to prevent further injury. Rest may be all that is needed for mild tendinitis. Activity should be restricted by confining the dog to a small area. Application of cold packs for the first 24 hours, followed by the use of warm, moist compresses over the next 24 hours, may relieve pain and inflammation. The vet may prescribe painkillers, one caution being that this may allow the dog to continue to use the injured leg while the injury is still healing. Tendon injuries take time, often more than six weeks, to heal. Incomplete healing is associated with increased risk of degenerative joint disease in the future.

BROKEN BONES

A break in a bone is called a fracture. Most fractures in dogs are caused by road accidents or falls from a height. The bones most commonly broken are the femur, pelvis, jaw, and spine. The extent of injury may vary from a barely visible crack to a complete shattering of the affected bone.

The most common types of fracture cause the two or more parts of broken bone to separate. These breaks are called complete fractures. A compound fracture is obvious: bone sticks through the skin. Compound fractures are prone to contamination by dirt and bacteria because the wound is exposed. In a simple fracture, the break is not visible but it causes pain and swelling. Other types of fracture split or compress the bone without separation. Young dogs can break their bones in much the same way as a young tree branch cracks but does not separate when you bend it. This break is called a greenstick fracture.

TYPES OF FRACTURE

This X-ray shows a simple fracture of the femur, which occurred a result of a road traffic accident. Surgical repair of such injuries involves pulling and rotating the two ends of the fracture back into perfect union. This union is maintained with a metal pin inserted in the hollow centre (medulla) of the bone. The pin emerges at the top of the femur by the hip, where it is cut off and remains under the skin. The surrounding heavy muscle provides limited support but a good blood supply, which helps healing. Six weeks later, when repair is complete, a small incision is made at the top of the femur and the pin is then pulled out.

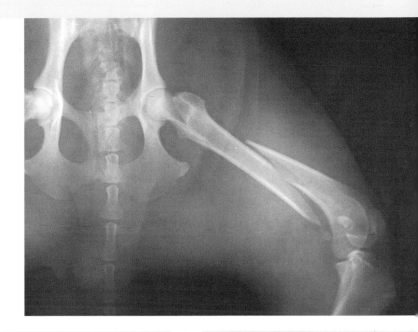

Signs of any type of bone fracture include pain and localized swelling. In a long bone, signs include inability to bear weight on a leg and deformity with shortening of a leg.

DIAGNOSIS AND TREATMENT Your vet will first make sure that there are no serious or life-threatening injuries, then give medications to control shock and pain, and intravenous fluids or blood as necessary, before attending to the fracture. X-rays reveal the degree of damage. Some fractures can be realigned and simply splinted with a cast; others need surgical correction with metal plates, pins, wires, screws, or even by external devices called fixators.

The injury site normally repairs itself by growing new bone. Broken bones heal faster in younger dogs. Healing also occurs quickly in well-muscled dogs, where there is already an efficient blood vessel supply around the injury site. Healing is more problematic, or may even fail, in thin bones with little muscle mass around them, such as the lower forelimbs of whippets or Italian Greyhounds.

ACQUIRED ARTHRITIS

The term "arthritis" simply means joint inflammation. It is used to describe a variety of painful conditions that can develop in any joint in a dog of any age. Inherited or developmental joint disorders that affect puppies are discussed on pp.366–86. There are many types of joint disease, but degenerative joint disease, also called osteoarthritis, is the most common.

DEGENERATIVE JOINT DISEASE (DJD)

Degenerative joint disease (DJD) affects about one out of five dogs during their lifetime. Large-breed dogs are affected more often than smaller breeds, and the disease usually develops as a dog grows older. DJD is progressive, and the damage that it causes is not reversible.

DJD occurs because the joint cartilage is unable either to maintain a healthy state or to repair itself after damage. This fault in joint cartilage may occur because of abnormal

Q **WHAT SHOULD I DO IF MY DOG HAS A BROKEN BONE?**

A A dog that has broken a bone should receive urgent veterinary attention. Remove the dog from danger and control blood loss (see First Aid, p392–97). Cover any open wounds, preferably with sterile dressing, but if that is not available use a clean towel. Try to restrain the dog to avoid movement at the site of the fracture. Heavy towelling usually provides sufficient support for the dog while travelling to the vet in the car. If splinting is necessary – for example, for a limb bone – do not try to straighten the break in the bone. Just wrap plenty of newspaper or other material around the leg, above and below the fracture, and hold the splint in place with tape, shoelaces, or similar items. Transport the dog immediately to the vet, who will assess the dog's condition, evaluate the injury, and perform X-rays to determine the severity of damage.

CONTROLLING DJD

There is no cure for degenerative join disease (DJD): the damage cannot be reversed. Treatment consists of alleviating pain, preventing or slowing further damage, and minimizing the impact of the condition on your dog's life. The mainstay of treatment for DJD is a change in lifestyle, focusing on diet and exercise, rather than veterinary intervention alone.

• Control weight

If a dog is overweight, alter the diet to bring weight back to within the normal range. If your dog's weight is "normal", discuss with your vet whether there is any value in reducing weight down to "lean". Do not give in to mournful brown eyes pleading hunger. If you cannot stop giving treats, reduce the calories supplied by meals, either by limiting the amount of food or by using a special low-calorie brand of prepared food.

• Control exercise

Rest is vital, but so is controlled, sensible exercise to maintain good muscle tone. Avoid running and retrieving games, because these put too much pressure on joints. In addition, avoid doing anything that encourages your dog to jump up. Forget about the dog going with you on a five-mile jog; instead, take your dog for a short to moderate walk several times a day, every day. Swimming is one of the best forms of exercise because it tones muscles while relieving pressure on the joints. Exercise in hydrotherapy pools is ideal; ask your vet for advice.

physical force on a normal joint or because of normal force on an abnormal joint. It may also occur seemingly for no reason.

The first sign of DJD, and indeed of most other joint disorders in dogs, is a reduced ability to carry out normal physical activities. An affected dog may not be as agile when exercising, for example, or may not bound up stairs as it used to do. It may step into a car rather than leap into it. The first signs of DJD are often subtle.

With time, DJD causes obvious stiffness or lameness after robust or prolonged physical activity, and then after shorter periods of activity. As the degeneration progresses, there may be stiffness or lameness even at rest. A dog's lying down position may change. At this stage, the stiffness upon arising can be "worked out" by a little physical activity. Eventually, the stiffness or lameness cannot be worked out, so that the dog is permanently stiff and lame.

Lameness is more apparent when DJD is more severe in joints on one side of the dog's body than on the other. If there is symmetrical DJD, there may not be limping as such but only stiffness and a reduced ability to perform previous physical tasks or manoeuvres.

DIAGNOSIS The vet will flex, extend, and rotate joints to assess their range of motion and the severity of any pain. He or she may flex the joint and listen for any sign of crepitus: a dry, grating sound from within the joint that indicates that the joint cartilage has worn away.

X-rays may show a narrowing of the joint space, new bone formation or calcium deposits in the joint cavity, or other pathological changes. The degree of change gives the vet a good idea of how advanced the DJD has become. Arthroscopy to view directly inside the affected joint, and analysis of the joint fluid, may also be undertaken.

TREATMENT Regardless of cause, there is a universal treatment for DJD. Most importantly, the dog's weight should be controlled and gentle exercise maintained (*see box, left*).

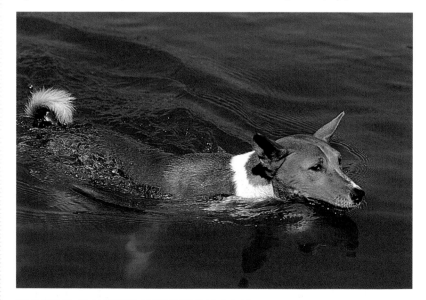

SWIMMING IS AN IDEAL EXERCISE FOR DOGS WITH DJD
Although dogs with degenerative joint disease may no longer be able to enjoy strenuous exercise, they can benefit from regular, gentle exercise, such as swimming. Swimming tones the muscles, while supporting the joints. It is ideal for any dog with joint problems.

Pain is controlled by various means. Non-steroidal anti-inflammatory drugs (NSAIDs) are effective and safe for long-term use in most dogs with DJD. Meloxicam and carprofen are the veterinary NSAIDs of choice. The availability of these and other advanced NSAIDs has dramatically enhanced pain control for DJD. All NSAIDs, however, are associated with gastrointestinal and other problems. If an NSAID is the only way to control pain but causes stomach irritation, the vet may recommend medications such as misoprostol or sucralfate to protect the stomach lining and prevent ulcers. Dogs having long-term treatment with carprofen should have periodic blood tests to assess their liver function, because carprofen may be associated with liver damage.

PREVENTION There are many products marketed as joint cartilage protectors (chondroprotectants). The most widely used are glucosamine and chondroitin. The dog food company Iams has been sufficiently impressed by its own research and other nutritional literature to add these natural chondroprotectants to their diets for large-breed pups and dogs. A more concentrated pharmaceutical-standard tablet form of these products is available as a veterinary nutritional supplement. These products will certainly do no harm, but because each individual dog with DJD is unique, double-blind effectiveness trials of nutritional supplements are very difficult to perform and sometimes inconclusive in their findings.

A variety of dietary nutrients are available that may reduce joint pain or even enhance joint health. There is good evidence that some essential fatty acids (EFAs) are "pro-inflammatory", while others are "anti-inflammatory". Translating this fact into a therapy should, at least in theory, be possible. The natural EFAs found in marine fish oil and linseed oil are high in "anti-inflammatory" EFAs, particularly two

---

WHAT HAPPENS INSIDE AN INFLAMED JOINT

The cartilage pads at the ends of the bones have a vital role in keeping the joints moving smoothly. When this cartilage is damaged or becomes unable to regenerate, the joint no longer moves smoothly. This causes wear and tear, and the joint tissues become inflamed.

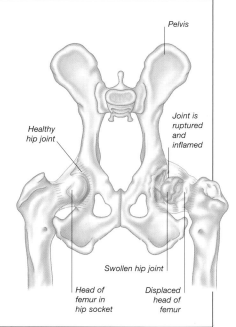

COMPARING THE TWO JOINTS
On the left is a healthy hip joint, with correctly positioned bones and smooth bone surfaces. On the right is a hip that has suffered damage. The head of the femur is not sitting firmly in the socket of the hip joint, and is causing wear and tear on the surrounding tissues.

Pelvis

Joint is ruptured and inflamed

Healthy hip joint

Swollen hip joint

Head of femur in hip socket

Displaced head of femur

---

substances called EPA and DHA. Adding these to your dog's diet may reduce joint inflammation and help alleviate pain. The question that still remains is how much EPA and DHA is necessary for a significant improvement. As yet, no one has produced an answer.

RHEUMATOID AND NON-DEFORMING ARTHRITIS

The autoimmune condition rheumatoid arthritis, while common in humans, is rare in dogs. It occurs mainly in the foot (carpal and tarsal) joints in toy or small breeds from about one to eight years old. Many dog owners think their dogs are "rheumatic" or have "rheumatism", when in fact what they have is degenerative joint disease.

Rheumatoid arthritic dogs are uncomfortable, may have a fever, and may be reluctant to eat. In the early stages of rheumatoid arthritis, there may be enlargement of the lymph nodes. More common than rheumatoid

---

Q **CAN ACUPUNCTURE RELIEVE THE PAIN OF DJD?**

A Acupuncture, and some other complementary therapies, may certainly make some dogs with DJD more comfortable. The exact reason for the beneficial effect remains elusive.

Q **IS SURGERY AN OPTION FOR TREATING DOGS WITH JOINT DISEASE?**

A In some cases of severe DJD, surgical fusion of painful joints, such as the hock or elbow, may relieve pain. This treatment may even restore some degree of movement in the affected joint – but the effects of surgery may not be permanent. Regular, gentle exercise, weight control, and painkillers such as non-steroidal anti-inflammatory drugs are the mainstays of treatment for DJD.

arthritis is a form of non-deforming autoimmune arthritis, usually seen in purebreds, causing intermittent cycles of fever, lethargy, and lameness involving more than one joint.

DIAGNOSIS Both rheumatoid arthritis and non-deforming arthritis are hard to diagnose. Blood tests that reveal an elevated level of a substance called rheumatoid factor may help a vet make the diagnosis, but are not conclusive. Other blood tests are also used.

TREATMENT Treatment is often difficult. Corticosteroid drugs give only temporary relief. More potent immunosuppressant drugs are usually needed to relieve clinical signs.

JOINT INFECTION (SEPTIC ARTHRITIS)

Infectious diseases can produce arthritis. Bacteria can enter the joint space through penetrating wounds, from local infection, but also from distant infection when bacteria are carried to one or more joints in the blood. Bacterial infections on the skin,

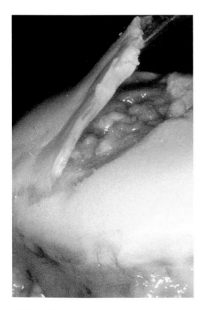

OSTEOCHONDROSIS
This picture shows the effects of the joint disorder osteochondrosis, in which flakes of cartilage detach from the bone.

in the mouth, the heart valves, the kidneys, or even the bladder can result in bacterial arthritis. *Borrelia burgdorferi*, the tick-borne organism that causes Lyme disease (*see p.154*), and other tick-borne disease organisms, such as rickettsia and ehrlichia (*see p.154–55*), can also reach joint cavities via the bloodstream. So can the sandfly-transmitted organism that causes leishmaniasis (*see pp.174–75*).

Fungal arthritis may occur as a rare complication of a systemic fungal infection.

DIAGNOSIS A diagnosis of bacterial arthritis, overwhelmingly the most common form of infectious arthritis, is made by analysing and culturing fluid withdrawn from the joints.

TREATMENT Infection is treated with appropriate antibiotics. Joint infection may be complicated by bone infection (*see p.368*) and frequently leads to degenerative joint disease.

POLYARTHRITIS

This disorder is inflammation affecting many joints. It is an increasingly diagnosed condition. It can be triggered by hypersensitivity to a variety of drugs, including the antibiotic trimethoprim sulfa. As well as joint inflammation, affected dogs may have a fever, skin rash, and swollen lymph nodes. The disorder spontaneously disappears when the drug is discontinued.

INHERITED OR DEVELOPMENTAL JOINT CONDITIONS

Some dogs are born with an inherited predisposition to develop a joint disease such as hip dysplasia, elbow dysplasia, osteochondrosis, or aseptic necrosis. This predisposition varies according to the breed. The conditions covered below are the most common inherited joint diseases. All of them cause lameness. Their treatment is often similar to that of degenerative

joint disease; the discomfort or lack of function associated with some of these conditions may also be alleviated by surgical intervention.

HIP DYSPLASIA

The hip bone (pelvis) cradles the heads of the two thigh bones (femurs) in deep, cartilage-lined, cup-like sockets. If the fit is not right – for example, if there is a slight misalignment and the femoral head is "lax," or loose – the cartilage of the femoral head rubs against the socket. Eventually, the cartilage wears through. This condition is called hip dysplasia; it is a common form of osteoarthritis. At first, hip dysplasia causes no clinical signs, but once there is sufficient wear and tear, there is pain and associated lameness.

Hip dysplasia is more common in large, fast-growing breeds (*see right*). Genetics, however, is only one of the predisposing factors leading to hip dysplasia. Experts say that heredity accounts for about 25 per cent of a dog's chance of developing this condition. Other important factors include diet, weight, and activity level.

DIAGNOSIS An initial diagnosis is made by breed history and feeling a hip joint for slackness (joint laxity). X-rays are used to grade the severity of hip dysplasia, but often there is no direct correlation between how badly affected the hips look on X-ray and how bad the dog feels.

TREATMENT Dogs are treated as for degenerative joint disease (*see p.363*). In most affected dogs, the condition is kept under control by weight management, moderate exercise, and pain medication such as the non-steroidal anti-inflammatory drugs (NSAIDs) meloxicam and carprofen. Natural joint nutrients such as chondroitin sulphate and glucosamine may also be beneficial.

When pain and lack of function is severe, there are a range of surgical interventions that may be used. For dogs weighing less than 20 kg (44 lb), the femoral head may be removed. A "false" joint consisting of fibrous scar tissue forms in the space left by the femoral head. Heavy individuals more often have total hip replacement. The surgeon removes the socket portion of the pelvis and, using screws and "cement", replaces it with a plastic cup. The ball at the top of the femur is removed and a titanium ball on a stem is inserted into the widened opening. New prostheses last the dog's lifetime.

PREVENTION The best prevention is selective breeding. Before breeding, dogs are X-rayed and their hips "scored" or "graded". An individual's score or grade can be compared to the breed average score. The lower the score or grade, the better. The vet takes X-rays according to the requirements of the hip-scoring body. The X-rays are also read by independent experts.

ELBOW DYSPLASIA

Most frequently seen in the Bernese Mountain Dog, Labrador Retrievers, Golden Retrievers, and Rottweilers, elbow dysplasia is really a constellation of different elbow conditions, including osteochondrosis and problems with the leg bones. It occurs during a pup's growth, generally from four to ten months of age, causing lameness that gets worse with exercise. In severe cases, the elbow feels swollen and is held away from the body. The joint may loose a lot of its range of motion.

DIAGNOSIS AND TREATMENT The condition is diagnosed by X-rays and is usually managed by weight control, careful exercise, avoiding games that stress the joints, and pain management using analgesics. Surgical repair of the affected bones or of osteochondrosis lesions may be beneficial.

OSTEOCHONDROSIS

This bone disorder is also called osteochondrosis dessicans, and abbreviated to OC or OCD. In OC, bits of poorly developing cartilage flake off as flaps within the joints of a growing puppy. The denuded areas of bone may become inflamed, while the chips of cartilage floating in the joint fluid simply get in the way of smooth joint function.

Technically, OC is a disease caused by a defect in the calcification process of the growth plates near the ends of the long bones. OC occurs most frequently in the shoulder joints but also in the elbows, stifles, and hocks. While it is usually bilateral, joint damage and associated lameness or altered gait may be more severe on one side than on the other. OC occurs most frequently in fast-growing, heavy dogs fed on high-energy diets.

DIAGNOSIS OC is diagnosed by physical examination and X-rays. A number of X-rays of the same joint may be needed to see the exact location of damage. Arthroscopy is useful for examining very large joints.

TREATMENT While simple rest is all that is necessary for some dogs, other dogs benefit from having the floating chips of cartilage surgically removed.

BREEDS AT RISK

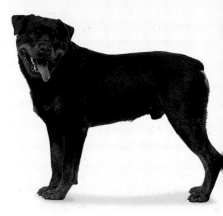

Breeds predisposed to hip dysplasia include:

- German Shepherd Dog
- Golden Retriever
- Labrador Retriever
- Newfoundland
- Rottweiler (above)
- Saint Bernard

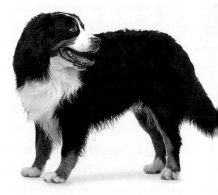

Breeds prone to elbow dysplasia include:

- Bernese Mountain Dog (above)
- Chow Chow
- German Shepherd Dog
- Golden Retriever
- Labrador Retriever
- Newfoundland
- Rottweiler
- Shar Pei

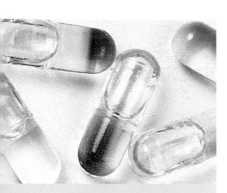

Q   DO DOGS NEED VITAMIN OR MINERAL SUPPLEMENTS?

A   Only if they are ill or elderly. Fast-growing pups do not need and should not be given calcium supplements. Research over a quarter of a century ago revealed that too much calcium is harmful to bone development. Diets formulated by the major pet food makers contain balanced amounts of vitamins and minerals. The best also contain high levels of beneficial anti-oxidants, making supplements unnecessary.

Q   ARE BONE GRAFTS USED IN DOGS?

A   Yes, they are, particularly as an alternative to amputation for dogs with bone cancer when the problem is diagnosed before the cancer has spread elsewhere. A bone graft does not just provide a superstructure to fill a gap. Even though all marrow is removed (to prevent rejection), the grafted bone still seems to contain substances that help stimulate new bone formation. As a limb-sparing technique for treating bone cancer, surgeons at Colorado State University's (USA) veterinary school have developed a biodegradable bone implant containing chemotherapy drugs. This implant has fewer side effects than whole-body chemotherapy treatment.

SLIPPING KNEECAPS

Common in toy breeds, particularly the Yorkshire Terrier, this inherited condition, also called patellar luxation, varies in severity. Being born with slightly rotated tibias (tibial torsion) leads to a slackness in the knee ligaments. This allows the kneecap to slip off inwards. Usually, there is no pain associated with the kneecap slipping (patellar luxation), but once it has come off, the leg no longer supports weight normally. An affected dog continues walking or running as if nothing has happened but hops along, not bearing weight on the affected hind leg. If the kneecap spontaneously slips back, which often happens, the leg again functions normally.

DIAGNOSIS AND TREATMENT   The disease is diagnosed by physical examination. For many individuals, no treatment is necessary. For others, especially those with severe luxations or individuals who have torn a lateral knee ligament, surgical correction is beneficial.

AVASCULAR NECROSIS

This condition, also called aseptic necrosis, Perthes disease, or Legg-Perthes disease, occurs in some toy breeds, the Poodle and the West Highland White Terrier in particular. In avascular necrosis, the blood vessels serving the head of the femur (in the hip joint) are prone to injury. If these vessels are damaged, the head of the femur effectively dies. This condition usually occurs between four and 12 months of age.

DIAGNOSIS   There is usually a loss of muscle mass on the affected leg, although if the disease occurs in both hips, which happens occasionally, the muscle loss is symmetrical. Avascular necrosis is diagnosed by X-ray.

TREATMENT   This painful condition is treated by surgically removing the dead (necrotic) head of the femur. This eliminates pain. In the following months, a "false" fibrous joint develops that is surprisingly efficient.

OTHER BONE DISEASES

Bone is prone to disease just like other parts of the body. When it is physically damaged it has a dynamic ability to repair itself.

BONE INFECTION (OSTEOMYELITIS)

Bone is usually quite resistant to infection. Although mycoplasma, rickettsia, and fungi can cause bone infection, staphylococcus bacteria cause about half of all cases. Bacteria enters bone from wounds (bites, foreign bodies, gunshots) but also from distant locations via the bloodstream. Acute infection is accompanied by high fever, loss of appetite and weight, lethargy, as well as heat and swelling in the muscles surrounding the site of infection.

DIAGNOSIS   Blood tests reveal the body is fighting an infection. X-rays show bony change consistent with infection-induced damage. Bacterial culture and sensitivity identifies the specific cause.

TREATMENT   Osteomyelitis is difficult to treat. Acute infections are treated for a month or more with antibiotics that penetrate bone tissue. Chronic infection requires additional surgical intervention to remove dead tissue.

BONE TUMOURS

Dogs can develop a variety of bone tumours, but the most common is the highly malignant osteosarcoma. These tumours are most likely to occur in the long bones of middle-aged or older large and giant breeds. The most common locations are in the radius, humerus, femur, and tibia.

The second most common type of tumour, a chrondrosarcoma, affects the flat bones. It, too, is highly malignant. The first sign of bone tumours is usually lameness and pain.

DIAGNOSIS AND TREATMENT   Diagnosis is confirmed by X-ray. Unfortunately, by the time osteosarcoma has been discovered there is a 90 per cent chance that it has spread to other parts of the body, the lungs and liver in particular. This development affects decisions about possible treatments. Amputation remains the treatment of choice for tumours in the long bones. Alternative limb-sparing techniques may also be used to control tumour-associated pain. With dramatic intervention, about one half of all affected dogs survive a year or more.

MUSCLE CONDITIONS

The skeletal muscles are kept toned by a steady flow of nerve impulses. If a muscle loses its nerve supply, it shrinks. Muscles also require a constant supply of blood, and if this is impaired stiffness may result. Muscles are more often injured than diseased, and are highly capable of self-repair. If one part of a muscle is damaged, the remaining parts compensate by growing larger and stronger.

Strains, bruising, and tearing are overwhelmingly the most common muscle injuries in dogs. Tendons sometimes tear, but because of the retraction caused by their natural elasticity, they do not repair as well as muscles. If tendons tear off bones, repair may be very difficult.

Disorders such as myasthenia gravis and tick paralysis are conditions affecting muscle–nerve junctions, while some rare infectious and autoimmune conditions such as polymyositis affect the muscles themselves.

BRUISING AND TEARING

Bruising, stretching, or tearing of muscle fibres is difficult to see, especially in dogs with full coats of hair. These forms of damage occur not only after injuries from falling, road accidents, or abuse, but also after excessive work or exercise. Racing greyhounds are particularly prone to muscle bruising and tears.

The signs vary with the degree of injury. Minor injuries produce local sensitivity and tenderness, while major damage from muscle tears causes more swelling and greater pain.

DIAGNOSIS Parting the hair may reveal reddening caused by bruised muscle below. Blood tests to measure muscle enzyme level can indicate the degree of damage. X-rays may be performed to confirm that the damage is restricted to the muscle tissue rather than affecting the bones and joints.

TREATMENT Treatment is the same as for muscle strains (*see above*). The most important element of treatment is rest, for at least three weeks when damage is severe, during which time full healing usually takes place.

CRAMP

Cramp occurs when muscle filaments, the components of muscle fibres, remain permanently contracted. It occurs most frequently in canine athletes as a result of muscle overuse, and causes painful muscle spasm.

Most cramps last only a few minutes, and can be relieved by massaging or stretching the muscles involved. If a dog appears to be in pain for longer than about an hour, there may be a more serious problem.

NATURAL WEAR AND TEAR

Over time, a dog's muscles naturally shrink and gradually lose their power. This process of natural wear and tear occurs more slowly if a dog is kept fit and healthy by frequent gentle exercise as it grows older.

In some cases, however, metabolic disorders elsewhere in the body (*see p.99*) may affect muscle mass. Certain metabolic disorders reduce the amount of nutrients available to the muscles or produce toxins that damage the muscle fibres. If your dog is losing muscle mass for no apparent reason, there may be a medical problem elsewhere in the body, and you should seek veterinary advice.

INHERITED BONE PROBLEMS OF YOUNG DOGS

A variety of painful but self-limiting bone problems commonly occur in a number of breeds. Non-steroidal anti-inflammatory drugs are used as needed to control pain caused by these conditions, which can persist for two to nine months.

DISEASE AND AGE	BREEDS AFFECTED	SIGNS
Craniomandibular osteopathy 3–8 months	Terriers, especially Scottish Terrier, West Highland White Terrier	Drooling, pain on opening mouth, swelling of the jaw
Panosteitis 6–18 months	Large and giant breeds especially German Shepherds, and males more than females	Acute but intermittent lameness in one or more legs; fever, lethargy, weight loss
Metaphyseal osteopathy (Hypertrophic osteodystrophy) 3–4 months	Large breeds	Painful swelling at ends of long bones, depression, loss of appetite

MYASTHENIA GRAVIS

Myasthenia gravis is a deficiency in the chemical called acetylcholine that transfers information from a nerve fibre to a muscle fibre. The condition can be congenital or acquired.

The rare congenital form of myasthenia gravis has been reported in Airedales, Jack Russells, Smooth Fox Terriers, and Springer Spaniels, with earliest signs usually appearing at about seven to eight weeks of age. Generalized muscle weakness progresses quite rapidly in juvenile myasthenia gravis to full paralysis.

Signs of acquired myasthenia gravis occur later in the dog's life and are more varied. Muscle weakness may be generalized in this form of the disorder, but it is just as likely to be local – for example, just affecting the oesophagus, causing it to relax and enlarge.

VET'S ADVICE

Exercise is of prime importance in maintaining the skeleton and the muscles. Most dogs need at least one, and preferably two, sessions of daily exercise that include trotting and galloping. This not only promotes muscle strength, but also helps to increase the density and strength of the bones. Regular, gentle exercise is particularly important for dogs with disorders affecting the joints and muscles. As a dog ages, its endurance diminishes but its need for regular exercise does not. Do not overexercise a mature dog. Walking and trotting is better than galloping. After a dog has been incapacitated by illness or injury, reintroduce exercise gradually say over a three-week period. For all dogs, ensure that exercise includes mental as well as physical stimulation.

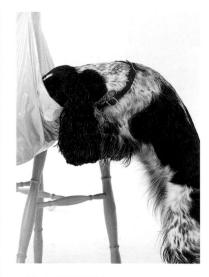

DOG SCAVENGING
Dogs that scavenge may come into contact with substances contaminated with botulism bacteria, which can cause paralysis.

DIAGNOSIS AND TREATMENT Myasthenia gravis is diagnosed by injecting a drug (edrophonium) that temporarily protects the chemical transmitter substance acetylcholine from breakdown. A transient improvement in muscle activity, or a lessening in weakness, is then diagnostic of myasthenia gravis. An antibody test (for antibodies to acetylcholine receptors) is another highly specific means of diagnosis. Long-term treatment with an acetylcholine inhibitor may be helpful, but the outlook for affected dogs is poor.

BOTULISM AND TICK PARALYSIS

Both botulism and tick paralysis are conditions that prevent acetylcholine, which transfers information from a nerve fibre to a muscle fibre, from being released by nerve fibres at their junction with muscle fibres.

Certain types of tick, such as *Dermacentor andersoni* (the Rocky Mountain wood tick), *Dermacentor variabilis* (the American dog tick), and

Ixodes holocyclus (the Australian paralysis tick), produce a toxin similar to that produced by botulism bacteria, which can cause poisoning.

Progressive paralysis without loss of consciousness occurs in both of these diseases.

DIAGNOSIS AND TREATMENT Botulism and tick paralysis are diagnosed on the basis of having eaten contaminated food, having contaminated wounds, or having ticks. Removing the source of the paralysis leads to improvement. During recovery, affected dogs may need antiserum and additional supportive care.

PRIMARY MUSCLE DISORDERS (MYOPATHIES)

All inherited myopathies, conditions affecting muscle fibres themselves, are rare in dogs. Most involve deficiencies in particular muscle cell proteins.

DIAGNOSIS AND TREATMENT Blood tests, muscle electrical tests, and physical examination are usually diagnostic. Genetic tests are available (or in development) that can determine carrier status for a variety of inherited disorders. At present, there are no effective treatments for these inherited conditions, but genetic testing and selective breeding can be used as a preventive measure.

POLYMYOSITIS

Polymyositis is, as its name suggests, an inflammation of many muscles. For unknown reasons it occurs most frequently in large, adult dogs.

While parasitic organisms such as *toxoplasmosis*, *neospora*, and *ehrlichiosis* (see pp.166–75) are said to cause polymyositis, the clinical disease is really caused by over-reaction of the immune system, producing widespread muscle inflammation varying from mild to excruciatingly painful. Other triggers for disease include drugs such as trimethoprim-sulfa.

INHERITED MYOPATHIES

CONDITION	BREEDS AFFECTED	SIGNS
X-linked muscular dystrophy	Golden Retriever Greenland Husky Rottweiler Samoyed Schnauzer (miniature)	Only affects males. Muscle weakness in pups, chewing and swallowing problems, splayed paws
Labrador myopathy	Labrador Retriever	General weakness, shrinking of head muscles in growing pups
Myotonia	Chow Chow	Excessive muscle mass in pups, a stiff gait, and a tendency to fall forwards
Phosphofructokinase deficiency	English Springer Spaniel	Anaemia and muscle weakness

DIAGNOSIS AND TREATMENT
Polymyositis is diagnosed by finding the underlying trigger for the condition, blood tests to detect elevated muscle enzyme activity, and muscle tissue biopsies. The underlying cause is treated. In addition, corticosteroid drugs are given both to relieve pain and to control the overactive immune system.

IMMUNE-MEDIATED JAW MUSCLE DISEASE

This rare condition is also called masticatory muscle myositis. It is seen more in German Shepherds than in other breeds, and begins with swelling of the chewing (masseter) muscles. As the condition progresses, the muscles shrink and it becomes painful for the dog to open its mouth.
DIAGNOSIS AND TREATMENT A muscle biopsy confirms the diagnosis. Early treatment with corticosteroid drugs is very beneficial.

OTHER CONDITIONS THAT CAN AFFECT THE BONES, MUSCLES, AND JOINTS

Certain disorders of the nervous system or of the metabolism can cause signs that are similar to those of muscle, bone, or joint disorders.

NERVE CONDITIONS

The demyelinating condition chronic degenerative myelopathy (*see p.371*) causes a progessive loss of use of the hind legs, particularly in German Shepherds but also in other breeds. There is no cure for this condition.

METABOLIC DISORDERS

Metabolic diseases affecting the bones, such as rickets, caused by a shortage of vitamin D, or nutritional secondary hyperparathyroidism (*see p.332–33*), caused by an excess of phosphorus or a lack of calcium in the diet, are very rare in dogs.

Q **MANY PEOPLE WITH CHRONIC JOINT PAIN BENEFIT FROM COMPLEMENTARY THERAPIES SUCH AS SHIATSU, CHIROPRACTIC, OSTEOPATHY, AND MASSAGE. ARE THESE PRACTICES HELPFUL FOR DOGS?**

A Anything that works is beneficial, even if we don't know why it works. In people, "mind over matter" is vital for pain control. A contentious question is whether we can influence a dog's attitude towards pain. There are good indications that we can.

Over 40 years ago, some very unpleasant research studies showed that a dog felt less pain from an electric shock when it was petted at the time of the shock than it felt when it received the shock in the absence of human contact. Physical touch helped to reduce the intensity of pain.

In the late 1990s, far more benign research conducted at the Ontario Veterinary College in Canada pointed in the same direction. This research involved dogs with DJD. Owners gave "painkillers" to their dogs; some dogs received capsules containing aspirin in rice flour, while others received a placebo containing only rice flour. Forty per cent of the dogs given placebo improved. (Almost 70 per cent of dogs receiving aspirin improved.) The significant improvement in mobility and reduction in pain from a placebo may be a consequence of touch, especially in a touch-sensitive, sociable species like the dog.

For "humanized" dogs – raised from puppyhood in our homes – any form of touch from petting or massage to acupressure, acupuncture, or osteopathy, may be rewarding and reduce pain.

CANCER

Cancer is the most common cause of death in older dogs. Almost 42 per cent of dogs succumb to one form of cancer or another. But do not assume that all lumps and bumps on older dogs are cancers. They are not. Many of these lumps are simply cysts or blocked sebaceous glands. Others are unsightly but benign warts.

One of the most common tumours to affect an older dog is a lipoma, a lump of fat usually between the skin and underlying muscle. Lipomas are not dangerous but can grow from the size of a bean to a baseball or larger.

TREATMENT Lipomas and warts (papillomas) are unsightly but only need attention when located in areas where they cause physical problems. Your vet will discuss the best treatment for more serious tumours.

If your dog has any form of cancer, but especially if it has a lymphoma, a cancer of the lymphatic system, avoid a high-carbohydrate diet. There is ample evidence that carbohydrate gives cancer cells extra energy. Instead, feed your dog a diet of high-quality fat and protein, supplemented with extra micronutrients. Your vet will guide you on what diet is best for your dog.

EUTHANASIA

Euthanasia means ending the life of an individual who suffers from a terminal illness or another incurable condition to relieve suffering. The word comes from the Greek *eu* ("good") and *thanatos* ("death") – a good death.

Euthanasia is almost certainly the most emotional decision you will ever make for your dog. The ethical aspects of euthanasia relate to the part your dog plays in your life and how much enjoyment it still gets from its own life. They are discussed in Your Family Dog (*see p.50*). There are also practicalities to consider when euthanasia is chosen as the best treatment.

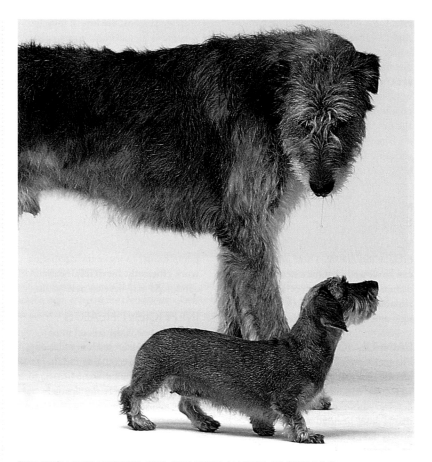

THE IRISH WOLFHOUND AND THE WIRE-HAIRED DACHSHUND
These two dogs illustrate the general rule about large dogs having a shorter life expectancy than small dogs. The Irish Wolfhound has a life expectancy of 6.2 years, while the Wire-haired Dachshund has a life expectancy of 12.2 years.

LETTING GO

An extensive survey of the records of a large pet insurance company revealed that euthanasia was the most common cause of death in dogs and was carried out because owners and vets felt it was in a dog's "best interests".

CAUSE OF DEATH	PERCENTAGE OF INSURED DOGS
Natural causes	8%
Accidents	5%
Illness	35%
Euthanasia due to behaviour problems	2%
Euthanasia due to illness	29%
Euthanasia due to old age	21%

PERFORMING EUTHANASIA

Euthanasia is a painless procedure in which a dog is given an overdose of an anaesthetic. The drug phenobarb is the most commonly used agent. It is administered intravenously in a more concentrated form than is normally the case for anaesthesia.

A dog loses consciousness within seconds, as happens with anaesthesia. Within another few seconds, while the dog is unconscious, its heart stops. Depending on the circumstances, a sedative may be given before the barbiturate and then a cannula is inserted into a vein to ensure that all goes smoothly.

While brain death occurs within seconds, electrical activity continues in the muscles and may cause some of the body's muscles to twitch. If the respiratory muscles are affected there can be a reflex "gasp" as if the dog were still alive. This kind of reflex muscle activity may take place up to ten minutes after death.

AFTERWARDS

Where I practise, all the bodies are routinely cremated after euthanasia unless the owners prefer burial. In this case, the body is kept in cold storage if it cannot be taken home immediately.

If you choose to bury your dog, as I have done with all of mine, make sure the body is enclosed in a material that is biodegradable, not synthetic. I have wrapped my dogs in cotton sheets. A grave should be deep enough so that wild animals cannot dig it up. This usually means 1 m (3 ft) or more.

YOUR NEXT DOG

At the time of euthanasia vets are frequently told by owners that they will never again keep a dog. Statistics, however, tell a different story. While we find the loss of a canine companion deeply distressing, most of us – over 75 per cent – bring a new dog into our lives within months.

LIFE EXPECTANCY IN VARIOUS BREEDS

What truly complicates comparing a dog's life expectancy with ours is that it varies tremendously from breed to breed. Listed below are the average life expectancy statistics for 65 breeds as collected by the world's largest pet health insurer, Pet Plan. As a general rule of thumb, the larger the dog the shorter its life expectancy. Old age in one breed is early middle age in another. It is important to remember that a dog's real biological age is determined by not only the breed but also its nutrition, the stresses it faces, and the care it is given.

14 YEARS AND OVER

Miniature Poodle (14.8)
Miniature Dachshund (14.4)
Toy Poodle (14.4)
Tibetan Terrier (14.3)
Bedlington Terrier (14.3)
Whippet (14.3)

13 YEARS AND OVER

Border Terrier (13.8)
Jack Russell Terrier (13.6)
Chow Chow (13.5)
Shih Tzu (13.4)
Beagle (13.3)
Pekingese (13.3)
Shetland Sheepdog (13.3)
Cairn Terrier (13.2)
Greyhound (13.2)
Random-bred / Mongrel (13.2)
Border Collie (13.0)
Chihuahua (13.0)
Dalmatian (13.0)
English Springer Spaniel (13.0)
Wire Fox Terrier (13.0)

12 YEARS AND OVER

Bull Terrier (12.9)
Irish Red and White Setter (12.9)
Basset Hound (12.8)
West Highland White Terrier (12.8)
Yorkshire Terrier (12.8)
Labrador Retriever (12.6)
Lurcher (12.6)
Cocker Spaniel (12.5)
Hungarian Viszla (12.5)
Bearded Collie (12.3)
German Shorthaired Pointer (12.3)
Dachshund (12.2)
Rough Collie (12.2)

Afghan Hound (12.0)
Golden Retriever (12.0)
Scottish Terrier (12.0)
Standard Poodle (12.0)

11 YEARS AND OVER

English Cocker Spaniel (11.8)
Irish Setter (11.8)
Old English Sheepdog (11.8)
Welsh Springer Spaniel (11.5)
Corgi (11.3)
Gordon Setter (11.3)
Airedale Terrier (11.2)
English Setter (11.2)
Samoyed (11.0)

10 YEARS AND OVER

Cavalier King Charles Spaniel (10.7)
Boxer (10.4)
German Shepherd (10.3)
English Toy Spaniel (10.1)
Norfolk Terrier (10.0)
Staffordshire Bull Terrier (10.0)
Weimaraner (10.0)

UNDER 10 YEARS

Doberman (9.8)
Rottweiler (9.8)
Scottish Deerhound (9.5)
Flat-coated Retriever (9.5)
Rhodesian Ridgeback (9.1)
Bullmastiff (8.6)
Great Dane (8.4)
Bernese Mountain Dog (7.0)
Bulldog (6.7)
Irish Wolfhound (6.2)

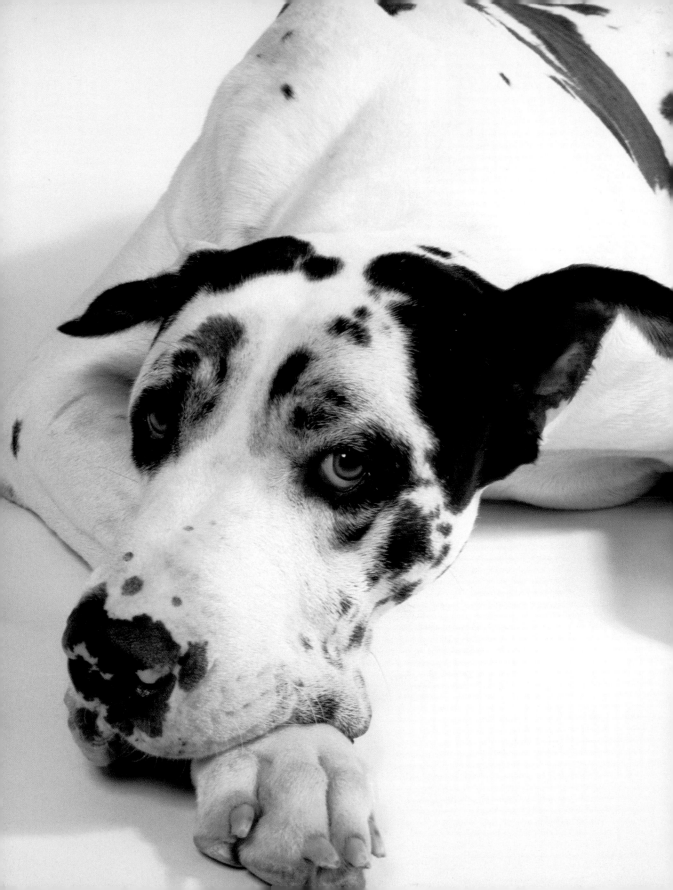

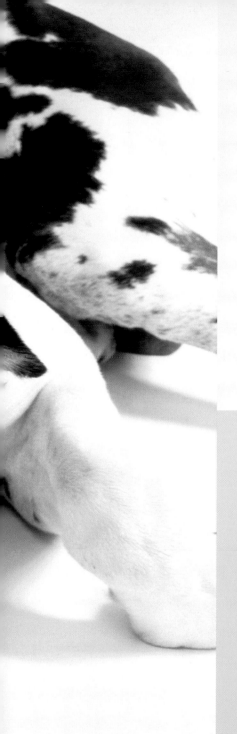

FIRST AID
AND
EMERGENCIES

Good veterinary care is usually within easy reach of most dog owners. However, there are occasions when emergencies happen and your dog depends on you for help. By planning ahead and practising how to restrain your dog, examine it, and carry out basic first aid, you will find that you are prepared for most eventualities. In any emergency your responsibility is to quickly assess the situation, restrain your dog if necessary, and then give it emergency first aid. In serious emergencies your aim is to prevent further damage to any injuries that your dog may have sustained, reduce its pain and distress and, of course, sustain life. When it is safe and practical to do so, you should then contact a vet and arrange for further professional help.

GENERAL EMERGENCIES
useful first aid equipment

The most common emergency affecting dogs is trauma – physical injury. Such accidents are most common during pleasant weather and most often occur outdoors. They can be as minor as a cut pad or as major as a severe road traffic accident. A dog's natural curiosity also predisposes it to other emergencies, such as choking on objects, contact with poisons, and near-drowning. Unfortunately, humans are responsible for many incidents, such as heatstroke, gunshot wounds, and malicious poisoning. This section describes what to do in any potentially life-threatening situation.

EMERGENCY ACTION PLAN
This plan outlines the sequence of actions to take for any medical emergency.

Ensure safety
Look for hazards. Are you or dog in danger?

YES → Deal with hazard, if possible, before you approach dog.

NO ↓

Restrain dog (see pp.384–85).

↓

Check response (see p.386)
Assess consciousness. Is dog conscious?

YES →
- Look for and treat any signs of choking (see pp.390–91).
- Check gums for shock (see p.388).
- Look for and treat severe bleeding (see p.392) or other conditions.
- Take dog to vet.

NO ↓

Check airway (see p.387)
Keep airway open. Remove any debris. Keep neck straight. Is breathing apparent?

YES →
- Check gums for shock.
- Look for and treat severe bleeding or other conditions.
- Take dog to vet.

NO ↓

Check breathing (see p.387)
Signs of breathing may be very slight or almost invisible. Is dog breathing?

YES →
- Check gums for shock.
- Look for and treat severe bleeding or other conditions.
- Get dog to vet ASAP. Monitor breathing and circulation (see p.387).

NO ↓

Give artificial respiration (see p.389) until breathing resumes.

↓

Check circulation (see p.387)
Feel for pulse. Look for signs of shock. Are there signs of circulation?

YES →
- Look for and treat severe bleeding or other conditions.
- Get dog to vet ASAP. Monitor breathing and circulation.

NO ↓

- Give CPR (chest compressions followed by artificial respiration) until pulse and breathing return (see p.389).
- Get dog to vet ASAP. Monitor breathing and circulation.

FIRST AID EQUIPMENT FOR YOUR DOG

Roller bandage	Non-sting antiseptic swabs or spray	Gauze	Adhesive bandage
Water-soluble lubricating jelly	Styptic pencil	Cotton wool	Stretchy bandage
Sterile wound dressings	Adhesive tape		Hydrocortisone cream
			Rectal thermometer
3% hydrogen peroxide or washing soda crystals	Activated charcoal powder	Antihistamine tablets	Tweezers
			Blunt-ended scissors

It is impossible to prevent all accidents, but you can dramatically reduce risks by simple means. It is also important to be prepared for emergencies.

- Train your dog to obey commands promptly, and keep it under control.
- Keep a first-aid kit containing basic dressings and medications, a muzzle, a secure dog carrier (if your dog is small), and a bottle of clean water. Store it in a cool, dry, safe place.
- Keep the telephone numbers of your veterinary surgeon, back-up veterinary help, and the emergency services in a convenient place.

VET'S ADVICE

If you live in an area prone to floods, hurricanes, or earthquakes, make sure that all personal and official emergency plans include provisions for your dog.

- If there are existing evacuation plans for your area, find out if they include designated locations for you to leave your dog for emergency kennelling. If contingencies for pets are not included in local disaster plans, ask your local authority to take this matter into consideration.

- If you are at risk of being isolated in your home for prolonged periods, make sure that you have all the food and equipment that you are likely to need for your dog. These supplies should include the following items: dry complete dog food; water-sterilization tablets; and airtight bags for disposing of faeces.

RESTRAINING DOGS

If a dog has had an accident but is still conscious, you will need to catch and restrain it so that you can examine it. Approach and handle the dog with care. Do not make sudden movements or restrain it too tightly, otherwise you could upset the animal and cause it to panic or struggle.

As you approach an injured dog, speak reassuringly to it. Avoid direct eye contact, which might intimidate or frighten it. Assess the expression of the face and body to determine how frightened it is; watch for unusually submissive or aggressive behaviour, which can be a sign of fear. Slip a lead around the neck, and stroke the dog under its chin. If no lead is available, use a tie or belt looped over the neck. Hold the dog gently but firmly.

You should use the minimum level of restraint necessary to ensure safety.

If the dog is very frightened or in severe pain, however, its behaviour may be unpredictable, so you will need to muzzle it to avoid being bitten. If you do not have a muzzle, you can make one from a length of soft fabric; if required, you can improvise an Elizabethan collar for extra protection. Once you have the dog under control, you can start to assess the injuries following a logical plan (see p.382).

Q WHY IS IT SO IMPORTANT FOR ME TO KEEP MY DOG UNDER CONTROL?

A This is the easiest and most effective way to protect your dog. As an example of this principle, when I began practising veterinary medicine I mended broken bones at least twice a week. Today, it is rare if I see more than one traumatic fracture a month. The difference? Today, most dog owners understand their responsibilities and keep their dogs on leads.

Q WHY DO I NEED TO PROTECT MYSELF AS WELL AS MY DOG IN AN EMERGENCY?

A If you are hurt or bitten, you will be less able to help the dog. Always approach and handle an injured dog with care. If you cannot safely manage the dog, call for emergency veterinary help.

Q WHAT SHOULD I DO FIRST – BEGIN EMERGENCY FIRST AID OR CALL FOR HELP?

A Assess the dog's condition and give essential aid such as resuscitation (see p.389), then call for veterinary help. If there is anyone else around, ask them to call for help while you treat the dog.

RESTRAINING DOGS

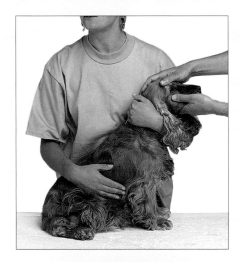

RESTRAINING A SMALL DOG

Gently but firmly grip the dog's muzzle. Apply a little pressure against the body with the elbow of your free hand while you carry out your examination. If the dog has a short muzzle or is very small, wrap a towel around its neck. If necessary, you can secure the towel with a safety pin while you proceed with your examination.

If the dog is being examined by someone else, grasp the animal gently but securely around the neck and body, and hold it close to you to give it reassurance.

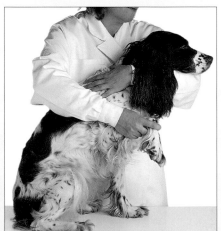

RESTRAINING A LARGE DOG

Wrap your arm as far as possible around the dog's neck and hold the head and shoulders close to your body. This leaves your other hand free for examining the dog.

If the dog is being examined by someone else, restrain it as specified above. Use your forearm and hand to hold the body securely. Alternatively, if the dog is on the ground, stand close behind it and hold it against your legs.

EMERGENCY MUZZLES

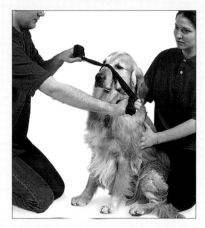

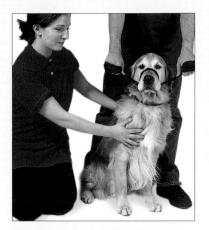

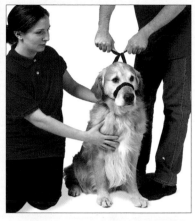

1 Take a 50–75 cm (2–3 ft) length of soft, strong material such as gauze bandage, a tie, or a pair of tights. Make a loop that is large enough for you to slip over the dog's muzzle. If you have only a short length of material, however, simply draw the material up under the dog's chin, quickly loop it, and tie it in a knot or bow. (Bear in mind that this type of muzzle can be easily removed by a dog because it is not secured behind the neck.)

2 Move behind the dog, letting its body rest against your legs. Speak to it calmly and reassuringly, using commands that the animal understands, such as "sit" and "stay". Quickly slip the loop of material over the dog's muzzle, with the crossed ends underneath the lower jaw, and tighten the loop. Do not tie a knot.

3 Bring the ends of the material behind the dog's ears. Tie a secure bow. Ensure that the muzzle does not interfere with breathing. If you are not familiar with the dog, keep the muzzle securely in place until you reach the vet; handling or movement may induce fear or pain, with consequent attempts to bite.

VET'S ADVICE

Use as little restraint as you can, because overly firm restraint upsets many dogs. Muzzle the dog if it is frightened or has obviously painful injuries.
• Approach any injured dog with great care – when frightened or in pain, a dog is likely to bite.
• Do not muzzle a choking dog or one with breathing difficulties.
• Do not muzzle a dog using harsh material such as rope, except in an extreme emergency: you could injure its face.
• Do not handle unknown dogs in areas where rabies is endemic without taking full precautions to avoid being bitten.

ELIZABETHAN COLLARS

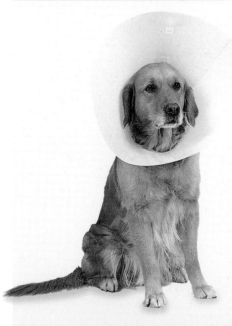

MAKING AN ELIZABETHAN COLLAR
This item is usually used to prevent a dog from chewing itself, especially at wounds or suture lines. A home-made collar can also be used to protect you from being bitten. To make an Elizabethan collar, you need a soft plastic or rubber flower pot, at least 5 cm (2 in) longer than the dog's face, or a piece of heavy corrugated cardboard; a sharp item for making holes; fabric strips; and strong adhesive tape.

If using a flower pot, cut the bottom out of it; if using cardboard, cut out a large crescent shape, then tape it along one side to form a cone. Tape over all of the cut edges to protect the dog from sharp surfaces. Make three or four holes near the narrower end, and thread fabric through them. Slip this end over the dog's head, then tie it to the dog's collar.

EMERGENCY ASSESSMENT

When a dog is injured or ill, you will need to assess it quickly to see if it is conscious; check the airway, breathing, and circulation (the "ABCs"); and look for signs of shock. The greatest threat to life is clinical shock (circulation failure); this condition may develop either rapidly or slowly and insidiously (*see p.388*). If there is no sign of breathing or heartbeat, or the dog is in shock, you may need to take urgent action to preserve the animal's life.

Always get veterinary help after any accident, even if the dog's injuries seem minor or respond immediately to first aid. What may appear to be no more than frightening, such as a seemingly small bump from a car, can quickly turn into a life-threatening emergency. Never underestimate the risks of internal damage (*see p.392*) and shock.

IS YOUR DOG CONSCIOUS OR UNCONSCIOUS?

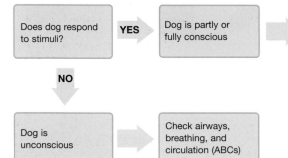

Does dog respond to stimuli? → **YES** → Dog is partly or fully conscious → Check for other conditions

NO ↓

Dog is unconscious → Check airways, breathing, and circulation (ABCs)

CONTROLLING PANIC

A dog that is unconscious may suddenly come round and may panic as a result of pain or shock. Take care that the animal does not injure itself further by trying to get up, and be very careful that it does not bite you. If the dog is in shock, keep it quiet and warm, and speak to it soothingly.

NATURAL REFLEXES

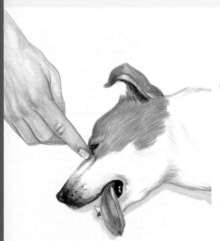

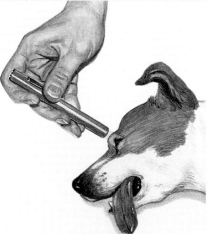

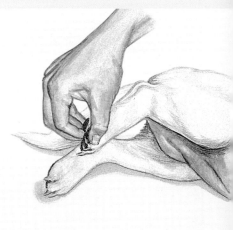

CORNEAL REFLEX
Gently touch the eyelids at the inner corner of the eye. If the dog is conscious, it will automatically blink. If it is unconscious, the eyelids will remain open and still even when your finger touches the eye.

LIGHT REFLEX
Shine a beam of light (for example, from a small torch) into the dog's eye. The pupil should constrict. If it does not, this may indicate that the heart has stopped beating. If the pupil is already constricted, this may be a sign of brain damage.

PEDAL REFLEX
Pinch one of the dog's toes or the web of skin between two toes. A conscious dog will withdraw its foot immediately. A dog that is lightly unconscious will retract its foot. If there is no movement, the dog is deeply unconscious.

AIRWAYS, BREATHING, AND CIRCULATION (ABCs)

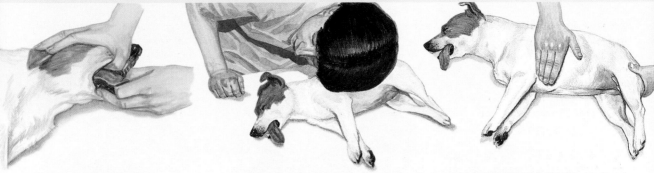

CHECKING THE AIRWAY

First, ensure that the airway is clear. Look for any debris. If the dog is unconscious, straighten the neck, then open the mouth and remove any debris. Gently pull the tongue forwards to keep the airway open; this action is most important in breeds with flat faces, because in these dogs the tongue can easily block the airway.

CHECKING BREATHING

To check the breathing rate, time the chest movements for 15 seconds and multiply the number by four. If you cannot see the chest move, hold a tissue in front of the nose to see the breaths, or put your hand on the chest to feel it move. Large dogs normally breathe about ten times a minute, while the smallest may breathe 30 times.

CHECKING CIRCULATION

Feel for a pulse by pressing behind the left elbow; squeezing both sides of the chest with one hand (on small dogs); or feeling the inside of the hind leg where it meets the body. Count the beats for 15 seconds and multiply by four to find the pulse rate. Normal rates vary from 50 beats a minute in large dogs to 160 beats in small dogs.

CHECKING GUM AND LIP COLOUR
What is the colour of your dog's gums and lips? What does this mean?

Pale	White	Blue	Red	Yellow
Early shock; anaemia; blood loss	Shock; severe blood loss	Lack of oxygen; shock	Carbon monoxide poisoning; haemorrhage	Liver problems (jaundice)
See vet ASAP	See vet ASAP	See vet ASAP	See vet ASAP	See vet within 24 hours

CHECKING CAPILLARY REFILL TIME
Press the gums; how long do the gums remain blanched when you lift your finger?

Over 4 seconds	Over 2 seconds	Less than 1 second
Deep shock	Mild shock	High blood pressure
See vet ASAP	See vet within a few hours	See vet within 24 hours

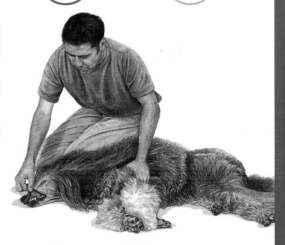

SHOCK

This condition is a potential killer. It develops when blood circulation fails and the body tissues are starved of oxygen. If emergency action is not taken, the dog will die.

A common cause of shock is severe external or internal bleeding. Another possible cause is a heavy loss of fluids (dehydration), which reduces the fluid level in the blood. Dehydration poses a severe risk; in extreme cases, it can lead to coma and death. It is a particular hazard for dogs that have metabolic disorders such as kidney failure, or have lost fluids due to severe vomiting, diarrhoea, or burns. A related disorder is anaphylactic shock (see p.427), caused by a severe allergic reaction.

Managing shock takes precedence over any other treatment. To detect shock, look at the gums and press them to assess the blood supply (see p.387). If you have a dog with naturally black gums, such as a Shar Pei, look inside the eyelid; alternatively, examine the inner lining of the vagina in bitches, or retract the prepuce (foreskin) and look at the colour of the penis in dogs.

Shock may either develop instantly or be delayed for several hours. The signs of early shock are:
- very fast breathing and heart rate;
- pale gums;
- cool ears and paws;
- anxiety or restlessness;
- lethargy and weakness;
- normal or sub-normal temperature;
- slow capillary refill in the gums; (more than 2 seconds).

The signs of advanced shock are:
- shallow, irregular breathing;
- irregular heart rate;
- very pale or blue gums;
- extreme weakness;
- unconsciousness;
- very low temperature – less than 36°C (98°F);
- very slow capillary refill in the gums (more than 4 seconds).

DEALING WITH SHOCK

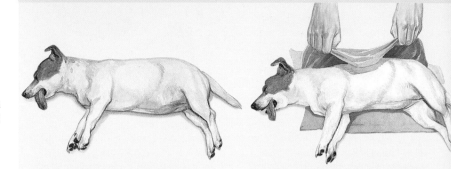

1 If your dog has signs of shock (see left), do not let it wander about or give it anything to eat or drink if it is still conscious. Check the ABCs – airway, breathing, and circulation (see p.387) – and give artificial respiration or cardiopulmonary resuscitation (see opposite) as necessary. Stop any external bleeding (see pp.392–93).

2 Wrap the dog in a blanket to prevent further loss of body heat. If it has lost consciousness, use pillows or towels to raise the hindquarters above the level of the head; this will ensure that sufficient blood reaches the brain. Keep the dog's head and neck extended. Transport it to your veterinary surgeon immediately.

CHECKING FOR DEHYDRATION

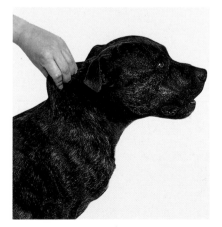

ASSESSING HYDRATION
The elasticity of the neck skin is a good indicator of hydration. Pull up a fold of skin, then let it go. It should almost instantly fall into place; if it takes a few seconds, the dog is dehydrated. In old or fat dogs it may be difficult to assess hydration this way, so feel the gums; they should be moist, not dry and sticky.

Pinch and release a fold of skin on the neck. In healthy dogs, the skin returns to normal almost immediately. What does it mean if the skin takes longer than one or two seconds to fall back into position?

Several seconds, in a dog of any age		A few seconds, in an old dog
⬇	⬇	⬇
Dehydration	Malnutrition	Natural, age-related loss of elasticity
⬇	⬇	⬇
See vet ASAP	See vet today	No action needed

ARTIFICIAL RESPIRATION AND CPR

Every living cell needs oxygen in order to survive. Oxygen is breathed into the lungs and picked up by red blood cells, then the heart pumps it around the body. Brain cells have a huge need for it – they use 20 per cent of the body's supply. If deprived of oxygen for even a few minutes, they will be damaged or die. If breathing has stopped, artificial respiration can supply oxygen to the lungs. Heart massage can restart a heart that has stopped beating. These techniques may be used together as cardiopulmonary resuscitation (CPR).

Only give artificial respiration if a dog has stopped breathing. First, check the gums (*see p.387*). If they are pink, it shows that the blood is carrying oxygen around the body. If they are blue or white, oxygen is not circulating.

Only give heart massage if the heart has stopped. First, look for a heartbeat. Check the eyes; the pupils dilate when the heart stops. Feel for a pulse (*see p.387*). Check the colour of the gums; if the heart has stopped, they will be dull pink or even white.

EMERGENCY ACTION

CPR may be needed in the following circumstances:
- blood loss;
- choking;
- concussion;
- diabetic coma;
- electrocution;
- heart failure;
- near-drowning;
- poisoning;
- shock;
- smoke inhalation.

If someone is helping, one gives heart massage for five seconds, then the other gives a breath. Continue until it is safe for one person to obtain veterinary help.

RESUSCITATION PROCEDURES

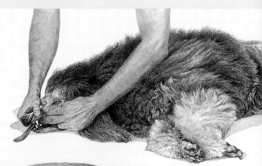

CLEARING AIRWAY
Place your dog on its right-hand side, if possible with its head lower than the rest of the body. Clear any debris from the nose and mouth, and pull the tongue forwards. Close the dog's mouth and ensure that the neck is aligned with the body.

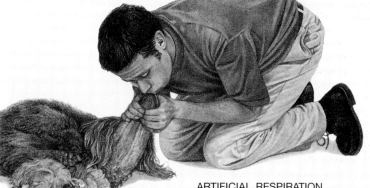

ARTIFICIAL RESPIRATION
Place your mouth over the dog's nose and blow in until you see the chest rise. If you prefer not to do this, seal your hand around the nose and give breaths through your hand. Lift your mouth. The lungs will deflate. Repeat 10–20 times a minute until the dog breathes on its own. Check the pulse (*see p.387*) every 15 seconds to make sure that the heart is still beating.

HEART MASSAGE
For a large dog: Place the heel of one hand behind the left elbow, and put the heel of your other hand on top of it. Press quickly and firmly towards the neck. Repeat 100 times a minute.

For a small dog: Grasp the chest, just behind the elbows, with one hand. Support the back with your other hand. Squeeze quickly and firmly, pushing towards the neck. Repeat 120 times a minute.

After 15 seconds of heart massage, give artificial respiration for 10 seconds. Continue until a pulse returns, then give breaths alone. Get emergency veterinary aid immediately. Note when you began CPR.

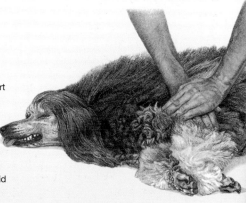

CHOKING

This condition is a potential killer. Choking can result from any injury or condition that causes the airway to become blocked. In most cases, it occurs when a dog swallows a foreign object. In unconscious dogs, it can occur if the dog vomits and the fluid blocks the throat. Choking can also result from an insect bite or sting in the mouth, or from an extreme allergic reaction called anaphylactic shock (see p.427), which can cause the throat tissues to swell. Another possible cause is injury to the muscles of the throat and neck; again, the bruised tissues may swell and press on the airway.

If your dog is choking, do not wait for veterinary help, because the dog is in danger of suffocating. Choking is frightening for dogs; even an otherwise calm dog is liable to struggle and bite. Take extra care to restrain the animal (see pp.384–85) so that it does not injure you.

LOOKING FOR SIGNS OF CHOKING

Obvious distress; choking sounds; pawing at the mouth; bulging eyes; blue tongue; agitation or unconsciousness → Completely blocked windpipe → Give immediate first aid for choking

Mild distress; gagging but no breathing difficulty; pawing at the mouth; rubbing face on ground; unpleasant breath → Partially blocked windpipe; foreign object stuck in the mouth → Look for any obstructions in the mouth

VET'S ADVICE

When treating a choking dog, take care that the object blocking the airway, and your first aid action, does not cause further damage.
• Take care when performing chest thrusts – extreme pressure on the belly can damage the liver and cause internal bleeding.
• If you can see thread, string, or fishing line in the mouth, do not pull it because it could be fixed to an object in the throat or stomach.

TREATING CHOKING IN AN UNCONSCIOUS DOG

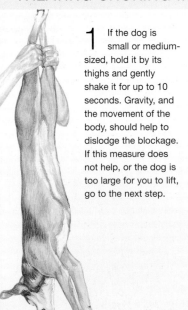

1 If the dog is small or medium-sized, hold it by its thighs and gently shake it for up to 10 seconds. Gravity, and the movement of the body, should help to dislodge the blockage. If this measure does not help, or the dog is too large for you to lift, go to the next step.

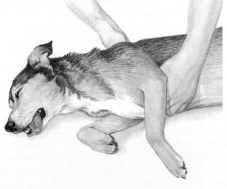

2 Lay the dog on its side. Using one hand to support its back, grasp the abdomen just behind the rib cage. If the dog is very large, lay it on its back and put both hands just under the rib cage. Thrust in and upwards twice, towards the throat. Do this carefully so that you do not put excessive pressure on the belly.

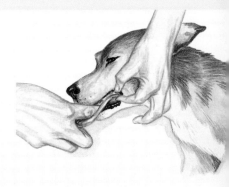

3 Check the dog's mouth. If the obstruction is visible, sweep your fingers through the mouth and remove the object. If there is thread, string, or fishing line in the mouth, however, do not pull it in case it is attached to an object lodged further down the digestive tract. If the dog is still choking, go to the next step.

CHOKING IN A CONSCIOUS DOG

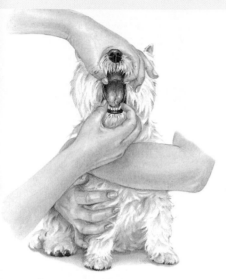

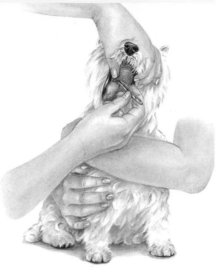

1 Restrain the dog. If the animal is small, wrap it in a towel with only its head visible. If the dog is large, restrain it by backing it into your legs (*see p.384*). Alternatively, ask someone else to hold on to the dog while you examine the mouth and remove the obstruction.

2 Open the mouth by grasping the upper jaw with one hand and pressing the upper lip over the upper teeth. Draw the lower jaw down with your other hand. Use tweezers or the blunt end of a spoon to pry the object off the teeth or away from the roof of the mouth.

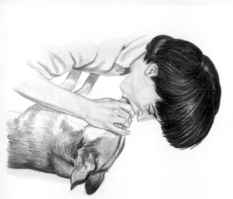

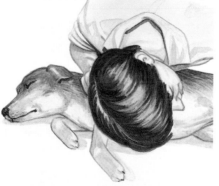

4 If debris remains in the windpipe, give two breaths of artificial respiration (*see p.389*), then two more thrusts to help dislodge it. Check inside the mouth again.

5 Check the pulse every few cycles (*see p.387*), and give CPR if necessary (*see p.389*). Repeat until the dog coughs out the obstruction and breathes. If artificial respiration or CPR is necessary at any stage, get immediate veterinary attention once you have finished treating the dog.

Q IF MY DOG IS GAGGING, IS IT IN DANGER OF CHOKING TO DEATH?

A Gagging may be one sign of choking, but the two conditions are actually different. A dog that is gagging will cough, splutter, and retch with its mouth open. This behaviour may be due to an object stuck at an awkward angle inside the mouth or throat. The dog will be in discomfort but is likely to remain alert. Choking, on the other hand, is always due to partial or complete obstruction of the airway. As well as gagging, the dog may have breathing difficulties; in severe cases, dogs lose consciousness and stop breathing altogether. If a dog is gagging on an object that is loose and easy to reach, the problem can easily be remedied by removing the object. Choking, however, is serious and needs emergency action.

Q HOW CAN I PREVENT MY DOG FROM CHOKING ON EVERYDAY OBJECTS?

A Inside the home, the easiest way to protect your dog is to make sure that it does not develop a habit of chewing everything. Take particular care if you have a puppy or an active, inquisitive dog. Train it not to chew (*see p.40*). Provide it with safe toys and dog chews that are large enough not to get lodged in the airway, and that will not splinter when the dog bites them. In addition, never leave small, chewable articles in any place where your dog can reach them, and never leave your dog alone for long periods so that it becomes bored and destructive. When exercising your dog outside, keep an eye on it and discourage it from picking up and chewing items such as pieces of bone or wood.

WOUNDS AND BLEEDING

ASSESSING BLEEDING

Blood spurting from wound	Bleeding does not stop after five minutes of pressure	Bleeding from penetrating wound (such as stab wound or gunshot)	Bright red blood in vomit or diarrhoea	Profuse bleeding from a body opening	Signs of shock	Bleeding wound larger than 2 cm (¾ in)	Bleeding area that is very dirty
⬇	⬇	⬇	⬇	⬇	⬇	⬇	⬇
Arterial bleeding	Severe damage to blood vessels	Internal injury along track of wound	Internal injury	Internal injury	Severe bleeding		
⬇	⬇	⬇	⬇	⬇	⬇	⬇	⬇
See vet ASAP	See vet ASAP	See vet ASAP	See vet ASAP	See vet ASAP	See vet ASAP	See vet today	See vet today

A wound is a break in the skin or internal tissues, and there is usually bleeding from damaged blood vessels. The main types are open wounds, in which the skin is broken, and closed wounds, in which the skin is intact.

Open wounds expose the underlying tissues to bacteria and carry a high risk of infection. The signs are:
• broken or punctured skin;
• pain;
• bleeding;
• increased licking of, or attention to, a specific area.

Although open wounds can look more serious, internal damage under closed wounds can be equally severe. The signs are:
• swelling;
• skin discoloration due to bruising;
• pain and increased heat in the area;
• superficial wounds such as scratches.

Heavy bleeding or slow, continuous bleeding can lead to shock (see p.388). Watch for pale or white gums; rapid breathing; weak, rapid pulse; cold extremities; and general weakness.

TREATING SEVERE OPEN WOUNDS

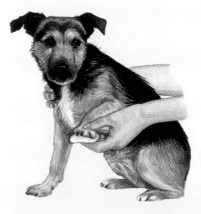

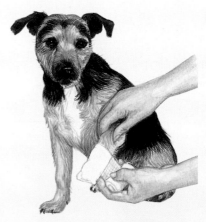

1 If you have first aid items available, apply pressure with a non-stick gauze pad. If you have no first aid equipment, use any clean, absorbent material, such as a tea towel. If you have nothing else to hand, use kitchen paper, toilet tissue, or facial tissue. Apply pressure to the area for at least five minutes, adding more absorbent material if necessary.

2 Secure the pad of material to the area with a bandage (see p.394). Do not remove the blood-soaked pad because it aids clotting. Do not apply hydrogen peroxide – it dissolves clots and causes further bleeding. Keep the injured area above the level of the heart, if possible, but do not elevate a leg if you suspect a fracture. Get immediate veterinary attention.

TREATING MINOR OPEN WOUNDS

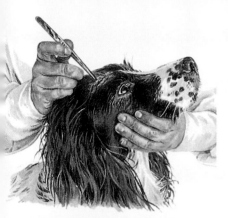

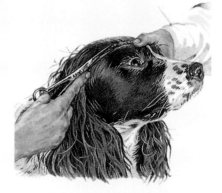

1 Use tweezers or clean fingers to remove loose dirt or other material from the wound. Flush the wound with 3% hydrogen peroxide, antiseptic fluid, or clean water. Pour the fluid over the wound, or use a clean hand-held plant spray with the nozzle turned to "jet".

2 If hair is getting into the wound, rub a little water-soluble jelly on to a pair of scissors and cut the hair away; the hair will stick to the scissors. Avoid using oil-based ointments, because these substances are particularly difficult for your vet to cleanse from around open wounds.

TREATING CLOSED WOUNDS

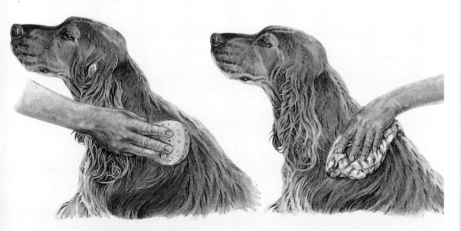

1 Take care when touching closed wounds. Touch may be painful and provoke a dog to bite. If there is superficial skin damage, such as scratches, cleanse the area with 3% hydrogen peroxide or use a non-stinging antiseptic liquid, cream, or spray. Look for hidden injuries, especially if your dog has been in a road traffic accident or has suffered other trauma.

2 Apply a cold pack to the wound. A bag of frozen peas wrapped in a tea towel makes an ideal cold pack because it thaws faster than ice and wraps itself to the contour of the injured area. The full extent of injuries from closed wounds may not be apparent for several days. Always contact your veterinary surgeon for advice, even if the injury appears to be minor.

VET'S ADVICE

Take the following precautions to prevent any further damage and minimize infection.

• Never pull large objects, such as arrows, pieces of wood, or metal, out of open wounds – uncontrollable bleeding could follow. Leave the object in the wound and get immediate veterinary attention.

• Do not rub an open wound; you could cause more damage.

• Do not underestimate the risks from small open wounds (such as puncture wounds); the injuries may be deep and severe.

• All wounds carry a risk of infection. After giving first aid, always see your veterinary surgeon as soon as possible.

Q WHAT DOES IT MEAN IF BLOOD IS SPURTING FROM A WOUND?

A Spurting blood shows that an artery has been damaged. This type of bleeding is difficult to stop because the blood travelling through arteries is being pumped from the heart at high pressure.

Q WHAT CAN I DO IF I SUSPECT INTERNAL BLEEDING?

A If a dog has collapsed and you suspect internal bleeding, place the dog on its side with its head and neck extended. Raise the hindquarters using a folded blanket, towel, or pillow. Keep the dog warm by wrapping it in coats or blankets, and get immediate veterinary attention.

BASIC BANDAGING TECHNIQUES

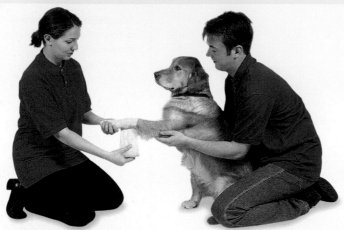

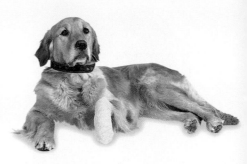

1 Clean and disinfect the wound, then place an absorbent pad over it. Sterile, non-stick pads are best, but if you have none, use any clean, absorbent material, such as a tea towel. Tissue paper can stick to the wound; if you must use it, apply water-soluble jelly to the wound first.

2 Starting at one edge of the pad, apply a gauze bandage. The first wrap is to secure the pad, then each layer covers about one-third of the previous one. Cover the whole pad as well as some of the fur on either side. Do not bandage too tightly; you could cut blood flow to the area.

3 Hold the end of the gauze, and apply the first wrap of adhesive bandage. Place two fingers under the bandage as you wrap, then remove them and continue wrapping at the same pressure. This stops you from bandaging too tightly. Extend the bandage beyond the ends of the gauze.

Q WHAT IS THE PURPOSE OF APPLYING A BANDAGE?

A Bandaging keeps wounds dry, protects injured areas from further injuries and contamination, and absorbs any seeping fluids. Bandages also provide constant, mild pressure on wounds to control pain or bleeding, and prevent pockets of serum (fluid from the body tissues) from building up under the skin.

Q HOW CAN I MAKE SURE THAT A BANDAGE IS NOT TOO TIGHT?

A A bandage should be sufficiently secure that the dog cannot remove it but not so tight that it impairs circulation. Take care if using elasticated bandages. Re-check the bandaging every few minutes, since wounds often swell and a correctly applied bandage may be too tight later on. Never let bandages get wet, because this increases the risk of wound infection.

Q HOW CAN I PREVENT OR DETECT INFECTION IN A BANDAGED AREA?

A Change the bandage every day, unless your veterinary surgeon tells you otherwise. If it is left on for too long, this increases the risk of infection or of tissue death from poor circulation. If a wound swells or discharges pus, it is infected; see your vet the same day. If it gives off an unpleasant smell, see the vet immediately.

Q HOW CAN I PREVENT A BANDAGE FROM GETTING DIRTY OR COMING OFF?

A Keep the bandage dry. When your dog goes outdoors, cover the bandage in a plastic bag. Keep the dog quiet, and restrict exercise until the area has healed and the bandage is removed. Do not let the dog chew the bandage; if necessary, your vet can fit an Elizabethan collar or a neck brace until the wound has healed.

VET'S ADVICE

A tourniquet is a tight band that is applied to a limb to stop life-threatening bleeding. If used properly it is effective, but when applied wrongly it cuts off the blood supply and can lead to the loss of the limb.
• Only use a tourniquet if there is profuse, dangerous bleeding that is not stopped by direct pressure.
• To make a tourniquet, wrap a strip of fabric above the wound and tie it in a releasable knot. Slip a pen into the knot, twist until bleeding stops, and secure it. Get immediate veterinary attention.
• A tourniquet should be applied for no more than 10 minutes.
• Do not use a tourniquet for a dog that has been bitten by a poisonous snake; instead, reduce blood flow by using a cold pack.

DRESSING BODY WOUNDS

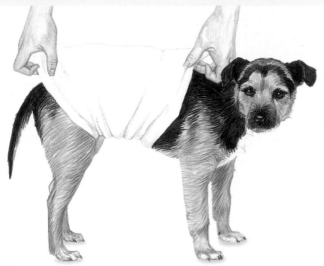

BANDAGING

For a wound to the torso, bandaging prevents further contamination and helps to stop the dog from licking the wound. First, flush dirt from the area with clean water. Wrap a clean towel or pillowcase around the dog's body, then secure it with pins on the opposite side to the wound. Contact a veterinary surgeon urgently.

Q WHAT WILL THE VETERINARY SURGEON DO IF MY DOG HAS A SERIOUS WOUND?

A Your veterinary surgeon will first clean any debris out of the wound by flushing (irrigating) it with sterile fluid. After thorough irrigation, the vet will use scalpel, forceps, and scissors to remove (debride) dead and dying tissue. Any blood vessels that are still bleeding will be tied off, then the wound is usually stitched to close it. (Other methods of closing a wound, such as metal clips, medical "superglue", or adhesive bandages, may also be used.) If there has been serious damage, interference with the wound, or infection under the skin, a thin rubber tube may be sewn into the suture line. This allows fluid to drain from the damaged area and accelerates healing.

DRESSING A BLEEDING EAR

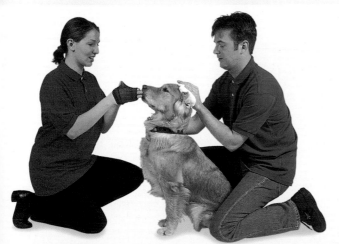

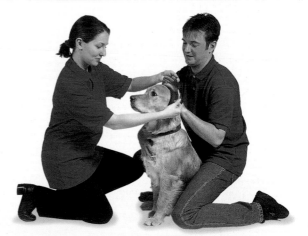

1 Using absorbent pads, apply direct pressure, on both sides of the ear, for several minutes. Sanitary pads are excellent for covering bleeding wounds. Leave the pads in place once you have finished applying pressure.

2 Speak calmly and soothingly to the dog to ensure that it does not object to the bandaging. Lay the ear back against the head, and secure it in position with stretchy bandage or a section cut from a pair of tights. Wrap the bandage around the head and under the jaw.

3 Make sure that the bandage will not interfere with the dog's breathing; you should be able to slip two fingers between the bandage and the chin, and the dog should be able to drink freely. Re-check the bandage routinely. See your veterinary surgeon within 24 hours.

TAIL WOUNDS

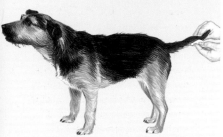

1 Place an absorbent pad on the wound and apply squeezing pressure to control bleeding. You can use both hands, or use just one, with your thumb below and your fingers above.

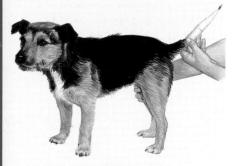

2 Wrap the pad to the wound with stretchy bandage. On dogs with sufficiently long fur, ensure that some of the tail hair is caught in the bandage to help prevent it from slipping off.

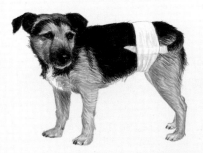

3 If the tail is long enough, bandage it to the side of the dog. This stops the dog from wagging the tail, which could cause further bleeding. See your veterinary surgeon the same day if possible.

TREATING A BLEEDING NOSE

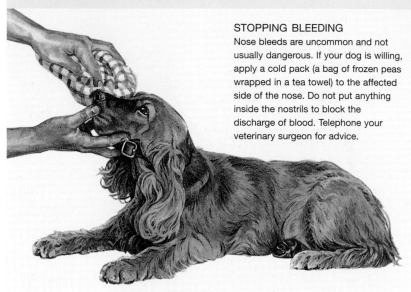

STOPPING BLEEDING

Nose bleeds are uncommon and not usually dangerous. If your dog is willing, apply a cold pack (a bag of frozen peas wrapped in a tea towel) to the affected side of the nose. Do not put anything inside the nostrils to block the discharge of blood. Telephone your veterinary surgeon for advice.

DRESSING A BLEEDING NAIL

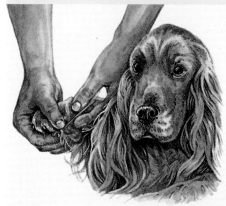

1 A torn nail may bleed so profusely that the injury appears to be life-threatening. It is not. In many cases, the nail is torn off completely, leaving a bleeding and sensitive stump. To stop the bleeding, apply a ferrous sulphate or silver nitrate stick (styptic pencil). Take care, because some dogs find this painful. Alternatively, place an absorbent pad on the wound and apply pressure to it for two minutes. Sometimes, the nail is broken but still attached. If it is "hanging by a thread", pull it off cleanly. If it is firmly attached, see your vet.

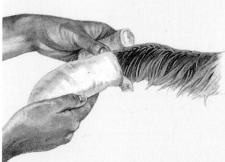

2 The blood clot that forms where a nail has been broken is easy to dislodge, either through licking or simply through normal walking. To prevent further damage and bleeding, apply a soft, secure non-slip bandage. Place non-stick material such as gauze on the wound, then lay cotton wool padding on top and secure it with stretchy bandage. Leave this bandage on for no more than 24 hours, because prolonged bandaging increases the risk of wound infection.

Q HOW CAN YOU TELL IF A DOG HAS FRACTURED A BONE?

A Fractures usually induce severe pain that causes your dog distress. If a limb is fractured, the dog will not be able to walk on it; if a rib or other bone inside the torso is affected, the dog may be reluctant to move. There is also swelling and bruising around the fracture site, and the bone may be positioned at an odd angle. In severe cases, the broken bone ends are dislodged; these ends may pierce through the skin (an "open fracture"). Broken bone ends inside the chest or abdomen may puncture organs or blood vessels inside the body, causing internal bleeding. For this reason, you need to look for any bleeding from the nose, mouth, anus, or genitals.

Q WHEN WOULD YOU NEED TO APPLY A SPLINT?

A Your dog is most likely to need a splint if it has fractured a limb and you cannot keep it completely still while you transport it to the vet. The splint will immobilize the fracture so that the broken bone ends do not move inside the injury site and cause any further damage. To make sure that the limb is kept completely still, you must apply a splint that is long enough to immobilize the joints above and below the fracture site.

Do not use a splint if the dog is struggling or if you are not sure that you can apply the splint correctly. Instead, place the animal in a suitably large container and pad around its body to keep it warm and still.

VET'S ADVICE

Fractures are serious injuries and in some cases can put the dog's life at risk. Life-threatening shock is a common complication of severe trauma. To prevent further damage, take the following steps.
• Before giving first aid, check for signs of developing shock and treat as necessary (see p.388).
• You must control bleeding (see p.392) to help prevent shock.
• Splinting a fracture is vital if you are a long way away from veterinary help. An improvised splint will reduce further damage, but do not spend needless time splinting the fracture, especially if there is help available. Instead, surround the damaged limb with soft material such as blankets and get local veterinary help.

SPLINTING A FRACTURED LIMB

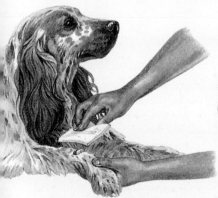

1 If you see bone protruding from a wound, cover it with a sterile pad or a clean dressing (such as a torn sheet) that extends well beyond the edges of the wound. Do not apply any ointment or cleansing fluid to the wound. Do not try to straighten a broken limb, but treat it in the position in which you find it.

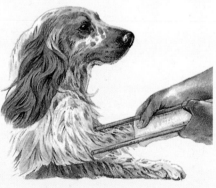

2 Place rigid items, such as garden canes, rolled magazines, or (for small dogs) pencils or pens, on both sides of the broken bone. Gently bind them to the limb, using strips of cloth or wide adhesive tape. Do not bind the splint too tightly otherwise you could cut off the circulation; poor splinting can make an injury much worse.

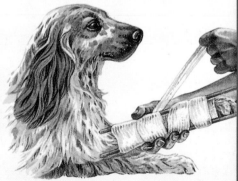

3 Transport the dog to a veterinary surgeon immediately. Every few minutes, re-check the circulation in the area beyond the splint by feeling the temperature of the toes. If they are cold, the splint may be too tight. In this case, you will have to undo the strips and re-fasten them more loosely.

REMOVING FOREIGN BODIES

Dogs taste life. They examine the world with their mouths much as we do with our hands. As world-class scavengers, some will try to eat almost anything. Objects such as splinters of bone and twigs can get stuck between the teeth or against the hard palate. Some environments contain particular hazards, such as discarded fish hooks, cans, and broken bottles. If any object obstructs the windpipe, a dog can choke (*see pp.390–91*) and will need emergency veterinary help.

Foreign bodies such as grass seeds can also enter the ears, nose, eyes, genitals, or skin, and especially the area between the toes. An affected dog may shake its head, sneeze, paw at the area, or lick it vigorously. If the object becomes firmly embedded in the skin or internal body tissues, the dog's body will try to eliminate it by forming an abscess (a sealed pocket of tissue filled with pus) around it; the abscess may eventually burst, releasing the object. There is a risk, however, that small, sharp objects may penetrate the tissues completely and then migrate further through the body.

REMOVING A FOREIGN BODY FROM A PAW

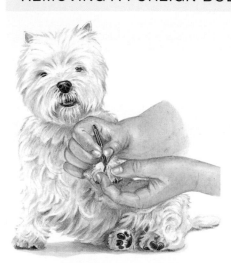

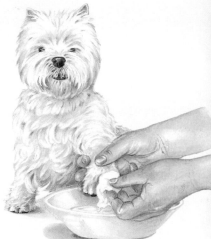

1 If your dog is limping or licking and worrying at its paw, check the pads of the paw for objects such as thorns or shards of glass, and look between the toes for grass seeds. Sterilize a pair of tweezers by passing the ends through a flame or dipping them in antiseptic, then remove any visible object with them. Clean the wound with mild antiseptic.

2 If an object is not visible, bathe the foot several times a day in a solution of one teaspoon of salt to one cup of water until the object comes to the skin surface. To remove an object just beneath the skin, gently scrape away the skin with a sterilized needle, then pull out the item with tweezers. Never try to remove a deeply embedded object; let your veterinary surgeon do this.

TAKING A FOREIGN BODY OUT OF AN EYE

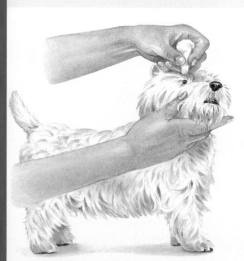

FLOATING OUT AN OBJECT
If your dog is pawing at its eye or rubbing the side of its head on the ground, first hold open the eyelids and look for objects such as pieces of grit and grass seeds. If you can see a foreign body on the eyeball, try floating it out by flushing the eye with clean water or eye drops. If an object has penetrated the eyeball, do not attempt to remove it, but take the dog to your veterinary surgeon immediately.

VET'S ADVICE

By taking the following simple steps you can lessen the risk of your dog suffering harm from foreign objects.
• Train your dog not to chew dangerous objects, such as twigs or bones that can easily splinter.
• Do not allow your dog to play with balls or other toys that are small enough to be swallowed.
• After exercising your dog, examine its coat and skin for foreign objects such as thorns, plant seeds, pieces of glass, needles, and fish hooks.

REMOVING A FOREIGN BODY FROM AN EAR

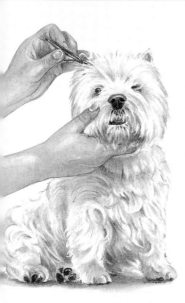

1 If your dog has been in grassy areas, or has been rubbing at its ear, examine the outside and inside of the ears for foreign bodies such as grass seeds. This is especially important in long-eared or lop-eared dogs such as spaniels. If the object is easily visible, remove it carefully with fingers or tweezers.

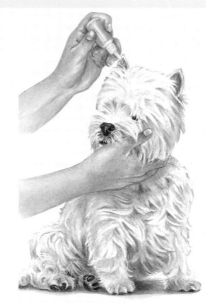

2 If the dog is worrying at its ear or shaking its head and you cannot see anything in the ears, there may be an object stuck in the ear canal. Take your dog to your veterinary surgeon to have the object removed. In the meantime, make the dog more comfortable by trickling a few drops of olive oil or mineral oil into the ear. In some cases, the oil can cause a foreign body to float up to the opening of the ear, and you may then be able to remove the object.

Q HOW CAN I PROTECT MY DOG FROM BEING INJURED BY FOREIGN BODIES?

A It is not possible to protect your dog completely, but you can minimize the possible risks. Look out for stinging plants and animals (see pp.424–27). Be aware of particular hazards in certain places, such as fish hooks discarded on river banks or pieces of glass and metal lying around waste bins. Make sure that your dog cannot get into domestic dustbins, and keep sharp items such as needles out of its reach.

Q WHY SHOULDN'T I REMOVE AN OBJECT THAT IS FIRMLY EMBEDDED IN A WOUND?

A If you attempt to pull out a firmly embedded object, you may cause further tissue damage and aggravate any bleeding. It is safer to leave the object alone and let your veterinary surgeon remove it.

REMOVING A FISH HOOK

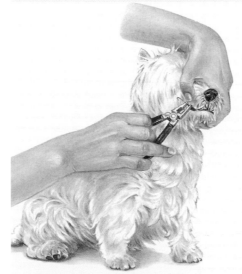

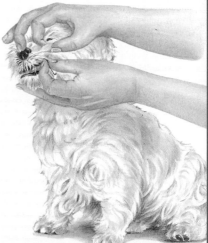

1 A dog that has been in an area used by anglers, such as a riverbank, could get a fish hook caught in its skin – most probably in a lip or a paw. If your dog has a fish hook embedded in its skin, first look at the area to see if the barbed end of the hook is sticking out. If you can see the barb, cut it off with wirecutters.

2 Gently ease the rest of the hook backwards out of the skin, then clean the wound with a mild antiseptic. (If you cannot see the end of an embedded hook, however, or if there is fishing line in the throat but no hook is visible, do not try to remove the objects.) Take the dog to your veterinary surgeon immediately.

EMERGENCY TRANSPORT

Take great care when moving an injured dog, because rough handling can cause pain and further damage. If the dog cannot walk, you will need to carry it. In this case, restrain the dog before moving it, so that it does not hurt itself. Pain may make a dog frightened or aggressive, so you may need to muzzle it (*see p.385*) to avoid being bitten. Do not use a muzzle, however, if the dog is vomiting, convulsing, has swallowed poison, or has obvious mouth or jaw injuries.

LIFTING AND CARRYING

The sequences below and opposite show how to lift and support a critically injured dog and how to pick up a dog with less serious injuries. Critical conditions include injuries in which a dog cannot move itself, and obviously serious conditions such as fractures and paralysis. The dog will probably be lying down, and may be unconscious. A dog with minor injuries, in contrast, may be sitting or standing up and may be able to walk.

TRANSPORTING BY CAR

When transporting your dog to the veterinary surgeon in a car or other vehicle, let the dog walk to the vehicle if it is able to do so; otherwise, carry it. Take extreme care when lifting a badly injured dog. Support the back. In addition, provide extra support for dogs with the following injuries.
• If there is a chest injury, lay the dog on the injured side, so that gravity will keep any blood seepage within the damaged lung. This will allow the uninjured lung to absorb oxygen as efficiently as possible and so maintain the oxygen supply to the brain.

• If the dog has a fractured leg, keep the limb supported in a raised position. If the dog also has a chest injury, however, supporting the chest injury should take priority.
• If the dog has suffered a head injury, transport it with the head higher than the hindquarters. This will help to prevent any increase in pressure inside the skull (intracranial pressure) from bleeding or swollen tissues.

Once the dog is inside the vehicle, let the animal find a position in which it can breathe comfortably. Make sure that the dog will be restrained and supported during the journey. If you are transporting it in a box or other container, put soft padding such as blankets around the animal's body to keep it warm and still. If you have a helper with you, ask this person to sit next to the dog and hold it still.

LIFTING A CRITICALLY INJURED DOG

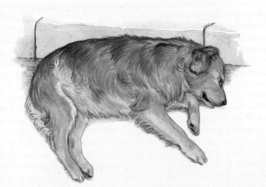 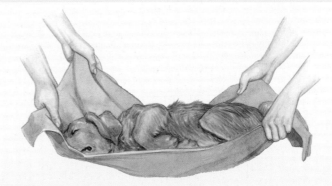

1 Transport the dog to your veterinary surgeon in the position in which it was found. If it is lying down, you will need to improvise a stretcher. Use a large, flat object such as an ironing board or a removable shelf; make sure that the object, together with the dog, will fit into your car. If no flat object is available, use a strong blanket or towel. You may need a helper to sit with the dog during the journey.

2 Keep the back towards you. Slip one hand under the chest and one under the rump, and gently pull the dog on to the stretcher. If you are using a board and have no helper to sit with the dog, place lengths of rope or cloth under the board, then slide the dog on and tie its body (but not its neck) to the board. If using a blanket or towel, wrap the dog in it if possible. If your dog is small, you could carry it in a box.

3 Ask for help if necessary, then carry the dog to the car. If using a blanket, grasp the fabric as close to the dog as possible before lifting. In the car, rest the dog with its back against the seat, and restrain it for the journey. If there is nobody to sit with it, support its body with pillows and blankets. Cover it with a blanket to keep it warm and reduce the risk of shock. In cold weather, turn on the car heater.

LIFTING A LESS INJURED SMALL DOG

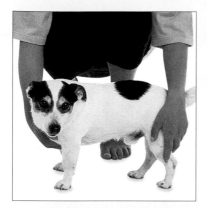

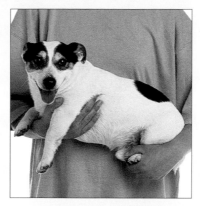

1 Reassure the dog and crouch down to its level. If it is lying down, hold its collar or neck with one hand and support its back and body with the other hand. If the dog is on its feet, place one hand under its chest, between the forelegs, and the other hand around the hind legs and rump. This will help you to control the dog and keep it from wriggling.

2 Lift the dog and cradle it against your body. If one side is obviously injured, keep that side away from you to minimize pain. In addition, keep the chest higher than the rump to reduce pressure inside the chest from any abdominal injuries. If the dog is alert, hold its chest and support its hind legs and rump, to prevent it from jumping out of your arms.

Q WHAT SHOULD I DO IF MY DOG STRUGGLES WHILE I AM CARRYING IT?

A A dog should be used to being picked up from an early age, and should learn not to struggle to get free. As part of its daily care, make sure that your dog is used to being lifted and carried, so that it will not be excessively worried in an emergency.

If an injured dog is nervous or stressed, you could ask a helper to hold its head gently and reassure it while you are carrying it. If the dog starts to panic, put it down so that it does not cause itself further injuries by struggling or jumping out of your arms. If you know that your dog is likely to bite, put a muzzle on it before lifting it up.

LIFTING A LESS INJURED LARGE DOG

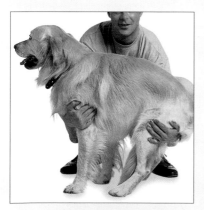

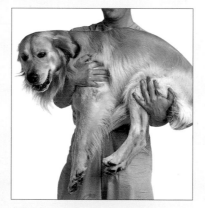

1 Crouch down to the dog's level. Slip one arm under the neck and grasp the foreleg on the side further from you. Make sure that you do not interfere with the breathing. Slip your other arm under the rump and grasp the further rear leg. On a medium-sized dog, or if you suspect that there is an injury to a hind leg, place your arm under the groin.

2 Bring your arms closer together to support the dog, and draw it closer to you. Stand up, keeping your back straight and using your leg muscles to support the dog's weight. By lifting in this way, you will avoid straining your back and the dog is less likely to struggle.

VET'S ADVICE

When lifting and transporting an injured dog, avoid bending or twisting its body or making sudden movements, otherwise you could cause further injury to the dog or to yourself.

• If you need to keep a dog flat on its side while carrying it, use an item such as a bulky blanket for small dogs or a large, flat object such as an ironing board or a removable shelf for larger animals. If your dog is seriously injured, however, do not waste time looking for suitable items; transport it to your veterinary surgeon as quickly as possible.

• Dogs can be bulky and difficult to lift. Try to keep your back straight while lifting and use your leg muscles to help you stand.

SPECIFIC EMERGENCIES
identifying and treating problems

To care for your dog, both in emergencies and in day-to-day handling, you need to know what is a normal state of health and what is abnormal for your animal. Noticing that something is wrong is far more important than knowing exactly what is wrong; if you need to take your dog to a vet, the details that you have already detected will help him or her to diagnose the problem.

This section explains how to assess your dog's health and detect unusual signs. It then shows how to manage specific emergencies, such as excessive heat or cold, electrocution, and poisoning.

If you get into the habit of observing your dog's habits and behaviour, assessing its health will soon become natural and you will quickly notice any deviations from the norm. What you see, hear, smell, and feel can provide important clues to possible problems.

When you give food or water, note how hungry or thirsty your dog is and whether anything is left over from the last time. Increased thirst, in particular, often indicates problems that may need medical attention. When the dog passes urine or faeces, watch for any change in the amount, colour, or consistency. While grooming, check for abnormal odours. Listen for very noisy breathing or any other abnormal sounds; such noises almost always signify problems needing veterinary attention within 24 hours. Weigh your dog regularly to detect any gain or loss in weight.

In addition, watch for changes in mood or level of activity. If your dog does not get up or go to sleep at the usual times, moves more slowly than normal, or is reluctant to play, contact your veterinary surgeon for advice. Even "attractive" changes, such as coming to you more often for comfort, can be a cause for concern. If your dog is normally aloof but now wants to be with you, it may have been frightened or may be feeling unwell.

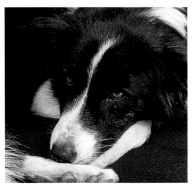

OBSERVING BEHAVIOUR
Be aware of any changes in your dog's behaviour, such as unusual docility, lethargy, or irritability. These may indicate that the animal is feeling ill.

RESPONSES AND ACTIVITY
Is there:

Glazed expression; drowsiness; depression; disorientation; bumping into things, staggering, or falling over	No response to commands	Heavy-footed or "sloppy" walking	Stiff or slow movement; limping for over 24 hrs; arched back; or walking in circles	Collapsing rather than lying down	Sudden increase or decrease in sleeping	Reluctance to move
Look for signs of shock (p.388)	Look for signs of shock (p.388)	See vet within 24 hours	See vet within 24 hours	See vet within 24 hours	See vet within 24 hours	Examine dog (p.406)

VISIBLE SIGNS
Is there:

Swollen abdomen and restlessness	See vet ASAP
Dilated eyes in bright light	See vet ASAP
Twitching, or sensitivity to light, sound, touch	See vet within 12 hours
Thread or fishing line hanging from mouth or anus	See vet within 12 hours
Visible swelling	See vet within 12 hours

Q WHY IS IT NECESSARY TO MAKE REGULAR CHECKS – WON'T IT BE OBVIOUS IF MY DOG IS ILL?

A Most dogs like to please their owners, so if they are unwell or in pain they may try to hide their discomfort and act normally. Your dog depends on you, so it is important to carry out regular health checks so that you identify any problems before they become distressing for the dog.

Q HOW DO I DECIDE WHEN MY DOG NEEDS TO SEE THE VET?

A The charts on pp.402–05 give general guidelines on the severity of various abnormal signs and the action needed in each case. If you are still unsure about what to do after consulting the relevant chart, telephone your veterinary surgeon for advice.

Q HOW CAN I FIND OUT IF MY DOG IS MORE HUNGRY OR THIRSTY THAN NORMAL?

A Develop a routine for checking and re-filling your dog's food and water bowls at regular times. Note how much you put in and how much is left when you come to re-fill them.

Q HOW CAN I WEIGH MY DOG ACCURATELY?

A The simplest way to weigh all but the largest dogs is to weigh yourself first and note your weight; pick up your dog and weigh the dog and yourself together, noting the combined weight; then subtract your own weight from the combined weight. A weight loss that is not related to any change in diet is worrying; unexpected weight gain can also be a sign of disease.

WEIGHT LOSS
Is there:

Fever, vomiting, or diarrhoea	See vet within 12 hours
Lethargy	See vet within 24 hours
Lameness	See vet within 24 hours
Increase or decrease in appetite or thirst	See vet within 48 hours
No other changes	See vet within 48 hours

WEIGHT GAIN
Is there:

Shivering and shaking, or vomiting	See vet within 24 hours
Lethargy	See vet within 48 hours
Increased thirst	See vet within 48 hours
Dull coat or hair loss	See vet within 48 hours
Reduced appetite	See vet within 48 hours

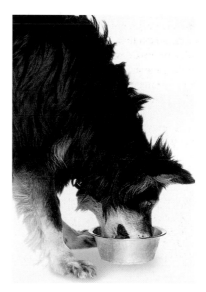

CHECKING APPETITE
When you feed your dog, make a habit of watching how it normally eats. Note abnormal signs such as excessive hunger, unusual reluctance or inability to eat, distaste for a particular food, vomiting after eating, or loss of appetite.

DRINKING AND THIRST
Is there:

Increased thirst, reduced appetite and lethargy in a female (with or without a vaginal discharge)	See vet ASAP
Increased thirst and fever	See vet within 24 hours
Increased thirst and weight loss	See vet within 24 hours
Increased thirst and increased urinating	See vet within 24 hours
Increased thirst and little urine passed	See vet within 24 hours

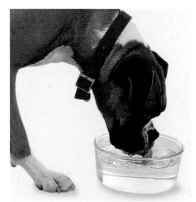

MONITORING DRINKING
Develop a routine for checking your dog's water bowl. Re-fill it at regular times, and fill it to roughly the same level each time. Monitor how much you put in and how much water is left over when you come to re-fill the bowl.

TOILET HABITS
Is there:

Straining but dog cannot urinate	See vet ASAP
Straining and passing only small amounts of urine	See vet within 12 hours
No urine passed, as far as you know, for 24 hrs	See vet within 12 hours
Blood in urine	See vet within 12 hours
Incontinence and lethargy	See vet within 12 hours
Incontinence but dog is otherwise normal	See vet within 48 hours
Urinating more often, or passing more urine, than normal	See vet within 48 hours
Straining but dog cannot defaecate	See vet within 12 hours
Blood in stool	See vet within 12 hours
No stool passed for 48 hrs	Phone vet
Soiling with normal urine or faeces	Examine dog (p.406)

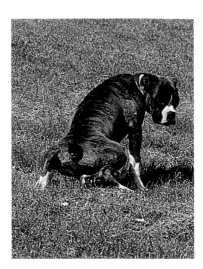

TOILET HABITS
Watch your dog whenever it passes urine or faeces. Note any changes in the dog's sanitary habits, such as urinating or defaecating more or less often than normal, diarrhoea or other changes in consistency, or difficulty in passing waste.

VET'S ADVICE

Dogs have highly accurate biological clocks. They also thrive on routine. As a result, they have a physical and psychological need to empty their bladders and bowels at set times. This is an advantage for owners, because it makes it easy for us to organize daily toilet routines. A typical dog passes stools twice each day and urine three or four times a day, although some individuals may need to do so slightly more or less often than average.

It is important to learn your dog's daily routines and rituals. Any change from normal habits or behaviour indicates a possible physical or even psychological problem. In either case, this warrants a call to the vet.

ABNORMAL SOUNDS
Is there:

Laboured or shallow breathing	Shock, pain, injury	See vet ASAP
Rapid or very slow breathing	Shock, pain	See vet ASAP
Choking or gasping	Blocked breathing	First aid (p.390)
Wheezing or coughing	Various causes	See vet within 24 hours
Intense, constant panting	Various causes	See vet ASAP
Crying, yelping, groaning	Pain	See vet ASAP
Grunting, sighing	Discomfort	See vet within 24 hours
Teeth chattering, shivering	Pain, fear, hypothermia	See vet ASAP
Unexpected barking	Pain, fear, brain disorder	See vet within 24 hours

ABNORMAL ODOURS
Is there:

Breath that smells sickly sweet	Kidney failure	See vet within 12 hours
Smoke, petroleum, antifreeze, or chemical smell	Possible poisoning	See vet ASAP
Anal gland smell	Dog is possibly frightened or injured	Examine dog (p.406)
Urine or faeces smell	Possible injury, urinary or gastrointestinal problem	Examine dog (p.406)

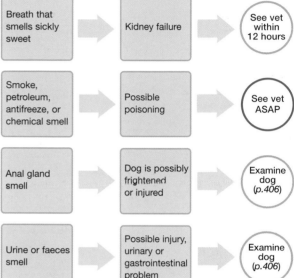

Q HOW CAN I TELL THE DIFFERENCE BETWEEN AN UNUSUAL SMELL FROM AN OUTSIDE SOURCE, SUCH AS MUD WALLOWING, AND A SMELL DUE TO ILLNESS?

A Try washing your dog with a tar-based shampoo. Such products are good at removing the smell from an oily coat as well as odours from wallowing. If your dog still has a whole-body odour after you have washed it, there is a strong possibility that it may have a generalized skin disease or a kidney problem. In this case, see your vet.

Q MY DOG'S FEET SOMETIMES MAKE A CRACKING SOUND – CAN DOGS CRACK THEIR KNUCKLES?

A Surprisingly, they can. They do not make this sound intentionally, however, as people do, and it is not always the knuckles that crack. Some dogs make unusual sounds when they stretch their bodies or even when they walk. The "knuckle-cracking" sound is caused by ligaments or tendons snapping back and forth over bony bits. There is no associated pain and no cause for concern. A change in weight may cause the sound to increase or decrease.

FULL PHYSICAL EXAMINATION

If observations alone are not enough to help you decide whether veterinary help is needed, the next stage is to carry out a full physical inspection.

An injured, ill, or frightened dog might resent being touched. Take care when approaching the dog, especially if it seems irritable or apprehensive, or tries to hide from you. Speak soothingly and touch it gently. If the dog does not object, check for hot, cool, sticky, tender, oversensitive, or numb areas.

While your dog is healthy, practise making regular inspections. In an emergency you will not have time for a full examination, but by knowing what to do, you can focus on vital checks. Assess the breathing rate and rhythm, heart rate or pulse, and the colour of the gums. Take the temperature, then check the body in sections from nose to tail. Start with the eyes, ears, nose, and mouth, then examine the head and neck; chest and abdomen; limbs and

tail; and the anus and genitals. Tell your dog to sit or stand for each part. Do not try to do all the checks in one session – it is too boring for most dogs. Reward your dog's obedience with a snack, touch, or praise after each step.

Training your dog from puppyhood to accept this procedure helps the dog, you, and the veterinary surgeon. Vets make faster, more accurate diagnoses if dogs willingly allow themselves to be examined.

CHECKS TO MAKE IN A FULL PHYSICAL EXAMINATION

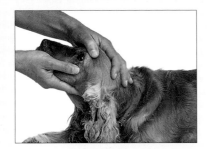

EYES
Look for discharge, cloudiness, redness, or injuries. Check for overly large (dilated) or small pupils; dilated pupils in good light can indicate fear, pain, or shock. Flick a finger at the eyes; the dog should see it and blink.

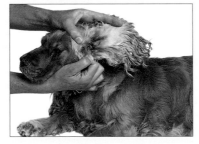

EARS
Examine the ears for bleeding in the ear canals and injuries to the ear flaps. Look at the way in which the dog holds its ears; flattened ears can indicate submission, but can also show pain, distress, or weakness.

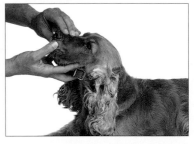

NOSE
Examine the nose for any bleeding or other abnormal discharge. Look for dryness, crusting, or loss of pigment. Watch how the nostrils flare as the dog breathes; excessive flaring could indicate breathing problems.

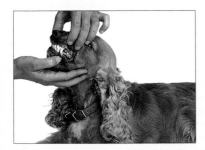

MOUTH
Look for inflamed gums and tooth decay. Check in the mouth for foreign objects and injuries to the tongue and hard palate. Such damage can be due to an injury occurring at speed, as in a fall or a road accident.

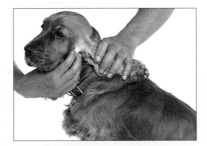

HEAD AND NECK
Run your hands over the head, jaws, and neck. Feel for swellings or heat, and for stickiness or scabs (which may indicate a puncture wound). Move the head from side to side and up and down, to check for pain.

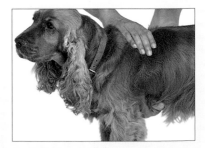

CHEST
Firmly but gently run your hands over the dog's back and chest, feeling for excess heat, stickiness, lumps, swellings, or sensitivity to touch. Part the hair and look for any skin discoloration.

TAKING TEMPERATURES SAFELY

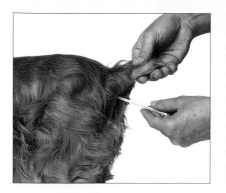

TAKING RECTAL TEMPERATURE

A dog's normal temperature is 38.1–39.2°C (100.5–102.5°F). Nervousness, exercise, heat, and infections raise the temperature. A low temperature may be due to shock or exposure to cold. When possible, use a digital thermometer, which is accurate and easy to read. Lubricate the end with water-soluble jelly, then insert it gently into the rectum, with a slight rotating action. Hold the thermometer, and the base of the tail, for 90 seconds, then remove it. Disinfect the thermometer after use.

°C	°F	Action
41+	106+	Cool dog; see vet ASAP
40.6	105	See vet within 24 hours
40	104	Fever; phone vet
39.4	103	Fever; phone vet
38.9	102	Normal
38.3	101	Normal
37.8	100	Normal
37.2	99	See vet within 24 hours
36.7	98	Warm dog; see vet ASAP

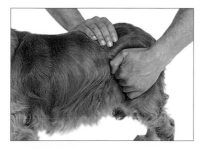

ABDOMEN

Feel the abdomen and groin for excess heat, stickiness, lumps, swellings, or sensitivity to touch. If you need to feel the femoral pulse, feel the middle of the inner thigh at the point where it meets the body.

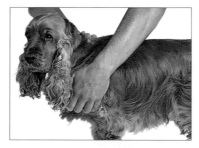

LIMBS

Run your hands down each leg. Examine both forelimbs first, then assess the hind limbs together, checking that they are symmetrical. Feel each joint for areas of excess heat or swelling.

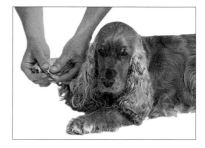

FEET

Examine the dog's feet for any abrasions, tears, or other injuries. Look at the tops and pads of the feet; check for broken nails; and examine the webs of skin between the toes.

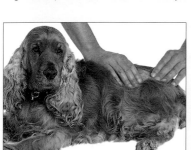

TAIL

Run your hand down the length of the tail. There should be no bumps or excess heat. If the tail hangs limp, pinch it to see if the dog reacts. A lack of response indicates an injury to the tail or lower spine.

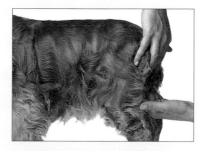

GENITALS

Examine the scrotum for swelling or injuries, and check the opening of the penis or vulva for inflammation or discharge. If a normally tidy dog's coat smells of urine, this is a sign of either illness or injury.

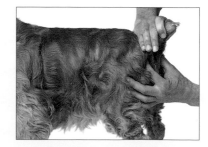

ANAL REGION

Lift the dog's tail. The anal region should be clean, with no signs of clinging faeces. If there is an intense and offensive smell, it indicates that the dog has been frightened or injured and has emptied its anal sacs.

HEATSTROKE

Dogs eliminate excess body heat by panting and, to a very limited extent, by sweating through their pads. If the environment is too hot, these processes become ineffective and the dog becomes overheated. The body temperature rises rapidly, causing heatstroke. If it gets above 40.5°C (105°F), the dog is in danger. Death follows quickly if the temperature is not immediately reduced.

The first priority is to remove the dog from heat. You then need to bring its temperature down using cool water; as the water evaporates, it will cool the skin. Take the rectal temperature (*see p.407*) every five minutes. Keep cooling the dog with water until the body temperature has fallen below 39.4°C (103°F). Do not worry if it falls to 37.8°C (100°F) or a little lower; a slightly low body temperature is less dangerous than a very high one.

WARNING
• Never put a dog's head under water.
• If the dog is unconscious, ensure that no water enters the mouth or nose.
• In severe cases, the brain can swell. Treat for shock if necessary and get immediate veterinary attention.

ASSESSING SIGNS OF HEATSTROKE

Coma; no breathing (life-threatening heatstroke)	Disorientation; collapse; pale gums; vomiting; diarrhoea (severe heatstroke)	Panting; glazed expression; frothing at mouth; bright red gums; increased heart rate; temperature above 40.6°C (105°F)

Reduce body heat; CPR

Reduce body heat ASAP

Reduce body heat ASAP

Q ARE CERTAIN TYPES OF DOG PARTICULARLY PRONE TO DEVELOPING HEATSTROKE?

A All dogs need to be protected from heatstroke, but certain animals are less efficient than others at ridding their bodies of excess heat. These individuals include flat-nosed breeds such as Pugs and Boxers; elderly dogs; and overweight dogs.

Q WHAT IS THE BEST WATER TEMPERATURE TO USE TO COOL MY DOG?

A Cool water is best. Avoid using freezing water; if the water is too cold, the blood vessels in the skin will contract in reaction to it. As a result, the blood will transport less of the "coolness" from the water into the interior of the body, where it is needed most.

PREVENTING HEATSTROKE

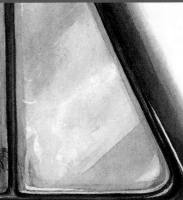

Heatstroke is a very common cause of avoidable death. You can prevent it by taking a few simple steps.
• Always provide good ventilation, access to shade, and plenty of water.
• In warm weather, ensure that flat-nosed, old, or fat dogs have access to cool rooms and plenty of water.
• Never leave your dog in a car on a warm day, even if you park in the shade and leave a window open.
• In cold weather, never leave your dog in a car in direct sunlight and with the heater switched on.

TREATING HEATSTROKE

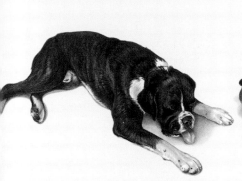

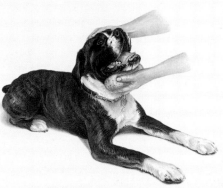

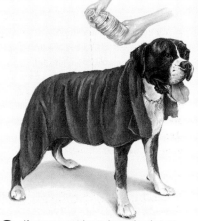

1 Remove the dog from the hot environment as quickly as possible. Take it to a cool, well-ventilated area. If you can, lay the dog on a cool surface to aid temperature reduction. Let the dog drink cool water with a pinch of salt added to replace salt lost from the body by panting.

2 Take special care to cool the head; this will lessen the risk of the brain overheating and can also aid breathing. Clear the mouth of saliva, and sponge the face with cool water. Place a bag of frozen peas, wrapped in a cloth, on the head to help reduce heat around the brain.

3 If you are outdoors, hose the dog or put it in a pool of water. If indoors, put it in a sink or bath with the plug in. Run a shower over the dog, or cover it with a wet towel and pour on more water to keep the towel cold. Massage the legs firmly to aid circulation and lessen the risk of shock.

NEAR-DROWNING

Regardless of how well your dog can swim, make sure that it is always safe whenever you are near water. Currents and cold are potentially just as lethal to dogs as they are to us, so keep the dog out of very cold, fast-flowing, or turbulent water that you would not swim in yourself. If you take your dog boating, put a life-jacket on it. If the dog does have a near-drowning accident, be sensible when attempting to rescue it; take care not to put yourself at serious risk.

Serious or even life-threatening problems can occur up to several hours after a near-drowning accident. After any such incident, get immediate veterinary attention for your dog.

SAVING A DOG FROM NEAR-DROWNING

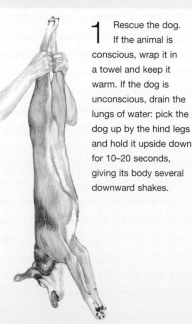

1 Rescue the dog. If the animal is conscious, wrap it in a towel and keep it warm. If the dog is unconscious, drain the lungs of water: pick the dog up by the hind legs and hold it upside down for 10–20 seconds, giving its body several downward shakes.

2 Lay the dog with its head lower than its chest, to help water drain from the lungs. Clear debris from the mouth and pull out the tongue to keep the airway open. Check the breathing and circulation. If there is a heartbeat but no breathing, give artificial respiration; if both breathing and heartbeat have stopped, give the dog CPR (see p.389).

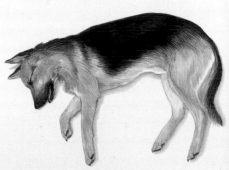

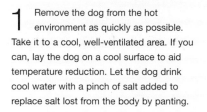

HYPOTHERMIA AND FROSTBITE

Exposure to extreme cold can chill the whole body. This abnormally low body temperature is called hypothermia. If the core temperature (in the centre of the body) drops very low, the dog may die. Many domestic dogs descended from breeds that originated in northern Europe, Asia, or North America, and have dense fur that protects them from extreme cold. In contrast, dogs with short, smooth hair or little body fat are highly susceptible to hypothermia.

This condition develops insidiously. Your dog may begin to shiver but may otherwise act normally; if this happens, move it to a warmer place or provide it with insulating clothing. Shivering leads to lethargy, and eventually to weakness and shallow breathing. The extremities (the tips of the ears, the tail, and, in males, the scrotum) have the least protection. These areas of the body can suffer from localized freezing (frostbite). Both hypothermia and frostbite are potentially very dangerous conditions and always warrant veterinary attention.

ASSESSING COLD-RELATED INJURIES
Has the dog been in cold water or been exposed to icy wind, snow, or cold, and is there:

Shivering; disorientation; drowsiness; exhaustion; rectal temperature below 36.7°C (98°F); convulsions or coma	Signs listed on the left occurring in a slim or thin-coated dog exposed to moderate cold, or in a pup or old dog recovering from shock or anaesthetic	Pale or red and puffy skin at tips of ears; pain in ears, tail, or paws when touched; skin that remains cold and is shrivelled
↓	↓	↓
Hypothermia; give first aid (*see opposite*)	Hypothermia; give first aid (*see opposite*)	Frostbite; give first aid (*see opposite*)
↓	↓	↓
See vet ASAP	See vet ASAP	See vet within 12 hours

VET'S ADVICE

Hypothermia may occur in any dog, even one with a dense coat, if it is exposed to cold for a long time. Vets see this condition most often, however, in puppies that are not kept sufficiently warm in the first week of life. Hypothermia in newborns develops insidiously. To avoid it, ensure that the room temperature is above 24°C (75°F).

Q HOW DO ARCTIC DOG BREEDS NATURALLY AVOID HYPOTHERMIA OR FROSTBITE?

A Breeds such as Siberian Huskies and Alaskan Malamutes grow dense, fine, downy insulating undercoats that prevent cold from penetrating to the skin. To rest, they settle into "snow dens", which act as insulation. Most Arctic breeds sleep with their faces tucked into their well-insulated tails. If you relocate your dog from a warm or temperate climate to a cold one, allow time for its coat to adapt to the new conditions.

Q SHOULD DOGS WEAR CLOTHES IN COLD WEATHER?

A Most breeds grow insulating winter fur, but some, such as the Boxer, Doberman, and Yorkshire Terrier, do not. These dogs should wear coats for extra body protection. In very cold, icy conditions, it is sometimes also useful for dogs to wear insulated boots.

TREATING HYPOTHERMIA

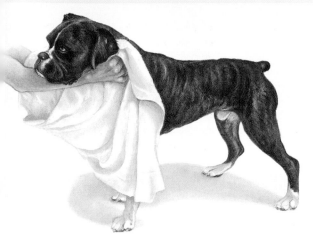

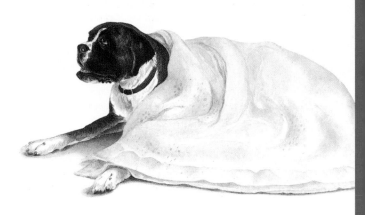

1 Wrap the dog in warm blankets. (You can warm blankets quickly by placing them in a tumble dryer and running it for a few minutes.) Place a hot water bottle wrapped in a towel against the abdomen. Do not use an unwrapped bottle because it will burn the skin.

2 If the dog is conscious, give it warmed fluids to drink. Take the temperature every 10 minutes. If it is below 36.7°C (98°F), get immediate veterinary help. Once it is above 37.8°C (100°F), remove the hot water bottle but keep the dog in a warm room. Avoid overheating the dog.

DEALING WITH FROSTBITE

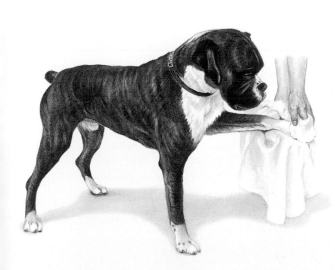

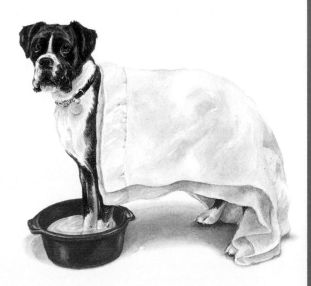

1 If your dog has been exposed to extreme cold, examine the feet, ears, and tail for pale skin and other signs of frostbite. Massage affected areas gently with a warm towel. Do not rub hard or squeeze because you could further damage the skin.

2 Warm any frozen areas with cool to lukewarm water. As the skin thaws it will become red. Take care not to use water that is too warm – if frostbitten areas are warmed too quickly, they become very painful. If the skin turns dark, get immediate veterinary help.

BURNS AND SCALDS

Burns can result from fire, direct heat, chemicals, and electricity. Hot liquids or steam can cause similar injuries (scalds). Burns are classified by depth. The least severe type, first-degree burns, affect only the skin surface. Second-degree burns damage underlying skin tissues. Third-degree burns penetrate all the skin tissues and affect underlying structures such as nerves and blood vessels. Second- and third-degree burns can lead to shock, even several days after the burning, and need immediate veterinary treatment, but even fairly small burns can be life-threatening.

ASSESSING BURNS AND SCALDS

Hair that has fallen out or can easily be pulled out; black or translucent skin; may or may not be pain	Hair still attached; skin that is red, swollen, or contracted, or singed and tan in colour; pain in burnt area	Hair still attached but singed; red, painful skin; burnt area that is blistered	Excessive dribbling; dog asks for food but then does not eat; unpleasant odour from mouth
↓	↓	↓	↓
Third-degree burn	Second-degree burn	First-degree burn	Possible burn in mouth
↓	↓	↓	↓
See vet ASAP	See vet ASAP	See vet within 24 hours	See vet within 12 hours

VET'S ADVICE

- Never leave your dog alone near a cooker or a barbecue while you are cooking. If you have an open fire, use a fire screen.
- Do not apply ointments, creams, butter, or margarine to burns; they may damage the skin tissues or increase the risk of infection.
- When treating a chemical burn, wear rubber gloves for protection.
- For a burn inside the mouth, lay the dog on its side and restrain it. Pour cool water through the mouth or flush with a garden hose.

TREATING BURNS

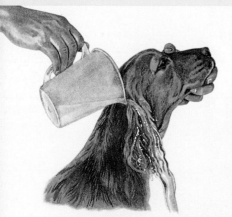

FIRST-DEGREE BURN
As soon as possible, flush the burn with cool water from a bath, hose, or shower to minimize further skin damage. Apply a cold pack (a bag of frozen peas wrapped in a cloth) for 20 minutes. Cover the burn with a non-stick bandage to protect it. See your veterinary surgeon the same day.

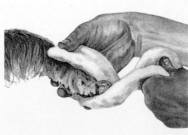

SECOND- OR THIRD-DEGREE BURN
Watch for and treat any signs of shock (see p.388). Apply water-soluble jelly and a clean, dry dressing. Avoid using cotton or other loose-fibred material, which will stick to the burn. Wrap torn sheeting or other soft material around the area. Take the dog to your veterinary surgeon immediately.

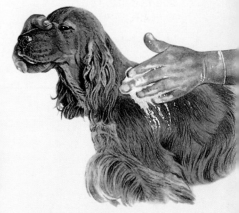

CHEMICAL BURN
Wear rubber gloves. Remove the collar if it is contaminated. Flush the burn with water for 20 minutes, keeping the run-off away from other areas; for acid burns, use a solution of bicarbonate of soda in water. Wash the skin with mild detergent or shampoo. For minor burns, apply a non-stick dressing.

ELECTRIC SHOCK

Contact with an electric current can cause burning and also cardiac arrest. Chewing on electric flex is the most common cause of electrocution in dogs. Occasionally, dogs may come into contact with power lines or suffer lightning strikes; these high-voltage forms of electricity are usually fatal.

Any electric shock damages the microscopic blood vessels in the lungs; this can lead to fluid accumulating in the lungs hours or even days after the injury. There may also be coughing and drooling. If the dog has chewed a flex, the shock may cause the jaw muscles to contract around the wire.

If your dog suffers an electric shock, get veterinary help immediately, even if it seems well. Monitor the breathing and pulse for the next 12 hours. Shock may occur up to several hours after a dog has apparently recovered.

ASSESSING ELECTRIC SHOCK
Has there been exposure to electric current, and is there:

Unconsciousness; convulsions; collapse; cardiac arrest; emptied bladder and bowels	→ Remove dog from source of electricity; give CPR (*see p.389*)	→ **See vet ASAP**
Burn with a pale centre surrounded by redness, especially in mouth; breathing rate that is slower or faster than normal	→ Treat burn	→ **See vet within 12 hours**

Q WHY SHOULD I NOT TOUCH A DOG THAT IS STILL IN CONTACT WITH AN ELECTRIC CURRENT?

A Your dog's body will be "live" and could electrocute you. This is why you must always ensure that the current is switched off or unplugged before starting first aid.

Q WHY SHOULD I AVOID ANY FLUIDS AROUND THE DOG?

A Fluids are highly effective conductors of electricity. If you come into contact with them, you could easily suffer a shock.

Q WHERE CAN I FIND PLASTIC SLEEVES TO FIT OVER FLEXES?

A These items can usually be obtained from hardware stores or computer stores.

VET'S ADVICE

Take the following measures to reduce the risk of electrocution.
• Examine your house and garden; reposition any electric flexes or cables that may be chewed by your dog.
• Always provide your dog with safe and appropriate chewing toys during puppyhood.
• Apply a bitter-tasting spray to electric flexes and cables to stop your dog from chewing them.
• Never leave a dog alone with live electric cords or terminals.
• If it is not possible to remove an electrical appliance, unplug it or turn it off at the plug when you are absent. Alternatively, cover the flex with a plastic sleeve.

EMERGENCY ACTION

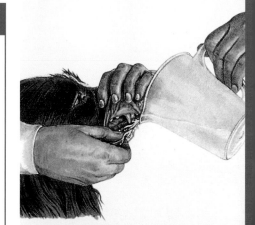

1 Turn off the current at its source. If this is not possible, put on rubber gloves, stand on a dry surface, and use a wooden broom handle to push the dog away from the current. Do not put your life at risk. If the dog is rigid, do not touch it until the current has been turned off. Keep away from fluids that are in contact with it.

2 Look for signs of breathing and circulation. Give artificial respiration if the dog's breathing has stopped, and give CPR if the heart has stopped (*see p.389*). Treat mouth burns by flushing with water, and treat skin burns with a cold pack (a bag of frozen peas wrapped in a cloth), to reduce further damage.

POISONING

Dogs are naturally curious; they sniff and taste almost anything in their environment, whether inside the home, in the garden, or outside during walks. In addition, in my experience, some dog owners are surprisingly careless about what they put down their dogs' throats or on their dogs' coats. The inevitable consequence is that poisoning is a common problem.

Often, the effects of ingesting or absorbing toxins are fairly minor, such as stomach irritation and vomiting caused by painkilling drugs that are designed for humans, not for dogs. In some cases, however, poisoning can have serious effects, such as seizures, internal bleeding, or even death.

Poisons can be swallowed, licked off the coat or absorbed through the skin, or inhaled. The following pages show a wide range of substances that are hazardous to dogs, and describe how to prevent and treat poisoning.

COMMON POISONS IN THE HOME

Cleaning fluids

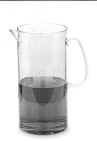
Antifreeze

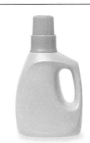
Fabric softener

Mothballs

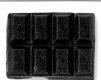
Dark chocolate

Cigarettes

Painkillers (such as aspirin, paracetamol)

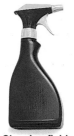
Dryer sheets

Marijuana

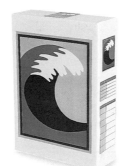
Dishwasher detergent

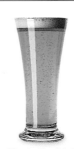
Alcoholic drinks

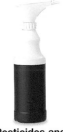
Pesticides and herbicides

Aromatherapy and pot pourri oils

Coffee grounds

DANGEROUS CHEMICALS

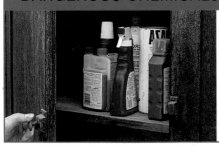

- Keep dustbins securely covered.
- Keep household chemicals to a minimum. Store them out of reach of dogs, in a lockable cupboard.
- Store all medicines out of reach of dogs. Do not give human medicines to a dog without first checking with your veterinary surgeon.

- Keep your dog out of your garden for at least 24 hours after chemicals are applied there. Never let a dog eat chemically treated grass.
- Never use a cleaning product on a dog if it is not safe for humans.
- When using insecticides, follow the manufacturer's instructions with care.

COMPOST HEAPS

A compost heap can be deadly. Coffee grounds, onions, stones from apricots, peaches, or plums, and apple or pear seeds are toxic. Moulds, fungi, and bacteria are also hazards. Fence off your compost heap securely and mix it regularly. Do not let your dog go near newly spread compost.

TOILET BOWLS

Do not let your dog drink from toilet bowls. As well as ingesting potentially hazardous bacteria, your dog may also swallow toilet cleaner, which almost always consists of dangerous acid or alkali solution. Train everyone in your household to put the lid down on the toilet after using it.

Q WHY CAN'T I GIVE HUMAN MEDICATIONS TO MY DOG?

A Medications for humans may be formulated differently from those for dogs. Some, such as aspirin, ibuprofen, and paracetamol, can be toxic to dogs. Always check with your vet before giving your dog any unprescribed medication.

Q ARE MEDICATIONS IN BOTTLES OR PACKETS SAFE?

A No. Glass bottles can shatter, and dogs can chew through plastic or cardboard packaging. Childproof caps are also ineffective deterrents. It is best to keep all medications in closed cabinets.

THE EFFECTS OF POISONS

Poisons are usually swallowed, absorbed through the skin, or inhaled. They are most likely to affect the systems with which they come into direct contact, such as the digestive system, skin, and respiratory system. If absorbed into the bloodstream, poisons may affect vital organs such as the heart, brain, and liver.

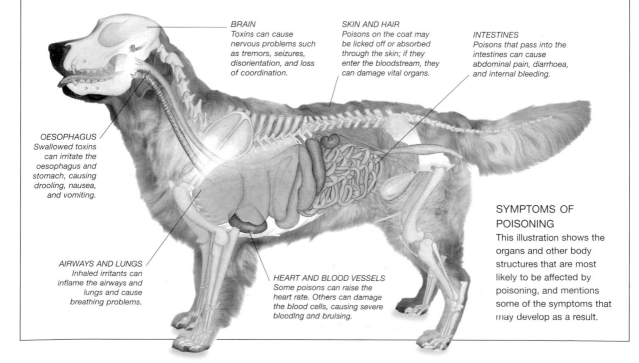

BRAIN
Toxins can cause nervous problems such as tremors, seizures, disorientation, and loss of coordination.

SKIN AND HAIR
Poisons on the coat may be licked off or absorbed through the skin; if they enter the bloodstream, they can damage vital organs.

INTESTINES
Poisons that pass into the intestines can cause abdominal pain, diarrhoea, and internal bleeding.

OESOPHAGUS
Swallowed toxins can irritate the oesophagus and stomach, causing drooling, nausea, and vomiting.

AIRWAYS AND LUNGS
Inhaled irritants can inflame the airways and lungs and cause breathing problems.

HEART AND BLOOD VESSELS
Some poisons can raise the heart rate. Others can damage the blood cells, causing severe bleeding and bruising.

SYMPTOMS OF POISONING
This illustration shows the organs and other body structures that are most likely to be affected by poisoning, and mentions some of the symptoms that may develop as a result.

COAT CONTAMINATION

A dog's coat can be contaminated by walking in or brushing against a toxic chemical. One common result is skin damage such as irritation or burns. If a dog tries to lick the chemical off, it may suffer burns in its mouth. Toxins that are swallowed or absorbed through the skin may cause general poisoning.

To clean the fur, you will need plenty of warm, soapy water and a mild detergent such as washing-up liquid or baby shampoo. Hand cleaners for use in DIY are also safe and non-irritating. To remove paint, tar, or motor oil, you will also need vegetable or mineral oil. Never use irritants or toxins such as paint stripper, turpentine, white spirit, or concentrated biological detergent.

POISONING BY SKIN CONTACT

Is there obvious chemical contamination of the fur or skin and is there:

Unconsciousness	Convulsions	Signs of pain or distress	Dribbling saliva	Drowsiness, loss of coordination	No other worrying signs
Give CPR (*see p.389*)	Wrap dog in a blanket	Look for chemical burns	Look for mouth burns		Follow instructions for cleaning coat
See vet ASAP	See vet ASAP	See vet ASAP	See vet ASAP	See vet ASAP	See below

CLEANING A CONTAMINATED COAT

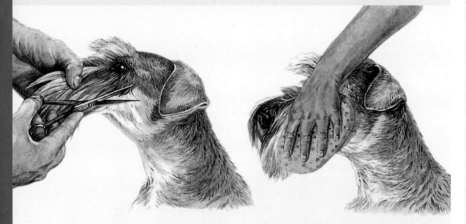

REMOVING PAINT, TAR, OR OIL
If the substance is hard, cut away affected hair. If it is soft, put on rubber gloves and rub in plenty of vegetable or mineral oil to loosen it. To clean a large area, add flour to the oil to help absorb the toxin, and remove the mixture with a wide-toothed comb. Wash the coat with warm, soapy water or mild detergent, and rinse, until it is clean.

REMOVING OTHER SUBSTANCES
Flush for at least five minutes with plenty of clean water to dilute the poison and stop any burning. To dilute alkali such as caustic soda, flush for 20 minutes. Pay attention to the eyes, and flush the groin and armpits as carefully as the rest of the body. Wash the fur with warm, soapy water or mild detergent, and rinse thoroughly.

Q **IS PAINT ON A DOG'S COAT DANGEROUS?**

A Although it is unsightly, paint is seldom dangerous, if only because it usually comes into contact with hair rather than skin. I see far more cases of damage due to people using paint remover or methylated spirit to remove the paint. Emulsion paint can be removed with mild detergent while still wet. Oil paint can be left to dry and then cut off (*see left*).

Q **IS IT DANGEROUS FOR A DOG TO ROLL ON GRASS TREATED WITH WEEDKILLER?**

A Assume that it is dangerous, although the degree of risk depends on the chemicals in the weedkiller. Never let your dog come into contact with grass that has just been treated with any chemical.

INHALED POISONS

Toxic substances that can be inhaled include smoke and fumes; chemical sprays (such as weedkillers and pesticides); chlorine and ammonia gas given off by cleaning substances; fumes from oil-based paints; or even sprays such as tear gas. Another common hazard is carbon monoxide gas, which is given off by propane gas heaters, cookers, or indoor barbecues that leak into unventilated areas. Older cars that are not fitted with catalytic converters also emit carbon monoxide. The gas causes weakness or unconsciousness, accompanied by cherry red gums.

Smoke, fumes, and carbon monoxide are most likely to pose a danger to humans and animals if they are trapped in confined spaces such as a closed room or a garage. Never leave your dog in an enclosed space contaminated with fumes, or with a vehicle or gas appliance that is turned on. If you take your dog camping, never leave it in a tent with a propane heater switched on.

Inhaled toxins most often interfere with breathing. Smoke and fumes cause obvious coughing and choking; you should assume that an affected dog's airways have been inflamed. Substances such as concentrated insecticide fumes cause neurological symptoms such as twitching and trembling, excessive salivating, and convulsions.

VET'S ADVICE

Be very careful when entering an area that is contaminated with smoke or chemical fumes.
• Do not put yourself at risk by entering an area containing toxic fumes. Use breathing apparatus if available, or call the fire brigade.
• Do not underestimate the risks from smoke or fumes; serious or possibly fatal swelling may affect the airways up to several hours later. After any inhalation incident, always get veterinary help.

POISONS THAT ARE INHALED

Has the dog been exposed to smoke, toxic or irritating fumes, or carbon monoxide and is there:

Unconsciousness and no breathing	Depressed state; loss of coordination; deep red gums; heavy panting; convulsions; breathing difficulties; coughing up blood; burns on the body; exposure to fire or smoke	Coughing but no exposure to serious fire and smoke	Smelly coat
Give CPR; see vet ASAP	See vet ASAP	See vet within 24 hrs	Clean coat; phone vet

TREATING A DOG THAT HAS INHALED POISON

1 Keep the dog's airway open, monitor breathing and circulation, and give artificial respiration or CPR (*see p.389*) as necessary. If the dog is still conscious, remove it from the area and get it into fresh air as quickly as possible.

2 If the dog is having convulsions, wrap it in a blanket and clear the area around it to prevent it from injuring itself. Get immediate veterinary help.

3 If there is time to do so, flush the eyes with plenty of clean, fresh water or with a proprietary eye wash fluid.

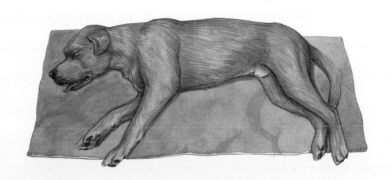

SWALLOWED POISONS

At one time or another I have treated dogs that have eaten women's tights, packets of birth control pills, a ten-inch rubber Donald Duck (whole), tennis balls, lead curtain weights, plastic bread bags, cat litter, tampons, socks, bottles of aspirin, bars of soap, bars of chocolate, underwear, and fruit stones. Most of these items are simply foreign bodies that do not belong in the dog's digestive system, but others, such as

lead, medicines, and – surprisingly – dark chocolate, are poisons.

If your dog has swallowed a toxic substance, your first objective is to save its life. If shock develops (*see p.388*) or the dog loses consciousness, keep the airway open and maintain the breathing and circulation (*see p.387 and p.389*). If the dog is having convulsions, prevent it from damaging itself and from biting you or other

people (*see pp.384–85*). In both cases, get immediate veterinary help.

If the poison has been swallowed in the previous two hours, it is usually best to induce vomiting by giving 3% hydrogen peroxide or a crystal of washing soda. You must not do this, however, if the dog has swallowed a corrosive or caustic chemical (*see below*), because vomiting could trigger further damage in the digestive system.

ASSESSING A DOG THAT HAS SWALLOWED POISON

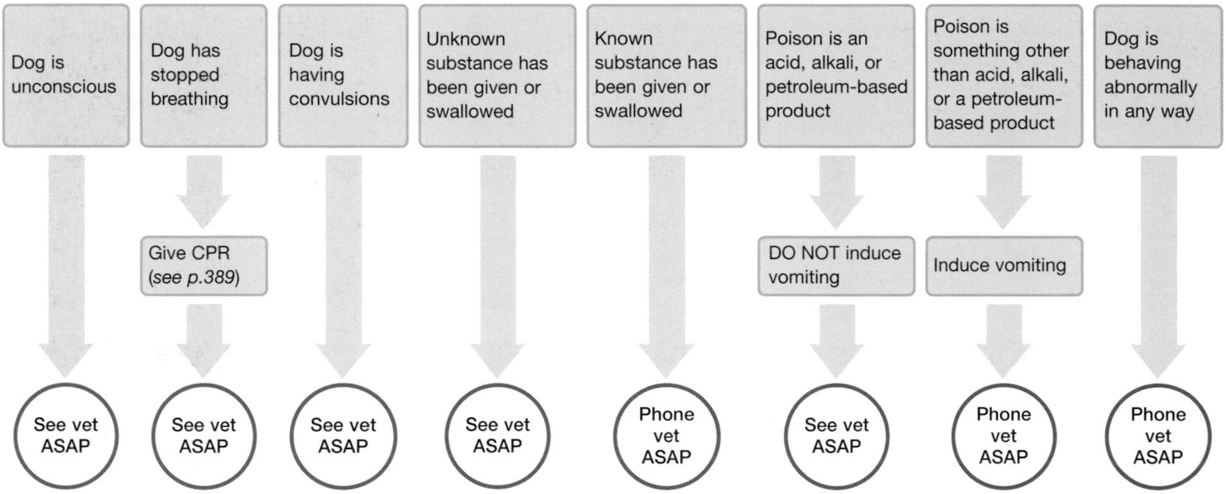

Dog is unconscious	Dog has stopped breathing	Dog is having convulsions	Unknown substance has been given or swallowed	Known substance has been given or swallowed	Poison is an acid, alkali, or petroleum-based product	Poison is something other than acid, alkali, or a petroleum-based product	Dog is behaving abnormally in any way
	Give CPR (*see p.389*)				DO NOT induce vomiting	Induce vomiting	
See vet ASAP	See vet ASAP	See vet ASAP	See vet ASAP	Phone vet ASAP	See vet ASAP	Phone vet ASAP	Phone vet ASAP

CORROSIVE OR CAUSTIC SUBSTANCES

The following items are acids, alkalis, or petroleum products. Do not induce vomiting if your dog has swallowed any of these substances because vomiting will cause further damage to the digestive tract.

- Battery acid
- Bleach
- Carbolic acid (phenol)
- Caustic soda
- Chlorine for swimming pools
- Dishwasher detergents
- Drain cleaner
- Fertilizer
- Furniture or floor polish
- Glue
- Household cleaning fluids
- Kerosene
- Laundry detergents
- Lye
- Motor oil
- Nail varnish
- Oven cleaner
- Paint stripper or remover
- Paint thinner
- Paintbrush cleaner
- Petrol
- Pine oil cleaners
- Plaster
- Putty
- Turpentine
- Wood preservatives

INDUCING VOMITING

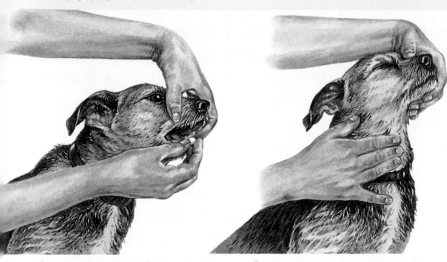

3% HYDROGEN PEROXIDE

This substance induces vomiting by fizzing in the stomach. It is available from chemists. If you buy a solution that is more concentrated, dilute it down to 3%. The dosage required to induce vomiting depends on the weight of your dog. The following chart shows dosages and approximate weights.

Dosage	Weight of dog
2.5 ml	Under 2 kg (5 lb)
5 ml	2–5 kg (5–10 lb)
10 ml	5–7 kg (10–15 lb)
15 ml	7–11 kg (15–25 lb)
20 ml	11–15 kg (25–35 lb)
25 ml	15–20 kg (35–45 lb)
30 ml	20–25 kg (45–55 lb)
35 ml	25–30 kg (55–65 lb)
40 ml	30–35 kg (65–75 lb)
45 ml	over 35 kg (75 lb)

1 If a dog has swallowed a non-caustic, non-corrosive substance such as rat poison, antifreeze, or dark chocolate, give a washing soda crystal. (You can also use 3% hydrogen peroxide; *see right*.) To give a crystal, lift the upper jaw with one hand, squeezing the lip on the teeth. With the other hand, drop the crystal in the throat.

2 Hold the mouth shut, and stroke the neck. When the dog licks its lips it has swallowed the soda and will vomit a few minutes afterwards. Mix activated charcoal with a little water to make a runny paste (slurry); give the dog 1–2 teaspoons of this mixture, which will help to absorb any remaining poison.

SEEKING VETERINARY HELP

If your dog has been exposed to an unknown poison, take the dog to the veterinary surgeon immediately. If the animal has vomited, take a sample of the vomit with you so that the poison can be identified.

If the poison is known, telephone your veterinary surgeon for advice. If possible, give the following details about the incident:
• product trade name and manufacturer;
• list of ingredients in product;
• amount of substance involved;
• type of exposure – mention any skin contact and inhalation as well as swallowing;
• duration of exposure;
• time passed since exposure;
• any signs shown by dog;
• any treatment given.

ACID OR ALKALI POISONING

These substances are corrosive. If your dog has swallowed an acid or alkali, do not induce vomiting, because the chemical will cause as much or more damage coming back up as it did going down. Instead, you need to neutralize the poison in the stomach.

For acid poisoning, give egg white, bicarbonate of soda, charcoal powder, or olive oil by mouth. To relieve mouth burns, apply bicarbonate of soda mixed with a little water to form a paste. To relieve skin burns, flush for 20 minutes with clean water (*see p.412*).

For alkali poisoning, give egg white, or small amounts of citrus fruit juice or dilute vinegar by mouth. Apply dilute vinegar to any mouth and skin burns. Epiotic ear wash (a salicylic acid solution) is also excellent for alkali burns to the skin.

VET'S ADVICE

If you need to induce vomiting, do so with care.
• Only try to induce vomiting if the dog is alert.
• Do not induce vomiting if the dog shows signs of neurological problems, such as disorientation or loss of balance. If a dog in this condition vomits, some of the vomit may enter the animal's windpipe, causing aspiration pneumonia (inflammation of the tiny air sacs inside the lungs).
• Do not attempt to induce vomiting by using salt because you could inadvertently cause salt poisoning.

COMMON HOUSEHOLD POISONS

The charts below and on the following pages deal with common household poisons. They cover a wide variety of substances, say where these items are usually found, and briefly explain how to treat poisoning in each case.

Your dog is most likely to risk being poisoned if it licks or swallows items such as cleaning fluids, or if it rolls in, brushes against, or walks through areas where chemicals have been applied or spilt. Take care to keep all

such items out of reach when you are not using them, and keep the dog away from any places where you have just applied a hazardous substance. If possible, use chemicals that are non-toxic to children and animals.

TREATING POISONING BY HOUSEHOLD ITEMS

POISON	SOURCE	SIGNS	ACTIONS
Food, drugs, and medications			
Chocolate (toxin: theobromine)	Fed as a treat; scavenging food.	Increased thirst; vomiting and diarrhoea; collapse. CAN BE FATAL.	• If excess chocolate has just been eaten, induce vomiting (see p.419). • If signs of poisoning develop, get immediate veterinary attention.
Tobacco (toxin: nicotine)	Scavenging in dustbins or ashtrays; eating cigars, cigarettes, pipe tobacco.	Vomiting; large amounts (e.g. from eating cigar butts) can also cause diarrhoea, abdominal pain, loss of coordination, collapse, death.	• Soothe stomach irritation by giving charcoal tablets. • For severe signs, get immediate veterinary attention.
Aspirin (toxin: salicylates)	Scavenging; given in error to relieve pain.	Appetite loss; depression; vomiting, possibly with blood; convulsions. VERY TOXIC IN LARGE AMOUNTS.	• Induce vomiting (see p.419). • Get veterinary attention.
Antidepressants, sedatives	Scavenging; given in error to relieve pain.	Depression; staggering; loss of coordination; coma.	• If just eaten, induce vomiting (see p.419). • Get immediate veterinary advice. (Most of these drugs are not life-threatening, but they are more toxic in small dogs.)
Cannabis	Scavenging; fed deliberately.	Loss of coordination; fear; agitation; biting; dilated pupils.	• Avoid sensory stimulation. • Give sedative recommended by your vet.
Paracetamol	Scavenging; given in error to relieve pain.	Vomiting; diarrhoea; restlessness; depression; abdominal pain; yellow gums. SYMPTOMS APPEAR SEVERAL DAYS AFTER POISONING.	• If item has just been swallowed, induce vomiting (see p.419). • Get immediate veterinary attention.
Flea repellents for dogs: chlorinated hydrocarbons	Skin treatments containing malathion or older chemicals such as lindane, gammexane, chlordane, toxophene.	Salivation; agitation; twitching; restlessness; convulsion; coma. CAN BE FATAL.	• If dog is not having convulsions, wash off as much of substance as possible. • If dog is twitching or convulsing, avoid light and take to vet immediately.
Flea repellents for dogs: organophosphates	Treatment with sprays, shampoos, flea collars, "spot-on" products, old-fashioned wormers.	Muscle tremors; drooling; difficulty breathing; increased urinating and/or defecating.	• Wash off substance thoroughly. • Take dog to vet immediately.
Insecticides for dogs: carbamates	Swallowing or contact with shampoos, collars, "spot-ons", or sprays.	Salivating; abdominal pain; loss of appetite; vomiting; diarrhoea; muscle tremors; convulsions; coma. CAN BE FATAL.	• Induce vomiting (see p.419). • Take dog to vet as soon as possible.

VET'S ADVICE

- Take particular care to keep young, curious, or active dogs away from any places in your home or surrounding area where they might find poisonous substances.

- Never use disinfectants to clean your dog's coat unless the product label says that it is safe to do so.
- Slug bait, strychnine, and arsenic may all be used by malicious

poisoners who target dogs. If you suspect that your dog has been deliberately poisoned, take a sample of the substance with your dog to your veterinary surgeon.

POISON	SOURCE	SIGNS	ACTIONS
Household cleaners			
Caustic soda; chlorine bleach	Walking in substance; licking; chemical wrongly applied to coat.	Inflamed skin; vomiting; diarrhoea; ulcers on tongue; possible convulsions.	• DO NOT INDUCE VOMITING. • Wash coat and skin with soap and water. • Feed milk and vegetable oil solution. • Get immediate veterinary attention.
Detergent concentrate	Licking or contact with cleaning solutions.	Foam or froth coming from mouth; itchy or inflamed skin.	• Wash mouth with clean water. • Wash skin with lots of fresh water.
Dishwasher detergent; oven cleaner; toilet cleaner	Licking, chewing, or swallowing substance; walking in it; drinking from toilet bowl.	Inflamed skin; vomiting; diarrhoea; ulcers on tongue; possible convulsions.	• DO NOT INDUCE VOMITING. • Wash coat and skin with soap and water. • Feed milk and vegetable oil solution followed by a purgative recommended by your vet (for example, sodium sulphate). • Get immediate veterinary attention.
Furniture or floor polish; paint stripper or remover; paint thinner. (These items usually carry a symbol showing that they contain acid or alkali.)	Licking, chewing, swallowing, or walking in substance.	Inflamed skin; vomiting; diarrhoea; ulcers on tongue; possible convulsions.	• DO NOT INDUCE VOMITING. • Wash coat and skin with soap and water. • Feed milk and vegetable oil solution followed by a purgative recommended by your vet (for example, sodium sulphate). • Get immediate veterinary attention.
Herbicides			
Arsenic	Ingesting herbicide or industrial waste; possible malicious poisoning.	Salivating; abdominal pain; vomiting; diarrhoea; weakness; collapse. CAN BE FATAL.	• Get immediate veterinary attention.
Chlorate	Contact with or ingestion of weedkiller in garden.	Depression; abdominal pain; loss of appetite; blood in urine; black faeces.	• Get immediate veterinary attention.
Dinitro compounds	Licked or absorbed through skin.	High body temperature; thirst; rapid breathing and heart rate; collapse, DEATH.	• Cool dog immediately in water (see p.409). • Get immediate veterinary attention.
Paraquat and Diquat	Licked off paws or swallowed.	Mouth or paw irritation; loss of appetite; loss of coordination; vomiting; depression; respiratory distress developing later.	• If substance has just been swallowed, give activated charcoal (see p.419).

TREATING POISONING BY HOUSEHOLD ITEMS (continued)

POISON	SOURCE	SIGNS	ACTIONS
Pesticides			
Insecticides: organochlorines	Skin contact or swallowing.	Apprehension; tremor; excitability; loss of coordination; convulsions; DEATH.	• Induce vomiting (see p.419). • Take dog to vet as soon as possible.
Insecticides: organophosphates	Contact with or ingestion of agricultural products such as sheep dip.	Loss of appetite; abdominal pain; vomiting; diarrhoea; loss of coordination; difficulty breathing; paralysis; convulsions. CAN BE FATAL.	• Induce vomiting (see p.419). • Take dog to vet as soon as possible.
Rodenticide: alphachlorulose	Eating rodent bait.	Drunken gait; coma; hypothermia. ESPECIALLY DANGEROUS TO SMALL DOGS.	• Keep the dog warm. • Avoid giving sedatives. • Induce vomiting ONLY if signs of poisoning have not yet developed.
Rodenticide: warfarin (also brodifacoum; chlorphacinone; coumachlor; difenacoum)	Eating rodent bait or poisoned rodent.	Lethargy; white or bleeding gums; blood in vomit and/or diarrhoea; bruising; difficulty breathing. CAN BE FATAL. NEWER PRODUCTS ARE MORE LETHAL.	• If poison has only just been ingested, induce vomiting. • Get immediate veterinary attention; vet will need to give vitamin K injections to stop the bleeding.
Calciferol	Swallowing commercial rodent bait.	Depression; excessive drinking and urinating; loss of appetite.	• Give plenty of fluids by mouth. • Keep dog out of sunlight. • Avoid giving calcium in diet.
Cyanide	Swallowing illegal poison.	Excitement; dilated eyes; salivation; difficulty breathing; convulsions; DEATH.	• Take dog to vet as soon as possible.
Phosphorus yellow	Swallowing or skin contact with commercial poison.	Garlic odour to breath; abdominal pain; vomiting; skin burns; convulsions; coma.	• Get immediate veterinary attention. • Avoid contact with vomit, because it may cause burns.
Slug and snail bait (metaldehyde)	Sometimes eaten; some dogs like taste.	Salivation; tremors; convulsions; coma. CAN BE FATAL.	• If bait has just been eaten, induce vomiting. • If there are clinical signs of poisoning (or you suspect malicious poisoning), get veterinary attention.
Strychnine	Contact with pesticide; eating illegal coyote bait (in USA).	Apprehensiveness; tension; stiffness; leads to seizures, convulsions; DEATH.	• Induce vomiting (see p.419). • Get immediate veterinary attention, especially if you suspect malicious poisoning.
Thallium	Swallowing commercial poison.	Salivation; loss of appetite; vomiting; diarrhoea; pain; convulsions; DEATH.	• Induce vomiting (see p.419).
Zinc phosphide	Swallowing commercial poison.	Loss of appetite; depression; abdominal pain; vomiting; convulsions; DEATH.	• Induce vomiting (see p.419). • Take dog to vet as soon as possible.

POISON	SOURCE	SIGNS	ACTIONS
Poisons in garage			
Antifreeze (ethylene glycol)	Licked from leaking car radiator. (Dogs like taste.)	Vomiting; wobbling; collapse; convulsions; coma. CAN BE FATAL.	• Induce vomiting (*see p.419*). • Get immediate veterinary attention.
Carbon monoxide	Breathing in car exhaust, fumes from faulty heating system or indoor barbecue.	Cherry-red gums; staggering; loss of consciousness.	• Get dog into fresh air. • Give artificial respiration (*see p.389*).
Chlorine	Chewing water sterilizers. (Chlorinated water in swimming pools is safe.)	Red eyes and mouth.	• Wash eyes thoroughly with water or saline solution. • Flush mouth with water or milk.
Drain cleaner	Walking in or licking item; contamination of coat.	Inflamed skin; vomiting; diarrhoea; ulcers on tongue; possible convulsions.	• DO NOT INDUCE VOMITING. • Wash coat and skin with soap and water. • Feed milk and vegetable oil solution. • Get immediate veterinary attention.
Gasoline (petrol)	Walked in; licked from pads; wrongly used to clean dog's coat.	Inflamed skin; vomiting; diarrhoea; ulcers on tongue; possible convulsions.	• DO NOT INDUCE VOMITING. • Wash coat and skin with soap and water. • Feed milk and vegetable oil solution. • Get immediate veterinary attention.
Kerosene oil (paraffin)	Swallowing or contact with heating fuel, lamp lighter, cleaning fluids, white spirit, diesel fuel.	Abdominal discomfort; weakness; depression; vomiting; collapse.	• DO NOT INDUCE VOMITING. • Feed milk and vegetable oil solution. • Get immediate veterinary attention.
Lead	Licking old paint or pipes; swallowing lead fishing weights, batteries, curtain weights, solder, putty, old linoleum, lubricants.	Vomiting; diarrhoea; abdominal pain followed by worried look; whining; nervousness; sensitivity to light; staggering; paralysis.	• If lead has been swallowed recently, induce vomiting. • Get immediate veterinary attention.
Phenol (Creosote, Cresol)	Swallowing or contact with wood preservatives; fungicides; disinfectants; photographic developer; tar; pitch; carbolic soap.	Local burns; thirst; abdominal pain; depression; loss of coordination; staggering; twitching; coma.	• Feed milk and vegetable oil solution . • Wash off any skin contamination. • Get veterinary attention.
Wood preservative	Walked in; spilt on coat; licked off coat or treated surface.	Inflamed skin; vomiting; diarrhoea; ulcers on tongue; possible convulsions.	• DO NOT INDUCE VOMITING. • Wash coat and skin with soap and water. • Feed milk and vegetable oil solution. • Get immediate veterinary attention.

POISONOUS PLANTS

Poisonous substances exist in nature as well as in man-made products. Natural toxins include sap or other substances in certain plants and venom or other poisons produced by some animals (*see pp.426–27*). Poisoning from plants is much less common in dogs than illness caused by ingesting medications or toxic chemicals; nevertheless, it is wise to protect your dog from any potential hazards posed by plants in your garden, house, or other frequently visited areas.

GARDEN PLANTS

Some of the plants found in gardens, or in similar places such as parks, can be toxic. Most just cause an upset stomach if the dog comes into contact with them or swallows plant material, but certain species are deadly. The chart below shows common garden plants that are toxic to dogs. If there are any of these plants in your garden, or in other areas where you exercise your dog, keep the dog well away from them. If possible, make sure that the

plants are out of reach – for example, by fencing them off and disposing of dead matter safely. In addition, keep your dog away from other poisonous plant matter in your garden, such as all fungi and bulbs.

The chemicals that are applied to many garden plants, such as fertilizers and weedkillers, can also pose a hazard to dogs. Keep all such chemicals locked away in a shed or garage when you are not using them. Whenever you are using these chemicals in your garden,

COMMON POISONOUS PLANTS

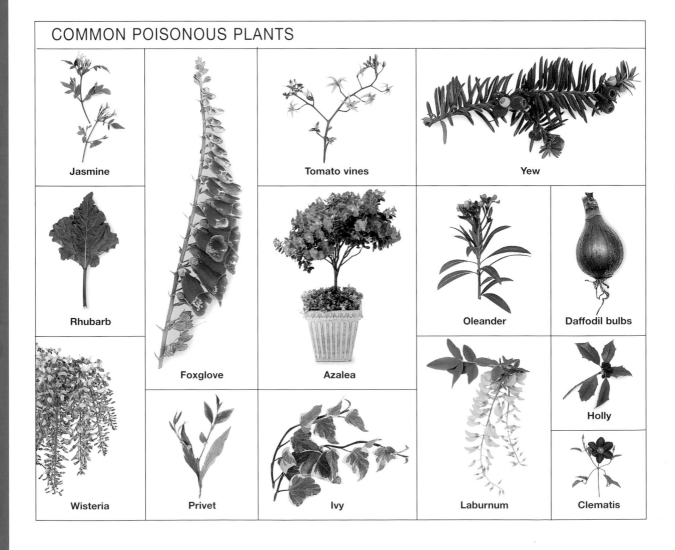

Jasmine

Rhubarb

Foxglove

Tomato vines

Azalea

Yew

Oleander

Daffodil bulbs

Holly

Wisteria

Privet

Ivy

Laburnum

Clematis

never leave the containers around unsupervised, and put them away as soon as you have finished with them. Keep your dog away from all plants that have just been treated with chemicals, including areas of lawn, for at least 24 hours.

Certain species of houseplants, such as dumb cane (*Dieffenbachia* species) and amaryllis, can also be poisonous to dogs. Dieffenbachia sap, for example, causes the tongue to swell enormously. It is, however, easy to minimize the risk of poisoning by keeping these plants out of reach and not leaving bored or active dogs alone with them.

WOODS, FIELDS, AND MEADOWS

Wild plants that are irritating to our skin have the same effect when they come into contact with a dog's skin. The surface chemicals of nettles, poison ivy, and poison oak most often cause inflammation to the skin of the abdomen, especially in dogs with short coats or little protective downy hair. In hot, humid grain-growing regions a toxin called aflatoxin can grow in contaminated grain, and is sometimes eaten by curious dogs. Aflatoxin from mouldy grain causes a loss of appetite, weight loss, and often fatal liver damage. Assume that any mouldy grain is potentially toxic. Take care when walking your dog in crop fields that have recently been sprayed with herbicides; while the plants themselves are not toxic, the sprayed chemicals may be dangerous.

SIGNS OF POISONING

The signs of plant poisoning vary enormously. Curious pups are most commonly affected. Most often, an affected dog vomits and may have diarrhoea. As a rough guide, assume until proven otherwise that any plant with a white sap is poisonous.

POISONOUS PLANTS

PLANT	TOXIC PARTS	PLANT	TOXIC PARTS
Irritant and toxic plants		Lupin (*Lupinus* species)	Stems, flowers, seeds
		Poinsettia (*Euphorbia pulcherrima*)	Leaves, stems, sap
Amaryllis (*Amaryllis*)	Leaves, flowers	Privet (*Ligustrum* species)	All parts
Autumn crocus (*Colchicum*		Rhododendron (*Rhododendron* species)	Stems, leaves
autumnale)	Bulbs	Rhubarb (*Rheum* species)	Leaves
Azalea (*Rhododendron*	All parts, especially	Skunk cabbage (*Symplocarpus foetidus*)	Leaves, flowers, roots
species)	leaves	Tomato (*Lycopersicon* species)	Vines
Bird-of-paradise flower (*Strelitzia*		Virginia creeper (*Parthenocissus*	
reginae)	Stems	*quinquefolia*)	Bark, stems
Bleeding heart (*Dicentra*		Wisteria (*Wisteria* species)	All parts
spectabilis)	Flowers, stems, roots		
Bloodroot (*Sanguinaria*		**Very toxic or deadly plants**	
canadensis)	All parts		
Box (*Buxus* species)	Bark, stems, sap, leaves	Castor-oil plant (*Ricinus communis*)	Seeds
Chinaberry tree (*Melia azedarach*)	Wood, branches	Cherry laurel (*Prunus laurocerasus*)	Wood, branches
Clematis (*Clematis* species)	Stems, leaves	Deadly nightshade (*Solanum nigrum*)	All parts, especially
Daffodils (*Narcissus* species)	Bulbs		berries
Delphinium (*Delphinium* species)	All parts	Dumb cane (*Dieffenbachia* species)	Leaves, roots, stems
Foxglove (*Digitalis* species)	All parts	Hemlock (*Conium maculatum*)	All parts, especially young
Holly (*Ilex* species)	Berries		leaves and berries
Ivy (*Hedera* species)	Leaves, berries	Jimsonweed/thorn apple (*Datura*	All parts, especially
Jasmine (*Jasminum* species)	Leaves	*stramonium*)	seeds
Jerusalem cherry (*Solanum*		Laburnum (*Laburnum* species)	All parts
pseudocapsicum)	Leaves, flowers, fruits	Mistletoe (*Viscum album*)	Berries
Larkspur (*Consolida ajacis*; syn.	All parts, especially	Oleander (*Nerium oleander*)	All parts
Consolida ambigua, Delphinium	stems, seeds, young	Precatory bean (*Abrus precatorius*)	Seeds
consolida)	leaves	Virginia pokeweed (*Phytolacca*	All parts, especially roots
Lily of the valley (*Convallaria*		*americana*, syn. *Phytolacca decandra*)	and seeds
majalis)	Leaves, flowers, seeds	Yew (*Taxus* species)	All parts

POISONOUS ANIMALS

In the UK, the only venomous wild animals are bees, wasps, ants, and adders. Insect stings often cause only mild symptoms, such as swelling and itching. In some dogs, however, a sting can cause life-threatening anaphylactic shock (*see opposite*).

Dogs in the UK may also be at risk from certain exotic creatures kept as pets, such as black widow spiders, scorpions, and venomous snakes. These animals can inflict severe bites or stings; the venom from some species is deadly.

In other parts of the world, dogs are more likely to meet venomous animals in the wild. They are also at risk of poisoning from licking or mouthing animals that exude toxins from their skins, such as certain species of toads and salamanders.

SPIDERS AND SCORPIONS

Venomous spiders (such as the brown recluse spider and the black widow in the United States and the funnel-web spider in Australia) give bites that can cause pain at the site of the wound. Later, an affected dog will become excitable, weak, and feverish, and show signs of muscle and joint pain. Convulsions, leading to shock (*see p.388*) and death, may occur if antivenin (a substance that counteracts the effect of venom) is not given. Scorpion stings cause intense pain and inflammation at the site, and the affected area heals only slowly.

SNAKES

While bites from non-poisonous species rarely cause any problems, poisonous snakes can badly harm or even kill a dog. Dangerous snake species include rattlesnakes and copperheads in the United States; the bushmaster and cord snakes in Central and South America; the puff adder, mambas, and the boomslang in Africa; cobras in Asia and Africa; and the taipan and death adder in Australia.

Signs of venom poisoning in dogs may include restlessness, panting,

POISONOUS ANIMALS

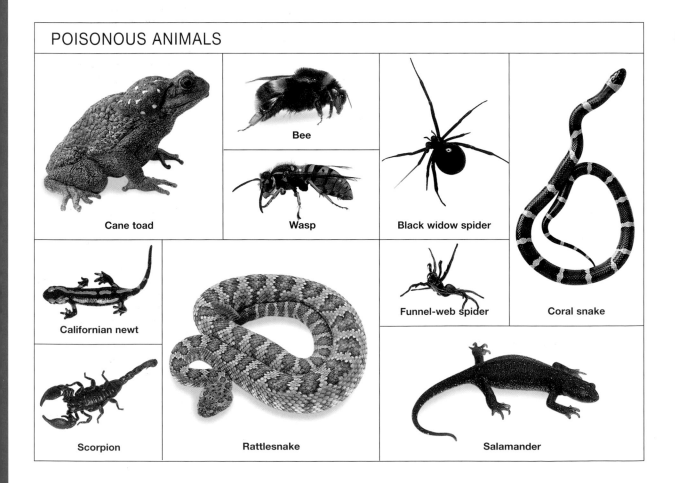

Cane toad

Bee

Wasp

Black widow spider

Californian newt

Funnel-web spider

Coral snake

Scorpion

Rattlesnake

Salamander

salivating, depression, vomiting and diarrhoea, loss of coordination, shock, and death. Coral snake venom has a potent nerve poison causing weakness, constricted ("pin-point") pupils, swallowing difficulties, and then rapid death from respiratory paralysis.

If you live in a country where any poisonous snakes are a hazard, find out what these species look like and where they live, so that in an emergency you can identify the species that caused the bite and the vet can provide the appropriate antivenin. If you plan to take your dog to an area where these snakes are found, and out of reach of vets, ask your vet if you should take an antivenin with you.

SNAKE BITES

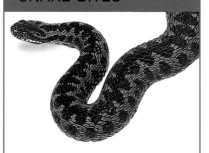

Dogs usually incur snake bites on the feet or head. If you suspect that your dog has been bitten by a venomous snake, keep it quiet and get immediate veterinary help. The earlier antivenin is given, the better the results. The vet may also give intravenous fluids and medications such as antihistamines.

• DO NOT wash the wound, because this will increase the absorption of venom.

• DO NOT cut the wound or try to suck out the venom; it will only make the injury worse and may even poison you.

INSECT BITES AND STINGS

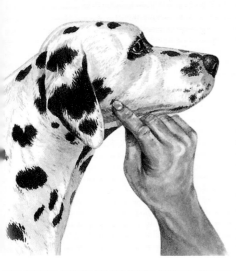

TREATING A BITE OR STING

If a bite or sting occurs, try to identify the insect if possible. Such wounds cause areas of swelling and itching. Apply a cold pack (a bag of frozen peas wrapped in a cloth) to the area to reduce swelling and treat with calamine lotion or hydrocortisone cream to relieve itching. If you have any antihistamine tablets from your vet, give these as well to help relieve the symptoms.

When bees sting, they leave their stings behind. A sting is a tiny spike with a venom sac at the end. Scrape it out of the skin with a fingernail or the edge of a credit card, taking care not to squeeze the sac. Mix bicarbonate of soda with water to form a paste, and apply it to the area.

ANAPHYLACTIC SHOCK

DIAGNOSIS AND TREATMENT

Anaphylactic shock is a life-threatening allergic reaction, usually caused by insect stings or reactions to medication. Signs include localized or general skin irritation, anxiety, and difficulty breathing. If not treated quickly, an affected dog may suffer weakness, collapse, coma, and death.

Treat as for shock (see p.388). Take the dog to the vet immediately; it will need vital treatment with corticosteroids, adrenaline, intravenous fluids, and oxygen.

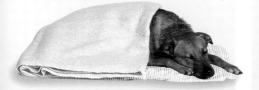

TOAD AND SALAMANDER POISONING

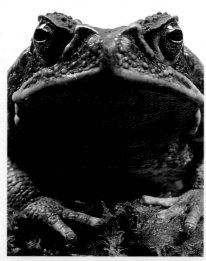

CAUSES AND TREATMENT

Amphibians such as the Florida marine toad, Colorado river toad, and the Californian newt in the United States, and the cane toad in Australia, are potentially poisonous if licked or tasted, or if a dog takes the animal in its mouth. An affected dog will drool saliva and will behave as if it has tasted something unpleasant (which it has), making faces and pawing at its mouth. Drooling may lead to convulsions and death, especially in small dogs and pups. If your dog has licked or mouthed a toad, flush its mouth repeatedly with fresh water from a garden hose or a shower.

GLOSSARY

A

ABSCESS A localized pocket of infection in body tissues

ACUTE Occurring suddenly, as in "acute pain"

ADENOMA Common, benign tumour in the glandular tissue

ADH Anti-diuretic hormone *see also* Diabetes insipidus

ADRENAL GLANDS Pair of endocrine gland, each composed of two fundamentally distinct tissues: an outer layer (cortex) and an inner layer (medulla)

AIHA *see* Autoimmune haemolytic anaemia

ALOPECIA Lack of hair

IMHA *see* Autoimmune haemolytic anaemia

ANAEMIA Reduced red blood cells or reduction in oxygen-carrying pigment (haemoglobin), associated with blood loss, bone marrow suppression, parasites, or immune-mediated disease that destroys red blood cells

ANALGESIA Pain control

ANAPHYLACTIC SHOCK An exaggerated, life-threatening allergic response to foreign protein or other substances

ANAPHYLAXIS *see* Anaphylactic shock

ANOESTRUS The phase of the oestrus cycle when the female dog is not sexually receptive to males.

ANOREXIA Lack of appetite

ANTHELMINTIC An agent that destroys worms

ANTIBODY Protein produced by specialized white blood cells in response to certain antigens. Antibody binds to antigen, a fundamental act of immunity

ANTICOAGULANT A drug, chemical, or other substance that prevents blood clotting

ANTIEMETIC An agent that relieves vomiting

ANTIGEN Any agent capable of inducing a specific immune response

ANTIGENICITY The capacity to stimulate the production of antibodies

ANTIOXIDANT A substance that prevents fats from going rancid

APNOEA No breathing

ARTHRITIS Inflammation of a joint; *see* Degenerative joint disease

ARTHROSCOPY Visual examination of the contents of a joint cavity using a fine fibre optic endoscope

ARTIFICIAL INSEMINATION The artificial introduction of live sperm into the female genital tract

ASCENDING PARALYSIS/PARESIS A complete or partial paralysis starting in the hindquarters and progressively moving forwards to the front limbs and head

ASCITES The accumulation or exudation of fluid in the abdominal cavity; *see also* Exudate

ATAXIA A lack of muscle coordination

ATOPY Allergy to external allergens such as pollens

ATROPHY Wasting

AUTOIMMUNE DISEASE Any condition in which the body's immune system erroneously attacks normal body parts

AUTOIMMUNE HAEMOLYTIC ANAEMIA (AIHA) A disorder in which the immune system attacks the red blood cells (also called immune-mediated haemolytic anaemia or IMHA)

AVASCULAR NECROSIS Cellular death because of a lack of blood supply

AVERSION THERAPY Treatment of a behaviour problem involving the use of mild physical or mental discomfort

B

BENIGN TUMOUR A local tumour that does not spread (is not malignant)

BIOPSY The collection of tissue for microscopic examination

BLOAT Dilation of the stomach, usually with gas or air; *see* Volvulus

BODY SCANS Examination of the interior of the body using radio waves or radioisotopes (radioactive substances)

BONE SCAN An imaging procedure using radioactive isotopes to picture bone and its surrounding tissue

BRACHYCEPHALIC Having a shortened muzzle and a wide head

BRACHYGNATHISM Protrusion of the lower jaw

BRONCHITIS Inflammation of the air passages

C

CAESAREAN SECTION The surgical opening of the uterus to deliver full-term puppies

CALCULUS A concretion of mineral salts deposited on tooth surfaces or hollow organs such as the bladder

CANINE COGNITIVE DYSFUNCTION (CCD) Another term for canine senile dementia

CARCINOGEN Any material, substance, or energy that potentially causes cancer

CARCINOMA A tumour originating in skin cells or cells that line internal organs

CARDIOVASCULAR Pertaining to the heart and circulation

CARNIVORE Meat-eater

CASTRATION Usually refers to the surgical removal of the testicles in males (in law it may refer to the sterilization of both male and female)

CATARACT Crystalline cloudiness in the lens of the eye

CCD *see* Canine cognitive dysfunction

CDRM *see* Chronic degenerative radiculomyopathy

CHOROID The membrane in the eye between the retina and the sclera; contains blood vessels supplying the eye

CHRONIC Having existed for some time, as in "chronic pain"

CHRONIC DEGENERATIVE RADICULOMYOPATHY (CDRM) An inherited

progressive deterioration to spinal transmission of signals, especially in the German Shepherd Dog

CHRONIC OBSTRUCTIVE PULMONARY DISEASE (COPD); a condition in which the structures within the lungs are inflamed or damaged, resulting in shortness of breath

CILIA Hair-like structures extending from some cells, such as those in the airways, that beat rhythmically to propel mucus and debris out of the area

CILIARY BODY Part of the eye connecting the choroid and iris; contains muscles that control the thickness of the lens

CLINICAL SIGNS What you observe your dog doing

CLINICAL SYMPTOMS How your dog is feeling

COCHLEA Spiral tube forming part of the inner ear

COLITIS Inflammation to the large intestine (the colon)

COLOSTRUM The first milk produced just after birth, containing passive protection against a variety of infectious diseases; may also, however, transmit intestinal parasites

COMA An unconscious state from which the dog cannot be aroused

CONCUSSION An unconscious state lasting from seconds to minutes, that kills brain cells

CONGENITAL A condition present at birth; congenital conditions may or may not be hereditary

CONJUNCTIVA The membranes lining the eyeballs and eyelids

CONJUNCTIVITIS Inflammation of the conjunctiva

CONSTIPATION Difficult, infrequent, or absent defaecation

CONTRAST X-RAY An X-ray image produced using a substance that absorbs X-rays, to improve the visibility of structures during radiography

CONTUSION Brain bruising; may or may not be associated with loss of consciousness, leading to temporary confusion and wobbliness

CONVULSION *see* Seizure

COPD *see* Chronic obstructive pulmonary disease

COPROPHAGIA Eating animal droppings

CORNEA The clear surface of the eyeball

CORTICOSTEROID Any of the hormones produced by the adrenal cortex (outer layer of the adrenal gland)

CPR Cardiopulmonary resuscitation; a life-saving technique involving heart massage to stimulate circulation and artificial respiration to supply air to the lungs

CRAMP The involuntary contraction of muscle filaments (the components of muscle fibres), occurring most frequently in canine athletes

CREPITUS Dry, grating sound when a joint extends or flexes

CRUSTS A consequence of skin inflammation, consisting of serum, blood, and inflammatory cells; also called "scabs"

CRYOSURGERY Destruction of cells through freezing

CT SCAN Computed tomography using X-rays to scan the body

CUSHING'S SYNDROME An overactive adrenal gland, causing thirst, hair thinning, and abdominal distension

CYANOSIS Purple-blue colour to mucous membranes, caused by lack of oxygen

CYST A sac within body tissues, filled with glandular secretions

CYSTOCENTESIS Removal of a sample of urine via a fine needle inserted through the abdominal wall into the bladder

CYTOKINES Body chemicals that exist in extremely minute quantities and control an extensive variety of cellular activities, such as stimulating or inhibiting cell growth

CYTOLOGY Examination of body cells under a microscope

D

DEGENERATIVE JOINT DISEASE (DJD) An inability to maintain healthy joint tissue or repair it after damage; often called "arthritis" or "osteoarthritis"

DEHYDRATION Loss of the natural level of liquid in body tissue

DEMODICOSIS Infection caused by *Demodex* mites, also called demodectic mange

DERMATITIS Inflammation of the skin

DERMATOPHYTOSIS Infection caused by fungal spores such as ringworm

DIABETES INSIPIDUS Deficiency in a pituitary hormone (anti-diuretic hormone or ADH) that controls urine concentration in the kidneys, causing excessive drinking and urinating

DIABETES MELLITUS OR SUGAR DIABETES High blood sugar, either because of a lack of insulin production or because body tissue cannot absorb circulating insulin

DIAPHRAGM Thin sheet of muscle separating the chest cavity from the abdomen

DIARRHOEA A change in the consistency, volume, or frequency of bowel movements; it may be acute or become chronic

DIOESTRUS The phase in the oestrus cycle when progesterone levels are high and oestrogen levels low; this is the physiological state most conducive to implantation and growth of the developing foetus

DISLOCATION The separation of a bone from its adjoining bone at a joint, often involving ligament tears; may be complete (luxation) or partial (subluxation)

DIURETIC A chemical, usually a drug, that increases the amount of urine passed

DJD *see* Degenerative joint disease

DNA Deoxyribonucleic acid; a complex molecule in cell nuclei that is the basic structure of genes

DYSPHAGIA Difficulty swallowing food or water

DYSPLASIA An abnormal development of tissue, usually associated with bone, as in hip dysplasia

DYSPNOEA Difficulty breathing

DYSTOCIA Difficulty in labour

DYSURIA Difficulty urinating

E

ECG *see* Electrocardiogram

ECHOCARDIOGRAPHY Imaging of the heart using sound waves bounced off the interior and exterior of the heart, then visualized on a monitor; *see also* Ultrasound

ECTROPION A slackness of the lower eyelid revealing visible conjunctiva

ELECTROCARDIOGRAM (ECG) Record of the electrical activity in the heart

ELECTROMYOGRAM (EMG) Record of the electrical activity in resting or working muscles

ELECTRORETINOGRAPHY (ERG) The study of the electrical changes in the retina in response to light stimulation

ELECTROSURGERY The use of an electrical impulse rather than a surgical blade to cut tissue

ELISA TESTING Enzyme-linked immunosorbent assay; a test used to detect or measure levels of an antigen or antibody

ELIZABETHAN COLLAR A coneshaped collar fitted around the neck that prevents a dog from licking or chewing its body

EMG *see* Electromyogram

EMETIC A drug, substance, or event that induces nausea and vomiting

EMPHYSEMA Pathological accumulation of air in tissues

EMPYEMA Accumulation of pus in a body cavity

ENCEPHALITIS Inflammation of the brain

ENDOCRINE GLAND A gland that manufactures hormones and secretes them directly into the blood stream

ENDORPHIN Naturally occurring brain chemical that diminishes pain perception

ENDOSCOPE An instrument for viewing the inside of an area of the body

ENTERITIS Inflammation of the intestines

ENTROPION Rolling in of the eyelids

EOSINOPHILS White blood cells that increase in the presence of internal parasites and allergy

EPIDERMIS The dead, cornified superficial layer of skin

EPILEPSY A disturbance in electrical activity in the brain that causes a seizure

ERG *see* Electroretinography

ESSENTIAL FATTY ACIDS Fatty acids that cannot be synthesized by the body and that must be acquired from the diet

EUTHANASIA The painless termination of life; may be active (by giving a substance that causes death) or passive (by withdrawing medical support that sustains life)

EXCLUSION DIET A diet that excludes all components of any previous diet, usually consisting of novel sources of protein, fat, and carbohydrate

EXOCRINE GLAND A gland that secretes its product through a duct

EXPLORATORY SURGERY An operation undertaken to find the cause of a medical condition

EXUDATE Fluid that has escaped from blood vessels and deposited either in or on tissues

F

FIBROMA A benign connective tissue tumour

FISTULA An abnormal channel from one body cavity to another; for example, from the anus to the vagina

FIT *see* Seizure

FOLLICULITIS Inflammation of hair follicles

FRACTURE A break in a bone, consisting of two or more parts of bone that separate, split, or compress

FREE RADICALS Naturally occurring atoms that destroy cells

G

GASTRIC DILATATION *see* Volvulus

GASTRITIS Inflammation of the stomach

GDV Gastric dilatation volvulus; *see* Volvulus

GENETIC DISEASE A medical condition known to be transmitted to an animal in a parent's genes

GINGIVITIS Inflammation of the gums

GLAUCOMA Increased fluid pressure inside the eye

GLUCOCORTICOIDS Corticosteroids that raise the concentration of blood sugar and of glycogen in the liver

GRANULOMA A benign connective tissue tumour associated with irritation or inflammation

H

HAEMATOMA A blood-filled swelling under the skin

HAEMATURIA Blood in urine

HALITOSIS Bad breath

HAW The third eyelid

HEAT *see* Oestrus

HEPATITIS Inflammation of the liver

HEREDITARY An inherited condition, passed on in the genes, that may occur at any time in life

HERNIA The protrusion of a body part out of the cavity in which it is normally located

HIP DYSPLASIA An abnormal development of hip joint tissue, usually leading to arthritis; in part a hereditary condition

HOMEOSTASIS Balance; the means by which the body maintains a constant internal environment despite external changes

HYPERSENSITIVITY An exaggerated immune response to a foreign agent

HYPERTHERMIA Unusually high body temperature

HYPOGLYCAEMIA Reduction in blood sugar

HYPOPLASIA Reduction in size

HYPOTHERMIA Reduction in core body temperature

I

IBD *see* Inflammatory bowel disease

IDIOPATHIC DISEASE A condition of which the cause is unknown

IMMUNE-MEDIATED DISEASE A condition caused by an overreaction of the immune system

IMMUNO-SUPPRESSED A term describing an animal with diminished immune system responsiveness

INCONTINENCE Uncontrolled dribbling of urine, especially when lying down; more common in older and neutered females

INCISORS Upper and lower front teeth

INCUBATION PERIOD The time between exposure to a

disease-producing agent and the development of clinical signs of disease

INFLAMMATORY BOWEL DISEASE (IBD) A group of intestinal diseases, each characterized by an increase in a specific type of inflammatory cell

INTERDIGITAL Between the toes

-ITIS An inflammation; for example, nephritis is an inflammation of the kidneys

J

JAUNDICE A yellow pigmentation of the mucous membranes or skin, usually associated with liver disease

JOINT FLUID ANALYSIS Examination of a sample of lubricating fluid from a joint; a test that helps vets to differentiate between infection, inflammation, and immune conditions

JOINT LAXITY How loose a joint feels when it is examined; particularly important with hip dysplasia and patella luxation

K

KERATIN Protein component of hair, nails, and tooth enamel

KERATITIS Inflamed cornea

KERATOCONJUNCTIVITIS Inflamed cornea and conjunctiva

KETOACIDOSIS Build-up of ketone bodies in the circulation as a result of kidney failure

KETONE BODIES Normal metabolic products (waste substances produced by chemical reactions in the body) such as acetoacetic acid and acetone

L

LAPAROSCOPY Examination of the abdominal cavity

using a viewing instrument called a laparoscope

LAPAROTOMY The surgical opening of the abdominal cavity

LARYNGITIS Inflammation of the opening of the windpipe (the larynx, or voice box)

LASER Light amplification by stimulated emission of radiation; a concentrated beam of light used as a tool in surgery

LESION A change to body tissue caused by disease or trauma

LIMBIC SYSTEM Brain system that is in control of the nervous and hormonal systems

LIPOMA A benign tumour of fat, particularly common in older, overweight large breeds

LUXATION see Dislocation

M

MACROPHAGES Large white blood cells that consume debris

MAGNETIC RESONANCE IMAGING (MRI) Diagnostic imaging showing detailed cross-sections of the internal anatomy of structures such as joints or the brain; particularly useful for brain scans

MALABSORPTION A condition in which insufficient amounts of nutrients are absorbed into the circulation from the small intestines

MALIGNANT TUMOUR A tumour that has the capacity either to invade the tissue that surrounds it or to spread via the blood or lymphatic circulation to other parts of the body, such as the lungs or the liver

MALOCCLUSION A bite that is

anatomically incorrect; see also Prognathism, Brachygnathism

MANDIBLE The lower jaw

MASTITIS Inflammation of mammary (breast) tissue

MAXILLA The upper jaw

MELAENA Black, tarry diarrhoea containing old blood

MELANOCYTES Pigment-containing cells

MENINGES Protective membranes surrounding the brain

MENISCUS Crescent-shaped cartilage in the stifle joint

METABOLISM The sum of all the chemical reactions that occur in the body

METASTASIS Spread of cancer cells from the area of origin to other parts of the body

METRITIS Inflammation of the uterus (womb)

MICROCHIP A small transponder injected under the skin, used for accurate identification of an animal

MICROFILARIA The larvae of heartworms, found in the bloodstream

MINERALOCORTICOIDS Corticosteroids with effects on sodium, chlorine, and potassium concentration

MRI SCAN see Magnetic resonance imaging

MUCOSA Another name for the mucous membranes, which line the hollow body structures such as the mouth and the small intestines

MUCUS Clear, lubricating secretion produced by cells in mucous membranes

MYCOSIS A disease caused by a fungus

MYELOGRAM X-ray of the spinal cord after the injection of contrast material (a substance opaque to X-rays)

MYOCARDITIS Inflammation of the heart muscle

MYOSITIS Inflammation of muscle

N

NECROSIS Cell death

NEOPLASIA Cancerous cell growth, which may be benign or malignant

NEPHRITIS Inflammation of the kidneys

NEURITIS Inflammation of nerve tissue

NICTITATING MEMBRANE Third eyelid

NSAID Non-steroidal anti-inflammatory drug; this group of drugs includes aspirin, carprofen, and meloxicam

NYSTAGMUS Rapid symmetrical eye movements, including rotations, in one direction

O

OEDEMA Excessive accumulation of fluid in body tissue; swelling

OESTROUS CYCLE The reproductive cycle in females

OESTRUS The period in the female's reproductive cycle when eggs are produced and released

OFF-LABEL USE OF DRUGS Therapeutic use of a drug in a species or for a purpose for which it is not licensed

OMNIVORE Animal that can eat both plant and animal matter

-OSIS A disease condition; for example, nephrosis is a disease condition of the kidneys

OSTEOARTHRITIS Inflammation of joint cells; *see* Degenerative joint disease

OSTEOARTHROSIS Pathological changes to joint cells

OSTEOCHONDROSIS Disease involving abnormal development of growth cartilage

OVARIOHYSTERECTOMY Removal of the ovaries and uterus, the normal "spaying" procedure

OVULATION Release of eggs from the ovaries

OXALATE Mineral sediment of stones produced in the bladder, as in "calcium oxalate"

P

PALLIATIVE TREATMENT Therapy that improves comfort but does not cure

PANCREATITIS Inflammation of the pancreas

PAPULE A small, elevated pimple filled solidly with inflammatory cells

PARALYSIS Temporary or permanent complete loss of muscle (motor) function

PARESIS An incomplete form of paralysis; for example, a dog with paresis can support itself, but needs help to get up from a lying position; *see* Ascending paralysis/paresis

PARTIAL SEIZURE *see* Seizure

PATELLA The kneecap

PATHOLOGY The study of damaging changes to tissue

PERIANAL Around the anus, as in "perianal adenomas"

PERINEAL Referring to the area between

the anus and the genitals

PERIODONTAL Around or near the tooth

PERIOSTEUM Specialized connective tissue covering all bones

PERITONITIS Inflammation of the lining of the abdominal cavity

PHARYNGITIS Inflammation of the back of the throat (pharynx)

PICA An appetite for unnatural and potentially dangerous substances

PINNA The ear flap

PITUITARY GLAND The "master gland" at the base of the brain, controlling all other hormone-producing glands and controlled by the hypothalamus (an area at the base of the brain)

PLAQUE Substance adhering to the enamel surface of teeth

PNEUMONIA Inflammation of the lungs

PNEUMONITIS Inflammation of lung tissue

PNEUMOTHORAX Loss of negative pressure in the chest cavity, causing the lungs to collapse

POLY- Excessive or multiple, as in "polyarthitis"

POLYARTHROPATHY Pathological change to many joints

POLYDYPSIA Excessive thirst

POLYPHAGIA Excessive hunger

POLYURIA Excessive urinating

PRA *see* Progressive Retinal Atrophy

PRO-OESTRUS The preparatory period

just before oestrus in the female reproductive cycle

PROGESTERONE A sex hormone produced in the ovaries after eggs are released

PROGNATHISM Protrusion of the upper jaw

PROGRESSIVE RETINAL ATROPHY (PRA) A hereditary eye condition that usually causes blindness

PROSTAGLANDINS Naturally occurring fatty acid substances with varied functions, including regulation of acid secretion in the stomach and control of inflammation

PROTEINUREA Protein loss in urine; often a sign of protein leakage in the kidneys as a consequence of kidney disease, or leakage elsewhere, for example from bladder inflammation (cystitis)

PRURITUS Itchiness

PSEUDOCYESIS False or phantom hormonal pregnancy

PSYCHOGENIC Originating in the mind, as in "psychogenic polydypsia"

PULMONARY Relating to the lungs

PULMONARY OEDEMA Fluid build-up in the lungs, often associated with heart failure

PURULENT Containing pus

PUS A mixture of bacteria and dead white blood cells, usually white or yellow and malodorous

PUSTULE A small, elevated, pus-filled pimple

PYO- Pus-related, as in "pyometra" (a pus-filled womb) or "pyoderma" (purulent skin disease)

R

REGURGITATION Backward flow: for example, regurgitated food comes from the oesophagus (as distinct from vomit, which comes from the stomach); regurgitated blood flows back from the heart's ventricles to the atria

RENAL Related to the kidneys

RETINA The light-sensitive layers of cells at the back of the eyes

RINGWORM A fungal infection of the skin (ringworm is not caused by worms)

RNA Ribonucleic acid; a complex molecule in all living cells, involved in cell protein synthesis; RNA is very similar in composition to DNA

S

SARCOMA A malignant tumour formed from body-tissue cells

SCALES Bits of the surface of the skin that may either flake off, as particles of dandruff, or remain, building up as calluses

SCLERA The tough white outer coat of the eyeball

SCLEROSIS Hardening of tissue, as a consequence of age or inflammation

SCOOTING Dragging the bottom on the ground

SEBACEOUS GLAND Oil-producing skin gland that adds water-proofing to the coat

SEBORRHOEA An increased activity of the skin's oil-producing sebaceous glands; in "dry seborrhoea" there is increased flaky scaling while in "wet seborrhoea" scale is retained in skin oil, producing a greasy, smelly coat

SEBUM Oily substance produced by sebaceous glands to make the coat waterproof and supple

SEIZURE Abnormal electrical activity in the brain, causing unusual nervous responses; also known as a "fit or "convulsion". A generalized seizure involves loss of consciousness accompanied by involuntary activities such as muscle contractions, paddling with the limbs, trembling, and facial twitching; frequently accompanied by salivation, urination and defaecation, and dilated pupils. A partial seizure involves only some of these changes and does not necessarily include loss of consciousness

SEPARATION ANXIETY An emotional problem resulting in destructive behaviour, barking or howling, urinating, or defaecating when left alone

SEPTICAEMIA Bacterial infection in the blood circulation

SHIVERING An involuntary, high-frequency contraction and relaxation of muscles

SHOCK A life-threatening emergency in which the cardiovascular system fails, causing physical collapse, rapid pulse, and pale mucous membranes

SIBO see Small intestine bacterial overgrowth

SMALL INTESTINE BACTERIAL OVERGROWTH (SIBO) An intestinal condition in which, for a variety of reasons, a pure culture of bacteria increases and displaces other beneficial bacteria

SMEGMA Normal discharge from the sheath of a dog's penis

SPHINCTER The usually circular tissue that constricts to control the flow of fluid or other material through an opening

SPRAIN An injury caused by over-stretching a ligament, resulting in lameness

STENOSIS The narrowing of a passageway, as in "windpipe stenosis"

STOMATITIS Inflammation of the mucosa of the mouth

STRAIN Damage to muscle fibres and tendons, often accompanied by slight bleeding and bruising

STRUVITE A mineral sand or sediment, otherwise called triple phosphate or magnesium ammonium phosphate hexahydrate, found in the bladder

STUPOR A condition during which a dog is unconscious; the animal can temporarily be aroused before falling back into the stupor

SUBCUTANEOUS Under the skin

SUBLUXATION Partial dislocation

SUGAR DIABETES see Diabetes mellitus

SYNOVIAL FLUID Lubricating joint fluid

SYNOVIAL FLUID ANALYSIS see Joint fluid analysis

T

TARTAR Yellowish film of mineral salts and food particles deposited on the teeth by saliva; see also Calculus, Plaque

TEAR Laceration of the skin, or rupture of ligaments, tendons, whole muscles, parts of muscles, or organs

TENOSYNOVITIS Inflammation of a tendon sheath

TESTOSTERONE Male sex hormone

THORACIC Pertaining to the chest cavity

THROMBOEMBOLISM Blockage of a blood vessel by an embolus (a detached piece of a thrombus)

THROMBUS A blood clot

THYROID GLAND The largest endocrine glands in the dog's body, producing hormones vital for growth and metabolism

TORSION Twisting

TOXOCARIASIS Infection with the roundworm *Toxocara canis*, a zoonotic disease common in dogs

TOXOPLASMOSIS Infection with *Toxoplasma gondii*, a rare, non-zoonotic condition in dogs

TRANSUDATE Fluid passed through a tissue membrane or extruded from tissue

TUMOUR Also called a neoplasm, a lump or bump, caused by multiplying cells, that can be benign or malignant

U

ULCER A lesion where surface tissue has been lost through damage or disease

ULTRASOUND Sound waves, inaudible to the human ear, used to examine structures inside the body or to treat various disorders of deep tissues

URAEMIA Build-up of waste in the blood as a consequence of kidney failure

UROLITHS Stones in the bladder

UVEITIS Inflammation to the uvea, the iris, ciliary body, and choroid in the eye

V

VESTIBULAR Pertaining to the organ of balance in the middle ear, as in "vestibular syndrome"

VILLI Microscopic, finger-like projections from the lining of the small intestine, that absorb nutrients from food

VISCERA The body's internal organs

VOLVULUS Abdominal distension and rotation, mainly in deep-chested large breeds, rapidly leading to clinical shock and requiring urgent emergency attention; also known as "gastric dilatation" or "bloat"

W

WHELPING Giving birth

WOBBLER SYNDROME Ataxia caused by compression of the cervical spinal cord due to vertebral instability

X

X-RAY High-energy electromagnetic radiation, and an image produced using this radiation; some body tissues such as bone absorb X-rays (radiopaque) and appear pale on X-ray images, while others allow X-rays through (radiolucent) and appear as dark areas

Y

YEAST General term for fungi that reproduce by budding, of which some are pathogenic

Z

ZOONOSES Diseases transmissible between vertebrates and humans

ZOONOSES

Zoonotic diseases are conditions that are passed from one species to another. Although zoonoses are always a matter for concern, almost all of them are rare. With uncommon exceptions, dogs do not get cat diseases, cats do not get human diseases, and humans do not get dog or cat diseases. The great exceptions are diseases caused by microbes that are passed through bites. Rabies, a viral infection, is the most serious. Other microbes may pass to us through dog faeces or may use parasites, such as ticks, as their method of spreading to us.

RABIES

Throughout Asia, Africa, and South America, rabies is by far the most serious zoonotic hazard from dogs. This almost always fatal disease is endemic in wildlife in large regions of North America. It most commonly affects raccoons, skunks, foxes, and bats, but in Texas the dog form of rabies has spread across the border from Mexico.

In Europe, the disease does not exist in the UK, Ireland, Scandinavia, mainland Spain, or Portugal. Elsewhere in western Europe, it is restricted to isolated pockets of wildlife, affecting mostly foxes. Australia, New Zealand, and Japan are all free of rabies.

In regions where rabies exists, humans are at risk when bitten by any dog that is not known to have been vaccinated against the disease.

Rabies virus can exist in a dog's saliva for up to two weeks before the dog shows clinical signs of the disease (see pp.144–45). An unvaccinated dog is quarantined for two weeks after biting a human to determine whether the dog develops rabies.

TREATMENT While quarantined dogs are not treated to see if the disease develops, bitten people are given post-exposure antiserum treatment.

DOG BITES

Not truly a zoonosis, dog bite injuries are the most common condition that we may experience as a result of contact with dogs. Most bites are not classified as serious, and less than five per cent become infected. When they do, *Pasteurella* bacteria are likely to be involved. Pathogenic strains of *Pasteurella*, carried in the mouth of one dog out of four, is the most likely cause of secondary infection from dog bites. (It is also carried by three out of four cats, and is the most likely cause of infection from cat bites.) *Pasteurella* infection associated with a bite is usually painful, swollen, and inflamed.

TREATMENT The antibiotic of choice is usually one from the penicillin group.

TICK-TRANSMITTED DISEASES

LYME DISEASE (BORRELIOSIS)

Dogs bring ticks into our vicinity, so dog owners are more at risk of contracting diseases transmitted through tick bites.

Lyme disease is caused by *Borrelia burgdorferi* bacteria, and is transmitted when ticks feed by sucking blood (see p.154). The bacteria are commonly carried by a variety of *Ixodes* species ticks, usually carried by deer.

A red rash develops where the tick was attached. Later, an individual may have a headache, fever, malaise, joint pain, and chills. The lymph nodes may also be enlarged.

TREATMENT The infection is treated with antibiotics from the tetracycline group.

ROCKY MOUNTAIN SPOTTED FEVER (RMSF) AND BOUTONNEUSE FEVER (BF)

These infections are caused by a specialized type of bacteria called rickettsia (see pp.154–155). RMSF is carried by wood ticks (*Dermacentor andersoni*) and the American dog tick (*Dermacentor variabilis*) in America. BF is carried by the brown dog tick (*Rhipicephalus sanguineus*) in Mediterranean Europe.

Both organisms cause a skin rash. RMSF causes a flu-like condition, while BF causes a black spot at the site of the tick and a fever.

TREATMENT Tetracycline group antibiotics are effective.

WORM INFESTATIONS

VISCERAL LARVA MIGRANS (TOXOCARIASIS)

Toxocara canis, the common dog roundworm, is inherited by many pups at birth. (It is also inherited by most fox cubs.) In most instances, affected puppies show few or no clinical signs of infestation. The worm is passed in faeces, contaminating ground where unwormed dogs (unwormed pups, in particular) defaecate. Embryonated eggs remain infectious in the environment for long periods, especially in warm weather (see p.168).

Humans, usually children, contract visceral larva migrans by accidentally consuming soil contaminated with worm eggs. The eggs hatch and develop into larvae, migrating through various parts of the body, including the intestines and the lungs, and sometimes ending up in the eye or central nervous system. Affected children usually have no symptoms, but some may show signs of allergy, coughing, blurred vision, and even convulsions.

TREATMENT Dogs and humans should be wormed if they contract the disease (*see p.168*). Dogs should not have access to children's play areas, and children should be taught to wash their hands after playing on the ground.

NOTE Toxocariasis is often confused with a zoonotic protozoal infection called toxoplasmosis. Canine toxoplasmosis does not pose a human health hazard. Feline toxoplasmosis, on the other hand, has serious hazards, particularly for pregnant women. (For the differences between toxocariasis and toxoplasmosis, *see p.173*.)

HYDATID DISEASE (ECHINOCOCCUS)

It causes few problems in dogs, but the tapeworm *Echinococcus granulosus* can be transmitted to humans, causing serious, sometimes fatal, disease. Dogs can also contract and transmit the fox tapeworm *Echinococcus multilocularis*.

Sheep ingest this tapeworm by accidentally consuming contaminated dog, fox, or (in Australia) dingo faeces. An affected sheep forms hydatid cysts in its viscera; hence, the illness is called hydatid disease. The cycle is completed when other dogs contract this tapeworm by eating raw viscera from sheep containing hydatid cysts. Humans can also act as intermediate hosts and develop cysts that cannot be destroyed by drugs.

TREATMENT All dogs in regions where hydatid disease occurs should be wormed regularly (*see p.171*). Dogs should also be prevented from scavenging dead sheep or eating sheep offal. The only effective treatment for

hydatid disease in humans is surgical removal of the hydatid cysts.

TAPEWORM DISEASE (DIPYLIDIASIS)

Another form of tapeworm, *Dipylidium caninum*, can cause dipylidiasis, a very rare disease. Tapeworm infestation may occur in children who accidentally eat dog fleas infected with tapeworm eggs. The symptoms in children are similar to those of human pinworms, namely itchy bottoms.

TREATMENT Effective flea control (*see pp.162–63*) together with dog worming (*see p.171*) to kill any adult tapeworms will minimize chances of a person contracting this disease. Children are treated for dipylidiasis with wormers that destroy tapeworms.

HOOKWORM DISEASE

Hookworms (*Ancylostoma caninum*) live in warm, moist soil. The larvae may pass on to humans by penetrating the skin, and temporarily cause itchy, inflamed skin known as creeping eruption or cutaneous larva migrans. This condition is rare.

TREATMENT Proper worming controls hookworms in dogs (*see p.169*). Antihistamine cream relieves itchiness in humans.

SKIN CONDITIONS

RINGWORM (DERMATOPHYTOSIS)

Ringworm is a superficial fungal skin infection of livestock, pets, and humans. Although Persian cats are the most common carriers of ringworm among pets, dogs occasionally also contract and transmit this infection by means of the fungus *Microsporum canis*. (Ringworm from rodents and livestock is *Trichophyton mentagrophytes*.)

Ringworm in dogs may cause moderate itchiness and local hair loss (alopecia) which starts as a raised pimple, then expands in a ring with a reddish border. In humans a round, red,

itchy patch appears, growing larger, with a red ring forming around it.

TREATMENT In dogs and humans, ringworm is treated with topical antifungal medication and an oral antibiotic (*see p.184*).

SARCOPTIC MANGE AND CHEYLETIELLOSIS

Sarcoptic mange, caused by the canine scabies mite, is slightly different from human scabies. While human scabies mites breed on us, dog scabies mites cannot, but they do affect humans – after contact with a dog that has scabies, humans may develop itchy, red skin, sometimes small blisters.

Cheyletiella yasguri is a puppy skin parasite, causing intense dandruff on a puppy's back and itchy pimples on us.

TREATMENT Antihistamines and insecticidal shampoos are used to treat humans when they contract either of these skin parasites.

GASTROINTESTINAL DISEASES

Several gastrointestinal bacteria can be transmitted from dogs to humans, but all are rare. The most common is *Campylobacter jejuni*, which causes fever, headache, abdominal cramps, and watery to bloody diarrhoea. The most common source of this bacterium is contaminated meat, especially chicken and unpasteurized milk, but a few instances of this infection can be traced back to dogs with diarrhoea.

Most cases of *Salmonella* infection come from contaminated food, but here, too, a small number of cases can be traced back to pets. *Salmonella* causes nausea, vomiting, cramps, and watery diarrhoea.

TREATMENT If anyone in your family has been diagnosed with either of these gastroenteric infections, it is sensible to have your pet examined to see if it is a carrier. Dogs are treated with antibiotics which, depending on culture and sensitivity, are effective at killing the bacteria.

INDEX

Page numbers in **bold** type refer to main entries; page numbers in *italic* type refer to captions.

ACKNOWLEDGMENTS

Author's Acknowledgments

The only way to manage an active veterinary clinic and still have time to write is to work with wonderful people who genuinely mean it when they say, "No problem". Bas Hagreis, who shares primary care responsibility with me said "No problem" more often than I hoped he would have to. So too did my veterinary nurses, Hester Small, Ashley McManus, Hilary Hayward, Manda Hackett and Suzie Gray.

The only way I can write authoritatively about disease is to take a little of my own clinical experience then add a lot of information from the most recent veterinary textbooks. There is one textbook, and one editor I am particularly indebted to. Stephen J. Ettinger created the *Textbook of Veterinary Internal Medicine*, now in its umpteenth edition. This book is a basic bible for clinical vets like me and what's most impressive is that Steve manages to do what he does while practising second opinion veterinary medicine in Los Angeles.

The only way to ensure that textbook advice has not already been superseded by the ever-changing advances in medicine is to ask clinicians at veterinary teaching hospitals. Dick White, Head of the Clinical Division at Cambridge University's Veterinary School and the best soft tissue surgeon I've met offered vital advice and read most of the chapters. Jane Dobson, Head of Oncology and Director of Cambridge's Veterinary Teaching Hospital and Mike Herrtage, Specialist in Cardiology and Diagnostic Imaging and the vet school's Vice Dean were equally generous with their chapter reading, time and advice. So, too, was Penny Watson, the vet school's Specialist in Internal Medicine who provided added insight on nutrition. Gary Clayton Jones, former Head of Orthopaedics at the Royal Veterinary College and the best orthopaedic surgeon I've ever watched operate reviewed muscles, nerves, bones and joints while Peter Bedford, Head of Small Animal Medicine and Surgery at the Royal Veterinary College offered advice in his Specialist field, ophthalmology. David Sutton, Head of Veterinary Services at Intervet provided his suggestions on infectious and parasitic diseases while Jo Stonehewer a Diplomate in Small Animal Medicine at Iams reviewed the section on nutrition. Simon Tai, a dermatologist I have worked with for years read the chapter on skin diseases. Peter Kertesz, who has carried out more root canal work on elephant tusks than anyone else in the world, and with whom I've worked for 25 years advised on dentistry. Hugh Wirth in Australia scrupulously read every single word, offering his experience and cogent suggestions throughout the book. In the US, Beth Adelman, who has edited countless dog care books, including previous ones by me, and her veterinary team ensured yet more learned eyes passed over the text. Thank you everyone.

Agency Photographs

4: Eyewire (c); **6:** N.H.P.A; Gerard Lacz (c); **6:** RSPCA; Geoff du Feu (cr); Mr Geoff du Feu (c); **7:** N.H.P.A; (cr); Mirko Stelzner (l); **7:** Eyewire (cl); **7:** RSPCA; Colin Seddon (cr); E A James c; **8:** Animal Photography; Sally Anne Thompson (cr); **8:** FLPA - Images of nature; David Dalton (cl); **8:** Photodisc/ Geostock (r); **9:** Kennel Club; Colin Seddon (cl); **9:** Eyewire (cr); **9:** Warren Photographic; Kim Taylor (r); **10-11:** Stone/Getty Images; Jeremy Walker (c); **14-15:** Stone/Getty Images; Alan & Sandy Carey (c); **16:** RSPCA; Geoff du Feu (cl); **17:** Eyewire (c); **19:** Photodisc/Geostock (bl); **19:** RSPCA; Colin Seddon (tr); **22:** RSPCA; Colin Seddon (bc); **23:** Oxford Scientific Films; Lon E Lauber (tr); **24:** Eyewire (tl); **25:** RSPCA; E A Janes (c); **30:** Eyewire (tl); **32:** FLPA - Images of nature; Foto Natura (tc); **33:** RSPCA; Angela Hampton (bl); **41:** Kennel Club; Colin Seddon (bl); **41:** FLPA - Images of nature; David Hosking (tr); **42:** FLPA - Images of nature; Foto Natura (c); **43:** RSPCA (tr); **44:** RSPCA; Dave Bevan (bc); **45:** FLPA - Images of nature; Gerard Lacz (cl); **46:** RSPCA; E A Janes (tl); **47:** FLPA - Images of nature; Albert Visage (tr); **48:** RSPCA; Angela Hampton (cr); **49:** Kennel Club; Colin Seddon (bl); **51:** FLPA - Images of nature; David Dalton (c); **52:** FLPA - Images of nature; Foto Natura cl; **53:** N.H.P.A (c); **62:** FLPA - Images of nature; Gerard Lacz (tl); **63:** RSPCA; E A Janes (bl); **66:** FLPA - Images of nature; Foto Natura (tl); **67:** RSPCA; Angela Hampton (bl); **68:** FLPA - Images of nature; Foto Natura (br); **72-73:** Powerstock Photolibrary; **74:** RSPCA; Geoff du Feu (tl); **75:** RSPCA; Stephen Oliver (tr); **77:** RSPCA; Geoff du Feu (bl); **79:** Science Photo Library; J;C;Revy (cl); **80:** Warren Photographic; Jane Burton (tl); **81:** N.H.P.A; Yves Lanceau (tr); **81:** Telegraph Colour Library/Getty Images; Jeffrey Sylvester (bc); **83:** Science Photo Library; Biology Media (br); **84:** N.H.P.A; Susanne Danegger (bl); **86:** FLPA - Images of nature; David T Grewcock (br); **86:** RSPCA; Angela Hampton (tl); **87:** FLPA - Images of nature; David Hosking (tl); **88:** RSPCA; Angela Hampton (bl); **89:** FLPA - Images of nature; Gerard Laci (c); **89:** RSPCA; Cheryl A Ertelt (cl); **90:** DK Picture Library; Tracy Morgan (cr); **93:** RSPCA; Colin Seddon (tl); **94:** RSPCA; Cheryl A Ertelt (br); **96:** DK Picture Library; Tracy Morgan (bl); **97:** RSPCA; Angela Hampton (bl); **99:** FLPA - Images of nature; Gerard Laci (bl); **110:** Animal Photography; Sally Anne Thompson (bl); **118:** RSPCA; Andrew Linscott (br); **124:** Science Photo Library; David Scharf (br); **125:** DK Picture Library; Tracy Morgan (br); **130:** Science Photo Library (cl); **132:** Science Photo Library; National Cancer Institute (cl); **133:** RSPCA; Angela Hampton (tr); **134:** RSPCA; Angela Hampton (br); **135:** DK Picture Library; Tracy Morgan (tr); **139:** Michael Herrtage, Queen's Veterinary School Hospital, University of Cambridge; (tl); **142:** Science Photo Library; CNRI (tl); **145:** Stone/Getty Images; Philip & Karen Smith (br); **146:** Warren Photographic; Jane Burton (cl); **147:** Warren Photographic; Kim Taylor (tl); **150:** Science Photo Library; CNRI (br); **152:** DK Picture Library; Tracy Morgan (bl); **154:** Science Photo Library; Eye of Science (tr); **155:** N.H.P.A; Mirko Stelzner (tr); **156:** Science Photo Library; Eye of Science (bl); **158:** Corbis; Michael S; Yamashita (br); **158:** Science Photo Library; Kent Wood (tl); **161:** RSPCA; Andrew Forsyth (tr); **165:** Science Photo Library; Eye of Science (br); **166:** Bayer plc (tl); **171:** Animal Photography; R;T; Willbie (br); **173:** Warren Photographic; Jane Burton (tr); **176-201:** DK Picture Library; Tracy Morgan, (running head); **176:** Science Photo Library; Alfred Pasieka (tl); **178:** N.H.P.A; Joe Blossom (cl); **180:** Dr Janet D Littlewood, Veterinary Dermatology Referrals (br); **181:** Science Photo Library; John Durham (tr); **184:** Dr Janet D Littlewood, Veterinary Dermatology Referrals (tr), (bl); **188:** Dr Janet D Littlewood, Veterinary Dermatology Referrals (tc); **189:** DK Picture Library; Tracy Morgan (tr); **192:** N.H.P.A;; Gerard Lacz (tr); **195:** Stone/Getty Images (tr); **196:** Dr Janet D Littlewood, Veterinary Dermatology Referrals (tr); **198:** Dr Janet D Littlewood, Veterinary Dermatology Referrals (br); **199:** N.H.P.A; Gerard Lacz (tl); **200:** DK Picture Library; Tracy Morgan (tl); **202:** The Wellcome Institute Library, London (tl); **204:** Dr Richard White, The Queens Veterinary School Hospital, University of Cambridge (bl); **206:** The Wellcome Institute Library, London (tr); **208:** DK Picture Library; Tracy Morgan (bc); **209:** David L Williams, Dept of Clinical Veterinary Medicine, University of Cambridge (tl); **211:** RSPCA; Tim Woodcock (br); **213:** Warren Photographic; Jane Burton (bl); **214:** David L Williams, Dept of Clinical Veterinary Medicine, University of Cambridge (tr); **215:** DK Picture Library; Tracy Morgan (tr); **216:** RSPCA; Angela Hampton (br); **218:** David L Williams, Dept of Clinical Veterinary Medicine, University of Cambridge (bl); **219:** David L Williams, Dept of Clinical Veterinary Medicine, University of Cambridge (tl); **219:** RSPCA; Tim Woodcock (br); **220:** Michael Herrtage, Queen's Veterinary School Hospital, University of Cambridge (tc), (tr); **220:** The Wellcome Institute Library, London; Royal Veterinary College (bl); **221:** DK Picture Library; Tracy Morgan (tr); **222:** RSPCA; Angela Hampton (bc); **226:** Science Photo Library; BSIP VEM (br); **227:** Dr Richard White, The Queens Veterinary School Hospital, University of Cambridge; (tc); **228:** Dr Richard White, The Queens Veterinary School Hospital, University of Cambridge (br); **231:** Dr Richard White, The Queens Veterinary School Hospital, University of Cambridge (tc); **232:** Science Photo Library; CNRI (tl); **236:** Michael Herrtage, Queen's Veterinary School Hospital, University of Cambridge (tr); **239:** RSPCA; Angela Hampton (r); **241:** DK Picture Library; Tracy Morgan (br); **242:** Michael Herrtage, Queen's Veterinary School Hospital, University of Cambridge (tr); **244:** Michael Herrtage, Queen's Veterinary School Hospital, University of Cambridge (br); **245:** Science Photo Library; David Scharf (tr); **246:** Science Photo Library (tl); **251:** Michael Herrtage, Queen's Veterinary School Hospital, University of Cambridge (bl); **252:** Michael Herrtage, Queen's Veterinary School Hospital, University of Cambridge (tr); **253:** DK Picture Library; Tracy Morgan (tr); **254:** Science Photo Library; Eye of Science (tl); **264:** Dr Richard White, The Queens Veterinary School Hospital, University of Cambridge (tl); **265:** Dr Richard White, The Queens Veterinary School Hospital, University of Cambridge (bl); **272:** Michael Herrtage, Queen's Veterinary School Hospital, University of Cambridge (bl); **275:** DK Picture Library; Tracy Morgan (br); **275:** RSPCA (bl); **276:** Michael Herrtage, Queen's Veterinary School Hospital, University of Cambridge (tr); **277:** DK Picture Library; Tracy Morgan (tr), (br); **278:** Science Photo Library; Andrew Syred (tl); **280:** Warren Photographic; Kim Taylor (cr); **283:** DK Picture Library; Tracy Morgan (tr), (br); **285:** DK Picture Library; Tracy Morgan (br); **291:** DK Picture Library; Tracy Morgan (tr); **292:** Science Photo Library; CNRI (tl); **297:** Corbis; Dale C. Spartas (tl); **300:** RSPCA; Colin Seddon (bl); **306:** Michael Herrtage, Queen's Veterinary School Hospital, University of Cambridge (br); **309:** DK Picture Library; Tracy Morgan (tr); **311:** Michael Herrtage, Queen's Veterinary School Hospital, University of Cambridge (tc); **312:** Warren Photographic; Jane Burton (br); **316:** Dr Richard White, The Queens Veterinary School Hospital, University of Cambridge (bl); **318:** Dr Richard White, The Queens Veterinary School Hospital, University of Cambridge (tr); **319:** Michael Herrtage, Queen's Veterinary School Hospital, University of Cambridge (br); **321:** Warren Photographic; Kim Taylor (br); **325:** DK Picture Library; Tracy Morgan (tr), (br); 328: Science Photo Library (tl); **334:** Corbis; Lowell Georgia (br); **336:** RSPCA; Angela Hampton (bc); **338:** DK Picture Library; Tracy Morgan (tr); **339:** DK Picture Library; Tracy Morgan (tr), (br); **340:** Science Photo Library; Tektoff-Merieux, CNRI (tl); **343:** Science Photo Library (tr); **345:** DK Picture Library; Tracy Morgan (tr); **349:** Animal Photography; Sally Anne Thompson (br); **350:** Science Photo Library; A;B; Dowsett (tl); **350:** Warren Photographic; Jane Burton (cl); **356:** Science Photo Library; Prof; P Motta/Dept of Anatomy, University of La Sapienza (cl); **362:** Michael Herrtage, Queen's Veterinary School Hospital, University of Cambridge (cl); 363: Warren Photographic; Jane Burton (tr); **364:** RSPCA; Cheryl A Ertelt (br); **366:** Michael Herrtage, Queen's Veterinary School Hospital, University of Cambridge (bl); **372:** RSPCA; Colin Seddon (tl); **380:** Stone/Getty Images; Jim Cooper (c); **383:** DK Picture Library; Stephen Oliver (bcl), (bcr); Tracy Morgan; **385:** DK Picture Library; Tracy Morgan (tl), (tc), (tr), (bc); **394:** DK Picture Library; Tracy Morgan (tl), (tr); **395:** DK Picture Library; Tracy Morgan (bl), (br); **424:** DK Picture Library; Guy Ryecart cl; Paul Goff (bl); **427:** DK Picture Library; Jerry Young (cr), (br).

All other images © Dorling Kindersley

For further information see: www.dkimages.com

Illustrations:

Medical artworks: Debbie Maizels

First Aid artworks: Andrew Beckett, Rowan Clifford, Angelica Elsebach, Chris Forsey